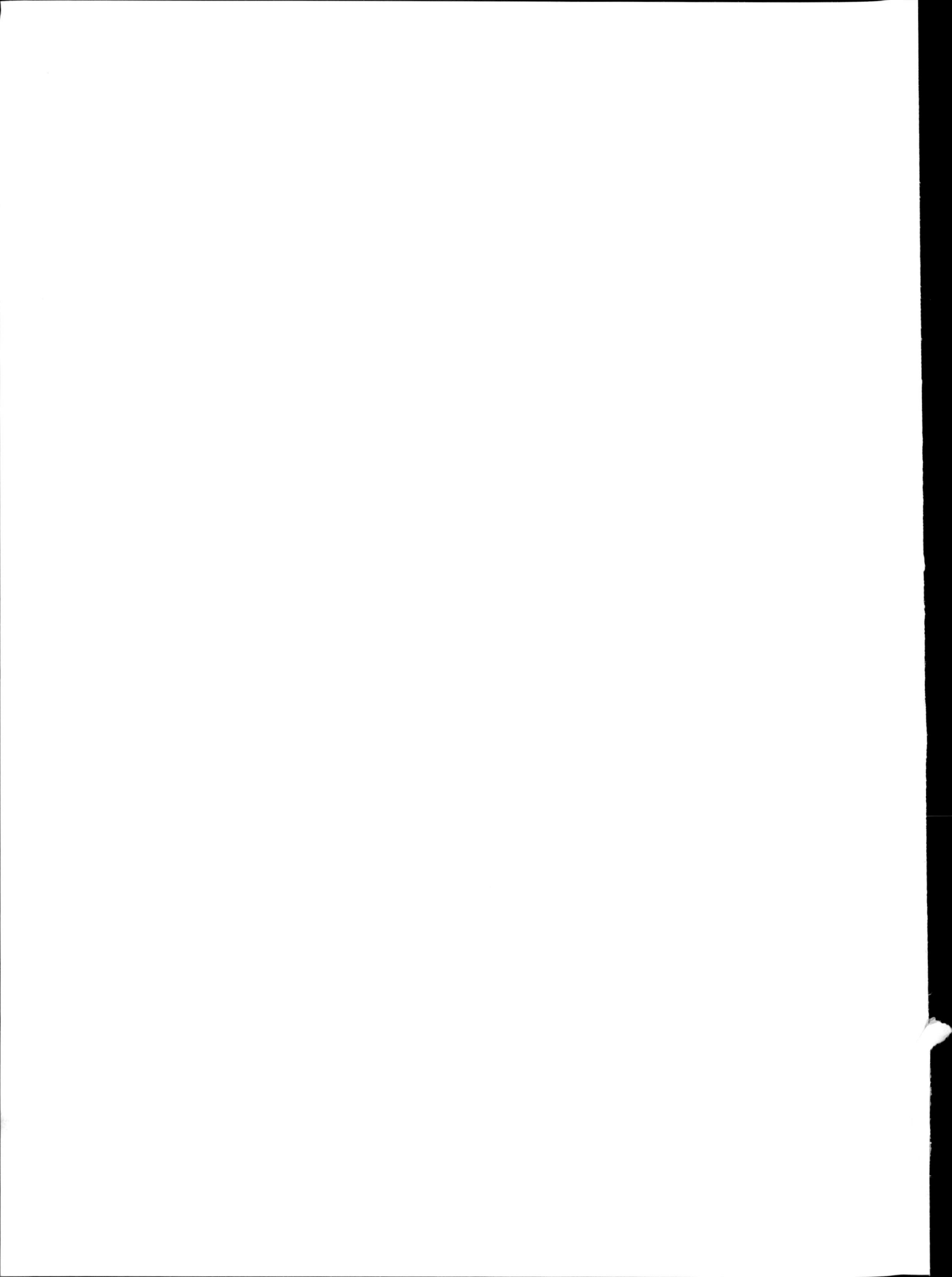

Endocrine Disorders: An Issue of the Endocrinology Clinics

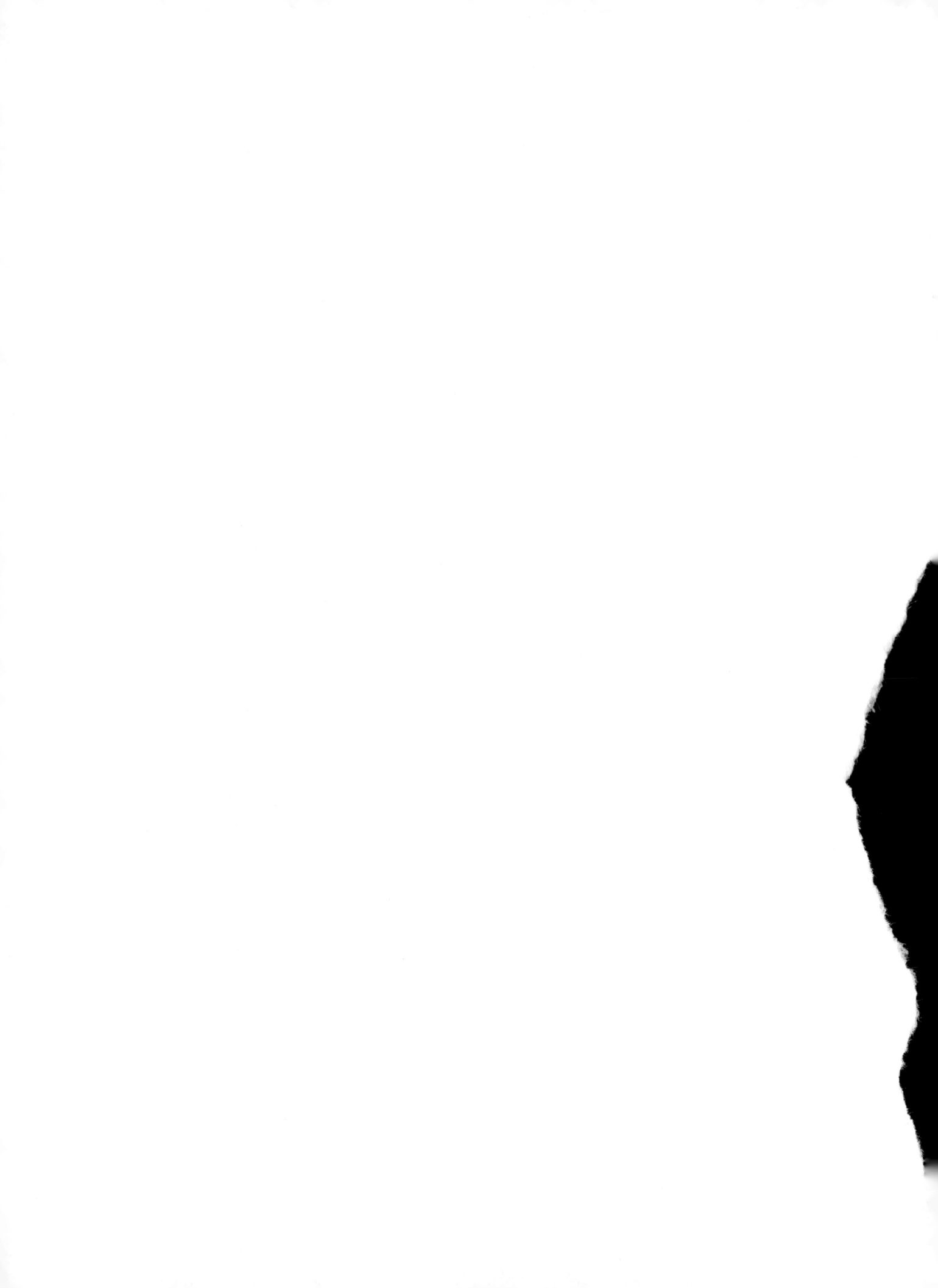

Endocrine Disorders: An Issue of the Endocrinology Clinics

Editor: Trever Quinn

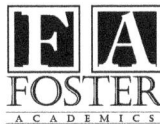

FA
FOSTER
A C A D E M I C S

www.fosteracademics.com

www.fosteracademics.com

FA
FOSTER
ACADEMICS

Cataloging-in-Publication Data

Endocrine disorders : an issue of the endocrinology clinics / edited by Trever Quinn.
    p. cm.
Includes bibliographical references and index.
ISBN 978-1-63242-647-5
1. Endocrine glands--Diseases. 2. Endocrinology. 3. Clinics. I. Quinn, Trever.
RC649.5 .E53 2019
6164--dc23

Foster Academics,
118-35 Queens Blvd., Suite 400,
Forest Hills, NY 11375, USA

ISBN 978-1-63242-647-5 (Hardback)

Contents

Preface

The main aim of this book is to educate learners and enhance their research focus by presenting diverse topics covering this vast field. This is an advanced book which compiles significant studies by distinguished experts in the area of analysis. This book addresses successive solutions to the challenges arising in the area of application, along with it; the book provides scope for future developments.

Endocrine disorders refer to the various disorders of the endocrine system. It may be classified into three groups, namely endocrine gland hypersecretion, endocrine gland hyposecretion and tumors. Some of the diseases falling within these groups include thyroid disorders such as hypothyroidism, hyperthyroidism and goiter, glucose homeostasis disorders like hypoglycemia and diabetes, various metabolic bone diseases, pituitary gland disorders and sex hormone disorders. Most endocrine disorders involve a complex combination of hyposecretion and hypersecretion. The branch of medicine that deals with all endocrine disorders is known as endocrinology. This book covers in detail some existing theories and innovative concepts revolving around endocrine disorders. Different approaches, evaluations, methodologies and advanced studies on endocrinology have been included herein. This book is a vital tool for all researching or studying endocrine disorders as it gives incredible insights into emerging trends and concepts.

It was a great honour to edit this book, though there were challenges, as it involved a lot of communication and networking between me and the editorial team. However, the end result was this all-inclusive book covering diverse themes in the field.

Finally, it is important to acknowledge the efforts of the contributors for their excellent chapters, through which a wide variety of issues have been addressed. I would also like to thank my colleagues for their valuable feedback during the making of this book.

Editor

Sex-related illness perception and self-management of a Thai type 2 diabetes population: a cross-sectional descriptive design

Wimonrut Boonsatean[1]* iD, Anna Carlsson[2], Irena Dychawy Rosner[2] and Margareta Östman[2]

Abstract

Background: Increased knowledge concerning the differences in the illness perception and self-management among sexes is needed for planning proper support programs for patients with diabetes. The aim of this study was to investigate the illness perception and self-management among Thai women and Thai men with type 2 diabetes and to investigate the psychometric properties of the translated instruments used.

Methods: In a suburban province of Thailand, 220 women and men with type 2 diabetes participated in a cross-sectional descriptive study. The participants were selected using a multistage sampling method. Data were collected through structured interviews and were analyzed using group comparisons, and psychometric properties were tested.

Results: Women and men with type 2 diabetes demonstrated very similar experiences regarding their illness perception and no differences in self-management. Women perceived more negative consequences of the disease and more fluctuation in the symptoms than men, whereas men felt more confident about the treatment effectiveness than women. Furthermore, the translated instruments used in this study showed acceptable validity and reliability.

Conclusions: The Thai sociocultural context may influence people's perceptions and affect the self-care activities of Thai individuals, both women and men, with type 2 diabetes, causing differences from those found in the Western environment. Intervention programs that aim to improve the effectiveness of the self-management of Thai people with diabetes might consider a holistic and sex-related approach as well as incorporating Buddhist beliefs.

Keywords: Type 2 diabetes, Illness perception, Self-management, Sex differences, Thailand

Background

Type 2 diabetes (T2D) has shown an increasing global prevalence in the latest decade [1, 2]. The worldwide prevalence was approximately 2.8% in 2000 [3] and increased to 9% in adults (20–79 years old) in 2014 [4]. The prevalence of T2D in Thailand has also increased annually to approximately 6.4% in 2013 [1], and is one of the five common chronic diseases in Thailand [5].

Various international studies have explored the biological risks in developing T2D between women and men [6, 7]. Additionally, there are also studies investigating the differences among sexes in psychological aspects such as distress, anxiety, and depression [8–10]. However, only few studies have investigated sex differences regarding the health perceptions and attitudes [11–14] or self-management [15] in a population with T2D.

The term "illness perception" is used both to describe a person's cognitive and emotional response pattern and coping styles when living with the disease as well as the experience and understanding of his or her situation [16]. Additionally, the perception of being discriminated against by society due to the disease is also included in the concept of illness perception [17]. As found in contemporary research, negative emotional responses can lead people with T2D to feel overwhelmed and to find it difficult to manage their life with diabetes [18].

* Correspondence: boonsatean@yahoo.com
[1]Faculty of Nursing Science, Rangsit University, Pathum Thani 12000, Thailand
Full list of author information is available at the end of the article

Self-management is often described as the way one is managing his or her life with the disease, a process of taking control of the disease through individual cognitive decision making by obtaining support from one's family and from healthcare professionals [19]. Western studies have shown that people that have been able to take control of their diabetes have adopted efficient and comprehensive ways of dealing with the disease [20], although dietary control was found to be difficult [15, 21]. Furthermore, demographic characteristics have been seen to influence individual management strategies [22]. While women with T2D are seen to more often strictly attend to medical recommendations and take advantage of social resources, men more often rely on themselves and search for new strategies to manage their disease [15].

Research has shown that only 28% of Thai people with diabetes can manage their disease well [23]. In order to increase the number of people that are able to effectively manage their T2D, more knowledge on the part of healthcare professionals concerning the influences of illness perception and self-management is needed. Studies conducted with Westerners with diabetes have found that some differences between women and men exist with regard to their perceptions and attitudes towards T2D [11, 12, 18] and the ability to handle the disease [15]. Because there is limited knowledge in Thailand concerning the differences in illness perception and self-management among women and men, a study comparing the sexes in these aspects would be appropriate.

The aim of this study was to investigate the illness perception and self-management among Thai women and men with type 2 diabetes. An additional aim was to investigate the psychometric properties of the translated instruments used.

Methods

A cross-sectional descriptive design [24] with a randomly-selected data collection at each level of the cluster sampling (district, sub-district, and healthcare facilities) was performed. Data were collected using questionnaires and each participant was measured one time.

Setting

The study site was located in a suburban province close to Bangkok, Thailand, with 1,005,760 residents, comprising 52.5% women and 47.5% men, and most of the residents were Buddhist (94.7%) [25]. The catchment areas received medical services from the Health Promoting Hospitals (HPHs), a frontline healthcare service, with free essential treatment cost. These services are provided by the staff of the HPHs in cooperation with the Village Health Volunteers (VHVs), community residents who act as mediators between the staff and the community inhabitants.

Procedures
Sampling method
A multistage sampling method [26] was used. One random sample was obtained at each respective level (district, sub-district, and HPH) (Fig. 1). All of the people with T2D that lived in communities within the responsibility of the sampled HPH were invited to participate in this study. If there were not enough participants available in the sampled

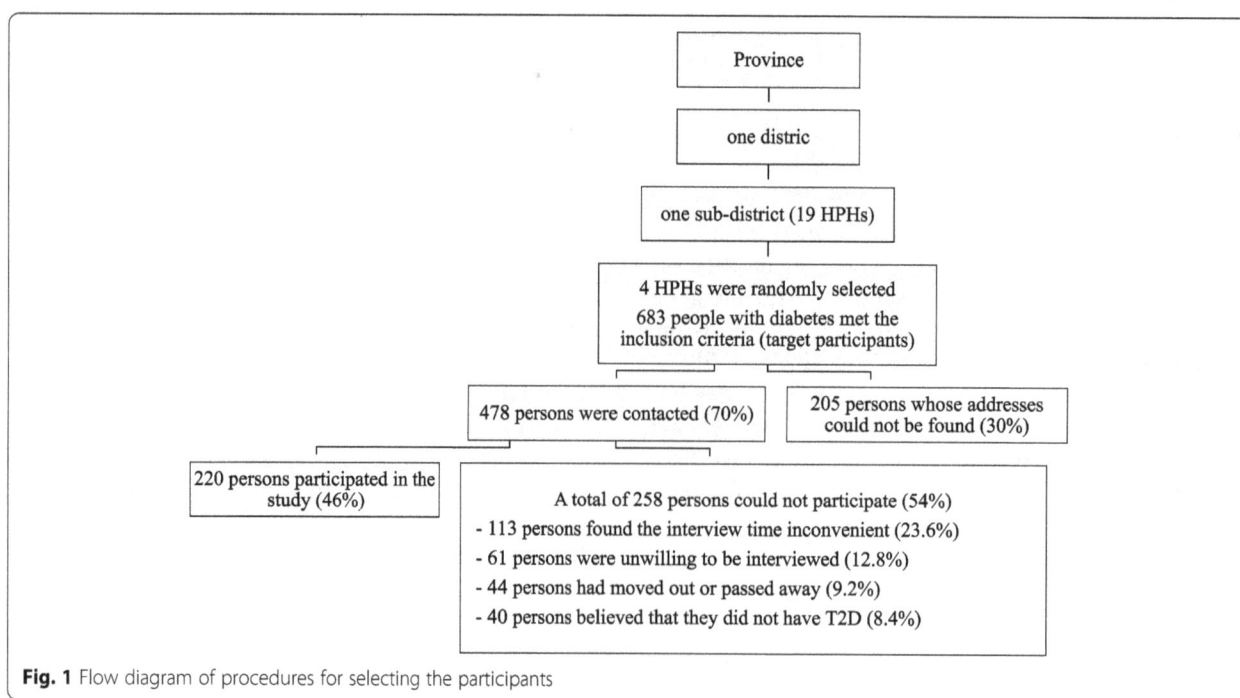

Fig. 1 Flow diagram of procedures for selecting the participants

HPH, another HPH was chosen, and four HPHs took part in this study. The sample size for this study was calculated using the estimated proportion of Thai people with diabetes (7.7%) with the absolute error of 5% and alpha, two-tailed, at 0.05 that the study would have power of 80% to detect the differences of illness perception and self-management among women and men [27]. The minimum sample size, including women and men, was 220 people.

Participants

All of the patients shown in the medical records of the HPHs were screened to fit the eligible inclusion criteria for participation: (1) Thai citizens that could converse in the Thai language, (2) individuals diagnosed with T2D by the physician for at least 1 year, and (3) those receiving anti-diabetic agent(s) or insulin until the day of the investigation. The people with T2D admitted to hospitals and those whose address could not be found were excluded from the study. A total of 478 people with T2D were contacted. Of this number, 61 people (12.8%) were not willing to participate in this study, 40 (8.4%) stated that they did not have T2D, 113 (23.6%) were not able to be reached for an interview because they had a daytime occupation (worked every day from 5 am to 8 pm), and 44 (9.2%) had moved out of the area or had died. In total, 220 people with T2D (46% of all contacts) participated in the study (Fig. 1).

Data collection

Data collection was run by three different qualified interviewers and supervised by a Thai researcher (first author) from June to August 2015. In order not to disqualify any person that was illiterate, all of the participants were interviewed face-to-face. All of the interviews took place at the participant's house or a place suggested by the participant. Before the interview began, the study, its purposes, assurance of confidentiality, and how to withdraw from the study were explained. When the participant decided to participate, a consent form was signed. Each interview lasted from 40 to 60 min. If omissions were found afterward, the interviewers visited the participants again to address the incomplete items.

Measurement tools

The measurement tools comprised a tool measuring the demographic characteristics developed by the researchers and two questionnaires which had earlier showed good psychometric properties: the revised diabetes illness perception (IPQ-R) questionnaire, developed by Moss-Morris et al. [16] (see the illness perception questionnaire website, http://www.uib.no/ipq/), and the 2015 revised diabetes self-management questionnaire (DSMQ-R), developed by Schmitt et al. [28]. Both questionnaires were originally developed in English, and then translated into the Thai language, inspired by the guidelines of the World Health Organization [29]. This main process included forward-backward translation between English and Thai language by two bilingual experts, discussion in a team of researchers to determine inadequate or different concepts of the translation, revision the concepts to be consistent with the original version, and a test of the translated questionnaires with a target population.

The IPQ-R questionnaire used to measure illness perception was divided into three main sections: identity, diabetes perception, and causal sections. The identity section included 14 common symptoms with a yes/no response format. The diabetes perception section consisted of 38 items of cognitive and emotional illness perception when living with T2D, which included seven subscales. Lastly, the causal section included 18 items that measured the participants opinion of what might have been the cause of T2D, focusing on the participants' own considerations. Both the diabetes perception and causal sections were designed using a five-point Likert scale as follows: 1 (strongly disagree), 2 (disagree), 3 (neither agree nor disagree), 4 (agree), and 5 (strongly agree). High scores for each subscale represented strongly-held or positive beliefs.

The DSMQ-R questionnaire was used to assess the self-care activities over the last 8 weeks of people with T2D. This instrument included 27 items of self-care activities (the first 20 items for non-insulin-treated participants and all 27 items for insulin-treated participants), comprising a sum scale and four sub-scales: glucose management, dietary control, physical activity, and healthcare use. The DSMQ-R was designed based on a four-point Likert scale, ranging from zero to three, with the responses "does not apply to me," "applies to me to some degree," "applies to me to a considerable degree," and "applies to me very much." The sum for each scale scores was computed and then transformed to a scale, ranging from 0 to 10 [28]. High scores indicated more effective self-management.

Psychometric properties of the measurement tools

Both Thai versions of the questionnaires were tested for validity and reliability [30]. The content validity was tested by three nursing experts specializing in diabetes. The process involved a team of experts considering if each item was conformed to the original versions, using 3-point rating scales as follows: 1 (not relevant), 2 (somewhat relevant), and 3 (highly relevant). Answer of each item was transformed into a dichotomous scale where highly relevant was considered as "relevant" and the others referred to "not relevant". The percentage of each relevant item, given by the experts, were calculated and documented as a content validity index for items (I-CVI) and for scales (S-CVI). [31]

The reliability of the questionnaires was tested for inter-rater, internal consistency, and test-retest. The inter-rater reliability was tested using three people with T2D to develop a consistent understanding among the three interviewers. Each participant was interviewed three times (each time by a different interviewer), and the three sets of questionnaires were checked for inconsistent answers, followed by a consensus discussion between the team of interviewers and the Thai researcher (first author). The internal consistency reliability was measured in a pilot study by interviewing 30 people with T2D. A re-interview was conducted 2 weeks after the initial interview to investigate the test-retest reliability.

Data analysis
The data were analyzed using SPSS for Windows version 21.0 [32] with a significance level of 0.05.

Analysis of the psychometric properties of the instruments
The content validity was established by calculating the content validity index (CVI) [31]. The proportion of each item rated as relevant by three experts, called the I-CVI, was computed, and the S-CVI was obtained by calculating the average of all I-CVIs of each instrument as reported in the Table 1. The percentage of the consistency of each set of questionnaires was calculated in order to determine the inter-rater reliability. The internal consistency reliability was examined using Cronbach's alpha coefficient [33]. The test-retest reliability was analyzed using Pearson correlation coefficient or the Spearman correlation coefficient, depending on the data distribution [34].

Statistical analysis
The categorical demographic characteristics of the participants were presented according to frequency and percentage, and the median was used for the continuous variables due to a skewed nature [34]. In order to compare the differences between the women and men, a chi-square test was used for the categorical variables, and the Mann-Whitney U test was used for testing the continuous variables [34].

The illness perception was presented according to each section in the IPQ-R scale using percentages, mean, and standard deviation (SD) Additionally, since a non-normal data distribution was found in the identity section and in each subscale of the diabetes perception section, the Mann-Whitney U test was used to compare the distribution of scores between the women and men [34]. In the

causal section, each item was transformed and grouped into a dichotomous variable (disagreement—strongly disagree, disagree, neither agree nor disagree; and agreement—agree and strongly agree). The percentage of agreement for each item was calculated to analyze the high respectively low rank of causal agreements.

Diabetes self-management was calculated using the mean score and SD of the sum scale and each subscale. The different scores of all subscales between the women and men were analyzed using the independent samples t test or Mann-Whitney U test, depending on the data distribution [34].

Results
Psychometric properties of the instruments
The Thai instruments, which were validated in this study, demonstrated acceptable validity and reliability (Table 1). The content validity of the DSMQ-R scale was high (0.91) and acceptable for all sections of the IPQ-R diabetic version scale (ranging from 0.75 to 0.98). Both instruments met the requirements for internal consistency (Cronbach's alpha >0.7). For the IPQ-R diabetic version scale, Cronbach's alpha of subscales were 0.81 for identity section, 0.76 for diabetes perception section, and 0.73 for causal section, and was 0.78 for the sum scale of the DSMQ-R instrument. The percentages of the consistency concerning inter-rater reliability ranged from 84.6 to 94.2%, which reflected consistent understanding in the team of interviewers. The results of the test-retest reliability showed a moderate association at the different significance level for both instruments, with the correlation coefficients ranking between 0.452 and 0.697, and the p-value in a range between less than 0.001 and less than 0.05. Results showing a moderate stability of the instruments obtained on two separate occasions.

Characteristics of the participants
The demographic characteristics are shown in Table 2. Of the total 220 participants, there were 150 women (68.2%) and 70 men (31.8%), and all were Buddhists. Most of the participants were married and had completed their education at the primary school level. More than half of the participants were unemployed. Men showed a higher percentage of marriage status ($\chi^2 = 5.344$, $p = 0.021$, df = 1),

Table 1 Validity and reliability test of the measurement tools

Measurement tools	Sum scale/Subscale	Validity and reliability test		
		Content validity index (CVI)	Cronbach's alpha	Test-retest reliability
Revised diabetes illness perception questionnaire (IPQ-R)	Identity section	0.98	0.81	$r_s = 0.697^{***}$ $p = 0.000$
	Diabetes perception section	0.75	0.76	$r = 0.502^{**}$ $p = 0.005$
	Causal section	0.96	0.73	$r = 0.452^{*}$ $p = 0.012$
Revised diabetes self-management questionnaire (DSMQ-R)	Sum scale	0.91	0.78	$r = 0.503^{**}$ $p = 0.005$

r = Pearson correlation coefficient, r_s = Spearman correlation coefficient $^{*}p < 0.05$ $^{**}p < 0.01$ $^{***}p < 0.001$

Table 2 Demographic characteristics of the participants

Demographic variables	Total ($n = 220$) n (%)	Women ($n = 150$) n (%)	Men ($n = 70$) n (%)	Statistical test	p-value
1. Socio-demographic characteristics					
Educational level					
Unschooled	27 (12.3)	24 (16.0)	3 (4.3)	$x^2 = 25.271$[***]	0.000
Primary school (Pratom 1 to 6)	146 (66.4)	107 (71.3)	39 (55.7)		
Secondary school (Mathayom 1 to 6)	30 (13.6)	14 (9.3)	16 (22.9)		
Higher than secondary school	17 (7.7)	5 (3.3)	12 (17.1)		
Marital status					
Married	146 (66.4)	92 (61.3)	54 (77.1)	$x^2 = 5.344$[*]	0.021
Not married	74 (33.6)	58 (38.7)	16 (22.9)		
Religion					
Buddhism	220 (100.0)	150 (100.0)	70 (100.0)	–	–
Occupation					
Employed	94 (42.7)	56 (37.3)	38 (54.3)	$x^2 = 5.605$[*]	0.018
Unemployed	126 (57.3)	94 (62.7)	32 (45.7)		
2. Illness-Related information					
Ordinary health service use					
Health Promoting Hospital	109 (49.5)	70 (46.7)	39 (55.7)	$x^2 = 1.742$	0.419
Other public hospitals	94 (42.7)	67 (44.7)	27 (38.6)		
Private Hospital	17 (7.7)	13 (8.7)	4 (5.7)		
Preferential treatment[a]					
Universal coverage	173 (78.6)	123 (82.0)	50 (71.4)	$x^2 = 3.213$	0.201
Other preferential treatment	37 (16.8)	21 (14.0)	16 (22.8)		
Self-payment	10 (4.5)	6 (4.0)	4 (5.7)		
Current treatment					
Oral anti-diabetic agent(s)	183 (83.2)	124 (82.7)	59 (84.3)	$x^2 = 0.089$	0.765
Oral pills in combination with other treatments	37 (16.8)	26 (17.3)	11 (15.7)		
Experience of diabetes complications					
No	53 (24.1)	30 (20.0)	23 (32.9)	$x^2 = 4.314$[*]	0.038
Yes	167 (75.9)	120 (80.0)	47 (67.1)		
Median (interquartile)					
Age (year)	64 (55-70)	62.5 (54-69.25)	67 (59.25-73)	$Z = -2.370$[*]	0.018
Duration of illness (year)	8 (4-14.5)	8 (4-14)	8.5 (3.75-15)	$Z = -0.515$	0.607
Level of Fasting Plasma Glucose (mg/dl)	144 (121.25-184)	147 (120-190)	141 (126-177)	$Z = -0.671$	0.502

[a] receive the treatment paid by the civil servants' medical benefits, social security, or universal coverage scheme

[*] $p < 0.05$, [**] $p < 0.01$, [***] $p < 0.001$, x^2 = Chi-square, Z = Mann-Whitney U test

had a higher educational level ($x^2 = 25.271$, $p < 0.000$, df = 3), were more often employed ($x^2 = 5.605$, $p = 0.018$, df = 1), and were significantly older than women ($Z = -2.370$, $p = 0.018$). Regarding the illness-related characteristics, most of the participants took oral anti-diabetic agents, used a universal coverage program as their preferential treatment, and received health services at the HPH and other public hospitals. There were no significant differences between men and women according to these illness-related characteristics,

except for a higher incidence of diabetic complications among women ($x^2 = 4.314$, $p = 0.038$, df = 1).

Illness perception

The 50th percentile (median) of symptoms experienced after being diagnosed with T2D was five (median (Mdn) 5, interquartile range (IQR) 3-7), six for women (Mdn 6, IQR 4-8) and three for men (Mdn 3, IQR 2-6). The most common symptoms that women experienced were dizziness, fatigue, pain, weight loss, sleep difficulties, and loss of strength, whereas men most often experienced fatigue, dizziness, and weight loss. Of these symptoms, both sexes believed that two symptoms were related to their diabetes (women: Mdn 2, IQR 1-4; men: Mdn 2, IQR 1-4), with no significant differences concerning the number of symptoms related to diabetes.

As seen in Table 3, women perceived to a higher degree negative consequences of T2D (Z = −2.204, p = 0.028) and a more fluctuating nature of their disease (Z = −3.441, p = 0.001) than men. Men felt more confident in the treatment given by the health professionals than women (Z = −2.031, p = 0.042).

Women and men presented a high percentage of agreement for possible causes of T2D. These causes were diet or eating habits (women: 85.3%, men: 92.9%), personal behaviors (women: 68.7%, men: 71.4%), and poor medical care in the past (women: 65.3%, men: 72.9%).

Self-management

There was no significant overall difference found in the self-care activities between women and men, although women demonstrated higher mean scores of glucose management and of healthcare use than men and men showed higher mean scores of dietary control and of physical activity than women (Table 4).

Discussion

Our findings showed that there were some differences in the illness perception between the Thai women and men with T2D, while they had similar experiences regarding self-management. Furthermore, the translated instruments used in this study showed acceptable content validity and internal consistency reliability, and moderate test-retest reliability.

The women in this study, in accordance with earlier studies, perceived to a higher degree negative consequences of the disease [12, 17, 18] as well as fluctuating symptoms than men [35]. They also showed a higher blood sugar level than the standard recommendations of glycemic control for

adults [36], implying poor glycemic control, which is known to lead to several symptoms connected with diabetes complications [37]. Furthermore, women in earlier studies were shown to be worried about their unpredictable future with diabetes [38] and expected everything to be under their control [9, 39], which may lead them to express negative perceptions when they detect something that does not align with their expectations.

On the other hand, men in this study showed higher confidence in the treatment effectiveness than women. This might be related to their higher educational level, corresponding to the findings in earlier research where it was seen that education may enhance the individual's sense of control, knowledge, and life skills [40, 41]. Furthermore, men in our study assessed their experiences of diabetes complications to a lower degree, which might give them a greater opportunity to develop confidence in the treatment, as seen in earlier studies [11, 12].

Our findings, that both women and men showed a low score on the "emotional representation" subscale for illness perception, is interesting since it might point to a less emotional response in a Thai diabetes population in comparison with Western populations [6, 8–10]. This might reflect that there is a different view of diabetes among people from diverse social contexts. While most Western people are shown to hold a strong belief in the biomedical model and to focus on self-responsibility [42], research conducted with Eastern people has found that they place a high value on a holistic view of health and illness, connecting with family closeness and religious beliefs [43] and social norms and values [44]. Corresponding to previous studies of Thai women with diabetes, the close attentiveness, encouragement, and understanding among the members in Eastern families [45] and their Buddhist beliefs [46] may have empowered our participants to improve their mental strength and have enabled them to accept their fate and to remain calm. This may also have increased their ability to cope with and manage their daily routines to suit their lives, in accordance with earlier Eastern research [47, 48].

Table 3 Tests for the different mean scores of illness perception between women and men

Subscales	Range	Total (n = 220) Mean (SD)	Women (n = 150) Mean (SD)	Men (n = 70) Mean (SD)	Mann-Whitney U test	p-value
Acute or chronic conditions[a]	5-30	24.53 (3.83)	24.75 (3.56)	24.07 (4.34)	Z = −0.516	0.606
Consequences	5-30	13.45 (3.88)	13.85 (3.96)	12.60 (3.60)	Z = −2.204*	0.028
Personal control	5-30	24.94 (2.71)	24.83 (2.74)	25.17 (2.67)	Z = −0.984	0.325
Treatment control	5-25	19.16 (2.52)	18.95 (2.55)	19.61 (2.41)	Z = −2.031*	0.042
Illness coherence	5-25	17.88 (3.43)	17.65 (3.60)	18.36 (3.00)	Z = −1.134	0.257
Fluctuating symptoms[b]	5-20	9.83 (2.82)	10.29 (2.73)	8.84 (2.76)	Z = −3.441**	0.001
Emotional representation	5-30	11.02 (5.16)	11.33 (5.38)	10.37 (4.63)	Z = −1.071	0.284

[a]Subscale name "timeline" was changed to "acute or chronic condition"
[b]Subscale name "timeline cyclical" was changed to "fluctuating symptoms"
* p < 0.05, ** p < 0.01

Table 4 Tests for the different mean scores of self-management between women and men

Subscales	Total ($n = 220$) Mean (SD)	Women ($n = 150$) Mean (SD)	Men ($n = 70$) Mean (SD)	Statistical tests	p-value
Sum scale	7.11 (1.24)	7.07 (1.16)	7.20 (1.41)	$t = -0.680$	0.498
Subscale					
- glucose management	6.80 (1.29)	6.83 (1.19)	6.73 (1.48)	$Z = -0.055$	0.956
- dietary control	7.34 (1.86)	7.26 (1.84)	7.51 (1.91)	$Z = -0.978$	0.328
- physical activity	7.13 (2.18)	6.97 (2.14)	7.46 (2.25)	$Z = -1.718$	0.086
- healthcare use	7.97 (1.34)	7.98 (1.21)	7.94 (1.58)	$Z = -0.784$	0.433

t = Independent samples t test, Z = Mann-Whitney U test

Another finding from this study, contrary to earlier Western research [15, 49], was the similarity in dietary control of women and men. A difference that might be explained by the influence earlier found from Buddhist teaching, the idea of using moderation and balance to accomplish goal existing in reality [50], and the strategy of "eating in moderation" in order to maintain acceptable levels of plasma glucose for most patients with T2D [47, 48]. Holding this view may have persuaded our participants with T2D to select proper food, reduce their intake of sweets, and to control their craving for harmful foods. Another explanation might be that patients with T2D in Thailand experience an inferior status to the healthcare professionals in the Thai healthcare system and tend to follow their advice [51]. Additionally, the personality of the Thai people, who choose avoidance or compromise rather than confrontation [52], may also have impelled the participants regardless of gender to comply with medical suggestions and to try to be consistent regarding the recommendations given to them.

The finding that both women and men demonstrated a low score on the glucose management subscale, which focused on self-monitoring of blood glucose levels (SMBG) and taking diabetes medications, was also interesting. Although SMBG was found to be a common self-care practice for managing diabetes among Western people [15], this procedure is not widely used among Thai people with T2D. In Thailand, healthcare professionals tend to take responsibility to monitor monthly plasma glucose, and SMBG seems to be inaccessible for Thai patients, at least our participants. Additionally, no formal patient education was provided at the HPHs; hence, the participants had less opportunity to learn about glucometers.

Being aware that the diabetes perceptions and the influences of the social context in the Thai population are gender based, might influence healthcare professionals to design clear, concise, and specific patient education programs. For an Eastern population with T2D, the concept of holistic care and belief in Buddhist teaching can be used to promote more effective self-management, particularly dietary control. Including assessments of diabetes perceptions and self-care activities, as well as considering the

preferences, needs, and beliefs of patients with T2D, might increase the compliance of supportive programs for individuals of both sexes in this population.

Strengths and limitations
Our findings were interpreted to have both strengths and limitations. The homogeneous socio-demographic characteristics of the participants, who were recruited from the same catchment areas of the HPH, were considered, and randomly selecting the HPHs was used to reduce bias and to provide an equal chance for each HPH to be chosen as a study sample [27]. This may allow our findings to be generalized to people with diabetes living in the suburban areas around Bangkok, Thailand. Additionally, our estimation of participating numbers of women and men calculated based on the likelihood ratio of developing T2D in Thai women and Thai men.

(2 : 1) [5] may also increase the possibility to generalize the findings to other populations.

The structured interview method provided an opportunity to obtain answers from all literate and illiterate participants. Furthermore, the researchers tried to reduce the errors in the data collected by selecting experienced interviewers, training them before the interview, and coaching them with the first author once a week. However, we lost one-fifth of the potential participants that were occupied with a daytime job, which would provide additional information. In addition, the relatively high degree of dropout participants (30%), with inaccurate addresses, might be a drawback to influence our results. However, it is a factor out of our control since finding accurate address in the Thai system is difficult and complex. The Thai version of the instruments used in this study showed acceptable validity and reliability, which showed that they were the proper tools for collecting the data, but these questionnaires still had some restrictions. For example, the glucose management subscale in the DSMQ-R questionnaire, which has three items focusing on SMBG activities, may not be suitable for assessing information from participants that do not use a glucometer. Furthermore, only 16 insulin-treated participants took part in this study, and these results should not be generalized to the insulin-treated population.

Conclusion

This study of women and men living with T2D in a suburban area of Bangkok, Thailand, showing that there are many similarities but also some differences between women and men in illness perception, might provide new knowledge in this area of research. Furthermore, the lack of differences between men and women with T2D regarding self-care activities in a Thai population is different from Western studies. The findings that women perceived more negative consequences of diabetes and more fluctuating symptoms of their disease, while men perceived more confidence in treatment effectiveness, are of interest and consistent with earlier research.

Abbreviations

SMBG: Self-monitoring of blood glucose levels; T2D: Type 2 diabetes

Acknowledgements

On particular, we wish to thank the directors of the sampled Health Promoting Hospitals and the Village Health Volunteers working in the catchment areas for their immense supports in the data collection phase.

Funding

This study was supported by Rangsit University, Thailand in terms of flight ticket, accommodation, and monthly expenses for the corresponding author when living in Sweden and by Malmö University, Sweden for educational materials and facilities.

Authors' contributions

WB and MÖ came up with the research idea. WB, MÖ, AC and IDR participated in the design and WB accomplished the data collection of the empirical studies. WB did the quantitative analysis. WB drafted the main part of the manuscript, with supervision of MÖ, AC and IDR. All authors read and approved the final version of the manuscript.

Authors' information

WB, the corresponding author is an Assistant Professor in nursing, Rangsit University, Thailand. AC and IDR are the senior lecturers and MÖ is the Professor. All co-authors are from the Faculty of Health and Society, Malmö University, Sweden.

Competing interests

The authors declare that they have no competing interests.

Author details

[1]Faculty of Nursing Science, Rangsit University, Pathum Thani 12000, Thailand. [2]Faculty of Health and Society, Malmö University, SE 205 06 Malmö, Sweden.

References

1. Guariguata L, Whiting DR, Hambleton I, Beagley J, Linnenkamp U, Shaw JE. Global estimates of diabetes prevalence for 2013 and projections for 2035. Diabetes Res Clin Pract. 2014;103:137–49.
2. Shaw JE, Sicree RA, Zimmet PZ. Global estimates of the prevalence of diabetes for 2010 and 2030. Diabetes Res Clin Pract. 2010;87:4–14.
3. Wild S, Roglic G, Green A, Sicree R, King H. Global prevalence of diabetes: estimates for the year 2000 and projections for 2030. Diabetes Care. 2004;27:1047–53.
4. World Health Organization. Diabetes. 2015. http://www.who.int/mediacentre/factsheets/fs312/en. Accessed 27 Sept 2015.
5. Thonghong A, Thepsittha K, Jongpiriyaanan P, Gappbirom T. Chronic disease surveillance report 2012. Wkly Epidemiol Surveill Report, Thail. 2013;44:800–8.
6. Tenzer-Iglesias P. Type 2 diabetes mellitus in women. Suppl to J Fam Pract. 2014;63:S21–6.
7. Nayak BS, Sobrian A, Latiff K, Pope D, Rampersad A, Lourenço K, et al. The association of age, gender, ethnicity, family history, obesity and hypertension with type 2 diabetes mellitus in Trinidad. Diabetes Metab Syndr. 2014;8:91–5.
8. Collins MM, Corcoran P, Perry IJ. Anxiety and depression symptoms in patients with diabetes. Diabet Med. 2009;26:153–61.
9. Gucciardi E, Wang SCT, DeMelo M, Amaral L, Stewart DE. Characteristics of men and women with diabetes: observations during patients' initial visit to a diabetes education centre. Can Fam Physician. 2008;54:219–27.
10. Svenningsson I, Björkelund C, Marklund B, Gedda B. Anxiety and depression in obese and normal-weight individuals with diabetes type 2: a gender perspective. Scand J Caring Sci. 2012;26:349–54.
11. Brown SA, Harrist RB, Villagomez ET, Segura M, Barton SA, Hanis CL. Gender and treatment differences in knowledge, health beliefs, and metabolic control in Maxican Americans with type 2 diabetes. Diabetes Educ. 2000;26:425–38.
12. Fitzgerald JT, Anderson RM, Davis WK. Gender differences in diabetes attitudes and adherence. Diabetes Educ. 1995;21:523–9.
13. Koch T, Kralik D, Taylor J. Men living with diabetes: minimizing the intrusiveness of the disease. J Clin Nurs. 2000;9:247–54.
14. Koch T, Kralik D, Sonnack D. Women living with type II diabetes: the intrusion of illness. J Clin Nurs. 1999;8:712–22.
15. Mathew R, Gucciardi E, De Melo M, Barata P. Self-management experiences among men and women with type 2 diabetes mellitus: a qualitative analysis. BMC Fam Pract. 2012;13:122.
16. Moss-Morris R, Weinman J, Petrie KJ, Horne R, Cameron LD, Buick D. The revised illness perception questionnaire (IPQ-R). Psychol Health. 2002;17:1–16.
17. Stuckey HL, Mullan-Jensen CB, Reach G, Kovacs-Burns K, Piana N, Vallis M, et al. Personal accounts of the negative and adaptive psychosocial experiences of people with diabetes in the second diabetes attitudes, wishes and needs (DAWN2) study. Diabetes Care. 2014;37:2466–74.
18. Svenningsson I, Marklund B, Attvall S, Gedda B. Type 2 diabetes: perceptions of quality of life and attitudes towards diabetes from a gender perspective. Scand J Caring Sci. 2011;25:688–95.
19. Richard AA, Shea K. Delineation of self-care and associated concepts. J Nurs Scholarsh. 2011;43:255–64.
20. de Alba Garcia JG, Rocha ALS, Lopez I, Baer RD, Dressler W, Weller SC. "Diabetes is my companion": lifestyle and self-management among good and poor control Mexican diabetic patients. Soc Sci Med. 2007;64:2223–35.
21. Mumu SJ, Saleh F, Ara F, Afnan F, Ali L. Non-adherence to life-style modification and its factors among type 2 diabetic patients. Indian J Public Health. 2014;58:40–4.
22. Weinger K. Psychosocial issues and self-care mental health concerns and family dynamics. Am J Nurs. 2007;107:34–8.
23. Sudchada P, Khom-Ar-Wut C, Eaimsongchram A, Katemut S, Kunmaturos P, Deoisares R. Diabetes and cardiovascular risk factor controls in Thai type 2 diabetes with no history of cardiovascular complications: situation and compliance to diabetes management guideline in Thailand. J Diabetes Complicat. 2012;26:102–6.
24. Mann CJ. Observational research methods. Research design II: cohort, cross sectional, and case-control studies. Emerg Med J. 2003;20:54–60.
25. Pathum Thani Provincial Health Office. แผนพัฒนาจังหวัดปทุมธานี 4 ปี (พ ศ. 2558-2561) ฉบับปรับปรง [revised version of the development plan for

4 years (2015-2018)]. 2013. http://123.242.173.131/pathumthani_news/attach_file/plan58_61_131256.pdf. Accessed 20 Oct 2015.

26. Sedgwick P. Multistage sampling. BMJ. 2015;351:h4155.

27. Naing NN. Determination of sample size. Malaysian J Med Sci. 2003;10:84–6.

28. Schmitt A, Gahr A, Hermanns N, Kulzer B, Huber J, Haak T. The diabetes self-management questionnaire (DSMQ): development and evaluation of an instrument to assess diabetes self-care activities associated with glycaemic control. Health Qual Life Outcomes. 2013;11:138.

29. World Health Organization. Process of translation and adaptation of instruments. 2014. http://www.who.int/entity/substance_abuse/research_tools/translation/en/. Accessed 20 Oct 2015.

30. Cook DA, Beckman TJ. Current concepts in validity and reliability for psychometric instruments: theory and application. Am J Med. 2006;119 doi: https://doi.org/10.1016/j.amjmed.2005.10.036

31. Polit DF, Beck CT. The content validity index: are you sure you know what's being reported? Critique and recommendations. Res Nurs Heal. 2006;29:489–97.

32. IBM corp. IBM SPSS statistics for windows, version 21.0. Armonk: IBM corp; 2012.

33. Pongwichai S. **การวิเคราะห์ข้อมูลทางสถิติด้วยคอมพิวเตอร์เน้นสำหรับงานวิจัย** [analysis of statistical data by the computer for the research project]. 24th ed. V-print company: Bangkok; 2013.

34. Kellar SP, Kelvin EA. Munro's statistical methods for health care research. 6th ed. Wolters Kluwer Health Lippincott Williams and Wilkins: Philadelphis; 2013.

35. Kacerovsky-Bielesz G, Lienhardt S, Hagenhofer M, Kacerovsky M, Forster E, Roth R, et al. Sex-related psychological effects on metabolic control in type 2 diabetes mellitus. Diabetologia. 2009;52:781–8.

36. American Diabetes Association. Standards of medical care in diabetes-2014. Diabetes Care. 2014;37:14–80.

37. American Diabetes Association. Implications of the diabetes control and complications trial. Diabetes Care. 2002;26:S25.

38. Boonsatean W, Carlsson A, Östman M, Dychawy Rl. Living with diabetes: experiences of inner and outer sources of beliefs in women with low socioeconomic status. Glob J Health Sci. 2016;8 doi: https://doi.org/10.5539/gjhs.v8n8p200

39. de Silva DM, Hegadoren K, Lasiuk G. The perspectives of Brazilian homemakers concerning living with type 2 diabetes mellitus. Rev Lat Am Enfermagem. 2012;20:469–77.

40. Mirowsky J, Ross CE. Education, personal control, lifestyle and health: a human capital hypothesis. Res Aging. 1998;20:415–49.

41. Slagsvold B, Sørensen A. Age, education, and the gender gap in the sense of control. Int J Aging Hum Dev. 2008;67:25–42.

42. Åsbring P. Words about body and soul: social representations relating to health and illness. J Health Psychol. 2012;17:1110–20.

43. Lundberg PC. Cultural care of Thai immigrants in Uppsala: a study of transcultural nursing in Sweden. J Transcult Nurs. 2000;11:274–80.

44. Sissons JM. Lay explanations of the causes of diabetes in India and the UK. In: Markova I, Farr RM, editors. Representations of health, illness and handicap. Chur Switzerland: Harwood Academic Publishers; 1995. p. 163–88.

45. Boonsatean W, Dychawy Rosner I, Carlsson A, Östman M. Women of low socioeconomic status living with diabetes: becoming adept at handling a disease. SAGE Open Med. 2015;3 https://doi.org/10.1177/2050312115621312.

46. Lundberg PC, Thrakul S. Religion and self-management of Thai Buddhist and Muslim women with type 2 diabetes. J Clin Nurs. 2013;22:1907–16.

47. Lundberg PC, Thrakul S. Type 2 diabetes: how do Thai Buddhist people with diabetes practise self-management? J Adv Nurs. 2012;68:550–8.

48. Sowattanangoon N, Kotchabhakdi N, Petrie KJ. The influence of Thai culture on diabetes perceptions and management. Diabetes Res Clin Pract. 2009;84:245–51.

49. Hjelm K, Nambozi G. Beliefs about health and illness: a comparison between Ugandan men and women living with diabetes mellitus. Int Nurs Rev. 2008;55:434–41.

50. Phromtha S. **พุทธปรัชญา: มนุษย์ สังคม และปัญหาจริยธรรม** [Buddhism philosophy: human being, social, and morality problem]. Bangkok: Chulalongkorn University Press; 1999.

51. Naemiratch B, Manderson L. Control and adherence: living with diabetes in Bangkok, Thailand. Soc Sci Med. 2006;63:1147–57.

52. Burnard P, Naiyapatana W. Culture and communication in Thai nursing: a report of an ethnographic study. Int J Nurs Stud. 2004;41:755–65.

2

Higher serum 25(OH)D level is associated with decreased risk of impairment of glucose homeostasis: data from Southwest China

Danting Li[1], Haoche Wei[2], Hongmei Xue[1], Jieyi Zhang[1], Mengxue Chen[1], Yunhui Gong[3] and Guo Cheng[1*]

Abstract

Background: Recent epidemiological studies have suggested inverse associations between vitamin D status and metabolic diseases including type 2 diabetes (T2DM). The aim of this study was to examine whether a higher serum 25-hydroxyvitamin D (25(OH)D) was associated with a more favorable glucose homeostasis among adults without diabetes in Southwest China.

Methods: Serum 25(OH)D concentration was measured in a cross-sectional sample of 1514 adults without diabetes aged 25–65 years recruited from Southwest China. Indices describing glucose homeostasis included fasting plasma glucose (FPG), fasting insulin, glycated hemoglobin (HbA_{1c}), the homeostatic model assessment 2-insulin resistance (HOMA2-IR) and odds of pre-diabetes. Data were analyzed by multivariable-adjusted regression models.

Results: The average serum 25(OH)D was 22.66 ng/ml, and percentages of vitamin D deficiency [25(OH)D < 20 ng/ml], insufficiency [20 ≤ 25(OH)D ≤ 30 ng/ml] were 47.6 and 32.2%, respectively. Serum 25(OH)D was inversely associated with fasting insulin ($P = 0.0007$), HbA_{1c} ($P = 0.0001$) and HOMA2-IR ($P = 0.0007$), but not with FPG, after adjusting for age, gender, monthly personal income, smoking status, energy intake, moderate-to-vigorous physical activity (MVPA) and waist circumference (WC). Compared with the lowest 25(OH)D tertile, the odds ratio for pre-diabetes in the highest tertile was 0.68 (95%CI: 0.47-0.99) after adjustment for cofounders. In the following stratified analyses according to weight status, we only observed this inverse association between serum 25(OH)D and pre-diabetes in overweight or obese adults ($n = 629$, $P = 0.047$), but not in their counterparts with BMI < 24 kg/m^2.

Conclusions: Our results advocate that a higher serum 25(OH)D level is associated with decreased risk of impairment of glucose homeostasis among adults without diabetes in Southwest China. Further studies are warranted to determine the role of vitamin D in glucose homeostasis.

Keywords: Vitamin D, Glucose homeostasis, Pre-diabetes, Adult

Background

Over the past decades, the prevalence of type 2 diabetes (T2DM) among Chinese adults has increased from 2.5% in 1994 [1] to 11.6% in 2013 [2]. Additionally, almost half of the adult population had pre-diabetes [2], a major risk factor for the development of T2DM [3].

* Correspondence: ehw_cheng@126.com
[1]Department of Nutrition, Food Safety and Toxicology, West China School of Public Health, Sichuan University, No.16, Section 3, Renmin Nan Road, Chengdu 610041, Sichuan, China
Full list of author information is available at the end of the article

It is becoming clear that vitamin D status is related to cancer [4], multiple sclerosis [5], cardiovascular disease [6], and diabetes [7–9], besides its role in the modulation of calcium absorption and bone metabolism. Moreover, Vitamin D deficiency has now recognized as a worldwide concern [10]. Zhen et al. [11]. reported that northwest Chinese adults exhibit high prevalence (75.2%) of vitamin D deficiency [25(OH)D < 20 ng/mL].

The associations between vitamin D and factors involved in glucose homeostasis have drawn a great deal of attention recently. 25-hydroxyvitamin D (25(OH)D), the sum of both 25(OH)D2 and 25(OH)D3, is a generally accepted biomarker of vitamin D status. Several observational studies have reported that serum 25(OH)D is negatively associated with fasting plasma glucose (FPG) and insulin among western populations [12–15]. In addition, patients with T2DM had lower serum 25(OH)D compared to control subjects without diabetes [16]. Notably, vitamin D metabolism and its nutritional status were found to differ by ethnicity [8], nonetheless evidence from Asian populations is limited. Available data from China report that 25(OH)D is negatively associated with insulin resistance in patients with T2DM [17], while studies conducted among participants without diabetes are much less [18]. Besides, existing studies mainly focus on the relation of vitamin D with partial indicators (e.g. FPG or insulin) which can not cover the general status of glucose homeostasis.

Therefore, using data from a representative study among Chinese adults without diabetes, we investigated whether a higher serum 25(OH)D was associated with a more favorable glucose homeostasis (a. relative lower level of FPG, fasting insulin, HbA$_{1c}$ and HOMA2-IR within their normal ranges; b. lower odds of prediabetes). Furthermore, our results may highlight the importance of improving vitamin D status in the general population.

Methods
Study population
We used data from an ongoing population-based prospective study conducted in Southwest China initiated in September 2013, which aimed to investigate the health impact of nutritional and lifestyle factors on the development of several chronic diseases, as described elsewhere [19]. Using a cluster random sampling design stratified by urban and rural locations, a representative sample of civilian aged 25–65 years was recruited from the general population in Chengdu, Southwest China. The participants were invited to the study center for interviews. Generally, each visit included anthropometric measurements, medical examinations, questionnaires and face-to-face interviews by trained investigators about nutrition-related behaviors, lifestyles and social status. However, the following participants were excluded from the study: a) if they had major organ diseases, including heart, liver or kidney disease; b) if they had mental diseases; c) if they were taking hormone-based drugs and other medicines that affect blood glucose and lipids; or d) if they were pregnant or lactating women. The study was approved by the Ethics Committee of Sichuan University, and all participants provided written informed consent.

For the reason that serum 25(OH)D concentration was not measured in 2013 and 2014, eligible data in the present analysis were identified from the baseline survey conducted from March to October, 2015. Participants in survey 2013-2014 did not differ in gender, age, location and educational status from those who were included in our study.

Laboratory methods
All participants were requested to have an overnight fast of at least 10 h. Peripheral venous blood samples were centrifuged, aliquoted and stored at – 80 °C until measurement. 25(OH)D, calcium^{2+} and insulin were assayed from serum samples, while plasma samples were used to measure the concentrations of FPG. Finally, HbA$_{1c}$ was quantified from resolved erythrocytes. Serum 25(OH)D was measured using high-performance liquid chromatography (Agilent 1260 HPLC, Shanghai, China) and the intra-assay Coefficient of Variation (CV) was less than 5%. Vitamin D nutritional status was assessed as "deficiency" (< 20 ng/ml), "insufficiency" (20-30 ng/ml) or "sufficiency" (> 30 ng/ml) [20]. Serum calcium^{2+}, which is closely related to serum 25(OH)D, was measured by automatic biochemistry analyzer. Serum insulin was assayed with chemiluminescence enzyme immunoassay within 4 h, and the intra-assay CV was 2.4%. Plasma glucose was measured by hexokinase assay on blood collected into fluoridated EDTA tubes within 2 h with an intra-assay CV of 2.5%. HbA$_{1c}$ was quantified with high-performance liquid chromatography (Bio-Rad D10 automatic analyzer, Shanghai, China) (intra-assay CV: 1.1%) at the clinical laboratory center in Chengdu, which was certified by the National Glycohemoglobin Standardization Program. Finally, the insulin resistance index (HOMA2-IR) was calculated using updated homeostasis model assessment methods (http://www.dtu.ox.ac.uk/homacalculator/) according to the Wallace formula [21].

Anthropometric measurements
Anthropometric measurements were performed by trained medical workers according to the standard procedures [22], with the participants dressed in underwear only, barefoot, and women's hair uncovered. Waist circumference (WC) was measured without clothes midway between the lower rib margin and iliac crest, to the nearest 0.1 cm, after inhalation and exhalation, using inelasticity tape. Height and weight were measured to the nearest 0.1 kg and 0.1 cm, respectively, with an ultrasonic meter (Weight and Height Instrument DHM-30, China). Weight, height and WC were each averaged based on two measurements. Body mass index (BMI) was calculated as weight (kg) divided by height squared (m^2) and was categorized as underweight (BMI < 18.5 kg/m^2), normal weight (18.5 kg/m^2 ≤ BMI < 24 kg/m^2), overweight (24 kg/m^2 ≤ BMI < 28 kg/m^2), or obese (BMI ≥ 28 kg/m^2) using the standard of Working Group on Obesity in China [23].

Definition of pre-diabetes

Pre-diabetes, based on glycaemic parameters above normal but below diabetes thresholds, is a high risk state for diabetes [24]. In our study, it was defined using the updated classification and diagnosis of diabetes of American Diabetes Association [3] as presentation of one or more of the following results: a) HbA_{1c} of 5.7-6.4%; b) Fasting blood glucose of 100-125 mg/dl (5.6-6.9 mmol/L).

Other covariates

Information on socio-demographic characteristics, lifestyle, dietary intake, and other potential confounders were collected by interviewer-administered questionnaires in a face-to-face interview.

For the present analysis, we assessed socio-demographic factors potentially associated with serum 25(OH)D level and glucose homeostasis, which included gender, age (years), education level (≤ 6, $6\sim 12$, or > 12 years of schooling), occupation (mental worker, physical worker, retired or unemployed) [25] and monthly personal income (≤ 1800 Yuan, $1800\sim 3200$ Yuan, or > 3200 Yuan) [26]. We also collected data on lifestyle, including smoking status (current smokers, ex-smokers and non-smokers), sleeping and stress, and physical activities. To quantify the intensity of physical activities, the energy cost of moderate-to-vigorous physical activity (MVPA) was measured in metabolic equivalents-hours per week (MET-hours/week) [27].

Dietary data were collected on two random days within a 10-day period by trained investigators using a validated 24-h dietary recall [19]. Participants were asked to recall all foods and beverages they consumed and the corresponding timing. Dietary intake data from 24-h dietary recall were converted into energy using the continuously updated in-house nutrient database based on China Food Composition 2009 [28]. And in this analysis, total energy intake for each participant was calculated as individual means of two-day 24-h dietary recall in kcal/day. Alcohol beverage consumption (cups/d) and coffee consumption (cups/wk) were accessed by food frequency questionnaire.

In addition, season of blood drawn (spring: March to May, summer: June to August; autumn: September to November; winter: December to February) was recorded.

Statistical analysis

All statistical analyses were performed with SAS software (SAS, version 9.3, 2011, SAS Institute Inc., Cary, NC, USA.). A P value < 0.05 was considered statistically significant, except for interaction tests, where $P < 0.1$ was considered significant. Normality of all continuous variables was examined using normal probability plots and the Kolmogorov-Smirnov test. Given their non-normality, all continuous variables were presented as median (25th percentile, 75th percentile). As the initial analysis indicated no interaction between gender and relations of serum 25(OH)D with FPG, HbA_{1c}, insulin levels, HOMA2-IR (range of P-value: 0.4–0.9), we pooled the sample in the follow-up analyses.

We cross-classified the study sample into categories of tertiles (T1-T3) of serum 25(OH)D to examine the distribution of baseline parameters. We tested differences in proportions using Student t-tests for normally-distributed continuous variables, the Wilcoxon rank-sum for non-normally distributed continuous variables and the Chi-square test for categorical variables, respectively.

To investigate the associations of serum 25(OH)D with glucose homeostasis, multivariable linear generalized regression models (PROC GLM in SAS) were performed. Serum 25(OH)D was defined as the independent variable in separate models. Glucose homeostasis including fasting insulin, FPG, HbA_{1c} and HOMA2-IR were dependent variables in separate models. The independent and dependent variables that enter the linear regression models were non-normally distributed continuous variables. To improve the fitting effect of the models, log-transformed values of insulin, FPG, HbA_{1c} and HOMA2-IR were used in the models.

In the basic models, the correlation analyses between serum 25(OH)D and glucose homeostasis (insulin, FPG, HbA_{1c}, HOMA2-IR) were carried out first. In a further analysis, the following variables potentially affecting these associations were added: gender, age (years), educational level (≤ 6 years, $6\sim 12$ years, or > 12 years of theoretical education), monthly personal income (≤ 1800 Yuan, $1800\sim 3200$ Yuan, or > 3200 Yuan), occupation (mental worker, physical worker, retired or unemployed), smoking status (current smokers, ex-smokers and non-smokers), MVPA (MET-hour/week), total energy intake (kcal/d), alcohol beverage consumption (cups/d), coffee consumption (cups/wk), serum $calcium^{2+}$ (mmol/L), season of blood drawn (spring, summer, autumn and winter) and WC (cm) or BMI (kg/m^2). Each variable was initially considered separately, and variables that had their own independent significant effect in the basic models or that substantially modified the association of serum 25(OH)D with each variable of glucose homeostasis were included in the multivariate analyses. Thus, age, gender, monthly personal income, smoking status and season of blood drawn were retained in model A. In a further step, we additionally adjusted for MVPA and energy intake (model B). WC was checked as a potential confounder in model C. The adjusted means were the least-squares means predicted by the model when the other variables were held at their mean values. Then the least-squares means and 95% confidence interval (95%CI) computed by the linear models were back transformed and then presented in the results.

Finally, multivariate logistic regression analyses were used to determine the association of serum 25(OH)D with the odds of pre-diabetes. To enhance comparability, models were constructed in analogy to the multivariable linear regression analyses. To explore interaction of weight status on this association, we divided the participants into two groups according to their weight status (overweight or not) and performed stratified analyses. Estimates are presented as odds ratios (ORs) with 95% CI.

Results

A total of 1710 adults (654 men and 1056 women) had their blood drawn, completing the anthropometric measurements and questionnaires initially in 2015. We excluded individuals who had already been diagnosed with diabetes mellitus ($n = 166$) and adults who had taken vitamin D supplements, calcitriol or calcium ($n = 21$). Furthermore, participants who had missing value on anthropometric or biological data, or information on relevant covariates were excluded ($n = 9$). Therefore, this analysis was based on a final sample of 1514 participants (Fig. 1).

General characteristics of the study sample are presented in Table 1. Participants (62.6% women) included in the present analysis had a mean age of 48.74 years. The average serum 25(OH)D concentration was 22. 66 ng/ml, and percentages of vitamin D deficiency and insufficiency were 47.6 and 32.2%, respectively. Almost 65.2% of the participants had pre-diabetes (Additional file 1: Table S1), and the prevalence of overweight or obesity was 41.5% in our study sample.

Across 25(OH)D tertiles, participants in higher serum 25(OH)D tertiles had significantly lower fasting insulin, HOMA2-IR, serum calcium^{2+} and monthly personal income, in addition, they were more likely to have their

blood drawn in summer and to engage in more physical activities than those in lower tertiles of serum 25(OH)D concentration. The differences in the associations (Vitamin D and glucose homeostasis) between the three proposed groups were not statistically significant in regard to FPG or HbA$_{1c}$ and several other variables. (Table 2).

The associations of tertiles of Vitamin D with glucose homeostasis are shown in Table 3. Multiple linear regression analysis showed that serum 25(OH)D concentration was inversely related to fasting insulin ($P = 0. 016$), HbA$_{1c}$ ($P = 0.0003$) and HOMA2-IR ($P = 0.016$) in these non-diabetic participants after adjustment for age, gender, monthly personal income, smoking status and season of blood drawn (model A), while association between vitamin D and FPG was not statistically significant ($P > 0.05$, after adjusting for confounders mentioned above). Further adjusting for MVPA, energy intake (model B), or including additional adjustment for WC (model C) did not materially change these inverse associations. Adults in the highest serum 25(OH)D concentration tertile had 12.4% lower fasting insulin ($P = 0. 0007$), 2.2% lower HbA$_{1c}$ ($P = 0.0001$) and 12.3% lower HOMA2-IR ($P = 0.0007$) than those in the lowest tertile.

Table 4 outlines the association of tertiles of Vitamin D with the odds of pre-diabetes. A significantly 32% lower odds of pre-diabetes was observed for adults in the highest tertile of serum 25(OH)D (OR: 0.68, 95%CI: 0.47-0.99) compared with those in the lowest tertile after adjustment for potential confounders. We further discovered an interaction of weight status on this association ($P = 0.06$). In stratified analyses, overweight individuals in the highest tertile of serum 25(OH)D had lowest risk of pre-diabetes ($P = 0.047$), but not in individuals with BMI < 24 kg/m^2. To compare these results with western adults, we conducted a sensitivity analysis using the criteria of World Health Organization to define overweight and observed similar result patterns (Additional file 2: Table S2).

Discussion

This study suggests that a higher vitamin D level was associated with a more favorable glucose homeostasis among non-diabetic adults in Southwest China. Moreover, a poor vitamin D status was significantly related with an increased risk of pre-diabetes especially in overweight or obese adults.

As indicated in previous studies [8, 12, 13], our findings suggested inverse associations of serum 25(OH)D with fasting insulin and insulin resistance. Of note, superior than the traditional assessment of HOMA1-IR, our study used HOMA2-IR to assess insulin resistance [29, 30]. The underlying mechanisms that may explain these associations have not been well understood, many

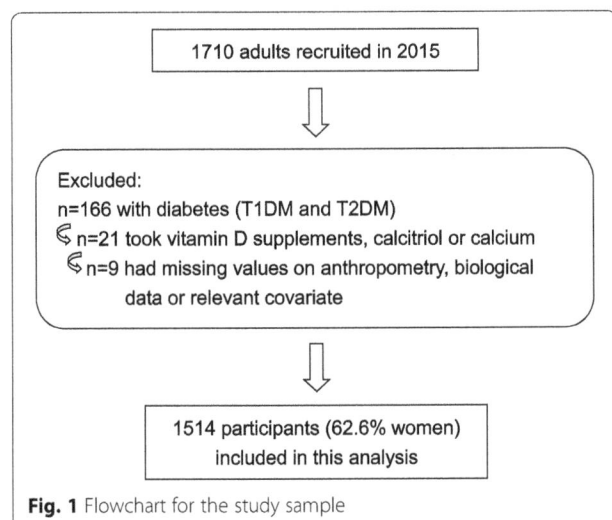

1710 adults recruited in 2015

⬇

Excluded:
n=166 with diabetes (T1DM and T2DM)
≲ n=21 took vitamin D supplements, calcitriol or calcium
≲ n=9 had missing values on anthropometry, biological data or relevant covariate

⬇

1514 participants (62.6% women) included in this analysis

Fig. 1 Flowchart for the study sample

Table 1 Characteristics[a] of study sample by gender ($n = 1514$)

Characteristics	Total	Male	Female
n (%)	1514 (100.0)	566 (37.4)	948 (62.6)
Age (yrs)	51.5 (37.9, 60.6)	46.7 (32.2, 60.4)	53.2 (42.1, 60.6)
Serum 25(OH) D (ng/ml)	20.7 (15.2, 27.9)	19.7 (14.6, 25.1)	21.8 (15.7, 29.9)
Pre-diabetes[b] (n (%))	987 (65.2)	383 (67.7)	604 (63.7)
Blood parameters			
Fasting plasma glucose (mmol/L)	5.20 (5.51, 5.85)	5.58 (5.28, 5.89)	5.46 (5.16, 5.84)
Fasting insulin (µIU/mL)	6.40 (4.13, 10.13)	6.70 (3.95, 10.00)	6.30 (4.20, 10.20)
HbA$_{1c}$ (%)	5.50 (5.20, 5.80)	5.50 (5.20, 5.80)	5.60 (5.30, 5.80)
HOMA2-IR[c]	0.87 (0.55, 1.35)	0.89 (0.52, 1.34)	0.84 (0.59, 1.37)
Serum calcium^{2+} (mmol/L)	2.42 (2.33, 2.51)	2.45 (2.36, 2.55)	2.40 (2.32, 2.50)
Anthropometric parameters			
Overweight[d] (n (%))	629 (41.5)	288 (50.9)	341 (35.9)
Overweight[e] (n (%))	442 (29.2)	212 (37.5)	230 (24.3)
Body mass index (kg/m^2)	23.2 (21.0, 25.4)	24.1 (21.9, 26.1)	22.7 (20.8, 25.0)
Waist circumference (cm)	84.1 (77.5, 91.0)	86.4 (80.5, 92.4)	82.5 (76.0, 89.1)
Social-demographic data			
High education level[f] (n (%))	676 (44.7)	311 (55.0)	365 (38.5)
High monthly personal income[g] (n (%))	576 (38.0)	319 (56.4)	257 (27.1)
Mental worker[h](n (%))	510 (33.7)	204 (36.0)	306 (32.3)
Lifestyles			
Smoking status (current, n (%))	217 (14.4)	192 (33.9)	25 (2.6)
MVPA (MET-hour/week)[i]	95.4 (60.6, 144.3)	78.5 (49.5, 122.1)	105.8 (69.5, 155.5)
Total energy intake (kcal/d)	1552.2 (1251.3, 1886.9)	1808.9 (1494.0, 2141.5)	1409.3 (1167.1, 1705.4)
Season of blood drawn (summer[j], n (%))	372 (24.6)	142 (25.1)	230 (24.3)

[a]Values are median (25th percentile, 75th percentile) for non-normally-distributed continuous variables and n (%) for categorical variables
[b]Pre-diabetes was defined using the updated classification and diagnosis of diabetes of American Diabetes Association (ADA) [3]
[c]HOMA2-IR, Homeostasis model assessment 2-insulin resistance, calculated by Wallace Formula [21]
[d]Body mass index ≥24.0 kg/m^2 [23]
[e]Body mass index ≥25.0 kg/m^2 [48]
[f]At least 12 years of school education
[g]Monthly personal income at least ≥3200 CNY (Chinese Yuan), which is moderate level among the general population in Southwest China [26]
[h]Mental worker includes professional and technical personnel (teacher/policeman/doctor etc), legislator & administrator, businessman and student [25]
[i]MVPA: moderate-to-vigorous physical activity (MET-hour/week) [27]. MET: Metabolic equivalent
[j]Summer in Southwest China is from June to August generally

possibilities being raised: a) vitamin D appears to exert effects on pancreatic β-cells secretory function and insulin sensitivity through direct modulation of gene expression via vitamin D receptors (VDRs) or regulation of calcium influx [31, 32]; b) VDR gene polymorphisms have been recently suggested to associate with variation in insulin secretion [33, 34]; and c) insufficient vitamin D usually results in increased serum parathyroid hormone which in turn has been found to be related to impaired glucose tolerance and decreased insulin sensitivity in healthy adults [35].

Serum 25(OH)D in the present study was shown to be negatively associated with HbA$_{1c}$, the longer-term marker of glycemic status, which was in line with a cross-sectional population-based survey from National Health and Nutrition Examination Survey (NHANES) 2003-2006 [36]. Liu et al. [12] reported an inverse association between serum 25(OH)D and FPG as well, whereas we did not observe that. One reason for the divergence might be that FPG is a short-term indicator of glycemic status susceptible to participants' diet and emotion at specific times. Moreover, evidence has suggested the decrease in HbA$_{1c}$ with increasing 25(OH)D was the steepest in levels < 65 nmol/L (26 ng/ml), with some small decreases with further increases [37]. In this scenario, the relative poorer vitamin D status of our study sample may lead to a more overt relation of serum 25(OH)D with HbA$_{1c}$ rather than with FPG.

Table 2 Characteristics of study sample by tertiles of serum 25(OH)D (n = 1514)[a]

	Tertiles of serum 25(OH)D (ng/ml)			P
	Tertile 1 12.6 (9.5, 15.1)[b]	Tertile 2 20.6 (18.6, 23.1)[b]	Tertile 3 31.9 (27.9, 38.9)[b]	
n (%)	504 (33.3)	505 (33.4)	505 (33.4)	–
Age (yrs)	58.9 (47.0, 64.9)	47.8 (34.9, 57.9)	57.7 (49.5, 62.2)	< 0.0001
Male (n (%))	203 (40.3)	222 (44.0)	141 (27.9)	0.0001
Pre-diabetes[c] (n (%))	323 (64.1)	334 (66.1)	330 (65.4)	0.847
Blood parameters				
Fasting plasma glucose (mmol/L)	5.51 (5.22, 5.82)	5.51 (5.17,5.84)	5.49 (5.20, 5.90)	0.929
Fasting insulin (μIU/mL)	7.00 (4.40, 10.86)	6.50 (4.20, 10.40)	5.80 (3.90, 9.35)	0.014
HbA$_{1c}$ (%)	5.50 (5.20, 5.80)	5.50 (5.20, 5.80)	5.60 (5.30, 5.80)	0.483
HOMA2-IR[d]	0.95 (0.59, 1.45)	0.87 (0.56, 1.39)	0.78 (0.52, 1.26)	0.018
Serum calcium^{2+} (mmol/L)	2.44 (2.36, 2.52)	2.43 (2.33, 2.51)	2.40 (2.30, 2.50)	0.006
Anthropometric parameters				
Overweight[e] (n (%))	208 (41.2)	202 (40.1)	219 (43.3)	0.707
Overweight[f] (n (%))	146 (29.0)	138 (27.4)	158 (31.3)	0.566
Body mass index (kg/m^2)	22.9 (20.9, 25.3)	23.3 (21.1, 25.2)	23.4 (21.1, 25.6)	0.372
Waist circumference (cm)	83.5 (77.4, 89.8)	84.1 (77.3, 90.0)	84.7 (78.1, 92.2)	0.119
Social-demographic data				
High education level[g] (n (%))	237 (47.0)	243 (48.1)	196 (38.8)	0.042
High monthly personal income[h] (n (%))	201 (39.9)	197 (39.0)	178 (35.3)	0.0005
Mental worker[i] (n (%))	188 (37.3)	196 (38.8)	126 (25.0)	< 0.0001
Lifestyles				
Smoking status (current, n (%))	72 (14.3)	79 (15.6)	66 (13.1)	0.539
MVPA (MET-hour/week)[j]	90.0 (54.6, 139.4)	89.24 (58.3, 137.4)	105.90 (66.6, 153.5)	0.019
Total energy intake (kcal/d)	1563.3 (1250.7, 1884.8)	1575.7 (1261.0, 1963.3)	1530.0 (1232.6, 1839.8)	0.361
Season[k] (summer, n (%))	84 (16.7)	138 (27.3)	150 (29.7)	< 0.0001

[a]Values are median (25th percentile, 75th percentile) for non-normally-distributed continuous variables and n (%) for categorical variables. For non-normally distributed data, Kruskal-Wallis test was used to test the differences of the parameters among the tertiles of 25(OH)D, and for categorical variables, chi-square test were used
[b]Values are median (25th percentile, 75th percentile) in tertiles of vitamin D (ng/ml)
[c]Pre-diabetes was defined using the updated classification and diagnosis of diabetes of American Diabetes Association (ADA) [3]
[d]HOMA2-IR, Homeostasis model assessment 2-insulin resistance, calculated by Wallace Formula [21]
[e]Body mass index ≥24.0 kg/m^2 [23]
[f]Body mass index ≥25.0 kg/m^2 [48]
[g]At least 12 years of school education
[h]Monthly personal income at least ≥3200 CNY (Chinese Yuan), which is moderate level among the general population in Southwest China [26]
[i]Mental worker includes professional and technical personnel (teacher/policeman/doctor etc), legislator & administrator, businessman and student [25]
[j]MVPA: moderate-to-vigorous physical activity (MET-hour/week) [27]. MET: Metabolic equivalent
[k]Summer in Southwest China is from June to August generally

In this study, low vitamin D status was associated with increased risk of pre-diabetes. Consistent relationships have been found among non-diabetic U.S. adults, using data from NHANES III [38, 39], as well as Kuwait adults [40]. In addition, above results suggest that vitamin D deficiency has important effects on insulin resistance and impaired β-cell function, which are the two critical factors that drive the development of T2DM. Remarkably, in the following stratified analyses, we only observed the association between serum 25(OH)D and pre-diabetes among overweight or obese adults.

Hypponen et al. [37] reported that obesity played an important role in the relation between serum 25(OH)D and glucose homeostasis. To some extent, our results were in agreement with the previous findings that overweight or obese adults had poorer vitamin D status [41, 42]. Nevertheless, another cross-sectional study among elder Brazilians indicated there was no association between 25(OH)D levels and pre-diabetes [43] due partly to their small sample size. Considering the higher prevalence of pre-diabetes among Chinese, a stage in the disease continuum where diabetes prevention has been

Table 3 Multiple linear regression least-squares means and 95% confidence interval for the association of tertiles of serum 25(OH)D (ng/ml) with glucose homeostasis ($n = 1514$)[a]

	Tertiles of serum 25(OH)D (ng/ml)			P for trend
	Tertile 1 12.6 (9.5, 15.1)[b]	Tertile 2 20.6 (18.6, 23.1)[b]	Tertile 3 31.9 (27.9, 38.9)[b]	
Fasting insulin (µIU/mL)				
Model A[c]	8.36 (7.59, 9.12)	8.00 (7.25, 8.75)	7.47 (6.68, 8.26)	0.016
Model B[d]	8.35 (7.58, 9.12)	7.98 (7.23, 8.73)	7.45 (6.66, 8.24)	0.015
Model C[e]	8.00 (7.31, 8.70)	7.63 (6.95, 8.31)	7.01 (6.29, 7.73)	0.0007
Fasting plasma glucose(mmol/L)				
Model A[c]	5.56 (5.48, 5.64)	5.55 (5.47, 5.63)	5.52 (5.44, 5.61)	0.331
Model B[d]	5.56 (5.48, 5.64)	5.55 (5.47, 5.63)	5.52 (5.43, 5.60)	0.291
Model C[e]	5.55 (5.47, 6.63)	5.53 (5.46, 5.61)	5.50 (5.42, 5.58)	0.197
HbA$_{1c}$ (%)				
Model A[c]	5.57 (5.51, 5.63)	5.53 (5.46, 5.59)	5.46 (5.40, 5.52)	0.0003
Model B[d]	5.57 (5.51, 5.63)	5.52 (5.46, 5.82)	5.45 (5.39, 5.52)	0.0002
Model C[e]	5.57 (5.50, 5.63)	5.52 (5.46, 5.58)	5.45 (5.39, 5.51)	0.0001
HOMA2-IR				
Model A[c]	1.11 (1.01, 1.21)	1.06 (0.97, 1.16)	0.99 (0.89, 1.10)	0.016
Model B[d]	1.11 (1.01, 1.21)	1.06 (0.96, 1.16)	0.99 (0.89, 1.10)	0.015
Model C[e]	1.06 (0.97, 1.16)	1.02 (0.93, 1.10)	0.93 (0.84, 1.03)	0.0007

[a]Values are models least-squares means and 95% confidence interval. Linear trends (P for trend) were obtained with vitamin D concentrations as continuous variables;
[b]Values are median (25th percentile, 75th percentile) in tertiles of Vitamin D (ng/ml);
[c]Model A: adjusted for age, gender, monthly personal income, smoking status and season of blood drawn;
[d]Model B: additionally adjusted for MVPA and energy intake;
[e]Model C: additionally adjusted for waist circumference

Table 4 Multiple logistic regression odds ratio (OR) and 95% confidence interval (CI) for the association of tertiles of serum 25(OH)D (ng/ml) with pre-diabetes[a]

	OR (95%CI)			P for trend
Pre-diabetes[c] (yes or no)	Tertile 1 12.6 (9.5, 15.1)[b]	Tertile 2 20.6 (18.6, 23.1)[b]	Tertile 3 31.9 (27.9, 38.9)[b]	
Total ($n = 1514$)				
Model A[d]	1.00	1.07 (0.75, 1.52)	0.70 (0.48, 1.01)	0.056
Model B[e]	1.00	1.07 (0.74, 1.52)	0.69 (0.47, 0.99)	0.049
Model C[f]	1.00	1.06 (0.74, 1.52)	0.68 (0.47, 0.99)	0.046
BMI < 24 kg/m^2 ($n = 885$)				
Model A[d]	1.00	1.32 (0.84, 2.08)	0.86 (0.53, 1.38)	0.182
Model B[e]	1.00	1.36 (0.87, 2.14)	0.86 (0.53, 1.39)	0.153
BMI ≥ 24 kg/m^2 ($n = 629$)				
Model A[d]	1.00	0.68 (0.36, 1.27)	0.45 (0.24, 0.85)	0.052
Model B[e]	1.00	0.65 (0.34, 1.22)	0.45 (0.23, 0.84)	0.047

[a]Values are odds ratio and 95% confidence interval. Linear trends (P for trend) were obtained with vitamin D concentrations as continuous variables;
[b]Values are median (25th percentile, 75th percentile) of in tertiles of Vitamin D (ng/ml);
[c]Using the Classification and Diagnosis of diabetes of American Diabetes Association to classify pre-diabetes [3];
[d]Model A: adjusted for age, gender, average personal income per month, smoking status and season of blood drawn;
[e]Model B: additionally adjusted for MVPA and energy intake;
[f]Model C: additionally adjusted for waist circumference

Higher serum 25(OH)D level is associated with decreased risk of impairment of glucose homeostasis: data...

17

shown to be effective [44, 45], identification and treatment of pre-diabetic individuals are therefore crucial.

In the meanwhile, our data indicated that vitamin D deficiency was fairly common in our study sample with an average age of 48.74 years (the prevalence of vitamin D deficiency or insufficiency was 79.8%), which was lower than another study focused on Chinese adults aged 50-70 years (93.6%, 2009) [46] perhaps owing to the fact that aging is associated with reduced capacity to produce vitamin D [20]. Notably, prevalence in this study was substantially higher than those observed among US population in 2009-2010 (64%) [47], which may lie in that fewer vitamin D fortified foods are available in China. Our results suggest that vitamin D deficiency might be universal in the general population in China and relevant measures might be taken to improve vitamin D status of Chinese adults.

Several limitations of our study merit consideration. Owing to the cross-sectional nature of the study design, a cause-effect relationship between serum 25(OH)D and glucose homeostasis cannot be inferred. The present study was completed within a relatively long period, from March to October, 2015, which may increase the seasonal variation in the biomarkers. However, data from the Ely Study (Cambridgeshire, U.K.) [13] and NHANES 2001-2006 [14] suggested that the associations between 25(OH)D and glucose homeostasis were independent of season. Finally, our analysis has excluded diabetic participants, many of whom were men due to the higher prevalence of diabetes in men than women among Chinese populations, generating an imbalanced sex proportion which could have potentially biased our results. Nonetheless, initial analysis indicated no interaction between gender and serum 25(OH)D, and we have adjusted gender in the multiple regression analyses. Furthermore, participants in the present analysis have been shown to be comparable to age-matched adults in the general population in Southwest China on sociodemographic and lifestyle characteristics [26].

Notwithstanding the limitations mentioned above, the present study had following strengths. Serum 25(OH)D allowed for objective measurement of vitamin D status rather than relying on self-reported vitamin D intake or sunlight exposure, which circumvented the recall bias. In addition, our analyses took into account many potential covariates that might confound the observed associations. Finally, we investigated participants aged 25-65 years with a range of quantitative indicators of glucose homeostasis (including FPG, fasting insulin, HbA$_{1c}$ and HOMA2-IR), providing more comprehensive results than the previous studies.

Conclusions

In conclusion, we have demonstrated inverse associations of serum 25(OH)D concentration with glucose homeostasis in Southwest Chinese adults without diabetes. Prospective studies and clinical trials are needed to confirm our findings.

Abbreviations

25(OH)D: 25-hydroxyvitamin D; BMI: Body mass index; CV: Coefficient of Variation; FPG: Fasting plasma glucose; HbA$_{1c}$: Glycated hemoglobin; HOMA2-IR: The homeostatic model assessment 2-insulin resistance; MVPA: Moderate-to-vigorous physical activity; NHANES: National Health and Nutrition Examination Survey; OGTT: Oral glucose tolerance test; T2DM: Type 2 diabetes mellitus; VDRs: Vitamin D receptors; WC: Waist circumference

Acknowledgements

All the participants in our study are gratefully acknowledged. We also thank the staff of the Department of Nutrition, Food Safety, and Toxicology for organizing this study and all the laboratorians involved in our study for providing technical support.

Funding

This study was supported by research grant from the National Nature Science Foundation of China (No.81472976). The funding agencies had no role in the design of study, data collection and analysis, or presentation of the results.

Authors' contributions

GC conceived the project and designed the study. DL conducted the analysis and wrote the manuscript. HW revised the manuscript critically for laboratory technique content. HX provided critical input on the calculation of physical activity. JZ and MC researched data. YG provided critical input on earlier versions of the manuscript. All authors had final approval of the final manuscript as submitted.

Competing interests

The authors declare that they have no competing interests.

Author details

[1]Department of Nutrition, Food Safety and Toxicology, West China School of Public Health, Sichuan University, No.16, Section 3, Renmin Nan Road, Chengdu 610041, Sichuan, China. [2]Center of Growth, Metabolism and Aging, Collage of Life Sciences, Sichuan University, Chengdu, China. [3]Department of Obstetrics and Gynecology, West China Second University Hospital, Sichuan University, Chengdu, China.

References

1. Pan X-R, Liu J, Yang W-Y, Li G-W. Prevalence of diabetes and its risk factors in China, 1994. Diabetes Care. 1997;20(11):1664–9.
2. Xu Y, Wang L, He J, Bi Y, Li M, Wang T, et al. Prevalence and control of diabetes in Chinese adults. JAMA. 2013;310(9):948–59.
3. American Diabetes A. Classification and diagnosis of diabetes. Diabetes Care. 2016;39(Suppl 1):S13–22.
4. van der Rhee H, Coebergh JW, de Vries E. Sunlight, vitamin D and the prevention of cancer: a systematic review of epidemiological studies. Eur J Cancer Prev. 2009;18(6):458–75.
5. Munger KL, Levin LI, Hollis BW, Howard NS, Ascherio A. Serum 25-hydroxyvitamin D levels and risk of multiple sclerosis. JAMA. 2006;296(23): 2832–8.
6. Wang TJ, Pencina MJ, Booth SL, Jacques PF, Ingelsson E, Lanier K, et al. Vitamin D deficiency and risk of cardiovascular disease. Circulation. 2008; 117(4):503–11.
7. Al-Daghri NM, Al-Attas OS, Alokail MS, Alkharfy KM, Yakout SM, Aljohani NJ, et al. Lower vitamin D status is more common among Saudi adults with diabetes mellitus type 1 than in non-diabetics. BMC Public Health. 2014;14(1):1–5.
8. Scragg R, Sowers M, Bell C. Serum 25-hydroxyvitamin D, diabetes, and ethnicity in the third national health and nutrition examination survey. Diabetes Care. 2004;27(12):134–9.
9. Pittas AG, Sun Q, Manson JE, Dawson-Hughes B, Hu FB. Plasma 25-hydroxyvitamin D concentration and risk of incident type 2 diabetes in women. Diabetes Care. 2010;33(9):2021–3.
10. Holick MF. Vitamin D deficiency. N Engl J Med. 2007;357(3):266–81.
11. Zhen D, Liu L, Guan C, Zhao N, Tang X. High prevalence of vitamin D deficiency among middle-aged and elderly individuals in northwestern China: its relationship to osteoporosis and lifestyle factors. Bone. 2015;71:1–6.
12. Liu E, Meigs JB, Pittas AG, McKeown NM, Economos CD, Booth SL, et al. Plasma 25-hydroxyvitamin d is associated with markers of the insulin resistant phenotype in nondiabetic adults. J Nutr. 2009;139(2):329–34.
13. Forouhi NG, Luan J, Cooper A, Boucher BJ, Wareham NJ. Baseline serum 25-hydroxy vitamin d is predictive of future glycemic status and insulin resistance: the Medical Research Council Ely prospective study 1990-2000. Diabetes. 2008;57(10):2619–25.
14. Ford ES, Zhao G, Tsai J, Li C. Associations between concentrations of vitamin D and concentrations of insulin, glucose, and HbA1c among adolescents in the United States. Diabetes Care. 2011;34(3):646–8.
15. Chiu KC, Chu A, Go VLW, Saad MF. Hypovitaminosis D is associated with insulin resistance and dysfunction. Amer J Clin Nutr. 2004;79(5):820–5.
16. Scragg R, Holdaway I, Singh V, et al. Serum 25-hydroxyvitamin D3 levels decreased in impaired glucose tolerance and diabetes mellitus [J]. Diabetes Res Clin Pract. 1995;27(3):181–8.
17. Zhang J, Ye J, Guo G, et al. Vitamin D status is negatively correlated with insulin resistance in Chinese type 2 diabetes:[J]. Int J Endocrinol. 2016; 2016(5):1–7.
18. Lin D, Wang C, Ma H, et al. The study of serum vitamin D and insulin resistance in Chinese populations with normal glucose tolerance [J]. Int J Endocrinol. 2014;2014(2014):870235.
19. Guo C, Xue H, Jiao L, et al. Relevance of the dietary glycemic index, glycemic load and genetic predisposition for the glucose homeostasis of Chinese adults without diabetes [J]. Sci Rep. 2017;7(1):400.
20. Holick MF. Vitamin D status: measurement, interpretation, and clinical application. Ann Epidemiol. 2009;19(2):73–8.
21. Wallace TM, Levy JC, Matthew DR. Use and abuse of HOMA modeling. Diabetes Care. 2004;27(6):1487–95.
22. Group CSCaHR. Reports on the physical fitness and health research of chinese school students. Beijing: Higher Education Press; 2010.
23. Working Group on Obesity in China. Guidelines for prevention and control of overweight and obesity in Chinese adults. Acta Nutrimenta Sinica. 2004; 26(1):1–4.
24. Tabák AG, Herder C, Rathmann W, Brunner EJ, Kivimäki M. Prediabetes: a high-risk state for diabetes development. Lancet. 2012;379(9833):2279–90.
25. Elias P, Birch M. SOC2010: revision of the standard occupational classification. Labour Gaz. 2010;4(7):48–55.
26. Statistical Bureau of Sichuan, NBS Survey Officie in Sichuan. SiChuan statistical yearbook. Beijing: China Statistic Press; 2015.
27. Ainsworth BE, Haskell WL, Herrmann SD, Meckes N, Bassett DR Jr, Tudor-Locke C, et al. 2011 Compendium of physical activities: a second update of codes and MET values. Med Sci Sports Exerc. 2011;43(8):1575–81.
28. Yuexin Y, Guangya W, Xingchang P. China food conposition: Peking University Medical Press; 2009.
29. Hermans MP, Levy JC, Morris RJ, Turner RC. Comparison of tests of β-cell function across a range of glucose tolerance from normal to diabetes. Diabetes. 1999;48:1779–86.
30. Hermans MP, Levy JC, Morris RJ, Turner RC. Comparison of insulin sensitivity tests across a range, of glucose tolerance from normal to diabetes. Diabetologia. 1999;42(6):678–87.
31. Tai K, Need AG, Horowitz M, Chapman IM. Vitamin D, glucose, insulin, and insulin sensitivity. Nutrition. 2008;24(3):279–85.
32. Pittas AG, Lau J, Hu FB, Dawson-Hughes B. The role of vitamin D and calcium in type 2 diabetes. A systematic review and meta-analysis. J Clin Endocrinol Metab. 2007;92(6):2017–29.
33. Reis JP, von Muhlen D, Miller ER 3rd. Relation of 25-hydroxyvitamin D and parathyroid hormone levels with metabolic syndrome among US adults. Eur J Endocrinol. 2008;159(1):41–8.
34. Hypponen E, Boucher BJ, Berry DJ, Power C. 25-hydroxyvitamin D, IGF-1, and metabolic syndrome at 45 years of age: a cross-sectional study in the 1958 British birth cohort. Diabetes. 2008;57(2):298–305.
35. Lee DM, Rutter MK, O'Neill TW, Boonen S, Vanderschueren D, Bouillon R, et al. Vitamin D, parathyroid hormone and the metabolic syndrome in middle-aged and older European men. Eur J Endocrinol. 2009;161(6):947–54.
36. Kositsawat J, Freeman VL, Gerber BS, Geraci S. Association of A1C levels with vitamin D status in U.S. adults: data from the national health and nutrition examination survey. Diabetes Care. 2010;33(6):1236–8.
37. Hypponen E, Power C. Vitamin D status and glucose homeostasis in the 1958 British birth cohort: the role of obesity. Diabetes Care. 2006;29(10):2244–6.
38. Shankar A, Sabanayagam C, Kalidindi S. Serum 25-Hydroxyvitamin D levels and prediabetes among subjects free of diabetes. Diabetes Care. 2011;34(5):1114–9.
39. Gupta AK, Brashear MM, Johnson WD. Prediabetes and prehypertension in healthy adults are associated with low vitamin D levels. Diabetes Care. 2011; 34(3):658–60.
40. Zhang FF, Hooti SA, Rao A, Jahmah NA, Saltzman E, Ausman LM. Low level of serum vitamin D is associated with elevated fasting glucose and prediabetes in Kuwait adults. FASEB J. 2013;27(1):lb376.
41. Gonzalez L, Ramos-Trautmann G, Diaz-Luquis GM, Perez CM, Palacios C. Vitamin D status is inversely associated with obesity in a clinic-based sample in Puerto Rico. Nutr Res. 2015;35(4):287–93.
42. Zhang Y, Zhang X, Wang F, Zhang W, Wang C, Yu C, et al. The relationship between obesity indices and serum vitamin D levels in Chinese adults from urban settings. Asia Pac J Clin Nutr. 2016;25(2):333–9.
43. Giorelli GV, Matos LN, Saado A, Soibelman VL, Dias CB. No association between 25-hydroxyvitamin D levels and prediabetes in Brazilian patients. A cross-sectional study. Sao Paulo Med J. 2015;133(2):73–7.
44. Knowler WC, Bar-rett-Connor E, Fowler SE, Hamman RF, Lachin JM, Walker EA, et al. Reduction in the incidence of type 2 diabetes with lifestyle intervention or metformin. N Engl J Med. 2002;346:393–403.
45. American Diabetes A. Standards of medical care in diabetes–2010. Diabetes Care. 2010;33(Suppl 1):S11–61.
46. Lu L, Yu Z, Pan A, Hu FB, Franco OH, Li H, et al. Plasma 25-hydroxyvitamin D concentration and metabolic syndrome among middle-aged and elderly Chinese individuals. Diabetes Care. 2009;32(7):1278–83.
47. Schleicher RL, Sternberg MR, Lacher DA, Sempos CT, Looker AC, Durazo-Arvizu RA, et al. The vitamin D status of the US population from 1988 to 2010 using standardized serum concentrations of 25-hydroxyvitamin D shows recent modest increases. Amer J Clin Nutr. 2016;104(2):454–61.
48. Pi-Sunyer F, Becker D, Bouchard C, Carleton R, Colditz G. Executive summary of the clinical guidelines on the identification, evaluation, and treatment of overweight and obesity in adults. Arch Intern Med. 1998;158(17):1855–67.

3

An international survey on hypoglycemia among insulin-treated type I and type II diabetes patients: Turkey cohort of the non-interventional IO HAT study

Rıfat Emral[1*], Tamer Tetiker[2], Ibrahim Sahin[3], Ramazan Sari[4], Ahmet Kaya[5], İlhan Yetkin[6], Sefika Uslu Cil[7], Neslihan Başcıl Tütüncü[8] and on behalf of the IO HAT investigator group

Abstract

Background: Limited real-world data are currently available on hypoglycemia in diabetes patients. The International Operations Hypoglycemia Assessment Tool (IO HAT) study was designed to estimate hypoglycemia in insulin-treated type I (T1DM) and type II (T2DM) diabetes mellitus patients from 9 countries. The data from Turkey cohort are presented here.

Methods: A non-interventional study to determine the hypoglycemia incidence, retrospectively and prospectively, in Turkish T1DM and T2DM patients using a 2-part self-assessment questionnaire.

Results: Overall, 2348 patients were enrolled in the Turkey cohort (T1DM = 306 patients, T2DM = 2042 patients). In T1DM patients, 96.8% patients reported hypoglycemic events (Incidence rate [IR]: 68.6 events per patient-year [ppy]), prospectively, while 74.0% patients reported hypoglycemic events (IR: 51.7 events ppy), retrospectively. In T2DM patients, 95.9% patients (IR: 28.3 events ppy) reported hypoglycemic events, prospectively, while 53.6% patients (IR: 23.0 events ppy) reported hypoglycemic events, retrospectively. Nearly all patients reported hypoglycemia during the prospective period.

Conclusions: This is a first patient-reported dataset on hypoglycemia in Turkish, insulin-treated diabetes patients. A high incidence of patient-reported hypoglycemia confirms that hypoglycemia remains under-estimated. Hypoglycemia increased healthcare utilization impacting patients' quality of life. Hypoglycemia remains a common side effect with insulin-treatment and strategies to optimize therapy and reduce hypoglycemia occurrence in diabetes patients are required.

Keywords: Diabetes, Turkey, Hypoglycemia, IO HAT, Insulin, Non-interventional

Background

Insulin therapy remains integral to treatment of type I diabetes mellitus (T1DM) and long-term type II diabetes mellitus (T2DM) [1]. A good glycemic control is essential to minimize development of microvascular complications and macrovascular events [2]. Hypoglycemia is the main hurdle for achieving optimal glycemic control in patients on insulin therapy [3]. Development of strategies or therapies to control hypoglycemia is important to help individuals achieve glycemic targets [4]. Achieving optimum glycemic control following the diagnosis of T2DM is vital to improving clinical outcomes, yet many patients and clinicians are hesitant to initiate and intensify insulin therapy. Reasons for this are manifold including lack of time, clinical expertise and patient understanding. However, considerable progress can be achieved with patient education and awareness programs soon after diagnosis [5].

* Correspondence: rifatemral@gmail.com
[1]Department of Endocrinology and Metabolic Diseases, Ankara University, Faculty of Medicine, İbn-i Sina Hospital, Academic Region M1/09, Samanpazarı, 06100 Ankara, Turkey
Full list of author information is available at the end of the article

Despite the apparent high risk of hypoglycemia, only a few studies have been conducted to evaluate the incidence rate of hypoglycemia in a real-world setting. Hypoglycemia is commonly reported in a clinical trial context; however, these studies seldom reflect real-life clinical practice due to rigorous inclusion and exclusion criteria involved, and continuous treatment and follow-up.

Increasing evidence on growing incidence of diabetes in low- and middle-income countries has been reported [6]. According to two population-based studies, the prevalence of T2DM in Turkey increased from 7.2% to 16.5% within 12 years [7, 8]. Current knowledge on hypoglycemia comes from a few studies in North American or European populations and very limited data are available on hypoglycemia in Turkish diabetes patients [9, 10].

This paper describes the results from the Turkey cohort of the International Operations Hypoglycemia Assessment Tool (IO HAT) study which was conducted in 9 countries. The IO HAT study builds on findings from the global HAT study that was conducted in 24 countries [11]. The IO HAT study is an observational study aimed at enhancing the clinical understanding of hypoglycemia, and its clinical, social and economic consequences. In turn, this will help to identify cost-effective solutions to improve blood glucose control and Quality of Life (QOL) for patients with diabetes. The current study aims to assess hypoglycemia retrospectively and prospectively among insulin treated patients with T1DM or T2DM.

Methods
Study design
The Turkey cohort of the IO HAT study was a non-interventional, multi-center, 6-month and 4-week retrospective and 4-week prospective study to assess hypoglycemia in insulin-treated diabetes patients.

The study was carried out at 92 sites in Turkey. The study design is described in Fig. 1. The study protocol and assessments were conducted in accordance with the Declaration of Helsinki (2013) and the Guidelines for Good Pharmacoepidemiology Practices (2007), and approved by an Ethics Committee. All study materials were translated into Turkish, and data obtained were translated back into English for analysis.

Study population
The study was conducted in male or female T1DM or T2DM patients treated with insulin for more than 12 months and who were 18 years or older, ambulatory, literate, and had given informed consent to participate in the study. To minimize selection bias, eligible patients were enrolled consecutively during routine clinic visits.

Assessments
This study comprised of a two-part self-assessment questionnaire (SAQ) including a retrospective cross-sectional evaluation (SAQ1) and a prospective observational evaluation (SAQ2).

SAQ1 assessed baseline demographic and treatment information, hypoglycemia unawareness and perceptions of hypoglycemia, history of severe hypoglycemia for 6 months before the baseline visit, and "any" and "nocturnal" hypoglycemia for 4 weeks before the baseline visit.

SAQ2 assessed severe and symptomatic hypoglycemia and its effect on productivity and healthcare utilization for 4 weeks from the baseline visit.

SAQ2 also included a validated diabetes-specific quality of life (DSQOL) questionnaire. To assist patients

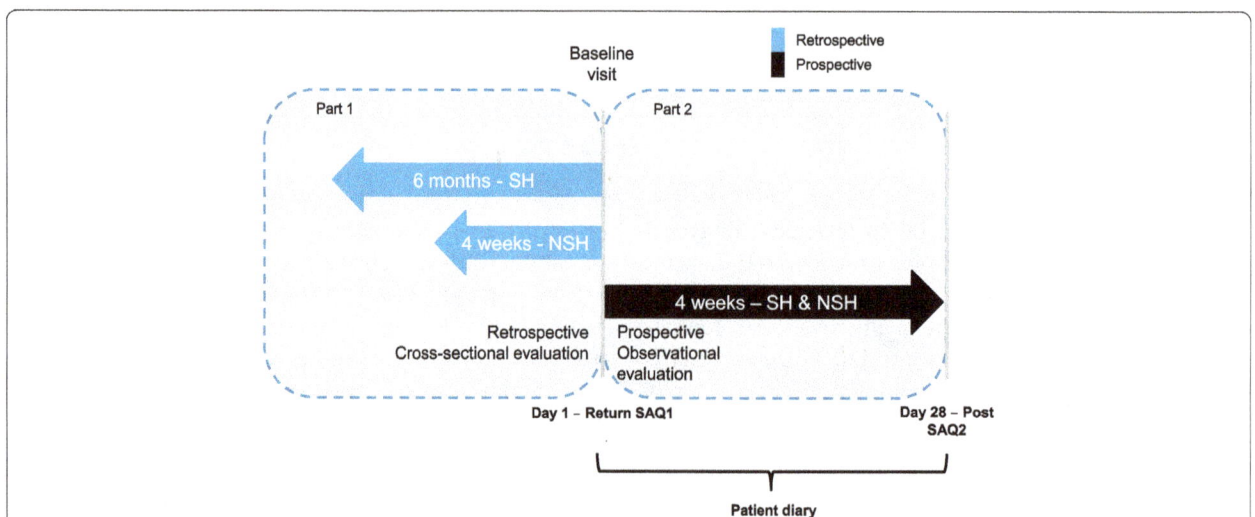

Fig. 1 IO HAT Study design. Severe hypoglycemia: an event requiring assistance of another person to actively administer carbohydrate, glucagon, or other resuscitative actions; Non-severe hypoglycemia: documented symptomatic (symptoms and blood glucose measurement ≤3.9 mmol/L [70 mg/dL]) and probable symptomatic (symptoms only). NSH = non-severe hypoglycemia; SH = severe hypoglycemia; SAQ = self-assessment questionnaire

recall, and as a reminder to complete SAQ2, patients were provided with a diary to capture hypoglycemic episodes. Paired responses to SAQ1 and SAQ2 were used to estimate the differences in the frequency of hypoglycemic episodes between the retrospective and prospective periods. The incidence of severe and symptomatic hypoglycemia (defined below) was calculated according to the frequency of episodes over the timeframe stated in the corresponding question. The diary which allowed patients to summarize hypoglycemia information on a daily basis over the 4-week period following the baseline visit was used to evaluate the incidence of hypoglycemia. If there were discrepancies between the diary and the SAQ2 questionnaire, the frequency of hypoglycemia was calculated using the highest recorded total frequency as stated on either of these forms.

Hypoglycemia unawareness was evaluated through the question: 'Do you have symptoms when you have a low sugar level?' where the response, 'occasionally' denoted impaired awareness and 'never' denoted severely impaired awareness [12]. Fear of hypoglycemia was reported as rated by the patient on a scale of 0 (not afraid at all) to 10 (absolutely terrified).

Study objectives

The primary objective of the study was to determine the percentage of patients experiencing at least 1 hypoglycemic episode during the 4-week prospective observational period among insulin-treated T1DM or T2DM patients.

The secondary objectives included: incidence of hypoglycemic episodes, difference in the incidence of hypoglycemic episodes before and after the baseline visit, relationship between patient demography, treatment, and hypoglycemia, use of health-care resources, and types of behaviors against hypoglycemia. Diabetes-related late complications, treatment regimen and glycemic control were ascertained from questions completed in the presence of the participant's health-care professional to improve accuracy.

All other study end-points including the primary end-point of interest were determined from questions completed by the patient.

Hypoglycemia classification

Severe hypoglycemia was defined as: requiring third-party assistance, based on the American Diabetes Association (ADA) definition [13]; non-severe hypoglycemia: managed by patient alone; any hypoglycemia: the sum of severe and non-severe hypoglycemia; nocturnal hypoglycemia: event occurring between midnight and 06:00 h.

Sample size

Sample size of the total cohort across 9 countries of the IO HAT study was determined to be 6000 patients assuming a worst case scenario proportion of patients (50%) reporting at least 1 hypoglycemic episode during the 4-week prospective observation period, and that the range of the 95% confidence interval was < 3 percentage point for the total cohort. Of these, 2000 patients were planned to be recruited from Turkey.

Evaluability of patients for analysis

Patients who returned any part of any SAQ or patient diary containing answers to any of the questions received was also included in the Full Analysis Set (FAS).

Statistical methods

All statistical tests were two-sided and regarded as exploratory, with the criterion for statistical significance set at $p < 0.05$. The p-values from 0.01 to 0.05 were taken to indicate a modest evidence of a difference, and p-values of < 0.01 were taken to indicate moderate evidence.

For the primary endpoint, the percentage of patients who experienced at least 1 hypoglycemic episode during the 4-week prospective observational period among T1DM or T2DM patients was calculated together with the confidence interval for this percentage. For secondary endpoints, the incidence of various types of hypoglycemia was calculated as number of episodes per patient-year (ppy) as expressed by the following formula (together with the 95% confidence interval).

Incidence rate = Total number of events / Total follow-up time (patient-years).

The incidence rate (IR) was reported by diabetes type: T1DM and T2DM patients. No imputation of missing data was performed except for calculation of Well-Being Questionnaire-5 summary scores where more than half the items were non-missing. All analyses were conducted in the FAS.

Relationship between HbA_{1c} at baseline and log-transformed number of hypoglycemia events reported by patients was shown by the scatter plot with regression line and 95% confidence interval (CI) and R-squared values were calculated.

Baseline refers to data collected using the Part 1 SAQ; follow-up refers to data collected using the Part 2 SAQ and, where applicable, patient diaries.

Results
Patient characteristics

Overall, 2348 patients (306 with T1DM and 2042 with T2DM) from Turkey enrolled and completed the Part 1 SAQ in the Turkey cohort constituting the FAS. Of these, 252 patients (82.4%) with T1DM and 1781 patients (87.2%) with T2DM completed the Part 2 SAQ; and 247 patients (80.7%) with T1DM and 1749 patients (85.7%) with T2DM completed the patient diary and were included in the completers analysis set (CAS).

Baseline characteristics for T1DM and T2DM patients in the FAS are presented in Table 1. Patients with T1DM were younger than those with T2DM (32.7 years vs. 58.0 years, respectively) and had a longer median duration of insulin use (11.2 years vs. 6.0 years, respectively). Mean HbA_{1c} was lower in patients with T1DM (8.4% [67.9 mmol/mol]) than in those with T2DM (8.8% [72.3 mmol/mol]).

Frequency of hypoglycemia

Any hypoglycemia

Any hypoglycemia rates in T1DM and T2DM patients are presented in Figs. 2 and 3, respectively. In T1DM patients, 96.8% patients reported hypoglycemic events (IR: 68.6 events ppy), prospectively, while 74.0% patients reported hypoglycemic events (IR: 51.7 events ppy), retrospectively. In T2DM patients, 95.9% patients (IR: 28.3 events ppy) reported hypoglycemic events, prospectively, while 53.6% patients (IR: 23.0 events ppy) reported hypoglycemic events, retrospectively.

The rates of any hypoglycemia were significantly higher in the prospective period compared with the retrospective period in both T1DM and T2DM patients (T1DM, $p = 0.005$; T2DM, $p < 0.001$).

Nocturnal hypoglycemia

Nocturnal hypoglycemia rates in T1DM and T2DM patients are presented in Figs. 2 and 3, respectively. Unlike, any hypoglycemia, the retrospective rates for nocturnal hypoglycemia were higher compared to the prospective rates in both T1DM and T2DM patients; 40.9% vs. 35.0% (IR: 18.0 ppy vs. 12.4 ppy) in T1DM, 15.2% vs. 10.6% (IR:5.0 ppy vs. 2.6 ppy) in T2DM; (T1DM, $p = 0.017$; T2DM, $p < 0.001$).

Severe hypoglycemia

Severe hypoglycemia rates in T1DM and T2DM patients are presented in Figs. 2 and 3, respectively. In T1DM patients, in the 6-month retrospective period, severe hypoglycemia was reported by 54.7% (IR: 8.9 events ppy) patients, while in the 4-week prospective period, severe hypoglycemia was reported by 53.3% (IR: 15.3 events ppy) patients. In T2DM patients, 50.1% (IR: 4.1 events ppy) and 61.9% (IR: 10.0 events ppy) patients reported severe hypoglycemia, retrospectively and prospectively. The rates of severe hypoglycemia were significantly higher in the prospective period compared with those in the retrospective period (T1DM, $p = 0.005$; T2DM, p < 0.001).

Use of health system resources

The impact of hypoglycemia on the medical system was higher in the 6-month retrospective period than in the 4-week prospective period for both T1DM and T2DM patients (Table 2).

Hypoglycemia requiring hospitalization

In T1DM patients, 10.2% patients (6-month retrospective period) and 3.3% patients (4-week prospective period) reported hypoglycemia requiring hospitalization. In T2DM patients, 6.1% patients (6-month retrospective period) and 1.9% patients (4-week prospective period) reported hypoglycemia requiring hospitalization (Table 2).

Requiring additional clinic appointments

In T1DM patients, 15.8% (6-month retrospective period) and 12.6% (4-week prospective period) patients required additional clinic appointments. In T2DM patients, 11.4% (6-month retrospective period) and 8.0% (4-week prospective period) required additional clinic appointments (Table 2).

Requiring number of additional telephone contacts made

In T1DM patients, 6.3% patients (6-month retrospective period) and 5.3% patients (4-week prospective period) made additional telephone contacts. In T2DM patients, 4.1% patients (6-month retrospective period) and 3.3% patients (4-week prospective period) made additional telephone contacts (Table 2).

Patient response to hypoglycemia

The overall patient actions resulting from hypoglycemia were more in the 6-month retrospective period than in the 4-week prospective period in both T1DM and T2DM patients (Table 2). For patients with T1DM, the 6-month retrospective and 4-week prospective data, respectively, were: the percentage of patients who consulted their doctor or nurse (47.4% vs. 32.9%), required any form of medical assistance (48.7% vs. 33.3%), increased calorie intake (35.3% vs. 28.6%), avoided physical exercise (17.6% vs. 13.1%), reduced insulin dose (35.0% vs. 18.7%), skipped insulin injections (23.9% vs. 10.3%), and increased blood glucose monitoring (52.3% vs. 46.4%).

In the T2DM patients, the 6-month retrospective and 4-week prospective data, respectively, were: the percentage of patients who consulted their doctor or nurse (39.3% vs. 32.6%), required any form of medical assistance (41.0% vs. 32.6%), increased calorie intake (27.6% vs. 17.6%), avoided physical exercise (11.3% vs. 9.2%), reduced insulin dose (18.8% vs. 13.0%), skipped insulin injections (18.0% vs. 9.8%), and increased blood glucose monitoring (28.9% vs. 20.9%).

Impact of hypoglycemia on work/studies

Higher percentage of patients took leave from work/studies, arrived late or left early from work/studies in the retrospective period than the prospective period (Table 2). In T1DM patients, the 6-month retrospective and 4-week prospective data, respectively were: 22.0% vs. 6.6% patients had taken leave from work/studies,

Table 1 Baseline characteristics

	T1DM (N = 306)	T2DM (N = 2042)
Age (years)	32.7 (11.6)	58.0 (10.5)
Median	30.5	58.0
Upper quartile, Lower quartile	39.0, 24.0	65.0, 51.0
Male/female (%)	44.1/55.9	40.9/59.1
Duration of diabetes (years)	12.1 (8.0)	12.5 (7.0)
Median	10.5	11.0
Upper quartile, lower quartile	17.0, 6.0	17.0, 7.0
Duration of insulin use (years)	11.2 (7.8)	6.0 (4.6)
Median	10.0	5.0
Upper quartile, lower quartile	16.0, 5.0	8.0, 3.0
HbA_{1c} (mmol/mol)	67.9 (18.1)	72.3 (20.4)
HbA_{1c} (%)	8.4 (1.7)	8.8 (1.9)
FBG (mmol/L)	8.6 (4.1)	9.6 (4.0)
FBG (mg/dL)	155.0	173.0
PPG (mmol/L)	11.1 (4.8)	12.5 (4.9)
PPG (mg/dL)	200.0 (86.5)	225.2 (88.3)
Weight (kg)	70.4 (16.2)	83.7 (14.9)
Median	68.0	82.0
Upper quartile, lower quartile	80.0, 60.0	92.0, 74.0
Height (cm)	167.8 (10.0)	164.2 (8.5)
Median	168.0	164.0
Upper quartile, lower quartile	174.0, 160.0	170.0, 158.0
BMI (kg/m^2)	25.0 (5.2)	31.2 (5.7)
Median	24.3	30.5
Upper quartile, lower quartile	27.2, 21.8	34.0, 27.3
Previous medical illnesses	% of patients	% of patients
Neuropathy	34.6	53.1
Retinopathy	20.6	39.6
Nephropathy	9.2	14.6
Peripheral vascular disease	14.7	20.2
Angina	9.8	17.4
Myocardial infarction	3.3	15.6
None	49.0	27.7
Symptoms of diabetes-related complications, %		
Any	98.4	95.4
Tremor	84.0	80.5
Sweating	85.6	79.4
Hunger	83.0	78.2
Tiredness	83.0	76.4
Weakness	78.4	72.9
Diabetes treatment regimen, %		
Short-acting insulin	12.1	5.5
Long-acting insulin	4.6	17.3

Table 1 Baseline characteristics *(Continued)*

	T1DM (N = 306)	T2DM (N = 2042)
Pre-mix	4.2	33.3
Both short- and long-acting	74.2	41.1
Both short-acting and pre-mix	0.3	0.6
Both long-acting and pre-mix	3.3	1.4
Short- and long-acting and pre-mix	0.0	0.0
Missing	1.3	0.8

Data are presented as mean (SD) unless otherwise stated
BMI = body mass index, FBG = fasting blood glucose, HbA1c = glycated hemoglobin, N = total number of patients participating, PPG = postprandial glucose, SD = standard deviation, T1DM = type I diabetes mellitus, T2DM = type II diabetes mellitus

24.5% vs. 9.0% patients had arrived late to work/studies, and 20.5% vs. 11.4% patients left early from work/studies. In T2DM patients, the 6-month retrospective and 4-week prospective data, respectively were: 10.8% vs. 3.1% patients had taken leave from work/studies, 6.4% vs. 2.5% patients had arrived late to work/studies, and 10.8% vs. 2.5% patients left early from work/studies.

Hypoglycemia awareness

More patients with T1DM than with T2DM had knowledge of hypoglycemia before reading the definition in the Part 1 SAQ (91.3% [T1DM] and 60.4% [T2DM]) and had a higher normal hypoglycemia awareness (71.6% [T1DM] and 53.3% [T2DM]) (Table 2). There were no notable differences between patients with T1DM or T2DM with respect to fear of hypoglycemia, with a mean (standard deviation) score of 5.3 (3.6) for patients with T1DM and 4.5 (3.6) for patients with T2DM (Table 2).

Hypoglycemia by insulin regimen

Incidence rates of any hypoglycemia in T1DM and T2DM patients in the 4-week retrospective and prospective assessment periods by insulin regimen (short-acting, long-acting, pre-mix, and short- plus long-acting) are shown in Figs. 4 and 5, respectively. Estimated IRs of any and severe hypoglycemia increased whilst estimated IRs of nocturnal hypoglycemia generally decreased in the prospective period versus the retrospective period in patients with T1DM and T2DM.

The estimated IRs of any hypoglycemic events in the 4-week retrospective and 4-week prospective assessment were highest in patients with T1DM using short-acting insulin in the prospective period (86.2 ppy) and lowest in patients with T2DM using long-acting insulin, in the retrospective period (11.9 ppy).

The IRs of nocturnal hypoglycemia were highest in patients with T1DM using short-acting insulin in the 4-week retrospective period (20.5 events ppy) and lowest

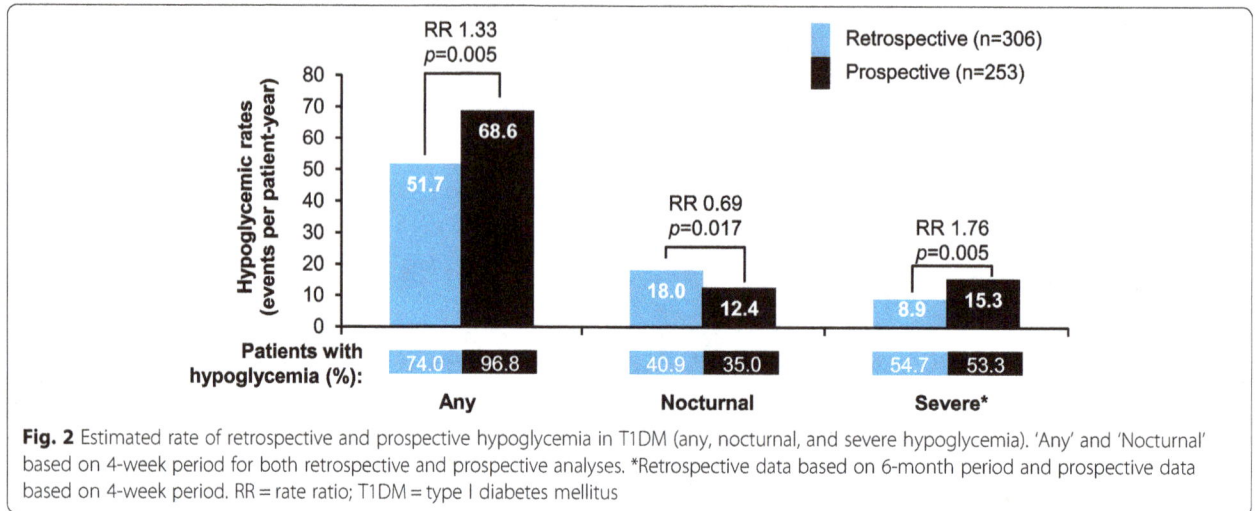

Fig. 2 Estimated rate of retrospective and prospective hypoglycemia in T1DM (any, nocturnal, and severe hypoglycemia). 'Any' and 'Nocturnal' based on 4-week period for both retrospective and prospective analyses. *Retrospective data based on 6-month period and prospective data based on 4-week period. RR = rate ratio; T1DM = type I diabetes mellitus

in the 4-week prospective period in T2DM patients using short-acting insulin (1.1 events ppy).

The IRs of severe hypoglycemia were highest in T1DM patients using pre-mix insulin in the 4-week prospective period (19.6 ppy) and lowest in T1DM patients using long-acting insulin in the 6-month retrospective period (1.2 ppy).

Associations between hypoglycemia and continuous or predictor variables

In this study, no correlation was observed between baseline HbA_{1c} and any hypoglycemia events in both T1DM and T2DM populations (Figs. 6 and 7, respectively). No significant association between hypoglycemia and duration of diabetes or duration of insulin therapy was seen (Additional files 1 and 2, respectively). Patients who measured their blood glucose levels more frequently reported higher rates of hypoglycemia compared to those who monitored their blood glucose levels less frequently (Fig. 8).

Discussion

This paper describes the results from the Turkey cohort of the international, non-interventional, multicenter, retrospective and prospective study to assess the incidence of patient-reported hypoglycemia in insulin-treated diabetes patients.

This is a first report of an observational study to assess hypoglycemia both retrospectively and prospectively in the Turkish T1DM and T2DM patients. While hypoglycemia has been reported from a few observational studies in Turkish population, the main aim of these studies were not to assess hypoglycemia. Minor hypoglycemia rates of 1.08 and 2.56 ppy were prospectively observed in the insulin detemir and insulin glargine group, respectively, in the Turkish T2DM cohort from the observational SOLVE study [10]. The lower hypoglycemic frequencies obtained in these studies could be explained by the fact that hypoglycemia assessment was not the primary objective of these studies and

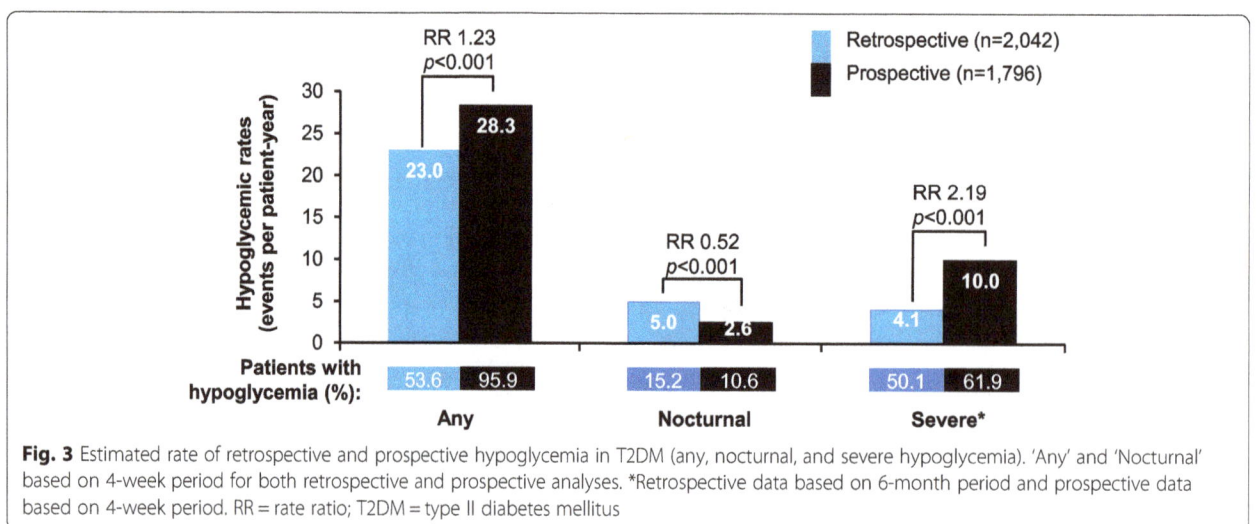

Fig. 3 Estimated rate of retrospective and prospective hypoglycemia in T2DM (any, nocturnal, and severe hypoglycemia). 'Any' and 'Nocturnal' based on 4-week period for both retrospective and prospective analyses. *Retrospective data based on 6-month period and prospective data based on 4-week period. RR = rate ratio; T2DM = type II diabetes mellitus

Table 2 Patient perspectives on hypoglycemia

	T1DM		T2DM	
Impact of hypoglycemic events on the medical system (%)	Retrospective (n = 306)	Prospective (n = 253)	Retrospective (n = 2042)	Prospective (n = 1796)
Events requiring hospital admission	10.2	3.3	6.1	1.9
Attended additional clinical appointments	15.8	12.6	11.4	8.0
Made additional telephone contacts	6.3	5.3	4.1	3.3
Patient response to hypoglycemia (%)	Retrospective (n = 306)	Prospective (n = 252)	Retrospective (n = 2042)	Prospective (n = 1781)
Consulted their doctor/nurse	47.4	32.9	39.3	32.6
Required any form of medical assistance	48.7	33.3	41.0	32.6
Increased calorie intake	35.3	28.6	27.6	17.6
Avoided physical exercise	17.6	13.1	11.3	9.2
Reduced insulin dose	35.0	18.7	18.8	13.0
Skipped insulin injections	23.9	10.3	18.0	9.8
Increased blood glucose monitoring	52.3	46.4	28.9	20.9
Impact of hypoglycemic events on work and study (%)	Retrospective (n = 200)	Prospective (n = 166)	Retrospective (n = 360)	Prospective (n = 321)
Taken leave from work or studies	22.0	6.6	10.8	3.1
Arrived late to work/studies	24.5	9	6.4	2.5
Left early from work/studies	20.5	11.4	10.8	2.5
	T1DM (N = 306)		T2DM (N = 2042)	
Knew what hypoglycemia was at baseline before Part 1 SAQ (%)				
	91.3		60.4	
Defined hypoglycemia based on (%)				
Symptoms only	54.6		52.4	
Blood glucose measurement only	2.3		3.5	
Either	15.4		15.2	
Both	24.2		18.8	
Hypoglycemia awareness (%)				
Normal	71.6		53.3	
Impaired	25.2		38.5	
Severely impaired	0.7		2.8	
Fear of hypoglycemia (Scale of 0 to 10; %)				
0 = no fear	19.9		24.3	
1	3.9		5.9	
2	2.3		5.8	
3	5.6		5.4	
4	5.6		4.6	
5	13.1		10.7	
6	6.5		6.6	
7	9.8		9.9	
8	10.1		8.7	
9	5.2		4.6	
10 = absolutely terrified	17.3		12.2	

Hypoglycemia unawareness was evaluated through the question: 'Do you have symptoms when you have a low sugar level?' where the response, 'occasionally' denoted impaired awareness and 'never' denoted severely impaired awareness

N = total number of patients participating; n = number of patients who responded to the set of questions; SAQ = self-assessment questionnaire; T1DM = type I diabetes mellitus; T2DM = type II diabetes mellitus

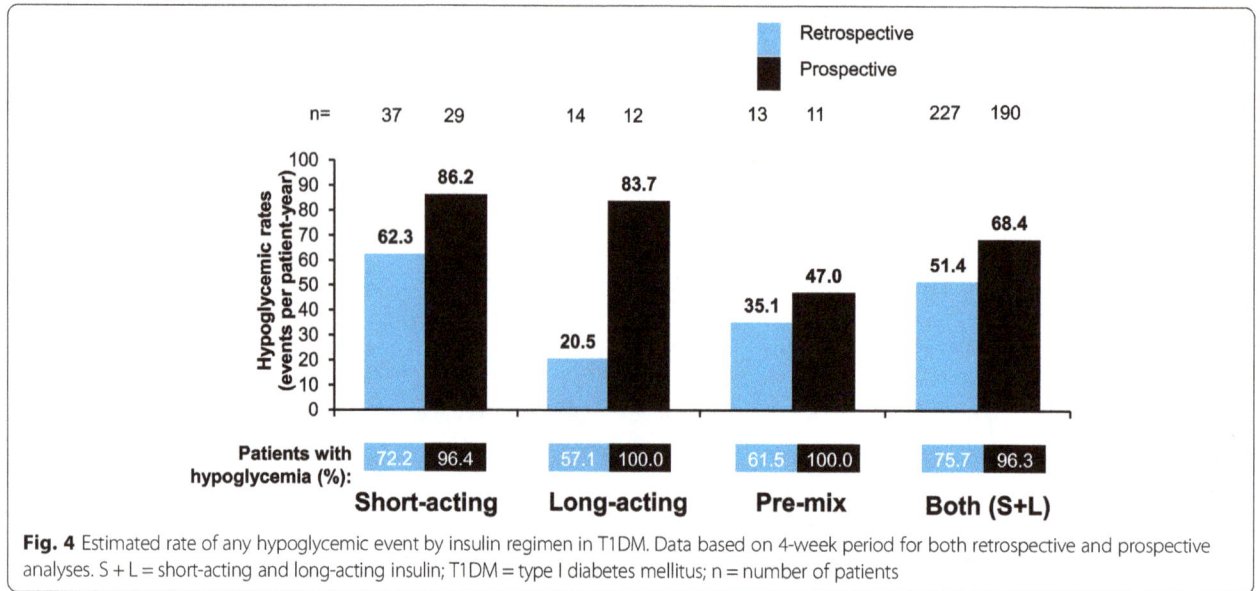

Fig. 4 Estimated rate of any hypoglycemic event by insulin regimen in T1DM. Data based on 4-week period for both retrospective and prospective analyses. S + L = short-acting and long-acting insulin; T1DM = type I diabetes mellitus; n = number of patients

the reported frequency is for minor hypoglycemia which may not encompass a total hypoglycemic rate. Total hypoglycemic episodes in the 4-week retrospective period in the PREDICTIVE study were 47.5 ppy in patients with T1DM and 9.2 ppy in patients with T2DM in the European cohort (Turkey population was included) [14], which are comparable to those for T1DM population but less compared to T2DM population observed in the current study (51.7 ppy and 23.0 ppy, respectively).

The hypoglycemia rates seen in the IO HAT Turkey cohort aligned with the overall IO HAT results [15]. The frequency of overall hypoglycemia in the prospective period in the Turkey cohort was comparable to global HAT in T1DM patients but was considerably higher in T2DM patients (28.3 events ppy) than the global HAT study (19.3

events ppy). The reason for this could be the country-specific variations in the prevalence and management of diabetes and hypoglycemia in the two studies.

Similar to the overall IO HAT results, higher frequency of patients reported hypoglycemia in the prospective period as compared to the retrospective period in both T1DM and T2DM patients in the Turkey cohort. The reason for this could be the use of patient diary during the prospective period. While a patient recorded data daily using patient diary during the prospective period, the data for the retrospective period was collected at baseline visit based on the patient's memory of the previous hypoglycemic events, possibly causing under-reporting. The patient education on hypoglycemia at the baseline visit could have also led to an improved reporting of

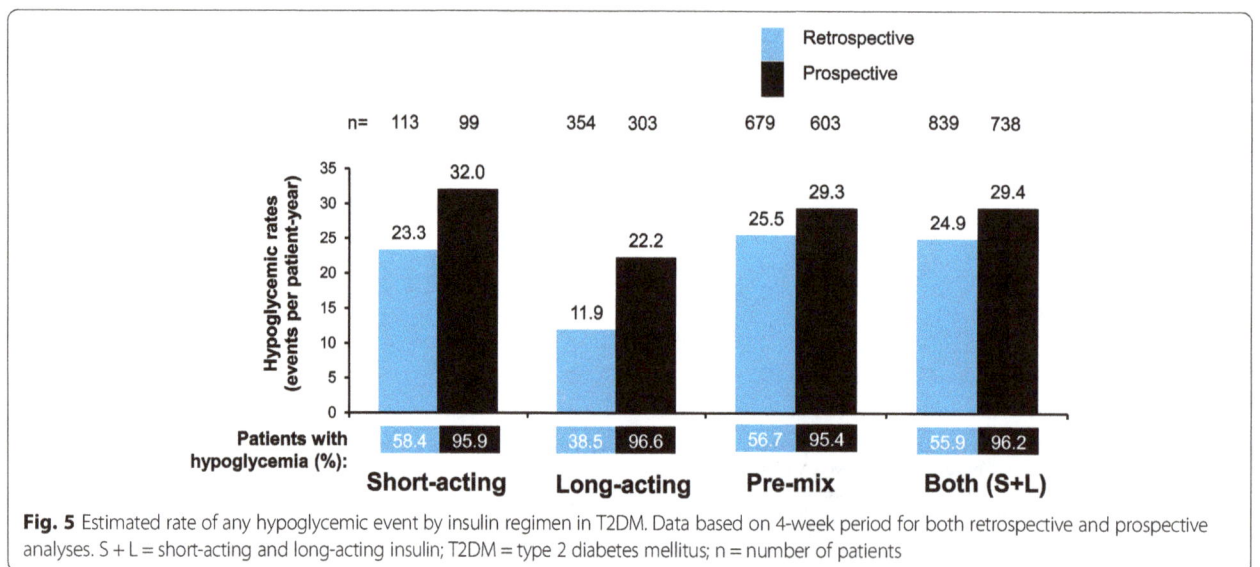

Fig. 5 Estimated rate of any hypoglycemic event by insulin regimen in T2DM. Data based on 4-week period for both retrospective and prospective analyses. S + L = short-acting and long-acting insulin; T2DM = type 2 diabetes mellitus; n = number of patients

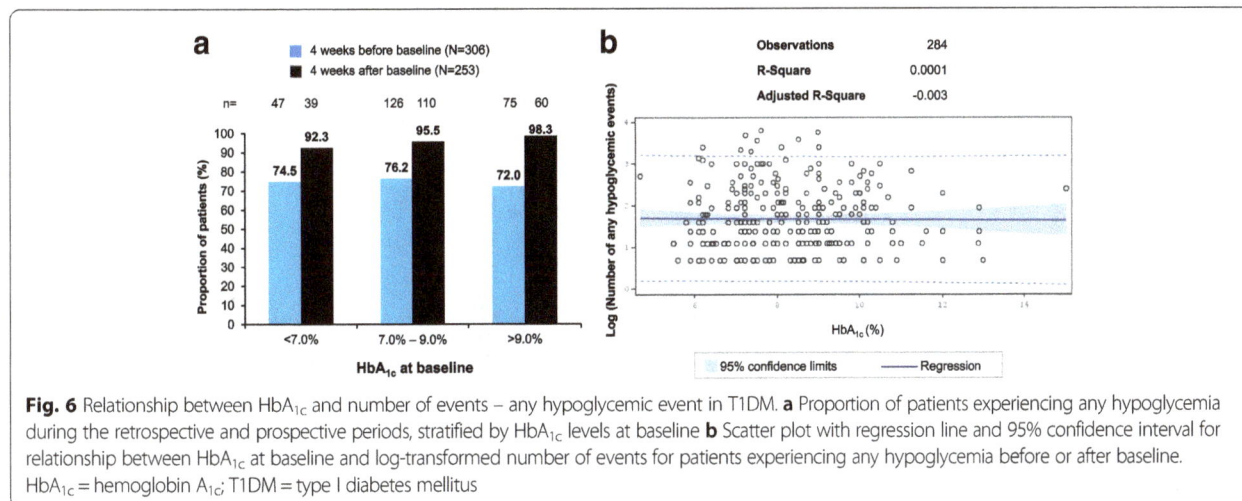

Fig. 6 Relationship between HbA$_{1c}$ and number of events – any hypoglycemic event in T1DM. **a** Proportion of patients experiencing any hypoglycemia during the retrospective and prospective periods, stratified by HbA$_{1c}$ levels at baseline **b** Scatter plot with regression line and 95% confidence interval for relationship between HbA$_{1c}$ at baseline and log-transformed number of events for patients experiencing any hypoglycemia before or after baseline. HbA$_{1c}$ = hemoglobin A$_{1c}$; T1DM = type I diabetes mellitus

hypoglycemia in the prospective period. On similar lines, the higher frequency of severe hypoglycemia observed during the prospective period over the retrospective period in both T1DM and T2DM patients could also be explained. However, a lower frequency of nocturnal hypoglycemia was reported in the prospective period over the retrospective period. This could be because of a well-defined cut-off for the nocturnal hypoglycemia, midnight to 06.00 am, during the prospective period. The perceived fear of nocturnal hypoglycemia could also probably cause an over-reporting of events during the retrospective period based on patient recall. Also, difficulty in using a diary during the night-time could have affected the reporting of nocturnal hypoglycemia during the prospective period. Interestingly, though the prospectively reported "any" and "severe" hypoglycemia rates were higher than retrospectively reported rates, a higher proportion of patients reported increased utilization of healthcare resources (hospital admissions, additional clinical appointments) in the retrospective period than the

prospective period. Similarly, a higher proportion of patients reported that the hypoglycemic events impacted their work and study in the retrospective period than in the prospective period. The reason for this could be because the patients were well-informed about hypoglycemia at the baseline visit leading to less impact on patients' quality of life in the prospective period. Another explanation could be that the assessment period for some of the parameters in the retrospective period was of 6 months compared to 4 weeks during the prospective period and hence the difference.

In the PREDICTIVE study, the frequency of hypoglycemia in insulin-treated patients showed a significant, positive association with duration of diabetes, and number of insulin injections but was inversely related to HbA$_{1c}$ [14]. Unlike the global HAT study [11], no significant correlation of hypoglycemia with duration of diabetes and insulin therapy was seen in the current study. Also, no significant correlation between HbA$_{1c}$ and hypoglycemia was observed which is in line with global

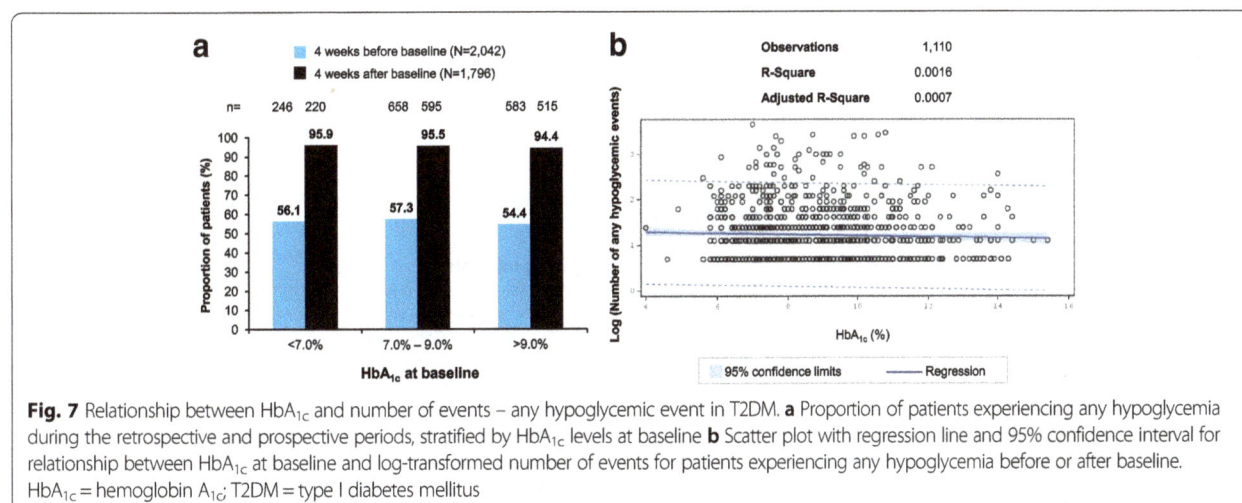

Fig. 7 Relationship between HbA$_{1c}$ and number of events – any hypoglycemic event in T2DM. **a** Proportion of patients experiencing any hypoglycemia during the retrospective and prospective periods, stratified by HbA$_{1c}$ levels at baseline **b** Scatter plot with regression line and 95% confidence interval for relationship between HbA$_{1c}$ at baseline and log-transformed number of events for patients experiencing any hypoglycemia before or after baseline. HbA$_{1c}$ = hemoglobin A$_{1c}$; T2DM = type I diabetes mellitus

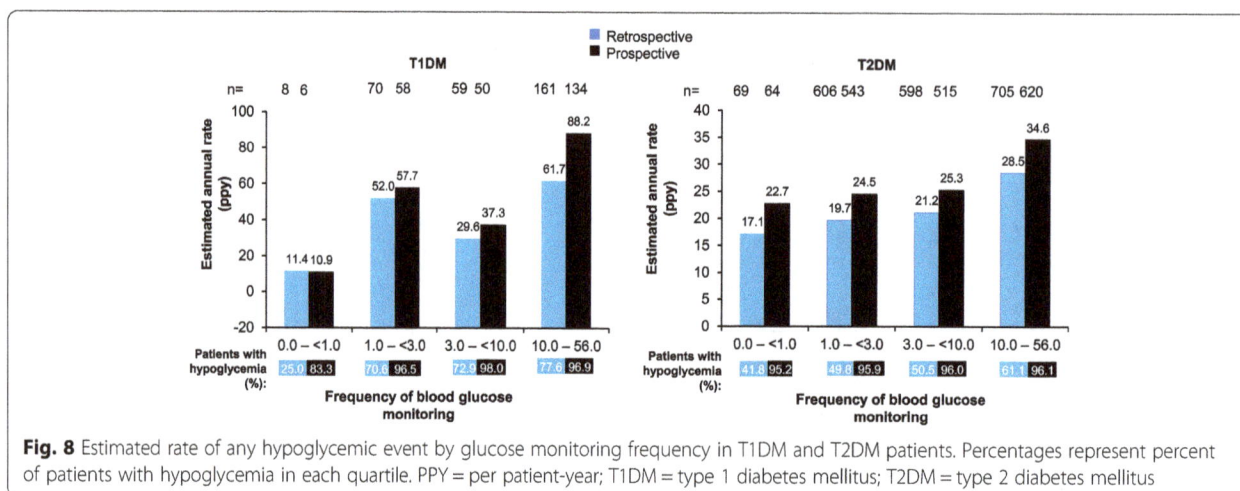

Fig. 8 Estimated rate of any hypoglycemic event by glucose monitoring frequency in T1DM and T2DM patients. Percentages represent percent of patients with hypoglycemia in each quartile. PPY = per patient-year; T1DM = type 1 diabetes mellitus; T2DM = type 2 diabetes mellitus

HAT study results [11] and recent findings that the inverse correlation between HbA$_{1c}$ and hypoglycemia has diminished due to advances in therapy in the recent years [16]. A regular self-monitoring of blood glucose is important to detect hypoglycemia and for overall diabetes management [17]. A positive correlation between frequency of blood glucose monitoring and reported hypoglycemia rates was seen in the current study which suggests its importance to detect hypoglycemia.

Conclusions

The current study has enabled to obtain real-world data on hypoglycemia rates from Turkey where very few data were available in spite of a high rate of diabetes prevalence. The results from this study confirms that hypoglycemia remains under-reported. The higher hypoglycemic rates observed in Turkish population could be because of higher burden of diabetes combined with lack of standard care and treatment as compared to European and North American population and needs to be investigated further. The hypoglycemia data in Turkish cohort is an important step towards a customized country-specific healthcare plan to control diabetes.

Additional file

Additional file 1: Estimated rate of any hypoglycemic event by duration of diabetes in T1DM and T2DM patients. Percentages represent percent of patients with hypoglycemia in each quartile. PPY = per patient-year; T1DM = type 1 diabetes mellitus; T2DM = type 2 diabetes mellitus. (PPTX 361 kb)

Additional file 2: Estimated rate of any hypoglycemic event by duration of insulin therapy in T1DM and T2DM patients. Percentages represent percent of patients with hypoglycemia in each quartile. PPY = per patient-year; T1DM = type 1 diabetes mellitus; T2DM = type 2 diabetes mellitus. (PPTX 362 kb)

Abbreviations

ADA: American Diabetes Association; CAS: Completers analysis set; CI: Confidence interval; DSQOL: Diabetes-related quality of life; FAS: Full analysis set; IO HAT: International Operations Hypoglycemia Assessment Tool; IR: Incidence rate; ppy: Per patient-year; QOL: Quality of life; SAQ: Self-assessment questionnaire; T1DM: Type I diabetes mellitus; T2DM: Type II diabetes mellitus

Acknowledgements

Statistical analysis was performed by Paraxel International. The authors acknowledge medical writing and submission support provided by Archana Gandhe from Cognizant Technology Solutions. Novo Nordisk was involved in the study design; collection, analysis and interpretation of data; and decision to submit the article for publication.

Funding

Financial support for the conduct of the research was provided by Novo Nordisk.

Authors' contributions

RE conceptualized the study design, was involved in acquisition of data, analyzed and interpreted the data, and finalized the manuscript. TT, IS, RS, AK, IY, and NT contributed towards study design, data acquisition, data interpretation, and preparation and finalization of the manuscript. SC contributed to study design, data interpretation, and preparation and finalization of the manuscript. All authors had input into the data interpretation and preparation of the final manuscript for publication, met the ICMJE criteria for authorship, and have approved the final article for submission.

Competing interests

RE: Speaker fees from Novo Nordisk, MSD, AstraZeneca, Boehringer, Sanofi; participation in advisory boards from Novo Nordisk, Sanofi, AstraZeneca.
TT: Speaker fees from Gen Pharmaceuticals, Novartis, Lilly, Novo Nordisk, MSD, AstraZeneca, Boehringer, Sanofi, Bilim; participation in advisory boards from Novo Nordisk, Sanofi, Lilly.
IS: Speaker fees from Novo Nordisk, MSD, AstraZeneca, Boehringer, Sanofi, Lilly and Novartis; participation in advisory boards from Sanofi, Lilly, Novo Nordisk and AstraZeneca.
RS: Speaker fees from Novo Nordisk, MSD, AstraZeneca, Boehringer, Sanofi, Lilly, Novartis; participation in advisory boards from Sanofi, AstraZeneca.

AK: Speaker fees from Novo Nordisk, AstraZeneca, Boehringer, Sanofi, Lilly, Novartis; participation in advisory boards from Sanofi, AstraZeneca, NovoNordisk.
IY: Speaker fees from Novo Nordisk, AstraZeneca, Boehringer, Sanofi, Novartis, Lilly; participation in advisory boards from Novo Nordisk, Sanofi, AstraZeneca.
SC: Employee of Novo Nordisk.
NT: Speaker fees from Novo Nordisk, MSD, AstraZeneca, Boehringer, Sanofi, Novartis, Lilly; participation in advisory boards from Novo Nordisk, Sanofi, AstraZeneca.

Author details

[1]Department of Endocrinology and Metabolic Diseases, Ankara University, Faculty of Medicine, İbn-i Sina Hospital, Academic Region M1/09, Samanpazarı, 06100 Ankara, Turkey. [2]Faculty of Medicine, Department of Endocrinology and Metabolic Diseases, Çukurova University, Adana, Turkey. [3]Endocrinology and Metabolism Department, Inonu University School of Medicine, Malatya, Turkey. [4]Division of Endocrinology and Metabolism, School of Medicine, Akdeniz University, Antalya, Turkey. [5]Division of Endocrinology and Metabolism, Meram School of Medicine, Necmettin Erbakan University, Konya, Turkey. [6]Division of Endocrinology and Metabolism, School of Medicine, Gazi University, Ankara, Turkey. [7]Medical Department, Novo Nordisk, Istanbul, Turkey. [8]Division of Endocrinology and Metabolism, School of Medicine, Baskent University, Ankara, Turkey.

References

1. Cryer PE. Managing diabetes: lessons from type 1 diabetes mellitus. Diabet Med. 1998;15(Suppl 4):S8–12.
2. Gumprecht J, Nabrdalik K. Hypoglycemia in patients with insulin-treated diabetes. Pol Arch Med Wewn. 2016;126(11):870–8.
3. Blumer I, Clement M. Type 2 diabetes, hypoglycemia, and basal Insulins: ongoing challenges. Clin Ther. 2017;39(8S2):S1–S11. https://doi.org/10.1016/j.clinthera.2016.09.020.
4. McCrimmon RJ. RD Lawrence lecture 2015 old habits are hard to break: lessons from the study of hypoglycaemia. Diabet Med. 2017;34(2):148–55.
5. Khunti K, Millar-Jones D. Clinical inertia to insulin initiation and intensification in the UK: a focused literature review. Prim Care Diabetes. 2017;11(1):3–12.
6. Whiting DR, Guariguata L, Weil C, Shaw J. IDF diabetes atlas: global estimates of the prevalence of diabetes for 2011 and 2030. Diabetes Res Clin Pract. 2011;94(3):311–21.
7. Satman I, Yilmaz T, Sengul A, Salman S, Salman F, Uygur S, et al. Population-based study of diabetes and risk characteristics in Turkey: results of the turkish diabetes epidemiology study (TURDEP). Diabetes Care. 2002;25(9):1551–6.
8. Satman I, Omer B, Tutuncu Y, Kalaca S, Gedik S, Dinccag N, et al. Twelve-year trends in the prevalence and risk factors of diabetes and prediabetes in Turkish adults. Eur J Epidemiol. 2013;28(2):169–80.
9. Besen BD, Sürücü HA, Koşar C. Self-reported frequency, severity of, and awareness of hypoglycemia in type 2 diabetes patients in Turkey. Peer J. 2016;4:e2700. eCollection 2016
10. Damci T, Emral R, Svendsen AL, Balkir T, Vora J, SOLVE™ study. Lower risk of hypoglycaemia and greater odds for weight loss with initiation of insulin detemir compared with insulin glargine in Turkish patients with type 2 diabetes mellitus: local results of a multinational observational study. BMC Endocr Disord. 2014;14:61. https://doi.org/10.1186/1472-6823-14-61.
11. Khunti K, Alsifri S, Aronson R, Cigrovski Berković M, Enters-Weijnen C, Forsén T, et al. Rates and predictors of hypoglycaemia in 27 585 people from 24 countries with insulin-treated type 1 and type 2 diabetes: the global HAT study. Diabetes Obes Metab. 2016;18(9):907–15.
12. Pedersen-Bjergaard U, Pramming S, Thorsteinsson B. Recall of severe hypoglycaemia and self-estimated state of awareness in type 1 diabetes. Diabetes Metab Res Rev. 2003;19:232–40.
13. American Diabetes Association Workgroup on Hypoglycemia. Defining and reporting hypoglycemia in diabetes: a report from the American Diabetes Association workgroup on hypoglycemia. Diabetes Care. 2005;28:1245–9.
14. Lüddeke HJ, Sreenan S, Aczel S, Maxeiner S, Yenigun M, Kozlovski P, et al. PREDICTIVE- a global, prospective observational study to evaluate insulin detemir treatment in types 1 and 2 diabetes: baseline characteristics and predictors of hypoglycaemia from the European cohort. Diabetes Obes Metab. 2007;9(3):428–34.
15. Emral R, Pathan F, Cortes C, El-Hefnawy MH, Goh S, Gómez AM, et al. Self-reported hypoglycemia in insulin-treated patients with diabetes: results from an international survey of 7289 patients from nine countries. Diabetes Res Clin Pract. 2017;134:17–28.
16. Karges B, Rosenbauer J, Kapellen T, Wagner VM, Schober E, Karges W, et al. Hemoglobin A1c levels and risk of severe hypoglycemia in children and young adults with type 1 diabetes from Germany and Austria: a trend analysis in a cohort of 37,539 patients between 1995 and 2012. PLoS Med. 2014;11(10):e1001742. https://doi.org/10.1371/journal.pmed.1001742.
17. Czupryniak L, Barkai L, Bolgarska S, Bronisz A, Broz J, Cypryk K, et al. Self-monitoring of blood glucose in diabetes: from evidence to clinical reality in central and Eastern Europe—recommendations from the international central-eastern European expert group. Diabetes Technol Ther. 2014;16(7):460–75.

4

Comparison of glycemic control and β-cell function in new onset T2DM patients with PCOS of metformin and saxagliptin monotherapy or combination treatment

Tao Tao[1]* , Peihong Wu[1], Yuying Wang[1] and Wei Liu[1,2]*

Abstract

Background: Impaired insulin activity in women with polycystic ovary syndrome might differ from that seen in type 2 diabetes mellitus without polycystic ovary syndrome. This study was designed to compare the effects of treatment with metformin, saxagliptin, and their combination in newly diagnosed women with type 2 diabetes mellitus and polycystic ovary syndrome in China.

Methods: A total of 75 newly diagnosed patients from Shanghai, China with type 2 diabetes mellitus and polycystic ovary syndrome were included in this randomized, parallel, open-label study. All patients received treatment for 24 weeks with metformin, saxagliptin, or their combination. Patients were allocated to one of three treatment groups by a computer-generated code that facilitated equal patient distribution of 25 patients per group. The primary outcome was a change in glycemic control and β-cell function.

Results: A total of 63 patients completed the study ($n = 21$, for each group). The reduction in hemoglobin A1c was significant in the combination group, compared to the monotherapy groups (saxagliptin vs. combination treatment vs. metformin: − 1.1 vs. -1.3 vs. -1.1%, $P = 0.016$), whereas it was comparable between the metformin and saxagliptin groups ($P > 0.05$). Saxagliptin, metformin, and the combination treatment significantly reduced the homeostasis model assessment- insulin resistance index and increased the deposition index ($P < 0.01$ for all). However, no significant change was observed in the homeostasis model assessment- β-cell function among the metformin and combination groups, and no significant changes were observed in the insulinogenic index among all three groups ($P > 0.05$ for all). In addition, saxagliptin and metformin treatments significantly reduced body mass index and high-sensitivity C-reactive protein levels ($P < 0.01$ for both).

Conclusions: Saxagliptin and metformin were comparably effective in regulating weight loss, glycemic control, and β-cell function, improving lipid profiles, and reducing inflammation in newly diagnosed type 2 diabetes mellitus patients with polycystic ovary syndrome.

Keywords: Polycystic ovary syndrome, Type 2 diabetes mellitus, Saxagliptin, Metformin

* Correspondence: taotaozhen@hotmail.com; sue_liuwei@163.com
[1]Department of Endocrinology and Metabolism, Renji Hospital, School of Medicine, Shanghai Jiaotong University, 160 Pujian Road, Shanghai 200127, China
Full list of author information is available at the end of the article

Background

Polycystic ovary syndrome (PCOS) affects 6–10% of reproductive-age women. Insulin resistance (IR) and hyperinsulinemia play a significant role in the predisposition to diabetes in PCOS [1]. About 30–40% of obese reproductive-age women with PCOS have impaired glucose tolerance (IGT) [1, 2], and approximately 10% have type 2 diabetes mellitus (T2DM) based on a 2-h glucose level > 200 mg/dL [3]. Notably, only a small fraction of women with PCOS and either IGT or T2DM display fasting hyperglycemia that is consistent with diabetes, based on the American Diabetes Association criteria.

The findings of Dunaif and coworkers [4] suggested that the impaired insulin activity in women with PCOS might differ from that seen in T2DM without PCOS, or in obese women, who did not exhibit the classical features of PCOS. Our previous study [5] reported early impairment of β-cell function in women with PCOS. Moreover, a more serious primary defect in insulin action has been detected in lean women with PCOS, compared to obese women with PCOS in China [5]. Therefore, reduced insulin secretion, particularly during the first phase of secretion, is the main characteristic of newly diagnosed women with PCOS and T2DM. However, the exact mechanism associated with this attenuated β-cell function in women with PCOS remains unclear. Recent studies have shown that an incretin defect might be related to β-cell dysfunction [6]. An important consideration is raised about the manner in which interventions might effectively treat hyperglycemia in women with T2DM and PCOS.

Metformin inhibits hepatic glucose production and increases peripheral glucose uptake and utilization [7]. Metformin can both improve insulin sensitivity in target tissues and directly influence ovarian steroidogenesis, and these effects do not appear to be primarily responsible for the attenuation of ovarian androgen production in women with PCOS [8, 9]. Although metformin benefits patients with diabetes by improving insulin sensitivity, whether it increases insulin secretion, particularly during the first phase of secretion, remains unclear.

Saxagliptin is thought to exert its effects by delaying the inactivation of incretin, through the inhibition of the dipeptidyl peptidase-4 (DPP-4) inhibitor, thereby enhancing and prolonging the action of incretin. This results in improved glucose-mediated insulin release and reduced postprandial glucagon secretion [6]. However, only a few studies have compared the effects of metformin and saxagliptin on glycemic control in patients with new-onset T2DM and PCOS. Therefore, an important question was raised of whether other medicines that modulate glycemic control might show more optimal effects than metformin in preventing the development of diabetes in Chinese women with PCOS.

This study therefore aimed to compare the effects of metformin and saxagliptin monotherapy, and metformin and saxagliptin combination therapy on blood glucose, hemoglobin A1c (HbA1c), anthropometric measurements, lipid profiles, and inflammation in newly diagnosed women with T2DM and PCOS.

Methods

Study design and patients

This study was an open-label prospective, randomized clinical trial conducted over 24 weeks, with three treatment groups. The primary outcome was a change in glycemic control and β-cell function. A total of 75 newly diagnosed patients with T2DM and PCOS were included in the study. They were recruited from the Outpatient Department of Endocrinology and Metabolism at Shanghai Renji Hospital. The PCOS diagnosis was based on the Rotterdam Criteria (2003), and T2DM was diagnosed based on the World Health Organization criteria (1998). Patients with coronary atherosclerotic heart disease, abnormal liver and renal function, diabetic ketoacidosis, chronic inflammatory disease, and severe gastrointestinal disease were excluded. All participants had a control diet for 2 weeks before treatment. Patients were allocated to one of three treatment groups by a computer-generated code that facilitated equal patient distribution of 25 patients per group. The study protocol was approved by the Human Research Ethics Committee of the Shanghai Renji Hospital, and written informed consents were obtained from all study participants (Clinical trial registration number: ChiCTR-IPR-17011120). All study evaluations and procedures were conducted in accordance with the guidelines of the Helsinki Declaration on human experimentation.

All participants were given advice on diet and exercise and were asked to follow a behavior modification program. Twenty-one patients received metformin (2000 mg/day), 21 patients received saxagliptin (5 mg/day), and 21 patients received combination therapy of metformin (2000 mg/day) and saxagliptin (5 mg/day). The administration of metformin or saxagliptin was fixed throughout the 24-week treatment period.

All patients were asked to presented to the Department of Endocrinology and Metabolism at Shanghai Renji Hospital at baseline and after the 24-week treatment period. Before the study day, patients were asked to have their dinner before 6 p.m. After the meal, patients were asked to fast for 14 h from solids and 12 h for liquids until the morning of the study day. On the study day, blood samples of the participants were collected at 8 a.m. for measurements of blood glucose, HbA1c, insulin, lipids, and high-sensitivity C-reactive protein (hsCRP). Height and weight were measured at baseline and at the end of treatment. Each patient completed a checklist and received weekly telephone contact to assess compliance after taking the medication.

Measurements

Anthropometric measurements

The height and weight of each subject were measured in light clothing to the nearest 1 cm and 0.1 kg, respectively. The waist circumference (WC) and hip circumference (HC) were measured by a particular investigator. The WC was measured at the narrowest circumference between the lower border of the rib cage and the iliac crest. The HC was measured at the level of the symphysis pubis and the greatest gluteal protuberance. Body mass index (BMI) = body weight (kg) / height (m) squared. The waist hip ratio (WHR) = WC (cm) / HC (cm). Weight, WC, and HC were measured at baseline and after the 24-week treatment.

Oral glucose tolerance test (OGTT) and relevant calculations

All study participants underwent a standard OGTT with 75 g glucose. The measurements for participants with PCOS were taken at baseline and at the end of treatment. After at least 8 h overnight fasting, blood samples were drawn to determine glucose and insulin levels before the glucose load, and they were again drawn at 30, 60, 120, and 180 min to determine the respective levels at those time points (marked as Gx, and Ix, where G was glucose and I was insulin).

Laboratory analysis

Blood glucose levels were measured by hexokinase method. Insulin concentrations were measured by a radioimmunoassay kit (Beijing Atom HighTech Co. Ltd., Beijing, China). The intra-assay coefficients of variation (CV) of insulin were 5.5%. The HbA1c levels were measured using high-pressure liquid chromatography. The lipid profile levels were measured on a clinical chemistry analyzer (Roche Original Reagents, Stockholm, Sweden). Analysis of the hsCRP was performed using immunonephelometric methods and a BN-II analyzer (Dade Behring, Deerfield, Germany). The inter- and intra-assay CV were 4.9 and 6.8%, respectively. Competitive electrochemiluminescence immunoassays on the Elecsys autoanalyzer 2010 (Roche Diagnostics, IN, USA) were used to quantify serum total testosterone (T), luteinizing hormone (LH), and follicle-stimulating hormone (FSH). The intra-assay CV of insulin and steroid hormone assays were < 10%. Sex hormone binding globulin (SHBG) levels were measured by chemiluminescent immunoassay (Elecsys autoanalyzer 2010, Roche Diagnostics), validated for plasma SHBG. The CV for SHBG using this methodology was 6%. Free androgen indexes (FAI) were calculated based on T and SHBG levels, i.e.: FAI = T / SHBG × 100.

Calculations

1) Insulin resistance was calculated by the homeostasis model assessment- insulin resistance index (HOMA-IR) [10] as follows:

   fasting insulin ($\mu IU/mL$)
   × fasting plasma glucose (mmol/L)/22.5.

2) Whole-body insulin sensitivity was calculated by the Matsuda index [11] as follows:

$$\text{Matsuda index} = 10\,000/\sqrt{[(\text{fasting glucose} \times \text{fasting insulin}) \times (\text{mean glucose} \times \text{mean insulin during OGTT})]}$$

3) Islet β-cell function was evaluated by the homeostasis model assessment- β-cell function (HOMA-IS) [10] as follows:

   20 × fasting insulin ($\mu IU/mL$)/
   (fasting plasma glucose (mmol/L)–3.5).

4) The insulinogenic index ($\Delta I_{30}/\Delta G_{30}$) (mIU/mmol) that is indicative of early-phase insulin secretion was calculated [11] as follows:

$$(I30–I0)/(G30–G0).$$

5) The responses in glucose and insulin to the glucose load were also assessed by calculating the area under the curve during the OGTT for glucose (AUC glucose) and insulin (AUC insulin), respectively, using the trapezoidal rule [12].

6) The deposition index (DI) was calculated to estimate the β-cell response, relative to the prevailing insulin sensitivity [13], i.e.:

$$DI = \Delta I30/\Delta G30 \ (mIU/mmol)/HOMA-IR = (I30–I0)/(G30–G0)/HOMA-IR.$$

Sample size and statistical analysis

To our knowledge, there were no previous studies using the DPP-4 inhibitor in the treatment of patients with PCOS when this clinical trial was first proposed. Thus, a non-inferiority trial was designed, with an average standard deviation (SD) of 0.22, that required 21 completers per treatment group, to yield a power of 90% to detect a statistically significant difference ($\alpha = 0.05$). The study was designed to recruit 25 patients in each group, based on an assumed dropout rate of 20%. Thus, 75 patients (25 per group) were required for random assignment.

The analysis was conducted in the per-protocol population (saxagliptin, $n = 21$; metformin, $n = 21$; and combination, $n = 21$). All statistical analyses were performed using SPSS version 21 (Statistical Package for the Social Sciences, USA). The normality of all variables was checked using the Shapiro–Wilk test. The results were presented as mean ± SD for variables of normal distribution, and mean (95% CI) for variables of skewed distribution. Statistical comparisons were made using one-way ANOVA for differences among the three groups, the paired t-test for changes observed in variables of normal distribution before and after treatment, and the Wilcoxon signed-rank test for variables of skewed distribution for differences between baseline and after the 24-week treatment. The Kruskal–Wallis test was used for variables of skewed distribution and one-way ANOVA was used for variables of normal distribution to evaluate differences among the three groups, and the Mann–Whitney U test was used to evaluate differences between the monotherapy groups. Statistical significance was set at $P < 0.05$.

Results

Clinical and biochemical patterns of target patients

Although 75 patients were randomly divided into three groups, 63 patients completed the 24-week treatment (saxagliptin, $n = 21$; metformin, $n = 21$; combination, $n = 21$), owing to migration, poor compliance, and adverse events. An additional file shows the numbers and characteristics of the various participants in more detail (see Additional file 1). The clinical characteristics and biochemical variables for the three groups according to the different therapies are summarized in Table 1. As expected, there were no significant differences in age, body weight, BMI, WC, WHR, or body fat (FAT)% among the three groups ($P > 0.05$ for all). Furthermore, the fasting blood glucose (FBG), 2-h glucose (2hBG), fasting insulin (FINS), 2-h insulin (2hINS), HbA1c, AUC glucose, and AUC insulin values showed no significant differences among the various groups ($P > 0.05$ for all). With respect to the lipid profile and inflammation, no significant differences were observed in triglyceride (TG), total cholesterol (TC), high-density lipoprotein cholesterol (HDL-C), low-density lipoprotein cholesterol (LDL-C), and hsCRP levels among the three groups ($P > 0.05$ for all). Moreover, sex hormone parameters, including LH, FSH, T, SHBG, and FAI showed no significant differences among the three groups ($P > 0.05$ for all).

Changes in parameters of glucose metabolism after saxagliptin, metformin, or combination treatment in patients with new-onset T2DM

Table 2 presents glucose metabolism parameters in the saxagliptin, metformin, and combination therapy groups.

Significant reductions in HbA1c were observed in all three groups after 24 weeks of treatment ($P < 0.001$ for all). The decline in HbA1c was more significant in the combination group, compared to the monotherapy groups, whereas differences between the monotherapy groups were not significant (saxagliptin vs. combination vs. metformin: – 1.1% vs. -1.3% vs. -1.1%, respectively, $P = 0.016$; saxagliptin vs. metformin: $P = 0.890$).

Parameters reflective of β-cell function are also presented in Table 2. The DI, insulinogenic index, and HOMA-IS, the parameters of β-cell function, were estimated both before and after the 24-week treatment. The insulinogenic index in the three groups and the HOMA-IS in the combination group and metformin group showed no significant change after the 24-week treatment ($P > 0.05$ for all), whereas the HOMA-IS in the saxagliptin group showed a significant decline ($P = 0.046$). Furthermore, an improvement was observed in the DI of all three groups after 24 weeks of treatment (saxagliptin group: $P = 0.004$; combination group: $P = 0.001$; metformin group: $P = 0.003$).

Patients in all three groups exhibited improved insulin sensitivity, which was indicated by the HOMA-IR and Matsuda index ($P < 0.001$ for all). Changes in the HOMA-IR and Matsuda index among all three groups were not significant ($P > 0.05$).

In the OGTT, glucose levels were significantly reduced in all three groups at 0, 30, 60, and 120 min following the 24-week treatment ($P < 0.05$ for all). Glucose levels at 180 min in the combination and metformin groups showed a significant decline (combination vs. metformin: – 1.24 vs. -0.83 mmol/L, $P = 0.001$ and 0.009, respectively); whereas in the saxagliptin group, this decline showed no significance ($P = 0.102$). Moreover, after 24 weeks of treatment, all three groups showed a significant decline in insulin levels at 0, 30, 120, and 180 min ($P < 0.01$ for all). Patients in the saxagliptin and metformin groups had significantly reduced insulin levels at 60 min (saxagliptin and metformin: – 15.49 and – 17.88 µIU/mL, $P = 0.042$ and 0.027, respectively). The differences in the AUC glucose and AUC insulin in all three groups were significant, compared to those evaluated 24 weeks earlier ($P < 0.001$ for all). Interestingly, the AUC insulin in the saxagliptin group showed significant improvement, but the FINS showed a greater decline in the metformin group (Fig. 1).

Changes in parameters of the lipid profile and inflammation after saxagliptin, metformin, or combination treatment in patients with new-onset T2DM

As shown in Table 3, TG, LDL-C, and hsCRP levels in the saxagliptin, metformin, and combination groups

Table 1 Baseline characteristics in PCOS patients with new-onset type 2 diabetes

Parameters	Saxagliptin	Saxagliptin + Metformin	Metformin	P-value
N	21	21	21	N/A
Age, years	30 ± 5	29 ± 5	28 ± 3	0.131
Weight, kg	70.4 (63.7–77.1)	69.3 (64.6–74.1)	67.9 (63.6–72.2)	0.886
BMI, kg/m^2	27.2 (24.94–29.46)	26.38 (24.66–28.1)	26.4 (24.63–28.18)	0.904
WC, cm	86.8 (81.2–92.4)	84.7 (80.0–89.4)	82.8 (79.0–86.6)	0.395
WHR	0.88 ± 0.08	0.86 ± 0.06	0.85 ± 0.06	0.256
FAT%	36.13 (32.74–39.53)	35.12 (32.19–38.05)	33.6 (31.21–35.98)	0.397
FBG, mmol/L	5.63 (5.31–5.96)	5.84 (5.62–6.06)	5.62 (5.39–5.84)	0.166
2hBG, mmol/L	14.73 (13.49–15.97)	15.59 (14.26–16.92)	14.64 (13.66–15.62)	0.482
FINS, µIU/mL	15.78 ± 6.7	16.18 ± 5.3	14.34 ± 4.85	0.546
2hINS, µIU/mL	100.24 (80.63–119.85)	111.82 (92.73–130.91)	100.26 (84.59–115.94)	0.298
HbA1c, %	7.4 ± 0.3	7.4 ± 0.3	7.3 ± 0.2	0.668
AUC glucose	16.63 (15.65–17.62)	17.18 (16.16–18.21)	16.5 (15.81–17.19)	0.586
AUC insulin	129.93 (105.47–154.39)	148.2 (128–168.41)	122.66 (104.04–141.27)	0.152
TG, mmol/L	1.44 (1.16–1.72)	1.34 (1.19–1.5)	1.32 (1.05–1.59)	0.634
TC, mmol/L	4.51 (4.2–4.81)	4.8 (4.44–5.15)	4.94 (4.57–5.31)	0.175
HDL-C, mmol/L	1.26 (1.16–1.37)	1.24 (1.14–1.35)	1.35 (1.26–1.43)	0.167
LDL-C, mmol/L	3.06 ± 0.7	3.4 ± 0.73	3.32 ± 0.69	0.273
hsCRP, mg/L	3.97 (3.1–4.84)	3.94 (3.09–4.8)	4.02 (3.23–4.8)	0.937
LH, IU/L	14.2 (11.28–17.12)	11.57 (9.76–13.37)	12.53 (10.14–14.92)	0.434
FSH, IU/L	6.51 ± 2.04	6.76 ± 1.44	7.33 ± 2.36	0.393
T, nmol/L	2.64 ± 0.69	2.65 ± 0.67	2.64 ± 0.69	0.999
SHBG, nmol/L	24.72 (17.14–32.29)	30.1 (20.48–39.72)	22.64 (15.73–29.54)	0.382
FTI	15.82 (11.06–20.58)	11.72 (8.36–15.08)	16.91 (11.22–22.6)	0.274

Data are presented as mean (95% CI); age, WHR, HbA1c, and LDL-C are presented as mean ± SD

P-values are based on one-way ANOVA for variables of normal distribution and the Kruskal–Wallis test for variables of skewed distribution for differences among three groups

BMI body mass index, WC waist circumference, WHR waist–hip ratio, FAT% body fat percentage, FBG fasting blood glucose, 2hBG 2-h glucose, FINS fasting insulin, 2hINS 2-h insulin, HbA1c hemoglobin A1c, AUC glucose glucose area under the curve during oral glucose tolerance test (OGTT), AUC insulin insulin area under the curve during OGTT, TG triglyceride, TC total cholesterol, HDL-C high-density lipoprotein cholesterol, LDL-C low-density lipoprotein cholesterol, hsCRP high-sensitivity C-reactive protein, LH luteinizing hormone, FSH follicle-stimulating hormone, T total testosterone, SHBG sex hormone binding globulin, FTI Free testosterone index

were all significantly reduced after the 24-week treatment, compared to baseline levels (saxagliptin group: $P < 0.001$, $P = 0.046$, and $P < 0.001$, respectively; combination group: $P < 0.001$ for all; metformin group: $P < 0.001$ for all). However, among the three groups, the metformin and combination groups showed significant reductions in TC ($P < 0.001$ and $P = 0.001$, respectively), whereas the saxagliptin group showed similar TC levels before and after treatment ($P = 0.223$). Regarding the HDL-C levels, a significant increase was observed in patients of the metformin group after the 24-week treatment ($P = 0.031$). Significant differences in TC and LDL-C levels were observed among the three groups (saxagliptin vs. combination vs. metformin groups: TC: – 0.09 vs. -0.27 vs. -0.38 mmol/L; LDL-C: -0.19 vs. -0.42 vs. -0.43 mmol/L; $P = 0.005$ and 0.027, respectively). In further comparisons between the monotherapy treatments,

the effects of metformin were superior to those of saxagliptin in modulating TC and LDL-C levels ($P = 0.002$ and 0.014, respectively).

Changes in anthropometric measurements after saxagliptin, metformin, or combination treatment in patients with new-onset T2DM

Table 4 shows the significant reductions observed in body weight, BMI, WC, WHR, and FAT% after saxagliptin, metformin, and combination treatments, in comparison to the respective values before treatment ($P < 0.01$ for all). Significant differences were observed in the reduction of weight, BMI, and FAT% among all three groups and between the two monotherapy groups (saxagliptin group vs. combination group vs. metformin group: weight: $P < 0.001$, BMI: $P < 0.001$, FAT%: $P = 0.026$; saxagliptin group vs. metformin group: weight: $P < 0.001$, BMI: $P < 0.001$, FAT%: $P = 0.043$).

Table 2 Parameters of glucose metabolism before and after treatment in PCOS patients

Parameters	Saxagliptin			Saxagliptin – Metformin			Metformin		
	Baseline	Treatment	Δ	Baseline	Treatment	Δ	Baseline	Treatment	Δ
FBG, mmol/L	5.63 (5.31 to 5.96)	5.39 (5.15 to 5.62)*	-0.25 (-0.49 to 0)	5.84 (5.62 to 6.06)	5.14 (5 to 5.27)**	-0.7 (-0.94 to -0.46)	5.62 (5.39 to 5.84)	5.01 (4.88 to 5.14)**	-0.61 (-0.86 to 0.35)
2hBG, mmol/L	14.73 (13.49 to 15.97)	7.23 (6.61 to 7.85)**	-7.5 (-8.62 to -6.38)	15.59 (14.26 to 16.92)	7.4 (6.93 to 7.86)**	-8.2 (-9.5 to -6.9)	14.64 (13.66 to 15.62)	7.78 (7.36 to 8.2)**	-6.86 (-8.02 to -5.7)
FINS, μIU/mL	15.78 ± 6.7	11.55 ± 4.57**	-4.23 ± 3.86	16.18 ± 5.3	10.67 ± 2.99**	-5.51 ± 2.92	14.34 ± 4.85	10.26 ± 1.74**	-4.08 ± 4.45
2hINS, μIU/mL	100.24 (80.63–119.85)	63.24 (49.57–76.91)**	-37 (-49.94 to -24.06)	111.82 (92.73 to 130.91)	69.49 (58.84 to 80.14)**	-42.33 (-57.39 to -27.27)	100.26 (84.59 to 115.94)	61.15 (49.87 to 72.43)**	-39.11 (-53.1 to -25.13)
HbA1c, %	7.4 ± 0.3	6.3 ± 0.2**	-1.1 ± 0.4*	7.4 ± 0.3	6.1 ± 0.2**	-1.3 ± 0.3*	7.3 ± 0.2	6.3 ± 0.3**	-1.1 ± 0.4*
AUC glucose	16.63 (15.65 to 17.62)	11.7 (10.82 to 12.57)**	-4.94 (-5.62 to -4.26)	17.18 (16.16 to 18.21)	11.53 (10.92 to 12.14)**	-5.66 (-6.44 to -4.87)	16.5 (15.81 to 17.19)	11.19 (10.72 to 11.66)**	-5.31 (-6.07 to -4.56)
AUC insulin	129.93 (105.47 to 154.39)	98.75 (83.41 to 114.1)**	-31.18 (-44.49 to -17.87)	148.2 (128 to 168.41)	120.77 (109.13 to 132.4)**	-27.44 (-41.07 to -13.81)	122.66 (104.04 to 141.27)	88.67 (76.72 to 100.62)**	-33.99 (-48.58 to -19.4)
HOMA-IR	4.03 (3.11 to 4.95)	2.82 (2.21 to 3.42)**	-1.21 (-1.71 to -0.71)	4.22 (3.55 to 4.89)	2.45 (2.1 to 2.8)**	-1.77 (-2.17 to -1.38)	3.56 (3.01 to 4.11)	2.29 (2.1 to 2.47)**	-1.28 (-1.82 to -0.74)
HOMA-IS	157.2 (123.12 to 191.28)	125.36 (101.75 to 148.96)*	-31.85 (-61.16 to -2.54)	141.38 (119.5 to 163.25)	133.3 (115.27 to 151.33)	-8.07 (-30.3 to 14.15)	143.91 (116.96 to 170.86)	141.32 (121.93 to 160.71)	-2.59 (-28.77 to 23.58)
Insulinogenic Index	21.04 (15.19 to 26.89)	20.32 (15.72 to 24.91)	-0.72 (-4.99 to 3.54)	23.65 (18.11 to 29.19)	22.57 (18.23 to 26.91)	-1.08 (-5.65 to 3.49)	19.35 (14.84 to 23.87)	18.76 (15.23 to 22.29)	-0.6 (-6.15 to 4.96)
Matsuda Index	50 (39.81 to 60.18)	78.6 (63.89 to 93.32)**	28.61 (21.58 to 35.63)	42.41 (35.12 to 49.7)	71.37 (62.45 to 80.29)**	28.96 (25.24 to 32.69)	50.12 (44.35 to 55.89)	84.82 (76.28 to 93.37)**	35.26 (27.86 to 42.66)
DI	6.1 (4.42 to 7.77)	8.7 (6.2 to 11.19)**	2.6 (0.59 to 4.62)	5.99 (4.5 to 7.49)	9.57 (8.11 to 11.03)**	3.57 (1.81 to 5.34)	5.63 (4.23 to 7.02)	8.71 (6.29 to 11.13)**	3.09 (0.53 to 5.64)

Data are presented as mean ± SD or mean (95% CI). P-values are based on the paired t-test for variables of normal distribution and the Wilcoxon signed-rank test for variables of skewed distribution, for differences between baseline and after the 24-week treatment; one-way ANOVA for variables of normal distribution and the Kruskal–Wallis test for variables of skewed distribution for differences among three groups. Δ denotes the changes after treatment compared with baseline. * $P < 0.05$ and ** $P < 0.01$ for changes before and after treatment in treatment columns, and for changes among three groups in Δ columns

FBG fasting blood glucose, *2hBG* 2-h blood glucose, *FINS* fasting insulin, *2hINS* 2-h insulin, *HbA1c* hemoglobin A1c, *AUC glucose* area under the curve during oral glucose tolerance test (OGTT), *AUC insulin* insulin area under the curve during OGTT, *HOMA-IR* homeostasis model assessment of insulin resistance, *HOMA-IS* homeostasis model assessment of insulin secretion, *DI* deposition index

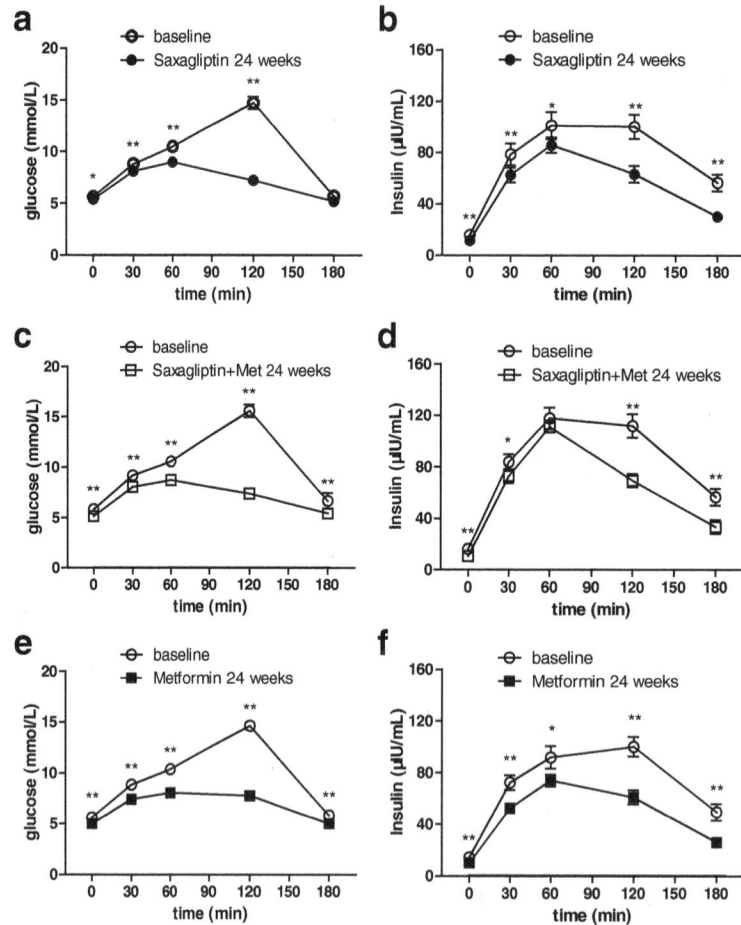

Fig. 1 OGTT-based glucose and insulin concentrations before and after treatment in PCOS patients with T2DM. **a, b** Glucose and insulin concentrations based on the OGTT in the saxagliptin group. **c, d** Glucose and insulin concentrations based on the OGTT in the saxagliptin + metformin group. **e, f** Glucose and insulin concentrations based on the OGTT in the metformin group. Data are presented as mean ± SEM. The AUC glucose and AUC insulin are shown in each figure. The P-values are based on the Wilcoxon signed-rank test for differences between groups. *$P < 0.05$; **$P < 0.01$. OGTT: oral glucose tolerance test; PCOS: polycystic ovary syndrome; T2DM: type 2 diabetes mellitus

However, no significant differences were noted in reductions of the WC and WHR among the three groups at 24 weeks ($P = 0.137$ and 0.161, respectively).

Changes in sex hormone levels after saxagliptin, metformin, or combination treatment in patients with new-onset T2DM

Table 5 shows the significant reductions observed in T levels after the saxagliptin, metformin, and combination treatments ($P = 0.03$, 0.02, and 0.013, respectively); whereas FSH levels showed a significant decline after metformin and combination treatments ($P = 0.009$ and $P < 0.001$, respectively). Following administration of the metformin treatment alone, the LH levels were significantly reduced ($P = 0.04$), and the FAI levels showed a decline only after the saxagliptin treatment ($P = 0.026$). No significant differences were observed in the reduction of sex hormone levels between the monotherapy

treatments ($P > 0.05$ for all). The saxagliptin treatment yielded greater improvements in T and FAI levels, compared to the combination treatment (T: − 0.52 vs. -0.34 nmol/L, $P = 0.049$; FAI: -6.94 vs. -2.35, $P = 0.015$). Moreover, the metformin treatment yielded a more significant increase in SHBG levels than the combination treatment (4.35 vs. 1.57 nmol/L, $P = 0.016$).

Discussion

The main findings of this study included the effects of saxagliptin to reduce glucose levels and improve β-cell function and their similarity to the effects of metformin in newly diagnosed patients with T2DM and PCOS. The HbA1c levels showed decline in all three groups after the 24-week treatment. The reduction in HbA1c was significant in the combination group, compared to the monotherapy groups, whereas differences between the monotherapies were not significant. Furthermore,

Table 3 Lipid profile and inflammation before and after treatment in PCOS patients with new-onset T2DM

Parameters	Saxagliptin			Saxagliptin + Metformin			Metformin		
	Baseline	Treatment	Δ	Baseline	Treatment	Δ	Baseline	Treatment	Δ
TG, mmol/L	1.44 (1.16 to 1.72)	1.01 (0.92 to 1.09)**	−0.43 (−0.67 to −0.2)	1.34 (1.19 to 1.5)	0.95 (0.86 to 1.04)**	−0.39 (−0.53 to −0.25)	1.32 (1.05 to 1.59)	0.9 (0.79 to 1)**	−0.43 (−0.62 to −0.23)
TC, mmol/L	4.51 (4.2 to 4.81)	4.41 (4.19 to 4.64)	−0.09 (−0.21 to 0.02)**	4.8 (4.44 to 5.15)	4.52 (4.29 to −4.75)**	−0.27 (−0.5 to −0.05)**	4.94 (4.57- to 5.31)	4.56 (4.28 to 4.84)**	−0.38 (−0.54 to −0.21)**
HDL-C, mmol/L	1.26 (1.16 to 1.37)	1.3 (1.24 to 1.36)	0.04 (−0.03 to 0.1)	1.24 (1.14 to 1.35)	1.32 (1.23 to 1.4)	0.07 (−0.03 to 0.18)	1.35 (1.26 to 1.43)	1.41 (1.35 to 1.46)**	0.06 (0 to 0.12)
LDL-C, mmol/L	3.06 ± 0.7	2.87 ± 0.48*	−0.19 ± 0.36*	3.4 ± 0.73	2.98 ± 0.41**	−0.42 ± 0.46*	3.32 ± 0.69	2.89 ± 0.45**	−0.43 ± 0.35*
hsCRP, mg/L	3.97 (3.1 to 4.84)	2.23 (1.84 to 2.63)**	−1.74 (−2.44 to −1.03)	3.94 (3.09 to 4.8)	2.51 (2.22 to 2.81)**	−1.43 (−2.08 to −0.78)	4.02 (3.23 to 4.8)	3.03 (2.57 to 3.49)**	−0.99 (−1.44 to −0.54)

Data are presented as mean ± SD or mean (95% CI). P-values based on the paired t-test for variables of normal distribution and the Wilcoxon signed-rank test for variables of skewed distribution, for differences between baseline and after the 24-week treatment; one-way ANOVA for variables of normal distribution and the Kruskal–Wallis test for variables of skewed distribution for differences among three groups. Δ denotes the changes after treatment compared with baseline. * $P < 0.05$ and ** $P < 0.01$ for changes before and after treatment in treatment columns, and for changes among three groups in Δ columns

TG triglyceride, TC total cholesterol, HDL-C high-density lipoprotein cholesterol, LDL-C low-density lipoprotein cholesterol, hsCRP high-sensitivity C-reactive protein

Table 4 Anthropometric measurements before and after treatment in PCOS patients

Parameters	Saxagliptin			Saxagliptin + Metformin			Metformin		
	Baseline	Treatment	Δ	Baseline	Treatment	Δ	Baseline	Treatment	Δ
Weight, kg	70.4 (63.7 to 77.1)	69.4 (62.8 to 76.1)**	−1.0 (−1.3 to −0.6)**	69.3 (64.6 to 74.1)	67.0 (62.4 to 71.6)**	−2.4 (−2.8 to 2.0)**	67.9 (63.6 to 72.2)	65.1 (61.0 to 69.3)**	−2.8 (−3.4 to −2.2)**
BMI, kg/m²	27.2 (24.94 to 29.46)	26.68 (24.51 to 28.85)**	−0.52 (−0.82 to −0.22)**	26.38 (24.66 to 28.1)	25.46 (23.79 to 27.13)**	−0.92 (−1.08 to −0.75)**	26.4 (24.63 to 28.18)	25.32 (23.63 to 27.02)**	−1.09 (−1.32 to −0.85)**
WC, cm	86.8 (81.2 to 92.4)	84.3 (79.1 to 89.5)**	−2.5 (−3.1 to −1.9)	84.7 (80.0 to 89.4)	81.5 (77.1 to 85.8)**	−3.2 (−3.9 to 2.6)	82.8 (78.9 to 86.6)	79.9 (76.4 to 83.3)**	−2.9 (−3.5 to 2.4)
WHR	0.88 ± 0.08	0.86 ± 0.08**	−0.02 ± 0.02	0.86 ± 0.06	0.83 ± 0.05**	−0.03 ± 0.02	0.85 ± 0.06	0.83 ± 0.05**	−0.02 ± 0.01
FAT%	36.13 (32.74 to 39.53)	33.89 (30.89 to 36.88)**	−2.25 (−2.98 to −1.52)*	35.12 (32.19 to 38.05)	31.59 (29.01 to 34.16)**	−3.53 (−4.36 to −2.71)*	33.6 (31.21 to 35.98)	30.5 (28.34 to 32.67)**	−3.2 (−3.81 to −2.59)*

Data are presented as mean ± SD or mean (95% CI). P-values based on the paired t-test for variables of normal distribution and the Wilcoxon signed-rank test for variables of skewed distribution, for differences between baseline and after the 24-week treatment; one-way ANOVA for variables of normal distribution and the Kruskal–Wallis test for variables of skewed distribution for differences among three groups. Δ denotes the changes after treatment compared with baseline. * $P < 0.05$ and ** $P < 0.01$ for changes before and after treatment in treatment columns, and for changes among three groups in Δ columns *BMI* body mass index, *WC* waist circumference, *WHR* waist hip ratio, *FAT%* body fat percentage

Table 5 Sex hormone levels before and after treatment in PCOS patients

Parameters	Saxagliptin			Saxagliptin – Metformin			Metformin		
	Baseline	Treatment	Δ	Baseline	Treatment	Δ	Baseline	Treatment	Δ
LH, IU/L	10.01 (6.21 to 13.81)	7.8 (7 to 8.61)	-2.21 (-5.54 to 1.12)	9.62 (7.24 to 12.01)	7.68 (6.86 to 8.5)	-1.94 (-4.27 to 0.39)	11.74 (8.59 to 14.89)	7.55 (6.65 to 8.45)*	-4.19 (-7.32 to -1.05)
FSH, IU/L	6.27 (5.24 to 7.3)	5.66 (5.16 to 6.16)	-0.61 (-1.62 to 0.4)	7.66 (6.94 to 8.38)	5.97 (5.57 to 6.37)**	-1.69 (-2.55 to -0.83)	8.18 (6.83 to 9.52)	5.92 (5.31 to 6.53)**	-2.26 (-3.86 to -0.66)
T, nmol/L	2.64 (2.33 to 2.96)	2.13 (1.94 to 2.32)**	-0.52 (-0.69 to -0.34)*	2.61 (2.35 to 2.86)	2.27 (2.09 to 2.45)*	-0.34 (-0.52 to -0.16)*	2.6 (2.33 to 2.86)	2.11 (1.97 to 2.26)**	-0.48 (-0.65 to -0.31)
SHBG, nmol/L	24.72 (17.14 to 32.29)	29.62 (23.77 to 35.48)	4.91 (1.56 to 8.25)	25.51 (19.98 to 31.04)	27.09 (22.76 to 31.41)	1.57 (-0.8 to 3.95)*	22.64 (15.73 to 29.54)	26.98 (21.55 to 32.42)	4.35 (1.72 to 6.97)*
FAI	15.82 (11.06 to 20.58)	8.88 (6.4 to 11.35)*	-6.94 (-9.83 to -4.06)*	11.72 (8.36 to 15.08)	9.37 (7.57 to 11.16)	-2.35 (-5.72 to 1.01)*	14.84 (9.06 to 20.63)	9.13 (7.38 to 10.88)	-5.72 (-10.79 to -0.64)

Data are presented as mean ± SD and mean (95% CI). P-values based on the paired t-test for variables of normal distribution and the Wilcoxon signed-rank test for variables of skewed distribution, for differences between baseline and the 24-week treatment; one-way ANOVA for variables of normal distribution and the Kruskal–Wallis test for variables of skewed distribution, for differences among three groups. Δ denotes the changes after treatment compared with baseline. * P < 0.05 and ** P < 0.01 for changes before and after treatment in treatment columns, and for changes among three groups in Δ columns
LH luteinizing hormone, *FSH* follicle-stimulating hormone, *T* total testosterone, *SHBG* sex hormone binding globulin, *FAI* Free androgen index

saxagliptin, metformin, and the combination treatment significantly reduced HOMA-IR and increased DI levels, whereas no significant changes were observed in the HOMA-IS of the metformin and combination groups, nor in the insulinogenic index of all three groups. In addition, saxagliptin and metformin treatments significantly reduced the BMI and hsCRP levels.

Impaired secretion and activity of the incretin hormone has been reported in women with PCOS, although the data are not consistent [14–16]. Vrbikova et al. [14] evaluated the relationship between incretin secretion and β-cell function in PCOS. They demonstrated that increased levels of total gastric inhibitory polypeptide (GIP) and lower concentrations of late phase active glucagon-like peptide-1 (GLP-1) were common characteristics observed during the OGTT in women with PCOS, who had higher levels of C-peptide secretion in comparison to healthy controls. Their study suggests that these peptides might be early markers of a pre-diabetic state [14]. Moreover, our previous study [5] showed that impaired β-cell function induced a primary defect in Chinese women with PCOS. It also suggested that impaired β-cell function in PCOS with T2DM might pose a more serious condition than that of those non-PCOS women with T2DM.

Studies in cell cultures and animal models have demonstrated that DPP-4 inhibitors have trophic effects on pancreatic β-cells [17–19] and can improve other metabolic characteristics, such as hyperlipidemia and low-grade inflammation. However, whether DPP-4 inhibitors play a unique role in women with T2DM and PCOS remains unclear. In the present study, we found that the effect of saxagliptin to reduce glucose levels was similar to that of metformin in newly diagnosed patients with T2DM and PCOS. The mean Matsuda `index values, whole-body insulin sensitivity evaluation derived from OGTTs, weight, lipid profile, and inflammation showed significant improvement after the 24-week saxagliptin treatment. Notably, we found that the reduction in HbA1c levels was significantly greater in the combination group, in comparison to the other groups of women with T2DM and PCOS. These enhanced effects of the combination therapy to reduce HbA1c levels suggest that β-cell dysfunction has a considerable impact on hyperglycemia in women with T2DM and PCOS in China. In a recent study, the effects of saxagliptin, metformin, and their combination were explored in pre-diabetic women with PCOS [20]. The combination treatment was found to be more effective at improving the insulin secretion-sensitivity index (IS-SI, which was derived by applying the concept of the DI to measurements obtained during the 2-h OGTT) in pre-diabetic women with PCOS [20]. In our study and study by Elkind-Hirsch et al., lipid parameters, such as TG, as

well as blood glucose were found to be reduced after saxagliptin and combination treatment. Thus, DPP-4 inhibitors evidently have a beneficial effect on metabolic disorders in both pre-diabetic and diabetic women with PCOS, especially if it is administered in combination with metformin.

When considered together, the above data infer that saxagliptin might be another favorable option to improve insulin sensitivity and sustain glycemic control in women with PCOS and T2DM. The mechanism by which these effects occur might be related to the activation of incretin and the increase in pancreatic β-cell insulin production.

In the present study, changes in the lipid profile (reduced TG and LDL-C levels) and reduced inflammation were both observed after all three treatments. Moreover, reductions were also observed in anthropometric measurements, such as weight, BMI, WC, WHR, and FAT%.

Metformin might be the most effective in long-term maintenance of PCOS, and it might exhibit favorable effects in preventing the progression to diabetes. However, the most common adverse reactions of metformin, the gastrointestinal symptoms (such as diarrhea, nausea, vomiting, abdominal bloating, flatulence, and anorexia), could limit its use in metformin-intolerant patients. Our previous findings suggest that the defect in ß-cell compensation for ambient IR, particularly in the stimulated state, already exists in women with PCOS. With respect to fasting glucose control, metformin treatment is prior to saxagliptin treatment. However, metformin monotherapy might be inadequate for 2-h control of glucose levels.

The conditions of T2DM and PCOS have special characteristics among different ethnic groups. In East Asians, T2DM is characterized by β-cell dysfunction, as opposed to IR due to increased adiposity. Thus, a preventative and therapeutic approach that precisely targets β-cell dysfunction is required [21]. As a result, the fact that saxagliptin enhances the glucose-dependent release of insulin by β-cells makes it an optimal choice for the treatment of T2DM in East Asians. Asian women with PCOS are no more likely to be obese than those without PCOS; however, when present, obesity still has metabolic effects [22]. Moreover, as women of some non-Caucasian ethnicities appear to have higher metabolic risks at a given adiposity, lower BMI and WC targets might be prudent in high-risk ethnic groups [22]. Thus, the effect of metformin on weight loss, as well as its ability to improve the uptake and utilization of glucose in peripheral tissue makes it an optimal choice for the treatment of PCOS in non-Caucasian ethnicities. Therefore, the combination of metformin and saxagliptin might have complementary effects on the treatment of patients with new-onset T2DM and PCOS.

Several limitations of the present study should be considered. Firstly, OGTT is less reliable than intravenous tests, possibly due to the increasing variability of DIx values (DI calculated by various methods). Nevertheless, the OGTT yields more favorable physiological expressions than those of intravenous tests, particularly because ubiquitous glucose sensors could actively participate in insulin activation and secretion [23]. Secondly, the samples of this study were relatively small and its duration was relatively short. Larger sample sizes and studies conducted over longer periods are required for future study. Finally, causality cannot be established with the cross-sectional design of the present study.

Conclusions
Both saxagliptin and metformin monotherapy treatments were effective in reducing blood glucose and HbA1c levels in women with PCOS and new-onset T2DM. It might be beneficial, during the earlier stages, to add a DPP-4 inhibitor to the treatment protocol for women with PCOS and T2DM.

Abbreviations
AUC glucose: Area under the curve during OGTT performance for glucose; AUC insulin: Area under the curve during OGTT performance for insulin; BMI: Body mass index; CV: Coefficients of variation; DI: Deposition index; FAI: Free androgen indexes; FAT: Body fat; FBG: Fasting blood glucose; FINS: Fasting insulin; FSH: Follicle-stimulating hormone; GIP: Gastric inhibitory polypeptide; GLP-1: Glucagon-like peptide-1; HC: Hip circumference; HDL-C: High-density lipoprotein cholesterol; HOMA-IR: Homeostasis model assessment insulin resistance index; HOMA-IS: Homeostasis model assessment β cell function; IGT: Impaired glucose tolerance; IR: Insulin resistance; LDL-C: Low-density lipoprotein cholesterol; LH: Luteinizing hormone; OGTT: Oral glucose tolerance test; PCOS: Polycystic ovary syndrome; SHBG: Sex hormone binding globulin; T: Testosterone; T2DM: Type 2 diabetes mellitus; TC: Total cholesterol; TG: Triglyceride; WC: Waist circumference; WHR: Waist hip ratio

Acknowledgements
We thank the women who participated in the study and gratefully acknowledge the assistance of the nursing staff at Shanghai Renji Hospital and the technical assistants who performed the biochemical analyses.

Funding
This work was supported by the National Natural Science Foundation of China [grant number 81200628]; the Chinese Medical Association Clinical Research and Special Funds - Squibb Endocrinology Diabetes Research projects [2012]; the Natural Science Foundation of Shanghai, China [grant number 12ZR1417800]; and the Shanghai Science and Technology Development Fund [grant number 08411953000].

Authors' contributions
TT and WL designed the study. TT, PW, and YW collected the data. TT and YW analyzed the data. All authors were involved in drafting the manuscript, and have read and approved the final version.

Competing interests
The authors declare that they have no competing interests.

Author details
Department of Endocrinology and Metabolism, Renji Hospital, School of Medicine, Shanghai Jiaotong University, 160 Pujian Road, Shanghai 200127, China. ²Shanghai Key laboratory for Assisted Reproduction and Reproductive Genetics, Center for Reproductive Medicine, Renji Hospital, School of Medicine, Shanghai Jiaotong University, 160 Pujian Road, Shanghai 200127, China.

References
1. Ehrmann DA, Kasza K, Azziz R, Legro RS, Ghazzi MN, PCOS/Troglitazone Study Group. Effects of race and family history of type 2 diabetes on metabolic status of women with polycystic ovary syndrome. J Clin Endocrinol Metab. 2005;90:66–71.
2. Legro RS, Kunselman AR, Dodson WC, Dunaif A. Prevalence and predictors of risk for type 2 diabetes mellitus and impaired glucose tolerance in polycystic ovary syndrome: a prospective, controlled study in 254 affected women. J Clin Endocrinol Metab. 1999;84:165–9.
3. Reaven GM. Banting lecture 1988. Role of insulin resistance in human disease. Diabetes. 1988;37:1595–607.
4. Dunaif A, Xia J, Book CB, Schenker E, Tang Z. Excessive insulin receptor serine phosphorylation in cultured fibroblasts and in skeletal muscle. A potential mechanism for insulin resistance in the polycystic ovary syndrome. J Clin Invest. 1995;96:801–10.
5. Tao T, Li SX, Zhao AM, Mao XY, Liu W. Early impaired β-cell function in Chinese women with polycystic ovary syndrome. Int J Clin Exp Pathol. 2012; 5:777–86.
6. Drucker DJ. The biology of incretin hormones. Cell Metab. 2006;3:153–65.
7. DeFronzo RA. Pathogenesis of type 2 diabetes: implications for metformin. Drugs. 1999;58(Suppl 1):29–30. discussion 75-82
8. Diamanti-Kandarakis E, Christakou CD, Kandaraki E, Economou FN. Metformin: an old medication of new fashion: evolving new molecular mechanisms and clinical implications in polycystic ovary syndrome. Eur J Endocrinol. 2010;162:193–212.
9. Nestler JE. Metformin for the treatment of the polycystic ovary syndrome. N Engl J Med. 2008;358:47–54.
10. Matthews DR, Hosker JP, Rudenski AS, Naylor BA, Treacher DF, Turner RC. Homeostasis model assessment: insulin resistance and beta-cell function from fasting plasma glucose and insulin concentrations in man. Diabetologia. 1985;28:412–9.
11. Seltzer HS, Allen EW, Herron AL Jr, Brennan MT. Insulin secretion in response to glycemic stimulus: relation of delayed initial release to carbohydrate intolerance in mild diabetes mellitus. J Clin Invest. 1967;46:323–35.
12. Drivsholm T, Hansen T, Urhammer SA, Palacios RT, Volund A, Borch-Johnsen K, et al. Assessment of insulin sensitivity and beta-cell function from an oral glucose tolerance test. Diabetologia. 1999;42(Suppl 1):A185.
13. Kahn SE, Prigeon RL, Mcculloch DK, Boyko EJ, Bergman RN, Schwartz MW, et al. Quantification of the relationship between insulin sensitivity and beta-cell function in human-subjects. Evidence for a hyperbolic function. Diabetes. 1993;42:1663–72.
14. Vrbikova J, Hill M, Bendlova B, Grimmichova T, Dvorakova K, Vondra K, et al. Incretin levels in polycystic ovary syndrome. Eur J Endocrinol. 2008;159:121–7.
15. Gama R, Norris F, Wright J, Morgan L, Hampton S, Watkins S, Marks V. The entero-insular axis in polycystic ovarian syndrome. Ann Clin Biochem. 1996; 33(Pt 3):190–5.
16. Pontikis C, Yavropoulou MP, Toulis KA, Kotsa K, Kazakos K, Papazisi A, et al. The incretin effect and secretion in obese and lean women with polycystic ovary syndrome: a pilot study. J Women's Health (Larchmt). 2011;20:971–6.
17. Meier JJ. GLP-1 receptor agonists for individualized treatment of type 2 diabetes mellitus. Nat Rev Endocrinol. 2012;8:728–42.
18. Farilla L, Bulotta A, Hirshberg B, Li Calzi S, Khoury N, Noushmehr H, et al. Glucagon-like peptide 1 inhibits cell apoptosis and improves glucose responsiveness of freshly isolated human islets. Endocrinology. 2003;144: 5149–58.

19. Crepaldi G, Carruba M, Comaschi M, Del Prato S, Frajese G, Paolisso G. Dipeptidyl peptidase 4 (DPP-4) inhibitors and their role in type 2 diabetes management. J Endocrinol Investig. 2007;30:610–4.

20. Elkind-Hirsch KE, Paterson MS, Seidemann EL, Gutowski HC. Short-term therapy with combination dipeptidyl peptidase-4 inhibitor saxagliptin/metformin extended release (XR) is superior to saxagliptin or metformin XR monotherapy in prediabetic women with polycystic ovary syndrome: a single-blind, randomized, pilot study. Fertil Steril. 2017;107:253–60.e1.

21. Yabe D, Seino Y, Fukushima M. Seino S. β cell dysfunction versus insulin resistance in the pathogenesis of type 2 diabetes in east Asians. Curr Diab Rep. 2015;15:602.

22. De Sousa SM, Norman RJ. Metabolic syndrome, diet and exercise. Best Pract Res Clin Obstet Gynaecol. 2016;37:140–51.

23. Holst JJ. The physiology of glucagon-like peptide 1. Physiol Rev. 2007;87: 1409–39.

5

The effects of synbiotic supplementation on hormonal status, biomarkers of inflammation and oxidative stress in subjects with polycystic ovary syndrome: a randomized, double-blind, placebo-controlled trial

Khadijeh Nasri[1], Mehri Jamilian[1], Elham Rahmani[1], Fereshteh Bahmani[2], Maryam Tajabadi-Ebrahimi[3] and Zatollah Asemi[2*]

Abstract

Background: To our knowledge, no reports are available indicating the effects of synbiotic supplementation on hormonal status, biomarkers of inflammation and oxidative stress in subjects with polycystic ovary syndrome (PCOS). This research was done to assess the effects of synbiotic supplementation on hormonal status, biomarkers of inflammation and oxidative stress in subjects with PCOS.

Methods: This randomized double-blind, placebo-controlled trial was conducted on 60 subjects diagnosed with PCOS according to the Rotterdam criteria. Subjects were randomly assigned into two groups to take either synbiotic ($n = 30$) or placebo ($n = 30$) for 12 weeks. Endocrine, inflammation and oxidative stress biomarkers were quantified at baseline and after the 12-week intervention.

Results: After the 12-week intervention, compared with the placebo, synbiotic supplementation significantly increased serum sex hormone-binding globulin (SHBG) (changes from baseline in synbiotic group: + 19.8 ± 47.3 vs. in placebo group: + 0.5 ± 5.4 nmol/L, $p = 0.01$), plasma nitric oxide (NO) (changes from baseline in synbiotic group: + 5.5 ± 4.8 vs. in placebo group: + 0.3 ± 9.1 μmol/L, $p = 0.006$), and decreased modified Ferriman Gallwey (mF-G) scores (changes from baseline in synbiotic group: − 1.3 ± 2.5 vs. in placebo group: − 0.1 ± 0.5, $p = 0.01$) and serum high-sensitivity C-reactive protein (hs-CRP) (changes from baseline in synbiotic group: − 950.0 ± 2246.6 vs. in placebo group: + 335.3 ± 2466.9 ng/mL, $p = 0.02$). We did not observe any significant effect of synbiotic supplementation on other hormonal status and biomarkers of oxidative stress.

Conclusions: Overall, synbiotic supplementation for 12 weeks in PCOS women had beneficial effects on SHBG, mFG scores, hs-CRP and NO levels, but did not affect other hormonal status and biomarkers of oxidative stress.

Keywords: Synbiotic, Hormonal status, Inflammation, Oxidative stress, Polycystic ovary syndrome

* Correspondence: asemi_r@yahoo.com
[2]Research Center for Biochemistry and Nutrition in Metabolic Diseases, Kashan University of Medical Sciences, Kashan, IR, Iran
Full list of author information is available at the end of the article

Background

Polycystic ovary syndrome (PCOS) is a common gynecological endocrine disorder related to irregular menstrual cycles and androgen excess affecting 6–12% of premenopausal women [1]. It was reported that several pro-inflammatory factors and mediators increase in subjects with PCOS, including C-reactive protein (CRP), leukocytes, cytokines, and reactive oxygen species [2]. Inflammation and oxidative stress are associated with obesity, type 2 diabetes mellitus (T2DM), hyperandrogenemia, insulin resistance as well as an increased risk of cardiovascular disease (CVD) [3].

Nowadays, there is a growing interest to use synbiotics and probiotics in diseases related to metabolic syndrome [4]. The basis of this interest derives mostly from the results of nutritional intervention studies suggest that synbiotics intake have beneficial effects on metabolic profiles, biomarkers of inflammation and oxidative stress among patients with gestational diabetes (GDM) [5], T2DM [6] and cancer [7]. In addition, gut microbiota may participate in the whole-body metabolism by affecting energy balance, insulin metabolism and inflammation related to metabolic disorders [8]. We have previously shown that consumption of the synbiotic bread for 8 weeks among participants with T2DM had beneficial effects on plasma nitric oxide (NO) and malondialdehyde (MDA) concentrations, but did not influence plasma total antioxidant capacity (TAC) and glutathione (GSH) values [9]. In another study by Ipar et al. [10], it was seen that synbiotic supplementation for 30 days in obese children had beneficial effects on lipid fractions and total oxidative stress. However, multispecies probiotics supplementation (10^{10} CFU/day) for 14 weeks did not affect biomarkers of inflammation and oxidative stress among trained men [11].

Synbiotics and probiotics may affect metabolic parameters through the effect on the production of short chain fatty acid (SCFA), decreased gene expression of inflammatory factors [12], and increased synthesis of GSH, apoptosis induction and up-regulation of oxidative pentose pathway activity [13]. To our knowledge, no reports are available indicating the effects of synbiotic supplementation on hormonal, inflammatory and oxidative parameters in subjects with PCOS. The objective of this study was to evaluate the effects of synbiotic supplementation on hormonal, inflammatory and oxidative parameters in these patients.

Methods

Trial design and participants

This randomized, double-blinded, placebo-controlled clinical trial, registered in the Iranian clinical trials website at: (http://www.irct.ir: IRCT201509115623N53). This study was conducted among 60 women with PCOS diagnosed according to the Rotterdam criteria [14, 15], aged 18–40 years who referred to the Kossar Clinic in Arak, Iran, from April to June 2016. Main exclusion criteria were: smokers, taking probiotic and/or synbiotic supplements, pregnant women, endocrine diseases including thyroid, diabetes and/or impaired glucose tolerance as well as gastrointestinal problems in the study.

Ethics approval and consent to participate

The study was followed the Declaration of Helsinki guideline and was approved by the ethics committee of the Arak University of Medical Sciences (AUMS), Arak, Iran. Informed consent was taken from all subjects.

Study protocol

At first, women were randomly allocated to receive either synbiotic supplements or placebo ($n = 30$ each group) for 12 weeks. Duration of the treatment was selected based on observed beneficial effects of probiotic supplementation on metabolic profiles in women with PCOS [16]. Randomization was done using computer-generated random numbers by a trained staff at the gynecology clinic. Randomization and allocation were concealed to the researchers and participants until the final analyses were completed. Synbiotic supplements were containing Lactobacillus acidophilus, Lactobacillus casei and Bifidobacterium bifidum (2×10^9 CFU/g each) plus 0.8 g inulin. Synbiotic supplements and the placebo were manufactured by Tak Gen Zist Pharmaceutical Company (Tehran, Iran) and Barij Essence Pharmaceutical Company (Kashan, Iran), respectively. The compliance rate during the intervention was monitored by a brief daily cell phone reminder to take the supplement and asking the subjects to return the supplement containers. All participants completed a 3-days food record and physical activity records as metabolic equivalents (METs) prior to intervention, at weeks 3, 6, 9 and 12 of the treatment. Daily macro- and micro-nutrient intakes were calculated by analyzing food data using nutritionist IV software (First Databank, San Bruno, CA) [17].

Anthropometric parameters

Anthropometric measurements were determined in a fasting status using a standard scale (Seca, Hamburg, Germany) at baseline and after the 12-week treatment. Body mass index (BMI) was calculated as weight in kg divided by height in meters squared.

Clinical assessments

Clinical parameters included determinations of hirsutism using a mFG scoring system [18].

Biochemical evaluation

At pre- and post-treatment, 10 mL blood were collected from each subject at Arak reference laboratory. Hormonal profiles were determined using an Elisa kits (DiaMetra, Milano, Italy) with inter- and intra-assay coefficient variances (CVs) lower than 7%. Free androgen index (FAI) was calculated based on suggested formulas. High sensitivity C-reactive protein (hs-CRP) and insulin values were assessed by ELISA kits (LDN, Nordhorn, Germany) and (Monobind, California, USA), respectively. The plasma NO [19], TAC [20], GSH [21] and MDA levels [22] were determined by the spectrophotometric method with inter- and intra-assay CVs less than 5%. To determine fasting plasma glucose, we used Pars Azmun kit, Tehran, Iran. The homeostatic model of assessment for insulin resistance (HOMA-IR) was determined according to suggested formulas [23].

Sample size

We used a randomized clinical trial sample size formula with type one (α) and type two errors (β) to be 0.05 and the power of 80% to calculate sample size. Based on a previous study [24], we used a standard deviation (SD) of 283.7 ng/mL and a difference in mean (d) of 230. 0 ng/mL, considering hs-CRP levels as the key variable. According to the calculation 25 women should be enrolled in each group. Assuming a dropout of 5 subjects per group, the final sample size was considered to be 30 per treatment group.

Statistical methods

The Kolmogorov-Smirnov test was performed to determine the normality of data. Outcome log-transformation was used if model residual has non-normal distribution (hs-CRP, MDA, SHBG and FAI). To detect differences in anthropometric parameters as well as in macro- and micro-nutrient intakes between the two groups, we applied independent t-test. To assess the effects of synbiotic supplementation on metabolic parameters, we used one-way repeated measures analysis of variance. Adjustment for changes in baseline values of biochemical parameters, age and baseline BMI was performed by analysis of covariance (ANCOVA). P-values < 0.05 were considered statistically significant. All statistical analyses were done using the Statistical Package for Social Science version 18 (SPSS Inc., Chicago, Illinois, USA).

Results

In this study, all 60 subjects [synbiotic and placebo ($n = 30$ each group)] completed the trial (Fig. 1). The compliance rate in this study was high; more than 90% of capsules were taken during the course of the trial in both groups. No side effects were reported following the intake of synbiotic supplements in patients with PCOS.

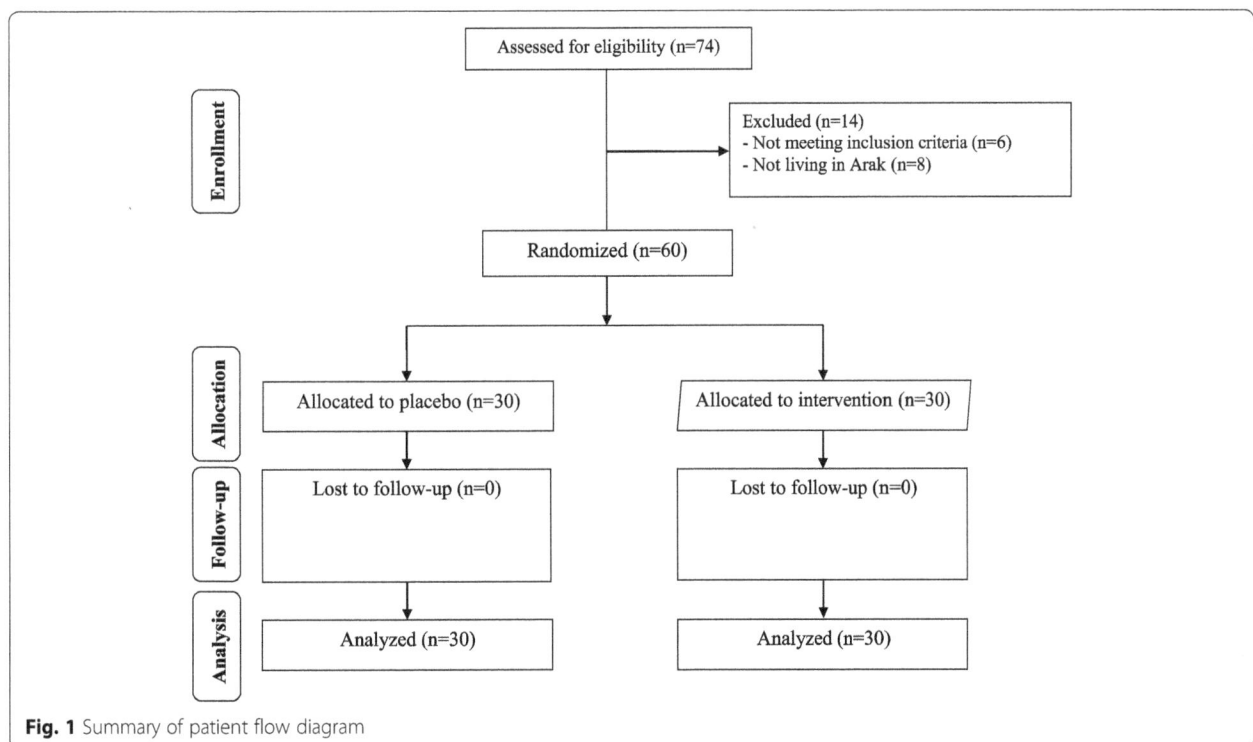

Fig. 1 Summary of patient flow diagram

Table 1 General characteristics of study participants

	Placebo group ($n = 30$)	Synbiotic group ($n = 30$)	p^a
Age (y)	25.9 ± 5.2	25.7 ± 5.5	0.90
Height (cm)	163.3 ± 6.6	161.4 ± 5.8	0.25
Weight at study baseline (kg)	72.4 ± 14.1	71.4 ± 11.6	0.79
Weight at end-of-trial (kg)	71.9 ± 14.4	71.2 ± 11.4	0.83
Weight change (kg)	−0.4 ± 1.0	− 0.3 ± 1.2	0.53
BMI at study baseline (kg/m^2)	27.2 ± 5.3	27.4 ± 4.0	0.84
BMI at end-of-trial (kg/m^2)	27.0 ± 5.4	27.3 ± 3.9	0.80
BMI change (kg/m^2)	−0.2 ± 0.3	− 0.1 ± 0.4	0.49
MET-h/day at study baseline	27.5 ± 2.0	27.7 ± 2.1	0.60
MET-h/day at end-of-trial	27.6 ± 2.2	27.8 ± 2.3	0.69
MET-h/day change	0.1 ± 0.6	0.04 ± 1.0	0.83

Data are means± SDs
[a]Obtained from independent t test. METs, metabolic equivalents

Mean age, height, and weight, BMI and METs at baseline and end-of-trial were not statistically different between the two groups (Table 1).

No significant difference in mean dietary macro- and micro-nutrient intakes between the two groups was seen (Data not shown).

Compared with the placebo, synbiotic supplementation significantly increased serum sex hormone-binding globulin (SHBG) (changes from baseline in synbiotic group: + 19.8 ± 47.3 vs. in placebo group: + 0.5 ± 5.4 nmol/L, $p = 0.01$), plasma NO (changes from baseline in synbiotic group: + 5.5 ± 4.8 vs. in placebo group: + 0.3 ± 9.1 μmol/L, $p = 0.006$), and decreased mF-G scores (changes from baseline in synbiotic group: − 1.3 ± 2.5 vs. in placebo group: − 0.1 ± 0.5, $p = 0.01$), FAI (changes from baseline in synbiotic group: − 0.12 ± 0.29 vs. in placebo group: − 0.01 ± 0.08, p

= 0.01) and serum hs-CRP (changes from baseline in synbiotic group: − 950.0 ± 2246.6 vs. in placebo group: + 335.3 ± 2466.9 ng/mL, $p = 0.02$) (Table 2). In addition, compared with the placebo, synbiotic supplementation resulted in a significant reduction in serum insulin levels (changes from baseline in synbiotic group: − 1.6 ± 2.9 vs. in placebo group: + 0.4 ± 2.3 μIU/mL, $p = 0.003$), HOMA-IR (changes from baseline in synbiotic group: − 0.4 ± 0.7 vs. in placebo group: + 0.1 ± 0.5, $p = 0.003$). A trend toward a greater decrease in total testosterone (changes from baseline in synbiotic group: − 0.4 vs. in placebo group: − 0.1 ng/mL, $p = 0.09$) and plasma MDA concentrations (changes from baseline in synbiotic group: − 0.2 ± 0.1 vs. in placebo group: + 0.5 ± 1.4 μmol/L, $p = 0.05$) was observed in synbiotic group compared with placebo group. We did not observe any significant effect of

Table 2 Hormonal status, biomarkers of inflammation and oxidative stress at baseline and after the 12-week intervention in subjects with polycystic ovary syndrome

	Placebo group ($n = 30$)			Synbiotic group ($n = 30$)			p^a
	Baseline	End-of-trial	Change	Baseline	End-of-trial	Change	
Total testosterone (ng/mL)	2.4 ± 1.2	2.3 ± 1.0	−0.1 ± 0.5	2.8 ± 1.3	2.4 ± 0.9	−0.4 ± 0.9	0.09
SHBG (nmol/L)	38.3 ± 17.3	38.8 ± 17.6	0.5 ± 5.4	37.3 ± 13.1	57.1 ± 48.6	19.8 ± 47.3	0.01
FAI	0.27 ± 0.21	0.25 ± 0.16	−0.01 ± 0.08	0.33 ± 0.36	0.21 ± 0.14	−0.12 ± 0.29	0.01
mF-G scores	15.1 ± 3.8	15.0 ± 3.7	−0.1 ± 0.5	15.3 ± 5.6	14.0 ± 4.9	−1.3 ± 2.5	0.01
DHEAS (μg/mL)	2.6 ± 1.3	2.5 ± 1.1	−0.1 ± 0.4	2.6 ± 1.5	2.2 ± 0.8	−0.4 ± 1.1	0.40
hs-CRP (ng/mL)	2990.7 ± 2510.7	3326.0 ± 2791.1	335.3 ± 2466.9	2920.0 ± 2251.2	1970.0 ± 1442.0	−950.0 ± 2246.6	0.02
NO (μmol/L)	40.5 ± 8.7	40.8 ± 9.3	0.3 ± 9.1	39.0 ± 3.1	44.5 ± 5.0	5.5 ± 4.8	0.006
TAC (mmol/L)	868.7 ± 158.4	877.9 ± 149.9	9.2 ± 119.3	773.1 ± 38.7	818.2 ± 57.5	45.1 ± 51.8	0.13
GSH (μmol/L)	494.2 ± 85.5	521.5 ± 117.2	27.3 ± 117.8	498.9 ± 56.8	523.5 ± 53.4	24.7 ± 58.7	0.91
MDA (μmol/L)	2.2 ± 0.7	2.7 ± 1.2	0.5 ± 1.4	2.3 ± 0.4	2.1 ± 0.4	−0.2 ± 0.1	0.05

All values are means± SDs
[a]P values represent the time × group interaction (computed by analysis of the one-way repeated measures ANOVA)
DHEAS dehydroepiandrosterone sulfate, FAI free androgen index, GSH total glutathione, hs-CRP high-sensitivity C-reactive protein, mF-G modified Ferriman Gallwey, MDA malondialdehyde, NO nitric oxide, SHBG sex hormone-binding globulin, TAC total antioxidant capacity

synbiotic supplementation on other hormonal status and biomarkers of oxidative stress.

Baseline levels of plasma TAC ($p = 0.002$) were significantly different between the two groups. Therefore, we controlled the analyses for the baseline levels, age and baseline BMI. When we adjusted the analyses for baseline values of biochemical variables, age and baseline BMI, significant changes in FAI ($p = 0.04$) were observed, but other findings did not alter (Table 3).

Discussion

In this research, which to our knowledge is the first of its kind, we assessed the effects of synbiotic supplementation on hormonal, inflammatory and oxidative parameters among subjects with PCOS. We shown that taking synbiotic supplements for 12 weeks among PCOS subjects had beneficial effects on SHBG, mFG scores, FAI, serum insulin, HOMA-IR, serum hs-CRP and plasma NO levels, but did not affect other hormonal, inflammatory and oxidative parameters. However, observed reduction at mFG scores after 12 weeks was statistically significant, it was clinically low. Long-term interventions and higher dosage of probiotic and inulin might result in greater changes in mFG scores.

Subjects with PCOS are susceptible to several metabolic complications including insulin resistance and inflammation [25, 26]. We found that synbiotic administration for 12 weeks among PCOS subjects led to a significant increase in serum SHBG values and FAI and a significant decrease in mFG scores, serum insulin levels and HOMA-IR, but did not affect hormonal profiles compared with the placebo. However, to our knowledge, no reports are available indicating the effects of synbiotic supplementation on hormonal status, biomarkers of inflammation and oxidative stress in subjects with PCOS; some studies have evaluated the effects of synbiotic supplementation on

markers of insulin metabolism among subjects without PCOS. We have previously shown that taking synbiotic supplements for 6 weeks among subjects with GDM had beneficial effects on markers of insulin metabolism [5]. Shoaei et al. [27] also indicated that probiotic supplementation for 12 weeks to women with PCOS significantly decreased fasting glucose and insulin concentrations. In another study conducted by Eslamparast et al. [28], it was seen that levels of fasting glucose and insulin resistance were improved significantly in the synbiotic group among subjects with metabolic syndrome after 28 weeks. In addition, the intake of synbiotic containing *Lactobacillus acidophilus*, *Bifidobacterium bifidum* and fructo-oligosaccharides in elderly people with T2DM resulted in a significant reduction in fasting glycemia [29]. Hyperinsulinemia and insulin resistance in women with PCOS directly stimulate ovarian steroidogenesis by acting on thecal cell proliferation and increasing secretion of androgens mediated by luteinizing hormone (LH), increased gene expression of cytochrome P450 and insulin-like growth factor 1 receptor [30]. In addition, androgens may regulate follicular atresia [31]. It was also reported that increased testosterone levels increase somatic cell atresia in rat ovaries [32]. Furthermore, hyperandrogenemia can induce inflammation in women with PCOS [33]. Therefore, synbiotic intake due to its useful effects on insulin resistance may be useful to control clinical and metabolic symptoms. Synbiotic intake might improve SHBG and mFG scores through improved insulin sensitivity, the modification of gut flora, the elevation of faecal pH [34] and the reduction of pro-inflammatory cytokine production [35].

Our previous study among subjects with T2DM has demonstrated that consumption of a synbiotic food for 6 weeks had significant effects on serum hs-CRP concentrations [24]. In addition, supplementation with a

Table 3 Adjusted changes in metabolic profile of the patients with polycystic ovary syndrome

	Placebo group ($n = 30$)	Synbiotic group ($n = 30$)	p^a
Total testosterone (ng/mL)	− 0.2 ± 0.1	− 0.3 ± 0.1	0.26
SHBG (nmol/L)	0.7 ± 6.1	19.5 ± 6.1	0.03
FAI	−0.04 ± 0.02	−0.10 ± 0.02	0.04
mF-G scores	−0.1 ± 0.3	−1.3 ± 0.3	0.007
DHEAS (μg/mL)	−0.1 ± 0.1	−0.3 ± 0.1	0.18
hs-CRP (ng/mL)	375.6 ± 339.8	−990.2 ± 339.8	0.006
NO (μmol/L)	0.6 ± 1.2	5.2 ± 1.2	0.009
TAC (mmol/L)	23.8 ± 16.3	30.5 ± 16.3	0.78
GSH (μmol/L)	26.3 ± 15.8	25.7 ± 15.8	0.98
MDA (μmol/L)	0.4 ± 0.2	−0.1 ± 0.2	0.02

All values are means± SEs. Values are adjusted for baseline values, age and BMI at baseline

[a]Obtained from ANCOVA

DHEAS dehydroepiandrosterone sulfate, *FAI* free androgen index, *GSH* total glutathione, *hs-CRP* high-sensitivity C-reactive protein, *mF-G* modified Ferriman Gallwey, *MDA* malondialdehyde, *NO* nitric oxide, *SHBG* sex hormone-binding globulin, *TAC* total antioxidant capacity

synbiotic among adults with nonalcoholic fatty liver disease over 28 weeks inhibited inflammatory markers [36]. Consumption of the synbiotic bread for 2 months in people with T2DM significantly increased plasma levels of NO and decreased MDA, but unchanged TAC, GSH, catalase concentrations [9]. These findings were similar in pregnant women [37] and patients with rheumatoid arthritis [38]. Furthermore, soy milk containing probiotic for 48 h increased NO production in human endothelial cells [39]. A significant decline in MDA values was also evidenced after the intake of probiotic in rabbits for 30 days [40]. However, synbiotic supplementation for 6 weeks did not influence CRP values [41]. In addition, NO status did not affect by probiotic in herpes simplex virus type 1 [42]. Supplementation with probiotic supplements for 7 days did not decrease MDA values [43]. Elevated inflammatory markers in subjects with PCOS would result in increased risk of atherosclerosis, diabetes and infertility [44]. In addition, oxidative stress is correlated with obesity and hyperandrogenism [45]. Increased oxidative stress could also induce directly genetic variation by DNA damage, and epigenetic change including elevated DNA methylation levels, which both play important roles in the pathogenesis of cancer [46, 47]. Upregulation of IL-18 by SCFA products [48] and elevated production of methylketones in gut by synbiotic [49] might decrease inflammatory markers. Decreased hydroperoxides by synbiotic intake may elevate NO levels [50, 51]. Moreover, synbiotic intake may reduce MDA because its impact on decreased lipid parameters [52] and inhibiting lipid peroxidation reactions [53, 54].

Limitations of our study include the absent of testing for a dose-response relationship between synbiotic intake and occurred changes in the metabolic profiles. Furthermore, we did not determine the effects of synbiotic on other metabolic parameters. However, duration of the treatment was too short to determine the effects of synbiotic on hormonal parameters and mFG scores; we believe that future studies with cross-over design and longer duration of the intervention are required to prove our findings. Furthermore, the high standard deviations (SDs) of dependent parameters in some cases might be due to the small number of participants in the study.

Conclusions

Overall, synbiotic supplementation for 12 weeks in PCOS women had beneficial effects on SHBG, mFG scores, FAI, hs-CRP and NO levels, but did not affect other hormonal status and biomarkers of oxidative stress.

Abbreviations

CVD: Cardiovascular disease; CVs: Coefficient variances; DHEAS: Dehydroepiandrosterone sulfate; FAI: Free androgen index; GDM: Gestational diabetes; GSH: Total glutathione; hs-CRP: High-sensitivity C-reactive protein; MDA: Malondialdehyde; mF-G: Modified Ferriman Gallwey; NO: Nitric oxide; PCOS: Polycystic ovary syndrome; SCFA: Short chain fatty acid; SHBG: Sex hormone-binding globulin; T2DM: Type 2 diabetes mellitus; TAC: Total antioxidant capacity

Acknowledgements

The present study was supported by a grant from the Vice-chancellor for Research, AUMS, Arak, and Iran.

Funding

The research grant provided by Research Deputy of Arak University of Medical Sciences (AUMS).

Authors' contributions

ZA contributed in conception, design, statistical analysis and drafting of the manuscript. KhN, MJ, ER, FB and MT-E contributed in data collection and manuscript drafting. All authors approved the final version for submission. ZA supervised the study.

Competing interests

The authors declare that they have no competing interests.

Author details

[1]Endocrinology and Metabolism Research Center, Arak University of Medical Sciences, Arak, Iran. [2]Research Center for Biochemistry and Nutrition in Metabolic Diseases, Kashan University of Medical Sciences, Kashan, IR, Iran. [3]Faculty member of Science department, Science Faculty, Islamic Azad University, Tehran Central Branch, Tehran, Iran.

References

1. Clark NM, Podolski AJ, Brooks ED, et al. Prevalence of polycystic ovary syndrome phenotypes using updated criteria for polycystic ovarian morphology: an assessment of over 100 consecutive women self-reporting features of polycystic ovary syndrome. Reprod Sci. 2014;21:1034–43.
2. Duleba AJ, Dokras A. Is PCOS an inflammatory process? Fertil Steril. 2012;97:7–12.
3. Boots CE, Jungheim ES. Inflammation and human ovarian follicular dynamics. Semin Reprod Med. 2015;33:270–5.
4. Akram Kooshki A, Tofighiyan T, Rakhshani MH. Effects of Synbiotics on inflammatory markers in patients with type 2 diabetes mellitus. Glob J Health Sci. 2015;7:1–5.
5. Ahmadi S, Jamilian M, Tajabadi-Ebrahimi M, et al. The effects of synbiotic supplementation on markers of insulin metabolism and lipid profiles in gestational diabetes: a randomised, double-blind, placebo-controlled trial. Br J Nutr. 2016;116:1394–401.
6. Saez-Lara MJ, Robles-Sanchez C, Ruiz-Ojeda FJ, et al. Effects of probiotics and Synbiotics on obesity, insulin resistance syndrome, type 2 diabetes and non-alcoholic fatty liver disease: a review of human clinical trials. Int J Mol Sci. 2016;17:928.
7. Tanaka K, Yano M, Motoori M, et al. Impact of perioperative administration of synbiotics in patients with esophageal cancer undergoing

esophagectomy: a prospective randomized controlled trial. Surgery. 2012; 152:832–42.

8. Cani PD, Delzenne NM. Involvement of the gut microbiota in the development of low grade inflammation associated with obesity: focus on this neglected partner. Acta Gastroenterol Belg. 2010;73:267–9.

9. Bahmani F, Tajadadi-Ebrahimi M, Kolahdooz F, et al. The consumption of synbiotic bread containing lactobacillus sporogenes and inulin affects nitric oxide and malondialdehyde in patients with type 2 diabetes mellitus: randomized, double-blind, placebo-controlled trial. J Am Coll Nutr. 2016;35: 506–13.

10. Ipar N, Aydogdu SD, Yildirim GK, et al. Effects of synbiotic on anthropometry, lipid profile and oxidative stress in obese children. Benef Microbes. 2015;6:775–82.

11. Lamprecht M, Bogner S, Schippinger G, et al. Probiotic supplementation affects markers of intestinal barrier, oxidation, and inflammation in trained men; a randomized, double-blinded, placebo-controlled trial. J Int Soc Sports Nutr. 2012;9:45.

12. Voltolini C, Battersby S, Etherington SL, et al. A novel antiinflammatory role for the short-chain fatty acids in human labor. Endocrinology. 2012; 153:395–403.

13. Matthews GM, Howarth GS, Butler RN. Short-chain fatty acid modulation of apoptosis in the Kato III human gastric carcinoma cell line. Cancer Biol Ther. 2007;6(7):1051.

14. Rotterdam ESHRE. ASRM-sponsored PCOS consensus workshop group. Revised 2003 consensus on diagnostic criteria and long-term health risks related to polycystic ovary syndrome. Fertil Steril. 2004;81:19–25.

15. Huang A, Brennan K, Azziz R. Prevalence of hyperandrogenemia in the polycystic ovary syndrome diagnosed by the National Institutes of Health 1990 criteria. Fertil Steril. 2010;93:1938–41.

16. Ahmadi S, Jamilian M, Karamali M, et al. Probiotic supplementation and the effects on weight loss, glycaemia and lipid profiles in women with polycystic ovary syndrome: a randomized, double-blind, placebo-controlled trial. Hum Fertil (Camb). 2017;20:254–61.

17. Asemi Z, Jamilian M, Mesdaghinia E, et al. Effects of selenium supplementation on glucose homeostasis, inflammation, and oxidative stress in gestational diabetes: randomized, double-blind, placebo-controlled trial. Nutrition. 2015;31:1235–42.

18. Hatch R, Rosenfield RL, Kim MH, et al. Hirsutism: implications, etiology, and management. Am J Obstet Gynecol. 1981;140:815–30.

19. Tatsch E, Bochi GV, Pereira Rda S, et al. A simple and inexpensive automated technique for measurement of serum nitrite/nitrate. Clin Biochem. 2011;44:348–50.

20. Benzie IF, Strain JJ. The ferric reducing ability of plasma (FRAP) as a measure of "antioxidant power": the FRAP assay. Anal Biochem. 1996;239:70–6.

21. Beutler E, Gelbart T. Plasma glutathione in health and in patients with malignant disease. J Lab Clin Med. 1985;105:581–4.

22. Janero DR. Malondialdehyde and thiobarbituric acid-reactivity as diagnostic indices of lipid peroxidation and peroxidative tissue injury. Free Radic Biol Med. 1990;9:515–40.

23. Pisprasert V, Ingram KH, Lopez-Davila MF, et al. Limitations in the use of indices using glucose and insulin levels to predict insulin sensitivity: impact of race and gender and superiority of the indices derived from oral glucose tolerance test in African Americans. Diabetes Care. 2013;36:845–53.

24. Asemi Z, Khorrami-Rad A, Alizadeh SA, et al. Effects of synbiotic food consumption on metabolic status of diabetic patients: a double-blind randomized cross-over controlled clinical trial. Clin Nutr. 2014;33:198–203.

25. Asemi Z, Foroozanfard F, Hashemi T, et al. Calcium plus vitamin D supplementation affects glucose metabolism and lipid concentrations in overweight and obese vitamin D deficient women with polycystic ovary syndrome. Clin Nutr. 2015;34:586–92.

26. Foroozanfard F, Jamilian M, Bahmani F, et al. Calcium plus vitamin D supplementation influences biomarkers of inflammation and oxidative stress in overweight and vitamin D-deficient women with polycystic ovary syndrome: a randomized double-blind placebo-controlled clinical trial. Clin Endocrinol. 2015;83:888–94.

27. Shoaei T, Heidari-Beni M, Tehrani HG. Effects of probiotic supplementation on pancreatic β-cell function and c-reactive protein in women with polycystic ovary syndrome: a randomized double-blind placebo-controlled clinical trial. International journal of preventive medicine. 2015;6:27.

28. Eslamparast T, Zamani F, Hekmatdoost A, et al. Effects of synbiotic supplementation on insulin resistance in subjects with the metabolic syndrome: a randomised, double-blind, placebo-controlled pilot study. Br J Nutr. 2014;112:438–45.

29. Moroti C, Souza Magri LF, de Rezende Costa M, et al. Effect of the consumption of a new symbiotic shake on glycemia and cholesterol levels in elderly people with type 2 diabetes mellitus. Lipids Health Dis. 2012;11:29.

30. De Leo V, Musacchio MC, Cappelli V, et al. Genetic, hormonal and metabolic aspects of PCOS: an update. Reprod Biol Endocrinol. 2016;14:38.

31. Walters KA, Allan CM, Handelsman DJ. Androgen actions and the ovary. Biol Reprod. 2008;78:380–9.

32. Azzolin GC, Saiduddin S. Effect of androgens on the ovarian morphology of the hypophysectomized rat. Proc Soc Exp Biol Med. 1983;172:70–3.

33. Gonzalez F, Sia CL, Bearson DM, et al. Hyperandrogenism induces a proinflammatory TNFalpha response to glucose ingestion in a receptor-dependent fashion. J Clin Endocrinol Metab. 2014;99:E848–54.

34. Compare D, Coccoli P, Rocco A, et al. Gut–liver axis: the impact of gut microbiota on non alcoholic fatty liver disease. Nutr Metab Cardiovasc Dis. 2012;22(6):471.

35. Li Z, Yang S, Lin H, et al. Probiotics and antibodies to TNF inhibit inflammatory activity and improve nonalcoholic fatty liver disease. Hepatology. 2003;37:343–50.

36. Eslamparast T, Poustchi H, Zamani F, et al. Synbiotic supplementation in nonalcoholic fatty liver disease: a randomized, double-blind, placebo-controlled pilot study. Am J Clin Nutr. 2014;99:535–42.

37. Asemi Z, Jazayeri S, Najafi M, et al. Effect of daily consumption of probiotic yogurt on oxidative stress in pregnant women: a randomized controlled clinical trial. Ann Nutr Metab. 2012;60:62–8.

38. Zamani B, Golkar HR, Farshbaf S, et al. Clinical and metabolic response to probiotic supplementation in patients with rheumatoid arthritis: a randomized, double-blind, placebo-controlled trial. Int J Rheum Dis. 2016;19:869–79.

39. Cheng CP, Tsai SW, Chiu CP, et al. The effect of probiotic-fermented soy milk on enhancing the NO-mediated vascular relaxation factors. J Sci Food Agric. 2013;93:1219–25.

40. Ghoneim MA, Moselhy SS. Antioxidant status and hormonal profile reflected by experimental feeding of probiotics. Toxicol Ind Health. 2016;32:741–50.

41. Holma R, Kekkonen RA, Hatakka K, et al. Low serum enterolactone concentration is associated with low colonic lactobacillus-enterococcus counts in men but is not affected by a synbiotic mixture in a randomised, placebo-controlled, double-blind, cross-over intervention study. Br J Nutr. 2014;111:301–9.

42. Khani S, Motamedifar M, Golmoghaddam H, et al. In vitro study of the effect of a probiotic bacterium lactobacillus rhamnosus against herpes simplex virus type 1. Braz J Infect Dis. 2012;16:129–35.

43. Ebrahimi-Mameghani M, Sanaie S, Mahmoodpoor A, et al. Effect of a probiotic preparation (VSL#3) in critically ill patients: a randomized, double-blind, placebo-controlled trial (pilot study). Pak J Med Sci. 2013;29:490–4.

44. Pawelczak M, Rosenthal J, Milla S, et al. Evaluation of the pro-inflammatory cytokine tumor necrosis factor-alpha in adolescents with polycystic ovary syndrome. J Pediatr Adolesc Gynecol. 2014;27:356–9.

45. Valmadrid CT, Klein R, Moss SE, et al. The risk of cardiovascular disease mortality associated with microalbuminuria and gross proteinuria in persons with older-onset diabetes mellitus. Arch Intern Med. 2000;160:1093–100.

46. Filippone EJ, Gupta A, Farber JL. Normoglycemic diabetic nephropathy: the role of insulin resistance. Case Rep Nephrol Urol. 2014;4:137–43.

47. Lu HJ, Tzeng TF, Liou SS, et al. Polysaccharides from Liriopes Radix ameliorate streptozotocin-induced type I diabetic nephropathy via regulating NF-kappaB and p38 MAPK signaling pathways. BMC Complement Altern Med. 2014;14:156.

48. Kalina U, Koyama N, Hosoda T, et al. Enhanced production of IL-18 in butyrate-treated intestinal epithelium by stimulation of the proximal promoter region. Eur J Immunol. 2002;32:2635–43.

49. Vitali B, Ndagijimana M, Cruciani F, et al. Impact of a synbiotic food on the gut microbial ecology and metabolic profiles. BMC Microbiol. 2010;10:4.

50. Komers R, Anderson S. Paradoxes of nitric oxide in the diabetic kidney. Am J Physiol Renal Physiol. 2003;284:F1121–37.

51. Szkudelski T. The mechanism of alloxan and streptozotocin action in B cells of the rat pancreas. Physiol Res. 2001;50:537–46.

52. Shakeri H, Hadaegh H, Abedi F, et al. Consumption of synbiotic bread decreases triacylglycerol and VLDL levels while increasing HDL levels in serum from patients with type-2 diabetes. Lipids. 2014;49:695–701.

6

Stem cells and beta cell replacement therapy: a prospective health technology assessment study

Klemens Wallner[1]*[ID], Rene G. Pedroza[2], Isaac Awotwe[1], James M. Piret[2], Peter A. Senior[3,4], A. M. James Shapiro[3,4,5] and Christopher McCabe[1]

Abstract

Background: Although current beta cell replacement therapy is effective in stabilizing glycemic control in highly selected patients with refractory type 1 diabetes, many hurdles are inherent to this and other donor-based transplantation methods. One solution could be moving to stem cell-derived transplant tissue. This study investigates a novel stem cell-derived graft and implant technology and explores the circumstances of its cost-effectiveness compared to intensive insulin therapy.

Methods: We used a manufacturing optimization model based on work by Simaria et al. to model cost of the stem cell-based transplant doses and integrated its results into a cost-effectiveness model of diabetes treatments. The disease model simulated marginal differences in clinical effects and costs between the new technology and our comparator intensive insulin therapy. The form of beta cell replacement therapy was as a series of retrievable subcutaneous implant devices which protect the enclosed pancreatic progenitors cells from the immune system. This approach was presumed to be as effective as state of the art islet transplantation, aside from immunosuppression drawbacks. We investigated two different cell culture methods and several production and delivery scenarios.

Results: We found the likely range of treatment costs for this form of graft tissue for beta cell replacement therapy. Additionally our results show this technology could be cost-effective compared to intensive insulin therapy, at a willingness-to-pay threshold of $100,000 per quality-adjusted life year. However, results also indicate that mass production has by far the best chance of providing affordable graft tissue, while overall there seems to be considerable room for cost reductions.

Conclusions: Such a technology can improve treatment access and quality of life for patients through increased graft supply and protection. Stem cell-based implants can be a feasible way of treating a wide range of patients with type 1 diabetes.

Keywords: Type 1 diabetes, Stem cells, Medical device, Transplantation, Disease simulation, Cost optimization, Cost modeling, Health technology assessment, Early technology assessment, Health economics

Background

Although islet cell transplantation is effective for treating certain type 1 diabetes patients, some hurdles are inherent to this and other donor-based transplantation methods [1–4]. Two hurdles are the limited graft supply and graft rejection. One solution for islet cell transplantation could

be to move from donor-harvested to stem cell-derived transplant tissue. That could involve production of pancreatic progenitor cells from human embryonic stem (hES) cells. Using stem cells in general may have some advantages compared to current islet cell transplantation. These advantages include the potential of producing stem cells in large quantities thereby eliminating the cell supply problem and possibly reducing the treatment cost per patient.

Research in that area of treatment has advanced from proof-of-principle studies in animals, to establishing

* Correspondence: wallner@ualberta.ca
[1]Department of Emergency Medicine Research Group, Department of Emergency Medicine, University of Alberta, 8303 - 112 Street, Edmonton, AB T6G 2T4, Canada
Full list of author information is available at the end of the article

controllable cell manufacturing processes, and the first clinical trials in humans [5–15]. As of 2017 clinical trials are ongoing in Canada and the United States that use a thin removable device which is implanted under the skin [7, 16]. This device has hES cell-derived pancreatic progenitor cells within a casing to shield the tissue from the immune system [15]. Those cells are expected to mature to functional endocrine cells which secrete insulin in a glucose-dependent manner [9, 14–16]. Further improvement in protection of transplant tissue could increase its viability and reduce graft rejection. The long term goal of research into beta cell replacement therapy is to reverse diabetes and completely avoid the need for immunosuppressive medication.

In 2011 Weir et al. mention, "due to the need for beta cell replacement therapy, much work has been done in the past decade to generate beta cells from a variety of cell sources" [13]. However, these efforts have had mixed success. A major barrier has been in the ability to direct cell lines to differentiate towards an endocrine lineage. That process was very inefficient and most cell lines could not be used. Further, technologies used in the preservation of graftable cells, for example through cooling to very low temperatures, have advanced considerably but are still difficult and costly [17, 18]. Use of simpler preservation technologies makes cell tissue more perishable but experiences in standard donor-derived transplantation may point towards greater affordability of such techniques. Still, those barriers add to existing complexities associated with supply logistics, regulatory frameworks and scaling out production to multiple cell manufacturing sites [19].

Given those developments and findings, stem cell-based beta cell replacement therapy is a case study for the necessity of prioritizing research resources when researching new healthcare technologies. In our study we aimed to explore the circumstances under which a stem cell-based graft tissue would be cost-effective, given its effectiveness is comparable to state of the art islet transplantation aside from immunosuppression drawbacks. Our core question is if and how such a new transplant option for beta cell replacement has a chance of being cost-effective.

Methods

To model the cost of hES cell-derived transplant doses we used a two part cost-effectiveness and manufacturing model (Fig. 1). This stochastic model is based on a previous treatment model of type 1 diabetes [20] and the work by Simaria and colleagues [21]. Presuming equal effectiveness with the current technology islet transplantation, aside from the immunosuppression drawbacks, we then ran the model to simulate marginal differences in clinical effects and costs, between the new

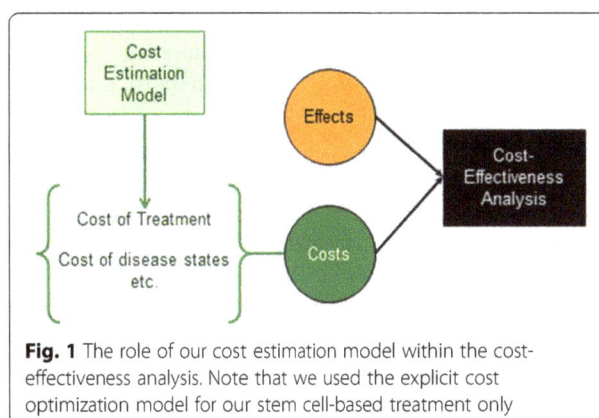

Fig. 1 The role of our cost estimation model within the cost-effectiveness analysis. Note that we used the explicit cost optimization model for our stem cell-based treatment only

stem cell-based technology and our comparator intensive insulin therapy. We used the models outputs to estimate the cost-effectiveness of this trial-stage therapy.

Compared treatments

The form of beta cell replacement therapy was modeled as a series of identical re-extractable subcutaneous implant devices ('sheets'). Each of these devices contain hES-derived cells, specifically pancreatic progenitors which were modified to attain the function of beta cells. Those cells are enclosed within a casing which shields them from the immune system but allows the transport of nutrients to and hormones from the encapsulated cells [14, 15]. In our study we make the important assumption that this shielding effect completely removes the need for immunosuppressive medication. Patients in our study can get up to four transplantations [20]. The average proportion of patients with full graft function after each transplantation was assumed to be increasing from first to third and fourth transplantation, i.e. from 15% to 70% and then 85% for the third and fourth ones [20].

The comparator treatment is intensive insulin therapy involves frequent self-monitoring of blood glucose and multiple daily insulin injections, further details are described elsewhere [20].

Cost-effectiveness analysis

We conducted a probabilistic and structural sensitivity analysis to investigate the cost-effectiveness of stem cell-based beta cell replacement therapy and to evaluate uncertainty around our results. Our simulation model was a discrete state-transition Markov model, which had a lifetime horizon. Its hypothetical cohort was composed of type 1 diabetes patients with hypoglycemia unawareness in the province of Alberta who fulfill the inclusion criteria to get an islet transplant. The model took the perspective of the provincial healthcare provider and its inputs were the same as in the pre-existing cost-effectiveness model

[20], except for the described variations. Effectiveness was expressed in quality-adjusted life-years (QALYs) to measure the impact of therapy on both quality of life and life expectancy. All monetary estimates are expressed in 2016 Canadian dollars, with necessary adjustments made using the Canadian consumer price index for health and personal care [22, 23].

We updated model parameters from our pre-existing model of unstable type 1 diabetes [20] as described below. We model a future technology functioning without the need of immunosuppression. Therefore we had to change the parameters that – even partially - had to do with this medication. For that we removed all disutilities, costs and probabilities that had only to do with immunosuppression. The parameters for rate, costs and disutility of initial complications were adjusted by lowering each by 40% because this portion was attributed solely to immunosuppression. Specifically the rate changed from 0.65 to 0.39, the cost from $600 to $360, and the disutility from 0.05 to 0.03. Further, a study of the impact of type 1 diabetes complications ($N = 2341$) served us to update our utility i.e. quality of life estimates [24]. Patients in that study were more comparable to our hypothetical cohort than the ones in our original. data sources. Yet they were still younger (39.3 vs. 47.0 years old) and with shorter diabetes duration (16.3 vs. 29.4 years) [20, 24]. Given that new evidence, we included neuropathy in the diabetes-related complications and adjusted our overall estimate for the complications state not only for multiple complications, but also to fit the actual age and duration of diabetes in our cohort [2, 24–29]. The utility parameter in the complications state was therefore adjusted from 0.57 to 0.47.

The cost-effectiveness model was constructed and run with the software TreeAge Pro 2016 (Williamstown, MA, USA). The cost of goods modeling was constructed and run using Microsoft Excel. Costs and benefits were discounted at 3%, and sensitivity analysis were performed at 0% and 5%. These were the rates that had been recommended by the Canadian Agency for Drugs and Technologies in Health [30]. Half-cycle correction was applied. Our probabilistic analyses used 64,000 iterations for each scenario. We estimated the value of further research reducing the decision uncertainty by way of value-of-information analysis [31, 32]. We calculated the expected value of perfect information (EVPI) and the expected value of partial perfect information (EVPPI) for the cost of goods group of parameters. For that EVPPI calculation we used nested Monte Carlo simulations with 600 'outer' and 600 'inner' loops. Additional information on our value of information approach, including choice of WTP thresholds, can be found elsewhere [20].

Integration of cost of goods results

To integrate the results of the cost of goods modeling into our cost-effectiveness model, we took the parameter representing the cost per transplantation within the transplant state in the original model, and split it up into non-dose costs and dose costs. Based on literature we assumed the non-dose costs, including the transplant procedure, to be about 38% of the costs per transplantation [33]. For that parameter of our model we used a Gamma distribution with a relative standard deviation of 10% (i.e. standard deviation as percentage of the mean). For the dose costs, based on our cost of goods (COG) model we used the following equation:

$$Dose\ costs = \mathrm{COG}_{upstream} \times \mathrm{factor}_{COG\ downstream} \\ \times \mathrm{factor}_{additional\ regulation} \qquad (1)$$

Here dose costs are calculated multiplying the cost of goods upstream by a cost of goods downstream factor and a factor that we called "regulatory burden factor". The cost of goods upstream came from the above described fitted distributions estimating the "pure" production cost of the cells. The downstream factor accounted for the so-called downstream processing, which is necessary after the cells are produced, e.g. cell harvesting, volume reduction, washing, formulation for storage or delivery (see Fig. 2). We used the regulatory burden factor to account for the possibility of additional regulatory burden due to stricter regulatory requirements for a new cell production process whose product is designed to enter regular healthcare practice.

The mean of the cost of goods downstream factor (multiplier) was assumed to be three, four and eight, depending on scenario, based on expert opinion and published literature [34]. The mean of the regulatory burden factor was assumed to be 1.2 and 1.8 depending on scenario (i.e. 20% and 80% additional costs respectively due to regulation). Both multipliers were made probabilistic using a Log-normal distribution and expert opinion on variation estimates.

Cost of goods modeling

We modeled the cost of goods in Microsoft Excel based on a report describing manufacture of pancreatic progenitors from single cell cultures of hES cells [6]. Briefly, the modeled process consisted of thawing one or more frozen hES cells vials and expanding them in adherent culture for about 14 days, passaging four times. Then, hES cells were cultured in suspension forming cell clusters, while a cocktail of molecular signals was added to the media to promote stepwise differentiation of hES cells into pancreatic progenitors.

The cost of goods was estimated by adapting a cost minimization decisional tool for this manufacturing

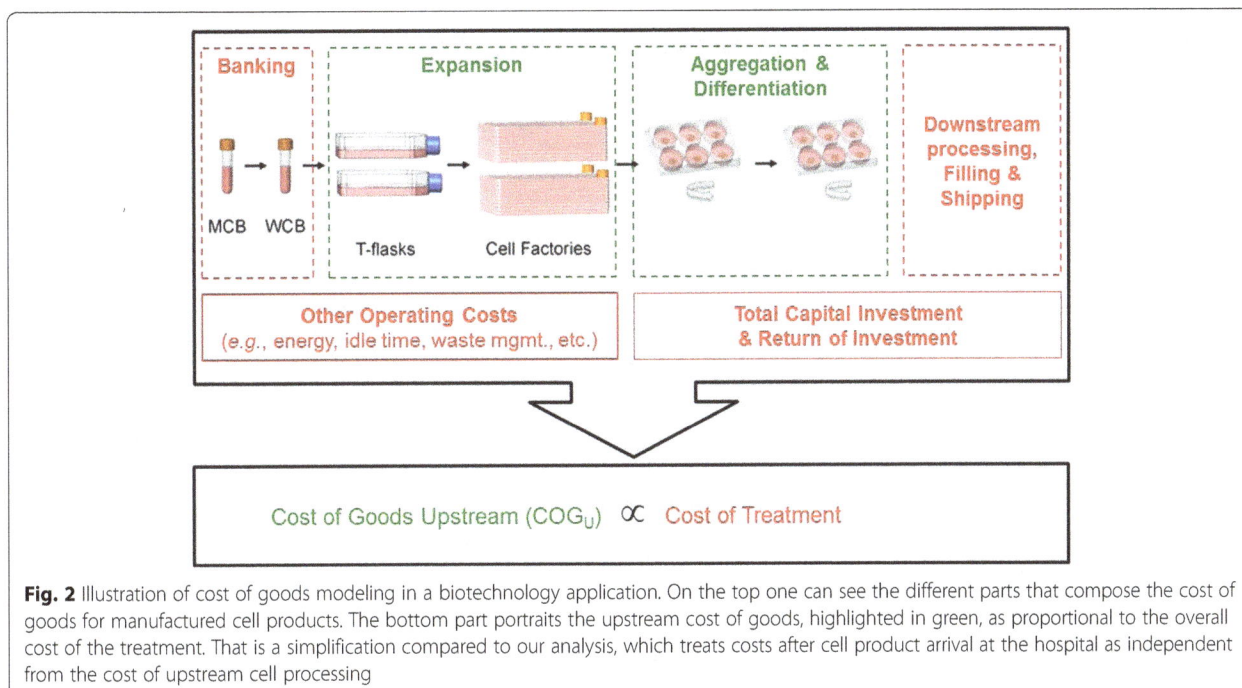

Fig. 2 Illustration of cost of goods modeling in a biotechnology application. On the top one can see the different parts that compose the cost of goods for manufactured cell products. The bottom part portraits the upstream cost of goods, highlighted in green, as proportional to the overall cost of the treatment. That is a simplification compared to our analysis, which treats costs after cell product arrival at the hospital as independent from the cost of upstream cell processing

process [21]. The tool selected the optimal set of disposable culture vessels for a user-specified annual demand, lot size, cell dose and user-specified manufacturing constraints, i.e. maximum allowed number of culture vessels per lot, which was set to 100. In its estimation process, the tool calculated the material (i.e. media, disposable culture vessels), labor, quality control and equipment costs involved in the expansion and differentiation stages of the process for a battery of sequential culture vessel combinations (see Fig. 2). Additional parameters utilized during the cost calculations were the overall yield of the manufacturing process and the expansion fold of the hES cells. In that way the upstream cost of goods were estimated.

The cost minimization decisional tool did not include the downstream component of the manufacturing process (e.g., finishing, packaging, shipping), therefore 95% credible ranges were derived for cost estimates in four different settings: two cell culture methods (adherent and suspension), and each with two supply levels (50 and 500 doses per year) (also see Table 1). The credible ranges were used to fit Gamma distributions, i.e. the lower and upper bounds of the credible ranges for every cost estimate were equated to the values of cumulative density functions (CDF) at values of CDF = 0.025 and CDF = 0.975. The distributions were then used directly in the health economic modeling software.

Scale of manufacturing

We simulated four manufacturing modes: local production (e.g. at one University only), large scale production (one central lab produces all the doses and then ships them to the hospitals), and two scale-out production modes (local and large scale). The scale-out scenarios involved a network of several labs producing their own doses at their respective location but collaborating with each other through sharing expertise and research resources. We simulated one scale-out scenario for local productions and one for large scale productions. The local and large scale production scenarios assume a demand of 50 and 500 doses per year respectively. In general, the scale out approach may engage the capabilities of multiple local institutions and companies. It could, however, also contribute to unequal product quality and an increased overhead costs.

We estimated the long-term capacity to perform device implants in Canada to be 10 clinical centers. That estimate was derived by counting the hospitals on the list of transplant centers by the Canadian Organ Replacement Register in which clinicians performed islet cell transplants or other transplants of at least three different kinds of organs [35, 36]. We took this as clinical capacity to carry out transplantations of beta cell replacement devices that *do not* require immunosuppression. In the short term there could be two centers, one for Western Canada and one Eastern Canada.

We describe the demand for and composition of the doses of beta cell replacement tissue as follows. The annual demand of beta cell replacement doses was based on the current number of islet cell transplants in Canada and assumed to be 50 per transplant center, which was derived as linear extrapolation of transplant numbers in at the

Table 1 Credible ranges and fitted distributions for cost of goods upstream

Production setting		Range		Gamma distribution			
Cell culture	Supply	Lower bound	Upper bound	Mean	RSD	Shape	Rate
Adherent	50	$21,300	$83,900	$47,443	34.00%	8.6505	0.0001823
Adherent	500	$14,700	$73,800	$38,585	39.60%	6.3769	0.0001653
Suspension	50	$16,900	$54,900	$33,193	29.42%	11.5535	0.0003481
Suspension	500	$10,300	$53,100	$27,535	40.20%	6.1880	0.0002247

University of Alberta Hospital. Further we presumed the number of lots produced per year is 10, i.e. about one per month, and a minimum of 500 million cells are required per dose. Those numbers were derived from considerations of cell quality loss over time and the production figures above. Based on experience in the biotechnology sector the production assumed one of two production technologies, adherent or suspension cell culture approach, each with optimized production set ups for the two demand options (50 or 500 doses per year).

As a substantial simplification due to the novelty of the membrane technology, we presumed the cost of the device casing without the cells is off-set by reductions in costs through increased ability to plan transplantation times and processes.

Results

Our analysis shows that the use of stem cells for beta cell replacement therapy can be an effective use of health budget funds. However, there is substantial uncertainty around the costs of this technology. We calculated the expected range of treatment costs for hES cell-based beta cell tissue. Our probabilistic results indicate that currently this technology could be cost-effective at a WTP threshold of $100,000 per QALY because three scenarios have ICERs substantially below that threshold (Tables 2 and 3). Specifically the ICERs of scenarios Adh20, Sus19 and Sus20 are $79,230, $89,173 and $60,111 per QALY respectivly. For the 95% Confidence interval values around our results please see in Additional file 1.

However, the results also indicate that large-scale production has the best chance of providing affordable graft tissue, as can be seen in scenarios ADh15, Adh16 and Adh20 in Table 2. These scenarios have the highest value for money for this method of cell culture. That means that for a given patient benefit the costs are minimized. For the suspension cell cultures the same scenarios also had the lowest ICERs (see scenarios Sus15, Sus16 and Sus20 in Table 3).

With adherent cell culture all scenarios have ICERs higher than $100,000 except scenario 'Adh20', which has a 0% discount rate and a supply of 500 doses per year. On the other side all suspension cell culture scenarios also have ICERs higher than $100,000 except for the scenarios 'Sus19' and 'Sus20', both use a 0% discount rate. Such a low discount rate does value small benefits with a long duration more favorable than a higher discount rate would.

Our finding that use of stem cells for beta cell replacement therapy can be an effective use of health budget funds can be confirmed by the value of information results. The value of information can be seen as both a measure of decision uncertainty as well as an indicator of research investment value [31, 32]. In Fig. 3 we show the expected value of research into the cost-effectiveness of the technologies under consideration. One can see all per-patient EVPI values do peak at high cost-effectiveness thresholds but there also is considerable value when using for instance a $50,000 threshold. That means that further research into the cost-effectiveness of this treatment can be worthwhile for Alberta up to these upper limits per patient, even if one uses a strict cost-effectiveness threshold of $50,000.

We found uncertainty around the mean outcomes and therefore the need to conduct further research in this kind of disease treatment. This becomes clear when we consider the results in Fig. 3 and the number of patients that could benefit. In Alberta alone there are more than 4000 patients with unstable type 1 diabetes [37–42]. Extrapolating this estimate, one can expect to have about 500,000 patients in North America [37–43]. When comparing those figures with the per patient values in Fig. 3, one can argue that further research in this area of technology can be a sound investment of health budget funds.

We report the treatment dose costs with the production settings we used for a set of example regulatory and cost of goods downstream factors (Table 4). In this comparison one can see the adherent cell culture with 50 dose per year setting has on average no chance of being cost effective because its mean is much higher than any of the maximum costs. The 'adherent 500' setting can only be cost effective with a 1% (or lower) discount rate, without immunosuppression and only at a less strict threshold of $100,000. At that threshold and discount rate both the suspension cell culture settings can be cost effective without immunosuppression.

Table 2 Results for different scenarios using adherent cell culture (means per patient)

Scenario Index	Production mode	Supply per facility	COGd factor	Regulatory factor	Variation (RSD[a])	Cost Strategy	Cost Difference	Benefit Strategy	Benefit Difference	ICER	EVPI WTP per QALY $50,000	EVPI WTP per QALY $100,000	Maximum Partial EVPI Dose Costs
Scenarios with 3% discount rate													
Comp1 (Comparator 3%)						74,230		11.12					
Adh1	Local	50	4	1.2	22.5%	629,181	554,951	13.85	2.73	203,203	18	4220	90,957
Adh2	Local	50	4	1.2	50.0%	628,936	554,707	13.85	2.73	203,114	677	19,749	135,128
Adh3	Local	50	4	1.8	22.5%	876,810	802,580	13.85	2.73	293,877	2	721	143,704
Adh4	Local	50	4	1.8	50.0%	873,510	799,281	13.85	2.73	292,669	169	8061	214,930
Adh5	Scale out local	50	3	1.2	22.5%	504,903	430,673	13.85	2.73	157,697	87	11,725	69,691
Adh6	Scale out local	50	3	1.2	50.0%	504,835	430,606	13.85	2.73	157,673	1493	32,911	106,144
Adh7	Scale out local	50	3	1.8	22.5%	690,050	615,819	13.85	2.73	225,492	11	2623	102,737
Adh8	Scale out local	50	3	1.8	50.0%	688,524	614,294	13.85	2.73	224,933	432	15,297	167,801
Adh9	Scale out local	50	8	1.8	22.5%	1,616,386	1,542,156	13.85	2.73	564,685	0	19	273,576
Adh10	Scale out local	50	8	1.8	50.0%	1,606,953	1,532,722	13.85	2.73	561,231	9	1052	443,892
Adh11	Large scale	500	4	1.2	22.5%	536,915	462,685	13.85	2.73	169,420	127	11,621	78,153
Adh12	Large scale	500	4	1.2	50.0%	536,730	462,501	13.85	2.73	169,351	1501	31,043	124,247
Adh13	Large scale	500	4	1.8	22.5%	738,478	664,248	13.85	2.73	243,225	24	3085	117,352
Adh14	Large scale	500	4	1.8	50.0%	736,541	662,311	13.85	2.73	242,516	499	14,700	192,416
Adh15	Scale out large	500	3	1.2	22.5%	435,777	361,548	13.85	2.73	132,386	453	24,792	63,732
Adh16	Scale out large	500	3	1.2	50.0%	435,661	361,432	13.85	2.73	132,344	3005	47,591	96,481
Adh17	Scale out large	500	3	1.8	22.5%	586,704	512,474	13.85	2.73	187,650	82	8143	93,084
Adh18	Scale out large	500	3	1.8	50.0%	585,166	510,936	13.85	2.73	187,088	1118	25,291	148,572
Scenarios with 0% discount rate													
Comp2 (Comparator 0%)						113,175		16.09					
Adh19	Local	50	4	1.2	22.5%	663,514	550,339	20.60	4.51	122,159	1395	52,620	90,906
Adh20	Scale out large	500	3	1.2	22.5%	470,111	356,936	20.60	4.51	79,230	11,315	30,540	63,752
Scenarios with 5% discount rate													
Comp3 (Comparator 5%)						58,559		9.09					
Adh21	Local	50	4	1.2	22.5%	616,693	558,134	11.18	2.09	267,339	0	614	90,973
Adh22	Scale out large	500	3	1.2	22.5%	423,290	364,731	11.18	2.09	174,701	32	6396	63,730

All scenarios used the base case assumptions with the described structural deviations. Cost measure is Canadian dollar (2016). Benefit measure is QALY. All result numbers are rounded and including sampling variation
[a]Relative standard deviation (RSD; i.e. SD as percentage of the mean) that was assumed for the two factors

Table 3 Results for different scenarios using suspension cell culture (means per patient)

Scenario Index	Production mode	Supply per facility	COGd factor	Regulatory factor	Variation (RSD[a])	Cost Strategy	Cost Difference	Benefit Strategy	Benefit Difference	ICER	EVPI WTP per QALY $50,000	EVPI WTP per QALY $100,000	Maximum Partial EVPI Dose Costs
Scenarios with 3% discount rate													
Comp1	(Comparator 3%)					74,230		11.12					
Sus1	Local	50	4	1.2	22.5%	480,575	406,346	13.85	2.73	148,790	56	12,126	59,158
Sus2	Local	50	4	1.2	50.0%	479,911	405,680	13.85	2.73	148,546	1541	35,232	92,836
Sus3	Local	50	4	1.8	22.5%	654,137	579,906	13.85	2.73	212,342	4	2464	88,524
Sus4	Local	50	4	1.8	50.0%	651,401	577,171	13.85	2.73	211,340	450	16,335	141,768
Sus5	Scale out local	50	3	1.2	22.5%	393,796	319,566	13.85	2.73	117,014	305	28,627	47,474
Sus6	Scale out local	50	3	1.2	50.0%	393,094	318,864	13.85	2.73	116,757	3215	53,937	76,931
Sus7	Scale out local	50	3	1.8	22.5%	523,705	449,475	13.85	2.73	164,582	33	8084	66,874
Sus8	Scale out local	50	3	1.8	50.0%	521,437	447,207	13.85	2.73	163,752	1084	28,588	113,389
Sus9	Scale out local	50	8	1.8	22.5%	1,172,878	1,098,648	13.85	2.73	402,287	0	50	169,848
Sus10	Scale out local	50	8	1.8	50.0%	1,163,974	1,089,744	13.85	2.73	399,026	35	2719	295,702
Sus11	Large scale	500	4	1.2	22.5%	421,724	347,494	13.85	2.73	127,240	590	28,370	59,316
Sus12	Large scale	500	4	1.2	50.0%	420,338	346,108	13.85	2.73	126,733	3399	51,260	83,398
Sus13	Large scale	500	4	1.8	22.5%	565,342	491,112	13.85	2.73	179,828	116	9785	86,421
Sus14	Large scale	500	4	1.8	50.0%	562,360	488,130	13.85	2.73	178,736	1294	27,942	124,381
Sus15	Scale out large	500	3	1.2	22.5%	349,649	275,419	13.85	2.73	100,848	1666	43,136	47,205
Sus16	Scale out large	500	3	1.2	50.0%	349,048	274,819	13.85	2.73	100,629	6192	64,312	64,826
Sus17	Scale out large	500	3	1.8	22.5%	457,207	382,977	13.85	2.73	140,232	384	21,505	67,653
Sus18	Scale out large	500	3	1.8	50.0%	455,948	381,718	13.85	2.73	139,772	2669	43,714	101,004
Scenarios with 0% discount rate													
Comp2	(Comparator 0%)					113,175		16.09					
Sus19	Local	50	4	1.2	22.5%	514,909	401,734	20.60	4.51	89,173	4389	40,830	59,131
Sus20	Scale out large	500	3	1.2	22.5%	383,981	270,808	20.60	4.51	60,111	26,451	7684	47,205
Scenarios with 5% discount rate													
Comp3	(Comparator 5%)					56,558		9.09					
Sus21	Local	50	4	1.2	22.5%	468,087	409,529	11.18	2.09	196,160	1	2042	59,162
Sus22	Scale out large	500	3	1.2	22.5%	337,161	278,602	11.18	2.09	133,447	172	16,410	47,207

All scenarios used the base case assumptions with the described structural deviations. Cost measure is Canadian dollar (2016). Benefit measure is QALY. All result numbers are rounded and including sampling variation
[a]Relative standard deviation (RSD); i.e. SD as percentage of the mean) that was assumed for the two factors

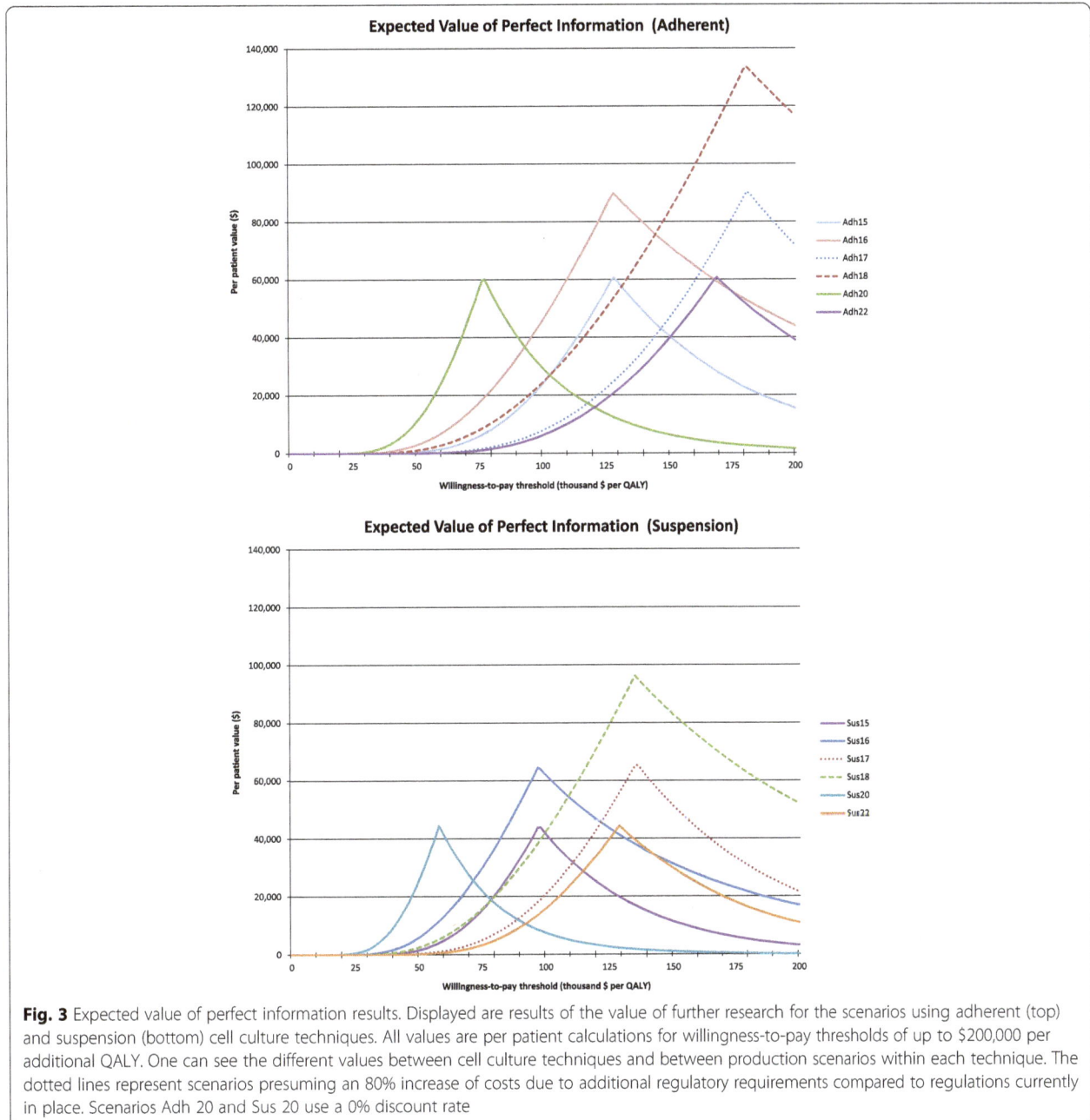

Fig. 3 Expected value of perfect information results. Displayed are results of the value of further research for the scenarios using adherent (top) and suspension (bottom) cell culture techniques. All values are per patient calculations for willingness-to-pay thresholds of up to $200,000 per additional QALY. One can see the different values between cell culture techniques and between production scenarios within each technique. The dotted lines represent scenarios presuming an 80% increase of costs due to additional regulatory requirements compared to regulations currently in place. Scenarios Adh 20 and Sus 20 use a 0% discount rate

Table 4 Full dose costs using example cost of goods downstream and regulator factors

Production setting		Factors		Full dose costs[a]		
Cell culture	Supply	Cost of goods downstream	Regulatory	Mean	Lower range	Upper range
Adherent	50	3	1.2	$170,795	$76,680	$302,040
Adherent	500	3	1.2	$138,906	$52,920	$265,680
Suspension	50	3	1.2	$119,495	$60,840	$197,640
Suspension	500	3	1.2	$99,126	$37,080	$191,160

[a]Means and values at the lower and upper 95% credible range

We report the full dose costs with the production settings we used for a set of example regulatory and cost of goods downstream factors (Table 4). In this comparison one can see that our results point towards an increased efficiency through a) high volume production, and b) use of adherent cell culture technique.

Discussion

Our results show that the use of stem cells for beta cell replacement therapy can be an effective use of health budget funds. Still, there is substantial uncertainty around the costs of this technology. Both of those findings confirm that methods of cost modeling combined with value-of-information analysis can be useful tools for aiding the prioritization. This especially applies to new healthcare technologies. Estimating the cost of transplant tissue we found it possible for the treatment to be cost-effective at commonly used cost-effectiveness thresholds if it greatly reduces the need for immunosuppression. The value of information as well as other results depend very much on the assumptions in the respective scenarios. Those assumptions include transplantations costs, especially transplant tissue cost of goods and immunosuppression, as well as discount rates.

In near future stem cell therapy could be expanded to a much broader population of type 1 diabetes patients. Currently the expansion of beta cell replacement therapy in general is limited by organ supply and risks of immunosuppression. If outcomes were better than for islet transplantation, i.e. long term euglycemia and insulin independence, the lifetime costs of conventional therapy due to management of diabetes complications would be avoided. That would include costs not considered in this analysis which would fall outside of the budget of the provincial health care service, e.g. costs covered by the federal health budget or costs for the patient's family or private insurance.

Challenges of donor-harvested transplants in Canada

Additional challenges of the donor-harvested approach in Canada could lead there to more readiness to adopt a stem cell based therapy approach even with initially higher costs. Among those challenges one needs to consider the relative shortage of organ donations, combined with great geographic distances between donors and the islet processing and transplantation site [44]. These factors can lead to two kinds of costs of timely organ transport. The monetary costs are sometimes covered by different regional health care services or air lines. Air transport companies are known to occasionally ship donor organs free of charge. Nevertheless non-monetary costs are unavoidable. An example is the cost of organ deterioration from with progressive cold ischemia can mar graft yield later on.

All those costs tend to be less for more densely populated countries, or even regions with different organ donation legislation, which can make a considerable difference in donor availability [45]. International coordination of donor organ availability could also further increase the efficient use available clinical resources. However, such coordination tends to come with substantial political and practical complexities, which require further research but are beyond the topic of this study.

On efficient treatment delivery

While high volume implant production can theoretically be cheaper one needs to weigh that with several considerations regarding demand, clinical capacity and other practical limitations. One of those considerations is that stem cell-derived doses are currently as perishable as the donor derived cells. This means they have to be used within about 12–36 h of completion of the production process.

The difference between stem cell derived tissue and harvested cells is here that one can determine the time when the tissue is ready. Instead of the cell dose coming into the hospital more or less randomly at any time of the day or night, one can time the production process so that the dose or doses arrive at the hospital at a predefined day and time of the day.

In that way one can avoid the additional costs involved in nightly or short notice transplantations. But graft doses still have to be transplanted as quickly as possible. If several doses arrive at the same time it is also the case that all need to be transplanted within a short period of time. That could be accomplished if for example every week or every month 10 doses arrive at a hospital and are then all transplanted into 10 patients within the same day.

For that reason the number of lots produced per year is important. Every time a lot is produced all the doses of the lot have to be used within about one day or else go waste. That is because currently it is not possible to preserve beta cell progenitors over long periods, e.g. via cryo-preservation. In this context, it is advantageous from an economic perspective to produce several lots per year with smaller lot sizes, since it is impossible to transplant for example 500 doses in one day – even if spread over 10 transplantation centers.

Given the nature of the cells, transporting the patients to a central location – as is done currently - might be a better idea than transporting the cells to multiple patient hospitals across Canada. That is because transport of patients may actually be more affordable than the sum of: a) the health lost through the certain quality loss in the highly perishable cells through transport duration, b) the monetary costs from transporting the cells on a punctual just-in-time basis, c) the costs of duplication of in-hospital infrastructure and staff training.

Limitations

Ongoing breakthroughs for example in current good manufacturing practice (cGMP) and mass cell expansion and limit the longevity of our estimates and modeling efforts. Breakthroughs include the genetic engineering technique CRISPR (Clustered Regularly Interspaced Short Palindromic Repeat) and the use of modern bioreactors which aid various kinds of bioprocessing [46, 47]. All those technologies have great influence on the capacities of researchers to generate new or more affordable ways of producing transplantable tissue.

We acknowledge that intensive insulin therapy as only comparator strategy to stem cell-based beta cell replacement therapy did limit the scope of our results. However, we consider the comparator and hypothetical patient cohort in our model to be appropriate because of the patient population under consideration. We explicitly limit our study population to patients who: 1) do not have the degree of major comorbidities which would justify risks of whole organ transplantation, 2) are on intensive insulin treatment and 3) are candidates for islet transplantation. Still, we think further studies in a North American context do need to include donor-base islet transplantation as one of the comparators. Other donor-based approaches to address type 1 diabetes could also be integrated.

The cost of the semi-permeable membrane in which the cells are enclosed had to be estimated doe to lack of data. This and the fact that we did not change the follow up costs and frequency compared to the study on islet transplantation are clear limitations of this study. However, in light of the technology under consideration being new and containing living cell tissue, the differences between the actual and our estimated follow-up costs are likely smaller than for a less complex implant device.

We expect that implantation would likely be an outpatient procedure with much more limited risks compared to islet transplantation, or even whole organ transplantation. In this study we presumed the new treatment technology would still be require an in-patient procedure including four days of hospital stay. Compared to that estimate, an out-patient procedure would further reduce the costs of stem cell-based beta cell replacement therapy while increasing patient quality of life.

One of the main goals of using re-extractable sheets for transplantation, instead of the standard cell injection into the liver, is to shield the cells from being attacked by the immune system. Since this is an early health technology assessment of a very new technology we made the assumption that this goal can be achieved without the use of imunosuppressive drugs. If future developments show that this is not the case then immunosuppression would be necessary and with it would come the usual costs and side effects as mentioned elsewhere [20].

Conclusions

Using new grafts substantially increased the value of research into beta cell replacement therapy, especially when also addressing the need for immunosuppression. Such a technology can improve treatment access and quality of life for patients through increased graft supply and protection. Stem cell-based implants can be a feasible way of treating a wide range of patients with type 1 diabetes.

Abbreviations
cGMP: Current good manufacturing practice; COG: Cost of goods; CRISPR: Clustered Regularly Interspaced Short Palindromic Repeat technology, a genome editing tool; EVPI: Expected value of perfect information; EVPPI: Expected value of partial perfect information; hES cells: Human embryonic stem cells; ICER: Incremental cost-effectiveness ratio; QALY: Quality-adjusted life-year; RSD: Relative standard deviation; SD: Standard deviation; Wtp: Willingness to pay per additional QALY

Acknowledgements
Not applicable.

Funding
This research was supported by grants from the Stem Cell Network, Alberta Innovates Health Solutions (Collaborative Research and Innovation Opportunities) and salary support: Endowed Chair in Emergency Medicine Research (CM), Faculty of Medicine & Dentistry at the University of Alberta (AMJS, CM, PAS), as well as the Canada Research Chairs Program (AMJS). The funders had no role in study design, data collection and analysis, decision to publish, or preparation of the manuscript.

Authors' contributions
KW and CM carried out data and cost-effectiveness and value-of-information analyses. RGP and JP performed the cost of goods analysis. KW, RGP and IA drafted the manuscript. CM, KW and RGP participated in research design. CM, KW, RGP, IA, PAS, AMJS and JP guided the framing of the research question, provided methodological and clinical insight, and supported the data collection. All authors had approval over the submitted manuscript and contributed substantially to its preparation.

Competing interests
The authors declare that they have no competing interests.

Author details
[1]Department of Emergency Medicine Research Group, Department of Emergency Medicine, University of Alberta, 8303 - 112 Street, Edmonton, AB T6G 2T4, Canada. [2]Michael Smith Laboratories and Department of Chemical & Biological Engineering, University of British Columbia, 2185 East Mall, Vancouver, BC V6T 1Z4, Canada. [3]Clinical Islet Transplant Program, Alberta Diabetes Institute, University of Alberta, 2000 College Plaza, 8215 - 112 Street, Edmonton, AB T6G 2C8, Canada. [4]Department of Medicine, University of Alberta, Edmonton, Canada. [5]Department of Surgery, University of Alberta, Edmonton, AB, Canada.

References

1. Barton FB, Rickels MR, Alejandro R, Hering BJ, Wease S, Naziruddin B, et al. Improvement in outcomes of clinical islet transplantation: 1999-2010. Diabetes Care. 2012; https://doi.org/10.2337/dc12-0063.
2. Senior PA, Kin T, Shapiro J, Koh A. Islet transplantation at the University of Alberta: status update and review of progress over the last decade. Can J Diabetes Elsevier Ltd. 2012; https://doi.org/10.1016/j.jcjd.2012.01.002.
3. Vantyghem M-C, Defrance F, Quintin D, Leroy C, Raverdi V, Prévost G, et al. Treating diabetes with islet transplantation: lessons from the past decade in Lille. Diabetes Metab. 2014; https://doi.org/10.1016/j.diabet.2013.10.003.
4. Chhabra P, Brayman KL. Overcoming barriers in clinical islet transplantation: current limitations and future prospects. Curr Probl Surg. 2014; https://doi.org/10.1067/j.cpsurg.2013.10.002.
5. Kroon E, Martinson L, Kadoya K. Pancreatic endoderm derived from human embryonic stem cells generates glucose-responsive insulin-secreting cells in vivo. Nat Biotechnol. 2008; https://doi.org/10.1038/nbt1393.
6. Schulz TC, Young HY, Agulnick AD, Babin MJ, Baetge EE, Bang AG, et al. A scalable system for production of functional pancreatic progenitors from human embryonic stem cells. PLoS One. 2012; https://doi.org/10.1371/journal.pone.0037004.
7. ClinicalTrials.gov. Identifier NCT02239354, A Safety, Tolerability, and Efficacy Study of VC-01TM Combination Product in Subjects With Type I Diabetes Mellitus. ClinicalTrials.gov. Bethesda (MD): National Library of Medicine (US), 2016.
8. Godfrey KJ, Mathew B, Bulman JC, Shah O, Clement S, Gallicano GI. Stem cell-based treatments for type 1 diabetes mellitus: bone marrow, embryonic, hepatic, pancreatic and induced pluripotent stem cells. Diabet Med. 2012; https://doi.org/10.1111/j.1464-5491.2011.03433.x.
9. Schulz TC. Enabling Technologies for Cell-Based Clinical Translation Concise Review: manufacturing of pancreatic endoderm cells for clinical trials in type 1 diabetes. Stem Cells Transl Med. 2015; https://doi.org/10.5966/sctm.2015-0058.
10. Soria B, Gauthier BR, Martín F, Tejedo JR, Bedoya FJ, Rojas A, et al. Using stem cells to produce insulin. Expert Opin Biol Ther. 2015; https://doi.org/10.1517/14712598.2015.1066330.
11. Rezania A, Bruin JE, Arora P, Rubin A, Batushansky I, Asadi A, et al. Reversal of diabetes with insulin-producing cells derived in vitro from human pluripotent stem cells. Nat Biotechnol. 2014; https://doi.org/10.1038/nbt.3033.
12. Pagliuca FW, Millman JR, Gürtler M, Segel M, Van Dervort A, Ryu JH, et al. Generation of functional human pancreatic β cells in vitro. Cell. 2014; https://doi.org/10.1016/j.cell.2014.09.040.
13. Weir GC, Cavelti-Weder C, Bonner-Weir S. Stem cell approaches for diabetes: towards beta cell replacement. Genome Med. 2011; https://doi.org/10.1186/gm277.
14. Desai T, Shea LD. Advances in islet encapsulation technologies. Nat Rev Drug Discov. 2016; https://doi.org/10.1038/nrd.2016.232.
15. Agulnick AD, Ambruzs DM, Moorman MA, Bhoumik A, Cesario RM, Payne JK, et al. Insulin-producing endocrine cells differentiated in vitro from human embryonic stem cells function in macroencapsulation devices in vivo. Stem Cells Transl Med. 2015; https://doi.org/10.5966/sctm.2015-0079.
16. Viacyte Inc. PEC-EncapTM (VC-01TM) – improving diabetes treatment. Viacyte Inc Available from: http://viacyte.com/products/pec%e2%80%90encap-vc-01. (Accessed 6 Jan 2017).
17. Lee JE, Lee DR. Human embryonic stem cells: derivation, maintenance and cryopreservation. Int J Stem Cells. 2011;4:9–17.
18. Karimi-Busheri F, Rasouli-Nia A, Weinfeld M. Key issues related to cryopreservation and storage of stem cells and cancer stem cells: protecting biological integrity. In: Karimi-Busheri F, Weinfeld M, editors. Biobanking and cryopreservation of stem cells. Cham: Springer International Publishing; 2016.
19. Hourd P, Chandra A, Medcalf N, Williams DJ. Regulatory challenges for the manufacture and scale-out of autologous cell therapies (June 30, 2014). In: The Stem Cell Research Community, editor. StemBook. StemBook, 2014.
20. Wallner K, Shapiro AMJ, Senior PA, Mccabe C. Cost effectiveness and value of information analyses of islet cell transplantation in the management of " unstable " type 1 diabetes mellitus. BMC Endocr Disord. 2016; https://doi.org/10.1186/s12902-016-0097-7.
21. Simaria AS, Hassan S, Varadaraju H, Rowley J, Warren K, Vanek P, et al. Allogeneic cell therapy bioprocess economics and optimization: single-use cell expansion technologies. Biotechnol Bioeng. 2014; https://doi.org/10.1002/bit.25008.
22. Statistics Canada. Table 326-0021 - consumer price index. Statistics Canada. Available from: http://www5.statcan.gc.ca/cansim/a26?lang=eng&retrLang=eng&id=3260021&pattern=&csid=. (Accessed 10 Jan 2017).
23. Statistics Canada. Consumer price index, by province (monthly). Statistics Canada Available from: http://www.statcan.gc.ca/tables-tableaux/sum-som/l01/cst01/cpis01a-eng.htm. (Accessed 10 Jan 2017).
24. Peasgood T, Brennan A, Mansell P, Elliott J, Basarir H, Kruger J. The impact of diabetes-related complications on preference-based measures of health-related quality of life in adults with type I diabetes. Med Decis Mak. 2016; https://doi.org/10.1177/0272989X16658660.
25. O'Reilly D, Hopkins R, Blackhouse G, Clarke P, Hux J, Guan J, et al. Development of an Ontario diabetes economic model (ODEM) and application to a multidisciplinary primary care diabetes management program. (Report prepared for the Ontario Ministry of Health and Long-term Care). Hamilton, Ontario: Program for Assessment of Technology in Health (PATH); 2006.
26. Clarke P, Gray A, Holman R. Estimating utility values for health states of type 2 diabetic patients using the EQ-5D (UKPDS 62). Med Decis Mak. 2002; https://doi.org/10.1177/0272989X0202200412.
27. Kirsch J, McGuire A. Establishing health state valuations for disease specific states: an example from heart disease. Health Econ. 2000; https://doi.org/10.1002/(SICI)1099-1050(200003)9:2<149::AID-HEC501>3.0.CO;2-N.
28. Tengs TO, Wallace A. One thousand health-related quality-of-life estimates. Med Care. 2000;38:583–637.
29. Palmer AJ, Roze S, Valentine WJ, Minshall ME, Foos V, Lurati FM, et al. The CORE diabetes model: projecting long-term clinical outcomes, costs and cost-effectiveness of interventions in diabetes mellitus (types 1 and 2) to support clinical and reimbursement decision-making. Curr Med Res Opin. 2004; https://doi.org/10.1185/030079904X1980.
30. Canadian Agency for Drugs and Technologies in Health (CADTH). Guidelines for the economic evaluation of health technologies. 3rd ed. Ottawa: Canadian Agency for Drugs and Technologies in Health; 2006.
31. Briggs A, Sculpher M, Claxton K. Decision modelling for health economic evaluation. Handbooks in health economic evaluation. 1st ed. New York and Oxford: Oxford University Press; 2006.
32. Edlin R, McCabe C, Hulme C, Hall P, Wright J. Cost effectiveness modelling for health technology assessment: a practical course. 1st ed. Heidelberg, New York, Dordrecht, London, Adis; 2015. http://www.springer.com/gp/book/9783319157436.
33. Institute of Health Economics. Islet transplantation for the treatment of type 1 diabetes. Edmonton, AB: Institute of Health Economics; 2013.
34. Hassan S, Simaria AS, Varadaraju H, Siddharth G, Warren K, Farid SS, et al. Allogeneic cell therapy bioprocess economics and optimization: downstream processing decisions. Regen Med. 2015; https://doi.org/10.2217/rme.15.75.
35. Canadian Institute for Health Information. Canadian Organ Replacement Register Annual Report: Treatment of End-Stage Organ Failure in Canada, 2003 to 2012. Canadian Organ Replacement Register Annual Report. 2014.
36. Canadian Institute for Health Information. Appendix B — Canadian Transplant Hospitals, Renal Programs and Independent Health Facilities Providing Dialysis to Chronic Renal Failure Patients as Reported to CORR. Canadian Organ Replacement Register Annual Report. 2015.
37. Daneman D. Type 1 diabetes. Lancet. 2006. https://doi.org/10.1016/S0140-6736(06)68341-4.
38. Canadian Diabetes Association. The cost of diabetes in Alberta. Canadian Diabetes Association. Available from: http://www.diabetes.ca/CDA/media/documents/publications-and-newsletters/advocacy-reports/cost-of-diabetes-in-alberta.pdf.
39. Merani S, Shapiro JAM. Current status of pancreatic islet transplantation. Clin Sci (Lond). 2006; https://doi.org/10.1042/CS20050342.
40. Cryer PE. The barrier of hypoglycemia in diabetes. Diabetes. 2008; https://doi.org/10.2337/db08-1084.
41. Skrivarhaug T, Bangstad H-J, Stene L. Long-term mortality in a nationwide cohort of childhood-onset type 1 diabetic patients in Norway. Diabetologia. 2006; https://doi.org/10.1007/s00125-005-0082-6.
42. Statistics Canada. Population by year, by province and territory (Number). Statistics Canada, CANSIM, table 051–0001. Available from: http://www.

statcan.gc.ca/tables-tableaux/sum-som/l01/cst01/demo02a-eng.htm. (Accessed 10 Jan 2017).

43. United Nations, Department of Economic and Social Affairs, Population Division. World Population Prospects: The 2015 Revision, Key Findings and Advance Tables. 2015. Working Paper No. ESA/P/WP.241. Available from: https://esa.un.org/unpd/wpp/Publications/Files/Key_Findings_WPP_2015. pdf. (Accessed 10 Jan 2017).

44. Canadian Institute for Health Information (CIHI). Organ donations continue to fall short of meeting demand. CIHI. Available from: https://www.cihi.ca/ en/types-of-care/specialized-services/organ-replacements/organ-donations-continue-to-fall-short-of. (Accessed 6 Jan 2017).

45. Abadie A, Gay S. The impact of presumed consent legislation on cadaveric organ donation: a cross-country study. J Health Econ. 2006. https://doi.org/ 10.1016/j.jhealeco.2006.01.003.

46. Pak E. CRISPR: a game-changing genetic engineering technique. Science in the news. Harvard University Available from: http://sitn.hms.harvard.edu/ flash/2014/crispr-a-game-changing-genetic-engineering-technique/. Accessed 16 Mar 2017

47. International Union of Pure and Applied Chemistry (IUPAC). In: AD MN, Wilkinson A, editors. Compendium of Chemical Terminology, (the "Gold Book"). 2nd ed. Oxford: Blackwell Scientific Publications; 1997. XML on-line corrected version: http://goldbook.iupac.org (2006-) created by M. Nic, J. Jirat, B. Kosata; updates compiled by A. Jenkins. https://doi.org/10.1351/ goldbook.

7

Pheochromocytoma as a rare cause of hypertension in a 46 X, i(X)(q10) turner syndrome: a case report and literature review

Ji Yeon Shin[1], Bo Hyun Kim[1,2,4*] ⓘD, Young Keum Kim[3], Tae Hwa Kim[1], Eun Heui Kim[1], Min Jin Lee[1], Jong Ho Kim[1], Yun Kyung Jeon[1], Sang Soo Kim[1] and In Joo Kim[1]

Abstract

Background: Cardiovascular disease (CVD) presents the most serious health problems and contributes to the increased mortality in young women with Turner syndrome. Arterial hypertension in Turner syndrome patients is significantly more prevalent than that in a general age-matched control group. The aetiology of hypertension in Turner syndrome varies, even in the absence of cardiac anomalies and obvious structural renal abnormalities. Pheochromocytoma is an extremely rare cause among various etiologies for hypertension in patients with Turner syndrome. Here, we reported a pheochromocytoma as a rare cause of hypertension in Turner syndrome patient.

Case presentation: A 21-year-old woman who has diagnosed with Turner syndrome with a karyotype of 46,X,i(X)(q10) visited for hypertension and mild headache. Transthoracic echography (TTE) showed no definite persistent ductus arteriosus shunt flow and cardiac valve abnormalities. Considering other important secondary causes like pheochromocytoma, hormonal studies were performed and the results showed increased serum norepinephrine, serum normetanephrine, and 24 h urine norepinephrine. We performed an abdominal computed tomography (CT) to confirm the location of pheochromocytoma. Abdominal CT showed a 1.9 cm right adrenal mass. I-131 meta-iodobenzylguanidine (MIBG) scintigraphy showed a right adrenal uptake. Laparoscopic adrenalectomy was performed and confirmed a pheochromocytoma. After surgery, blood pressure was within normal ranges and postoperative course was uneventful, and no recurrence developed via biochemical tests and abdominal CT until 24 months.

Conclusion: Our case and previous literatures suggest that hypertension caused by pheochromocytoma which is a rare but important and potentially lethal cause of hypertension in Turner syndrome. This case underlines the importance of early detection of pheochromocytoma in Turner syndrome. Clinicians should keep in mind that pheochromocytoma can be a cause of hypertension in patients with Turner syndrome.

Keywords: Hypertension, Turner syndrome, Pheochromocytoma

* Correspondence: pons71@hanmail.net
[1]Department of Internal Medicine, Pusan National University College of Medicine, Busan 49241, South Korea
[2]Biomedical Research Institute, Pusan National University Hospital, Busan 49241, South Korea
Full list of author information is available at the end of the article

Background

Turner syndrome is well known as a common chromosomal disorder with complete or partial absence of one X chromosome. Monosomy X is present in approximately 50% of cases. It occurs only in women between approximately 1/2500 and 1/5000 live female births. Turner syndrome represents an important cause of short stature and ovarian insufficiency in females [1]. In addition to these typical phenotypes, congenital and acquired cardiovascular disease (CVD), diabetes, hypothyroidism, impaired hearing, scoliosis, renal abnormalities and neurocognitive disorders are frequently associated with Turner syndrome [1, 2]. Among these diseases, CVDs such as cardiovascular malformation and coronary artery disease present the most serious health problems and contribute to the increased mortality rates. Importantly, arterial hypertension occurs frequently in Turner syndrome patients with an estimated prevalence of 13 to 58% in girls. Hypertension significantly increases the risk for CVD and aortic dissection [3–6]. Congenital malformation such as coarctation of the aorta and renal abnormalities, which can cause hypertension, can often be seen in patients. In addition, aortic dissection is a fatal complication in patients with Turner syndrome and often occurs at a young age [7]. Although the cause of hypertension in Turner syndrome is still not clear, structural etiology as well as heart autonomic innervations, increased plasma renin activity (PRA), and parasympathetic neuropathy, can cause hypertension in Turner syndrome patients. Thus, hypertension is the most important modifiable risk factor for aortic dissection and rupture that occurs in young women with Turner syndrome [3, 8–10]. Therefore, adults with Turner syndrome should undergo regular cardiac examinations and imaging studies to detect aortic root dilatation, cardiac valve disease, or other cardiovascular anomalies, as well as routine blood pressure (BP) monitoring [4]. However, according to the English literature, pheochromocytoma is an extremely rare cause among various aetiologies for hypertension in patients with Turner syndrome [11–13]. Here, we present a rare case of a female patient with 46 X, i(X)(q10) Turner syndrome and hypertension due to pheochromocytoma and review previous cases according to the literatures.

Case presentation

A 21-year-old woman was referred due to secondary amenorrhea. Her past medical history was significant for persistent ductus arteriosus (PDA), she underwent surgery when she was 11 months old, and she was diagnosed with type 2 diabetes mellitus (DM), which was incidentally detected at the age of 18 years. At that time,

the physical examination findings were as follows: height of 155 cm, body weight of 80 kg, body mass index (BMI) of 33.3 kg/m^2, and BP of 108/76 mmHg. After being diagnosed with type 2 DM, the patient took metformin for a few months, and she tried to lose weight through exercise and diet control. Recently, although she had not taken metformin for several months, her blood glucose was within normal ranges. At this visit, a physical examination showed a height of 155.3 cm and a weight of 53.7 kg, with a BMI of 22.3 kg/m^2. Her BP was 130/80 mmHg, with a regular heart rate of 80 beats/min, and her body temperature was 36.5 °C. The development of her breasts and her pubic hair were Tanner stage 2 and stage 3, respectively. The female internal genitalia were infantile. However, there was no webbed neck or skeletal deformities.

Laboratory tests revealed a fasting glucose level of 88 mg/dL, HbA1C 4.8%, C-peptide 6.34 ng /mL(reference range, 0.4–4 ng/mL), and anti-glutamate decarboxylase (GAD) antibody < 0.5 U/mL(reference range, 0–1.0 U/mL). Hormonal tests showed a thyroid-stimulating hormone (TSH) level of 2.45 μIU/mL (reference range, 0.3–5.0 μIU/mL), a T3 level of 169.8 ng/dL (reference range, 80–200 ng/dL), a free T4 level of 1.15 ng/dL (reference range, 0.75–2.0 ng/dL), a prolactin level of 8.18 ng/mL (reference range, 1.9–19.7 ng/mL), a luteinizing hormone (LH) level of 20.2 mIU/mL, a follicular stimulating hormone (FSH) level of 100 mIU/mL, a testosterone level of 0.01 ng/mL (reference range, 0–0.77 ng/mL), an oestradiol level of 1.06 μg/dL(reference range, 30–333 μg/dL). A small uterus was detected, and both ovaries could not be identified on pelvis ultrasonography and computed tomography (CT) (Fig. 1a, b). However, there was no renal abnormality (Fig. 1c). A chromosome study finally showed a karyotype of 46,X,i (X)(q10) Turner syndrome. Transthoracic echography (TTE) revealed no residual PDA shunt flow and bicuspid valve. Bone mineral density (BMD) using dual-energy X-ray absorptiometry showed an age-matched Z score of − 0.7 at the lumbar spine. She was regularly followed up for type 2 DM and took ethinyl oestradiol/drospirenone for regular menstruation.

Three years after the diagnosis of Turner syndrome, the patient complained of mild headache, intermittent palpitation, and dizziness without neurological deficit. Her measured BP was 166/100 mmHg at the doctor's office and 145/90 mmHg at home. Her BP at the time of the Turner syndrome diagnosis (3 years ago) was within normal ranges. There was no radio-femoral delay which meant delay between the radial pulse and femoral pulse suggesting coarctation of aorta. Recent TTE showed no residual PDA shunt flow and cardiac valve abnormality. There was no family history of hypertension. A thyroid function test and chemistry were within normal ranges.

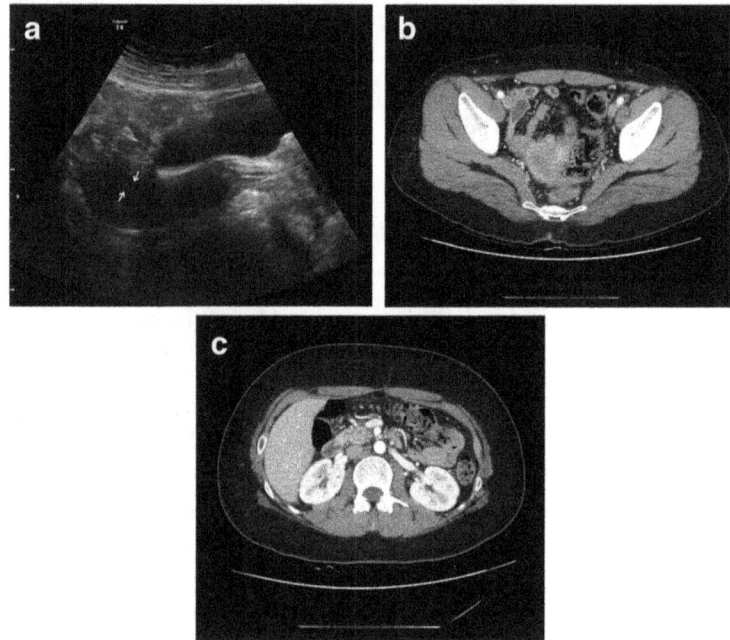

Fig. 1 Ultrasonography image (**a**) and abdomen computed tomography axial image with contrast enhancement (**b**) shows small uterus and both ovaries are not visible. There was no abnormalities of urogenital system (**c**)

We consider other important secondary causes of hypertension like a pheochromocytoma. Thus, hormonal studies were performed and the results showed increased serum norepinephrine, serum normetanephrine, and 24 h urine norepinephrine (Table 1). We performed an abdominal computed tomography (CT) to confirm the location of pheochromocytoma. Abdominal CT showed a 1.9 cm right adrenal mass, measuring 42 Hounsfield units pre-contrast, heterogenous contrast enhancement with a contrast wash-out ratio of 65% (Fig. 2a and b). According to her clinical manifestations, biochemical results and atypical CT phenotype, I-131 meta-iodo-benzylguanidine (MIBG) scintigraphy was performed to detect of extra-adrenal pheochromocytoma.

Table 1 Laboratory findings for adrenal gland mass on admission and post-operation

Parameters	Pre-operative value	Post-operative value	Reference ranges
Serum norepinephrine, pg/mL	1066.2	294.0	110–410
Serum epinephrine, pg/mL	17.5	14.4	< 50
Serum normetanephrine, nmol/L	3.32	0.5	< 0.9
Serum metanephrine, nmol/L	0.13	0.12	< 0.5
Urinary norepinephrine, μg/24hours[a]	282.6	34.4	0–97
Urinary epinephrine, μg/24hours[a]	4.35	3.6	0–27
Urinary normetanephrine, μg/24hours[a]	399.9	176.3	88–444
Urinary metanephrine, μg/24hours[a]	21.3	58.6	52-341
Urinary VMA, mg/day	4.72	2.04	1.2–6.52
Serum ACTH, pg/mL	10.38	16.15	10–60
Serum cortisol, μg/dL	45	40.0	2.5–12.5
24 h urine free cortisol, μg/24 hours[a]	49.7	45.4	7–96
Plasma renin activity, ng/ml/hr	9.14	5.16	0.15–2.33
Serum aldosterone, pg/mL	864.4	199.7	10–160
Aldosterone renin ratio	9.46	3.9	< 30
Serum Potassium, mmol/L	4.23	3.92	3.5–5.3

[a]24 hours urine total volume 1650 mL, urinary creatinine 1171.9 mg/24 h

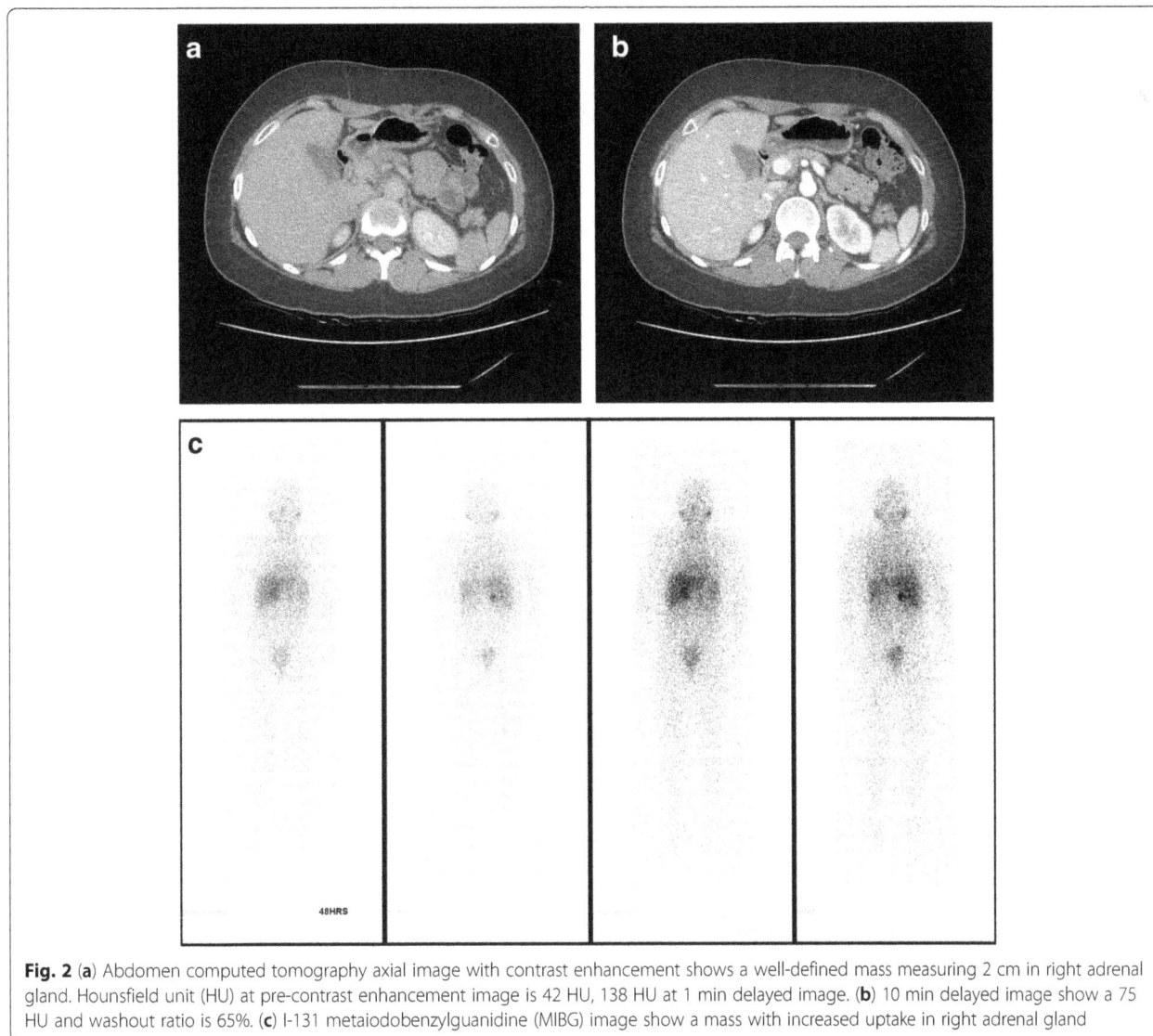

Fig. 2 (**a**) Abdomen computed tomography axial image with contrast enhancement shows a well-defined mass measuring 2 cm in right adrenal gland. Hounsfield unit (HU) at pre-contrast enhancement image is 42 HU, 138 HU at 1 min delayed image. (**b**) 10 min delayed image show a 75 HU and washout ratio is 65%. (**c**) I-131 metaiodobenzylguanidine (MIBG) image show a mass with increased uptake in right adrenal gland

The results showed MIBG uptake on the right adrenal gland (Fig. 2c). She had no family history of pheochromocytoma. After pre-operatively administering phenoxybenzamine, laparoscopic adrenalectomy was performed. Final pathology revealed that the pheochromocytoma extended to the adrenal cortex but was well-circumscribed. The cut surface of the tumour was tan and darkened with focal haemorrhage. The tumour showed characteristic "Zellballen" architecture. The tumour cells were larger than normal chromaffin cells, and their cytoplasm was granular. Immunostaining for S-100 protein demonstrates the sustentacular framework surrounding the tumour cells and positive for chromogranin (Fig. 3). Postoperative blood pressure was recorded as 120/70 mmHg without any anti-hypertensive drugs. Postoperative hormonal tests revealed decreased catecholamine levels (Table 1). The postoperative course was uneventful, and no recurrence developed via biochemical tests and abdominal CT until 24 months.

Discussion

In this article, we reported a rare case of hypertension caused by pheochromocytoma in a young woman with 46 X, i(X)(q10) Turner syndrome. Hypertension in Turner syndrome patients is significantly more prevalent than that in a general age-matched control group [4, 5, 10]. The aetiology of hypertension in Turner syndrome varies, even in the absence of cardiac anomalies and obvious structural renal abnormalities [3, 8–10]. Adults with Turner syndrome should undergo regular cardiac examinations and imaging studies to detect cardiovascular abnormalities, as well as routine check-ups of systemic BP, because CVD is the primary cause of mortality in Turner syndrome. Considering these points, hypertension is the

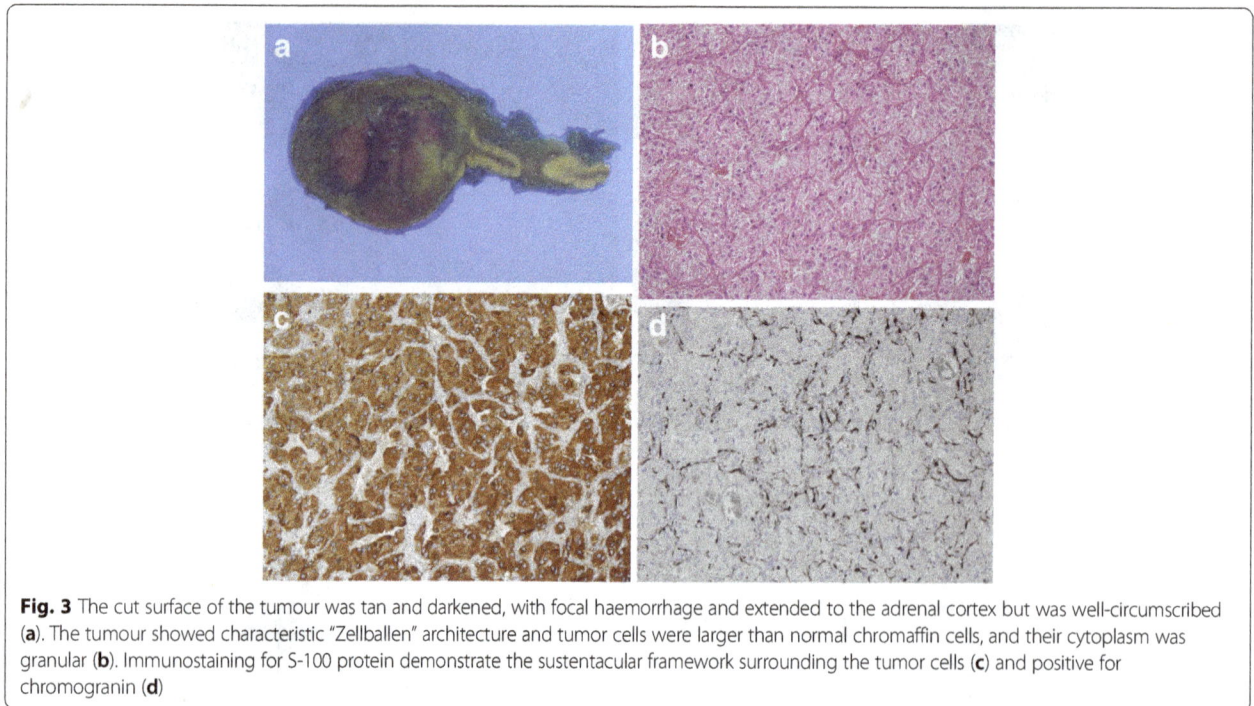

Fig. 3 The cut surface of the tumour was tan and darkened, with focal haemorrhage and extended to the adrenal cortex but was well-circumscribed (**a**). The tumour showed characteristic "Zellballen" architecture and tumor cells were larger than normal chromaffin cells, and their cytoplasm was granular (**b**). Immunostaining for S-100 protein demonstrate the sustentacular framework surrounding the tumor cells (**c**) and positive for chromogranin (**d**)

most easily detectable and treatable cardiovascular risk factor to prevent CVD [4].

Turner syndrome patients usually are overweight; have central obesity, truncal fat mass, short stature, and high BMI; and are at risk for diabetes, which can cause cardiovascular abnormalities [6, 14, 15]. Turner syndrome is also associated with vascular wall abnormalities that are both structural and functional. Although some factors in the pathogenesis of hypertension remain uncertain, the potential pathogenesis includes inappropriate activation of the renin–angiotensin–aldosterone system, oxidative stress, inflammation, impaired insulin-mediated vasodilatation, increased stimulation of the sympathetic nervous system and abnormal sodium processing by the kidney [6, 16]. PRA has been found to be elevated in approximately 50% of Turner syndrome patients compared to the general population [8]. Over-activated autonomic innervations of the heart in Turner syndrome can increase the heart rate and BP [3]. Increased C-reactive protein is observed in half of

Turner syndrome patients, which results in a chronic inflammatory state in the vascular endothelium and can likely lead to hypertension due to endothelial dysfunction [17]. In addition, hypertension with Turner syndrome is related to aortic stenosis, malformation of the urogenital system and other cardiac malformations [6]. High-dose growth hormone (GH) treatment causes hypertension due to sodium and water retention with increased levels of PRA and aldosterone levels [18]. However, in our case, the patient had no residual PDA shunt flow and cardiac valve abnormality and renal abnormalities and she did not receive GH treatment.

It is well-known that pheochromocytoma is one of the rare but important and potentially lethal causes of endocrine hypertension. Pheochromocytoma in patients with Turner syndrome is rarely reported, according to the English language literature [11–13]. Table 2 summarizes the clinical features and cardiovascular outcomes in previously reported cases. For the first time, Kinsely et al. reported an autopsy case with diagnosed

Table 2 The summary of the reported cases of pheochromocytoma in patient with Turner syndrome

Authors, year of publication (reference)	Age	Karyotype	Size of pheochromocytoma	Clinical manifestations	Cardiovascular outcomes
Knisely et al. (1988) [11]	27	45,XO	7.5 cm	Hemorrhagic cerebral infarct	Sudden death
Landin-Wilhelmsen et al. (2004) [12]	39	45,X[46]/46,X + mar [4]	3.0 cm	Chest pain hypertension	Aortic dissection
Fatma et al. (2016) [13]	48	46 X,i(Xq)/45X	6.0 cm	Adrenal incidentaloma hypertension	Curative hypertension
In our case	21	46 X, i(X)(q10)	1.9 cm	Hypertension	Curative hypertension

pheochromocytoma and sudden death caused by haemorrhagic cerebral infarction in Turner syndrome [11]. Landin-Wilhelmsen et al. also reported a case of aortic dissection and pheochromocytoma in a case of Turner syndrome [12]. Recently, Fatma et al. reported that Turner syndrome with 45,X/46,X,i(Xq) karyotype was associated with incidentally detected pheochromocytoma [13]. In our case, the size of the pheochromocytoma was the smallest compared with previous cases. Unfortunately, the former two cases showed that pheochromocytoma in Turner syndrome led to poor CVD outcomes due to delayed diagnosis. Therefore, early detection and treatment of pheochromoctyoma is very important to prevent CVD and reduce mortality in young women with Turner syndrome. In case of clinical suspicion of pheochromocytoma, biochemical testing including plasma free or urinary metanephrines should be measured. In our case, serum norepinephrine, serum normetanephrine, and urinary norepinephrine were increased. However, urinary normetanephrine was within normal reference value. It is well known that the very high diagnostic sensitivity of metanephrines is due to the continuous diffusion of intratumorally-produced metanephrines into the circulation, which contrasts with the episodic secretion of the parent catecholamines [19]. However, it is not clear why the value of urinary normetanephrine was normal in this case. Previous two studies also reported increased metanephrine and normetanephrine [12, 13], however, levels of catecholamines and their catabolic products in serum or urine had not been determined in Knisely et al. study [11].

Although cancer risks in Turner syndrome except having an increased gonadoblastoma have not been clearly established, high incidence of extragonadal neoplasms with a preponderance of neurogenic tumors has been reported [20–22]. Although the overall risk of cancer was not increased in a population-based study, women with Turner syndrome had an increase of site-specific risk for gonadoblastoma, meningioma, childhood brain tumors, bladder, and uterine cancer when compared with the general population [23]. However, the clinical importance of this result was unclear due to very small number of cases. Like this population-based study, the related mechanisms between Turner syndrome and pheochromocytoma remain unclear, and it is also uncertain whether pheochromocytoma is over-represented in Turner syndrome because coexistence of these two diseases is extremely rare. Pheochromocytomas are known to be hereditary in 30–40% of cases, and hereditary catecholamine-secreting tumors typically present at a younger age than sporadic tumors [24]. Genetic testing should be considered in all patients and is strongly indicated in specific patients such as those with unilateral adrenal pheochromocytoma onset at a young age, those with a positive family history of pheochromocytoma and

paraganglioma or carriers of tumor susceptibility gene mutations, and those with syndromic features or metastatic disease [19]. However, unfortunately, our patient had no family history of pheochromocytoma and she refused a genetic testing due to expensive cost of genetic testing. Further studies including genetic tests are necessary to define the mechanisms underlying association between Turner syndrome and pheochromcytoma.

Conclusion
Our case and data from previous literature suggest that hypertension caused by pheochromocytoma which is a rare but important and potentially fatal cause of hypertension in Turner syndrome. This case underlines the importance of early detection of pheochromocytoma for prevention of CVD and reduction of mortality in young women with Turner syndrome. Clinicians should keep in mind that pheochromocytoma can be a cause of hypertension in patients with Turner syndrome. Thus, adults with Turner syndrome should undergo regular cardiac examinations, as well as routine BP monitoring. Furthermore, the possible association between Turner syndrome and pheochromocytoma should be elucidated in future studies.

Abbreviations
BMD: Bone mineral density; BMI: Body mass index; BP: Blood pressure; CT: Computed tomography; CVD: Cardiovascular disease; DM: Diabetes mellitus; FSH: Follicular stimulating hormone; GAD: Glutamate decarboxylase; GH: Growth hormone; HU: Hounsfield unit; LH: Luteinizing Hormone; MIBG: Meta-iodobenzylguanidine; PDA: Persistent ductus arteriosus; PRA: Plasma renin activity; TSH: Thyroid-stimulating hormone; TTE: Transthoracic echography

Authors' contributions
JYS and THK drafted the manuscript and treated the patient. YKK reviewed pathology. EHK, MJL and JHK provided perioperative care of the patient and helped draft the manuscript. YKJ, SSK and IJK supervised drafting of the manuscript. BHK reviewed and modified the draft manuscript. All authors read and approved the final manuscript.

Competing interests
The authors declare that they have no competing interests.

Author details
[1]Department of Internal Medicine, Pusan National University College of Medicine, Busan 49241, South Korea. [2]Biomedical Research Institute, Pusan National University Hospital, Busan 49241, South Korea. [3]Department of Pathology, Pusan National University Hospital and Pusan National University School of Medicine, Busan 49241, South Korea. [4]Division of Endocrinology and Metabolism, Department of Internal Medicine, Pusan National University Hospital, 305 Gudeok-ro, Seo-gu, Busan 602-739, South Korea.

References

1. Stochholm K, Juul S, Juel K, Naeraa RW, Gravholt CH. Prevalence, incidence, diagnostic delay, and mortality in turner syndrome. J Clin Endocrinol Metab. 2006;91:3897–902.
2. Gravholt CH. Clinical practice in turner syndrome. Nat Clin Pract Endocrinol Metab. 2005;1:41–52.
3. Gravholt CH, Hansen KW, Erlandsen M, Ebbehoj E, Christiansen JS. Nocturnal hypertension and impaired sympathovagal tone in turner syndrome. J Hypertens. 2006;24:353–60.
4. Bondy CA. Turner syndrome study group. Care of girls and women with turner syndrome: a guideline of the turner syndrome study group. J Clin Endocrinol Metab. 2007;92:10–25.
5. Pedreira CC, Hameed R, Kanumakala S, Zacharin M. Health-care problems of turner syndrome in the adult woman: a cross sectional study of a Victorian cohort and a case for transition. Intern Med J. 2006;36:54–7.
6. De Groote K, Demulier L, De Backer J, De Wolf D, De Schepper J, T'sjoen G, De Backer T. Arterial hypertension in turner syndrome: a review of the literature and a practical approach for diagnosis and treatment. J Hypertens. 2015;33:1342–51.
7. Gravholt CH, Landin-Wilhelmsen K, Stochholm K, Hjerrild BE, Ledet T, Djurhuus CB, Sylvén L, Baandrup U, Kristensen BØ, Christiansen JS. Clinical and epidemiological description of aortic dissection in Turner's syndrome. Cardiol Young. 2006;16:430–6.
8. Virdis R, Cantu MC, Ghizzoni L, Ammenti A, Nori G, Volta C, Cravidi C, Vanelli M, Balestrazzi P, Bernasconi S. Blood pressure behaviour and control in turner syndrome. Clin Exp Hypertens A. 1986;8:787–91.
9. Nathwani NC, Unwin R, Brook CG, Hindmarsh PC. The influence of renal and cardiovascular abnormalities on blood pressure in turner syndrome. Clin Endocrinol. 2000;52:371–7.
10. Los E, Quezada E, Chen Z, Lapidus J, Silberbach M. Pilot study of blood pressure in girls with turner syndrome: an awareness gap, clinical associations, and new hypotheses. Hypertension. 2016;68:133–6.
11. Knisely AS, Sweeney K, Ambler MW. Pheochromocytoma and sudden death as a result of cerebral infarction in Turner's syndrome: report of a case. J Forensic Sci. 1988;33:1497–502.
12. Landin-Wilhelmsen K, Bryman I, Hanson C, Hanson L. Spontaneous pregnancies in a turner syndrome woman with Y-chromosome mosaicism. J Assist Reprod Genet. 2004;21:229–30.
13. Chaker F, Chihaoui M, Yazidi M, Bouyahia M, Slimane H. Pheochromocytoma in a 45 X, iso (Xq) turner syndrome. Ann Endocrinol. 2016;77:57–9.
14. Holl RW, Kunze D, Etzrodt H, Teller W, Heinze E. Turner syndrome: final height, glucose tolerance, bone density and psychosocial status in 25 adult patients. Eur J Pediatr. 1994;153:11–6.
15. Gravholt CH, Naeraa RW, Nyholm B, Gerdes LU, Christiansen E, Schmitz O, Christiansen JS. Glucose metabolism, lipid metabolism, and cardiovascular risk factors in adult Turner's syndrome. The impact of sex hormone replacement. Diabetes Care. 1998;21:1062–70.
16. Lastra G, Syed S, Kurukulasuriya LR, Manrique C, Sowers JR. Type 2 diabetes mellitus and hypertension: an update. Endocrinol Metab Clin N Am. 2014;43:103–22.
17. Ostberg JE, Attar MJ, Mohamed-Ali V, Conway GS. Adipokine dysregulation in turner syndrome: comparison of circulating interleukin-6 and leptin concentrations with measures of adiposity and C-reactive protein. J Clin Endocrinol Metab. 2005;90:2948–53.
18. Radetti G, Crepaz R, Milanesi O, Paganini C, Cesaro A, Rigon F, Pitscheider W. Cardiac performance in Turner's syndrome patients on growth hormone therapy. Horm Res. 2001;55:240–4.
19. Lenders JW, Duh QY, Eisenhofer G, Gimenez-Roqueplo AP, Grebe SK, Murad MH, Naruse M, Pacak K, Young WF Jr, Endocrine Society. Pheochromocytoma and paraganglioma: an endocrine society clinical practice guideline. J Clin Endocrinol Metab. 2014;99:1915–42.
20. Brant WO, Rajimwale A, Lovell MA, Travers SH, Furness PD 3rd, Sorensen M, Oottamasathien S, Koyle MA. Gonadoblastoma and turner syndrome. J Urol. 2006;175:1858–60.
21. Sivakumaran TA, Ghose S, Kumar H, Singha U, Kucheria K. Nongonadal neoplasia in patients with turner syndrome. J Environ Pathol Toxicol Oncol. 1999;18:339–47.
22. Kamoun M, Mnif MF, Rekik N, Belguith N, Charfi N, Mnif L, Elleuch M, Mnif F, Kamoun T, Mnif Z, Kamoun H, Sellami-Boudawara T, Hachicha M, Abid M. Ganglioneuroma of adrenal gland in a patient with turner syndrome. Ann Diagn Pathol. 2010;14:133–6.
23. Schoemaker MJ, Swerdlow AJ, Higgins CD, Wright AF, Jacobs PA. UK clinical cytogenetics group. Cancer incidence in women with turner syndrome in great Britain: a national cohort study. Lancet Oncol. 2008;9:239–46.
24. Neumann HP, Bausch B, SR MW, Bender BU, Gimm O, Franke G, Schipper J, Klisch J, Altehoefer C, Zerres K, Januszewicz A, Eng C, Smith WM, Munk R, Manz T, Glaesker S, Apel TW, Treier M, Reineke M, Walz MK, Hoang-Vu C, Brauckhoff M, Klein-Franke A, Klose P, Schmidt H, Maier-Woelfle M, Peçzkowska M, Szmigielski C, Eng C, Freiburg-Warsaw-Columbus Pheochromocytoma Study Group. Germ-line mutations in nonsyndromic pheochromocytoma. N Engl J Med. 2002;346:1459–66.

Prevalence of metabolic syndrome in Saudi Arabia - a cross sectional study

Khalid Al-Rubeaan[1*], Nahla Bawazeer[2], Yousuf Al Farsi[1], Amira M. Youssef[3], Abdulrahman A. Al-Yahya[4], Hamid AlQumaidi[1], Basim M. Al-Malki[1], Khalid A. Naji[1], Khalid Al-Shehri[1] and Fahd I. Al Rumaih[4]

Abstract

Background: The evaluation of metabolic syndrome in a society predisposed to the diabetes mellitus epidemic opens a new avenue to understanding this rapidly growing global metabolic problem. Although Saudi Arabia reports one of the highest prevalence levels of obesity and diabetes, a very limited number of epidemiological studies have examined the prevalence of metabolic syndrome. Therefore, the main aim of the current study was to estimate the prevalence of metabolic syndrome and its risk factors among the adult Saudi population in comparison to other countries.

Methods: A total of 12,126 Saudi subjects were randomly recruited from the 13 administrative regions, and evaluated for metabolic syndrome and its risk factors. This exercise was carried out by trained physicians, through clinical evaluations and overnight fasting blood glucose and lipid profile measurements. Both the International Diabetes Federation (IDF) and modified National Cholesterol Education Program and Adult Treatment Panel III (NCEP ATP III) Criteria were employed, and subjects with metabolic syndrome were identified using country-specific waist circumference cutoff values.

Results: The prevalence of metabolic syndrome in Saudi Arabia was found to be 39.8% (34.4% in men and 29.2% in women) and 31.6% (45.0% in men and 35.4% in women), according to the NCEP ATP III and IDF criteria, respectively. Metabolic syndrome was also observed to be more prevalent among men and older subjects. The most frequently observed component of metabolic syndrome was found to be low levels of high-density lipoprotein (HDL), followed by abdominal obesity. The most significant risk factors in the studied cohort included age ≥ 45, smoking history, low educational level, and living in urban areas.

Conclusions: This study shows a high prevalence of metabolic syndrome in Saudi Arabia, and thereby warrants urgent implementation of preventive health care strategies to reduce both morbidity and mortality related to this medical problem.

Keywords: Metabolic syndrome, Prevalence, Risk factors, Obesity, Diabetes, Cross-sectional survey, Saudi Arabia

Background

Metabolic syndrome was first recognized by the medical community during the late 1980s and was characterized by the clustering of abdominal obesity, elevated blood pressure, hyperglycemia, and dyslipidemia [1]. This syndrome has been redefined through several amendments by different scientific bodies, and was finally defined by either the ATP III [2] or IDF criteria [3], wherein the

IDF criteria mandates the presence of central obesity as one of the components of metabolic syndrome. Subjects with metabolic syndrome are at increased risk for coronary heart disease (CHD), and the presence of metabolic syndrome alone can predict approximately 25% of all new-onset cardiovascular disease (CVD) [4]. In addition, metabolic syndrome is associated with an increased risk of death from CHD, CVD, and all other causes [5]. It affects nearly one quarter of the adult population worldwide, and its prevalence varies, according to the definition used, ethnicity under study, and level of urbanization [6]. Among the most recent studies, the

* Correspondence: krubeaan@dsrcenter.org
[1]University Diabetes Center, College of Medicine, King Saud University, PO Box 18397, Riyadh, Riyadh 11415, Saudi Arabia
Full list of author information is available at the end of the article

prevalence of metabolic syndrome has been reported to be between 10% and 84% worldwide depending on the age, sex, and ethnicity of the population [7]. The National Health and Nutrition Examination Survey (NHANES), using the ATP III criteria, showed the prevalence of metabolic syndrome to be 34.5%, whereas this figure was 39.0% with the IDF criteria [8]. These findings are different from those observed in an Irish study that reported a prevalence at 21.4% and 13.2%, using the IDF and ATP III definitions, respectively [9]. The prevalence was even lower among Chinese individuals, reported at 7.9% and 15.1% using ATP III and IDF definitions, respectively [10].

The Middle East and North African (MENA) region is known for its high prevalence of metabolic syndrome, where it has been reported to be 45.5% and 24.3% in Tunisia, using the IDF criteria and ATP III definition, respectively [11]. Gulf countries, being part of the Middle East, have shown a prevalence of metabolic syndrome that ranges from 17% in Oman [12] to 40.5% in the United Arab Emirates (UAE) [13], according to the ATP III and IDF criteria, respectively. Although no recent nationwide survey has evaluated the prevalence of metabolic syndrome in Saudi Arabia, Al-Nozha et al. [14] reported it to be 39.3% in 2005, using the 2001 ATP III criteria.

This study is a part of the Saudi Abnormal Glucose Metabolism and Diabetes Impact Study (SAUDI-DM) [15] that investigates the prevalence of metabolic

syndrome and its risk factors in the adult Saudi society, in comparison to other societies.

Methods
Subjects
The SAUDI-DM is a nationwide, household cross-sectional population-based survey that uses a multistage stratified cluster sampling technique. The study recruited 87,417 Saudi nationals between 2007 and 2009 from the 13 administrative regions of Saudi Arabia. The data of all study participants were adjusted for age, area of residency (urban and rural, according to the definitions of the Ministry of Municipal and Rural Affairs), and sex distribution, using the Saudi national census for the year 2007 that led to the exclusion of 34,047 noncompatible participants [15]. For the current analysis, we further excluded 17,172 subjects with incomplete clinical data, or those who did not report for blood sampling. Subjects younger than 18 years of age (totaling 23,523) were also excluded. A total of 549 women from this cohort were found to be pregnant and had to be excluded. The final study cohort comprised of 12,126 Saudi subjects aged ≥18 years, with complete clinical and biochemical data, as shown in Fig. 1.

The current study was conducted by trained physicians and nurses, through primary healthcare centers, to secure accurate and complete data. The data that were collected consisted of general demographic and clinical information including age, sex, highest level of education

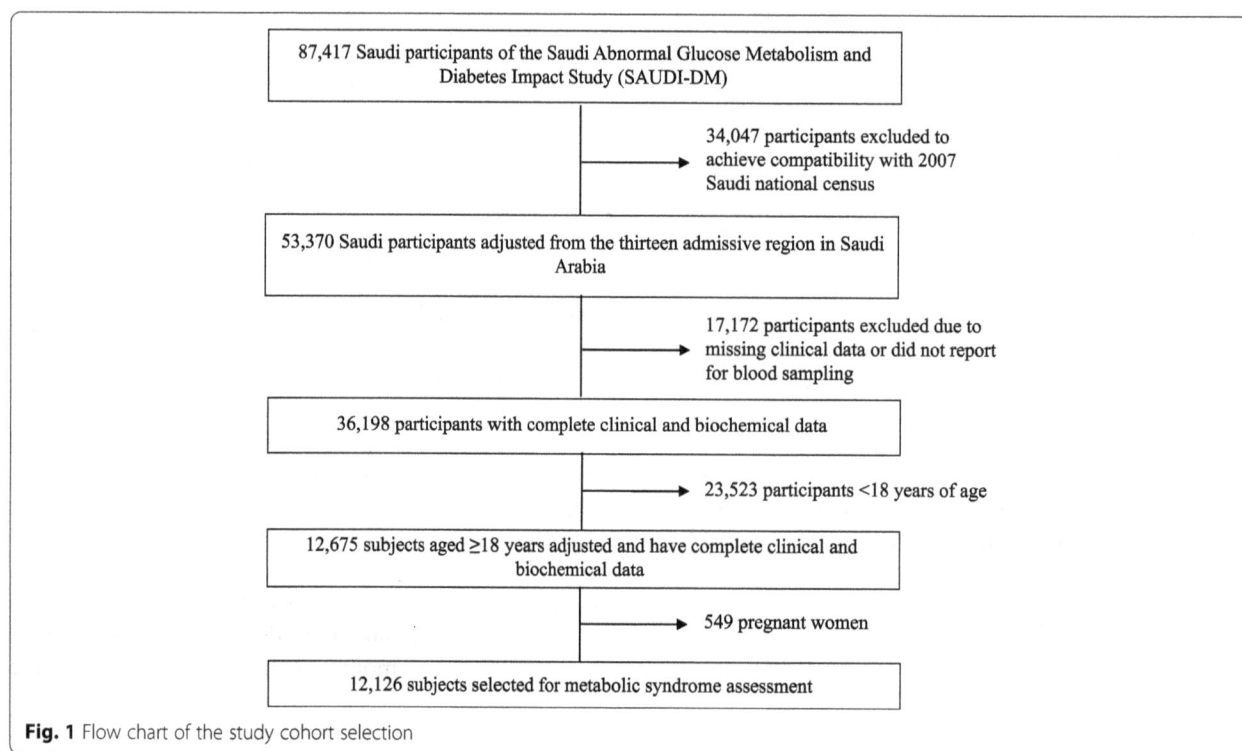

Fig. 1 Flow chart of the study cohort selection

attained, and monthly income, in addition to history of diabetes, hypertension, and dyslipidemia. The SAUDI-DM study was reviewed and approved by the Institutional Review Board at the College of Medicine, King Saud University.

Anthropometric measurements and vital signs

Anthropometric measurements, including weight, height, and waist circumference, were taken with the subjects in a standing position, wearing light clothing without shoes. Weight and height were assessed, using a weighing scale (Adam Equipment Oxford CT USA, model MDW-250 L) with a capacity of 250 kg and reliability of 0.1 kg. Waist circumference was measured at the midpoint between the top of the iliac crest and the lower margin of the last palpable rib. Hip circumference was measured at the widest part of the body below the waist. The waist-to-hip ratio (WHR) was calculated by dividing the waist circumference by the hip circumference. Systolic (SBP) and diastolic blood pressure (DBP) measurements were taken from the left arm, after at least 5 min of rest, with the subjects in a sitting position, using a standardized mercury sphygmomanometer (Baumanometer, Model 0320, W.A. Baum Co., Inc. USA).

Laboratory analysis

All subjects were asked to report to the nearest primary health care center (PHCC) after more than 10 h of overnight fasting, after which 10 mL of venous blood was collected using a sodium fluoride tube. All blood samples were sent to the central laboratory at the Strategic Center for Diabetes Research in the Riyadh, the capital city of the Kingdom, using portable refrigerators in which the temperature was maintained between 4 °C and 8 °C. Plasma was stored at − 20 °C at the central laboratory. The blood glucose assessment was conducted, using the glucose oxidase/peroxidase method; whereas blood cholesterol was measured using the esterase oxidase/peroxidase method; and levels of high-density lipoprotein (HDL), low-density lipoprotein (LDL), and triglycerides were determined, using the glycerokinase oxidase/peroxidase method.

Definition of metabolic syndrome

Metabolic syndrome was defined, using both the modified National Cholesterol Program Adult Treatment Panel III (NCEP ATP III) and the International Diabetes Federation (IDF) criteria, and implementing the new cutoff value for waist circumference in Saudi society [16]. Therefore, subjects were considered to have metabolic syndrome if they had central obesity that was defined by a waist circumference ≥ 92 cm in men and ≥87 cm in women, along with two or more of the following criteria, as per the IDF definition [3]: high fasting

glucose level ≥ 100 mg/dL (5.6 mmol/L), or patients known to have diabetes mellitus and/or on treatment for diabetes; hypertriglyceridemia - serum triglyceride level ≥ 150 mg/dL (1.7 mmol/L); low HDL cholesterol - serum HDL cholesterol < 40 mg/dL (1.0 mmol/L) in men and < 50 mg/dL (1.3 mmol/L) in women, or patients known to have dyslipidiema; high blood pressure - SBP ≥ 130 mmHg and/or DBP ≥ 85 mmHg, or patients known to have hypertension, and/or on treatment for hypertension. The NCEP-APT III criteria for metabolic syndrome were met if an individual had three or more of the aforementioned criteria [4].

Statistical analysis

Data were analyzed using the SPSS statistical package version 21. Continuous variables were expressed as mean ± standard deviation (SD), and categorical variables were expressed as percentages. The t- test was used for continuous variables and chi-squared test for categorical variables. Risk factors for metabolic syndrome were assessed using univariate, age- and sex-adjusted, and multivariate logistic regression models. The odds ratio and 95% confidence intervals were used to express different risk factors. A p-value less than 0.05 was used as the level of significance.

Results

The studied cohort of 12,126 subjects represents the Saudi population over 10-year age intervals, with a mean age of 35.7 ± 15.0 years, wherein men were significantly older than women, and both had similar distribution. More subjects lived in urban areas than in rural areas. The prevalence of obesity, particularly as morbid obesity (body mass index (BMI) ≥ 30 kg/m2), was higher among women versus men [(36.5% versus 29.4% ($p < 0.001$)]. Men had a significantly higher mean waist circumference; whereas women had a higher mean hip circumference. The mean WHR was significantly higher among men. Only 20.7% of the study cohort had a relatively high monthly income (> 8000 Saudi Riyals [SR]) and a higher proportion of men were smokers in comparison to women. Men had a significantly higher mean SBP and DBP, as well as higher mean fasting plasma glucose (FPG), mean LDL, and triglycerides. In contrast, mean HDL cholesterol was significantly higher among women. The prevalence of metabolic syndrome according to the IDF criteria was 31.6%; specifically, 34.4% in men and 29.2% in women. However, according to the ATP III criteria, the prevalence of metabolic syndrome was higher at 39.9%; specifically, 45.0% in men and 35.4% in women, as shown in Table 1.

The prevalence of metabolic syndrome and its components increased with age, except in the age group ≥70 years. The most frequently observed component of

Table 1 Baseline characteristics of the study cohort and the calculated metabolic syndrome prevalence

Total 12,126	Men 5571(45.94)		Women 6555(54.06)	P value
Discreptive analysis; mean (± SD)				
Mean age (years)	35.7 (±15.0)	36.1 (±15.2)	35.5 (±14.8)	P value
Mean WC (cm)	87.0 (±16.7)	89.71 ± 17.11	84.75 ± 16.03	0.035
Mean Hip (cm)	99.1 (±16.8)	98.7 (±16.8)	99.4(±16.8)	< 0.001
Mean W-H ratio	0.9 (±0.12)	0.9(±0.1)	0.9 (±0.1)	0.014
Mean Systolic Bp (mmHg)	117.7 (±13.8)	119.7 (±13.1)	↑16.0 (±14.1)	< 0.001
Mean Diastolic Bp (mmHg)	76.1 (±8.6)	77.3 (±8.9)	75.2 (±8.7)	< 0.001
Mean FPG (mmol/L)	5.7 (±2.4)	5.8 (±2.6)	5.6 (±2.3)	< 0.001
Mean LDL Cholesterol (mmol/L)	3.2 (±1.1)	3.2 (±1.1)	3.2 (±1.0)	< 0.001
Mean triglyceride (mmol/L)	1.6 (±1.2)	1.8 (±1.3)	1.5 (±0.1)	0.012
Mean HDL cholesterol (mmol/L)	0.1 (±0.3)	0.9 (±0.3)	1.0 (±0.3)	< 0.001
Frequancy anlysis; number (%)				
Age groups: 18-29 years	5196 (42.9)	2328(41.8)	2868(43.8)	< 0.001
30-39 years	2660 (21.9)	1276(22.9)	1384(21.1)	
40-49 years	2207 (18.2)	942(16.9)	1265(19.3)	
50-59 years	1086 (8.1)	524(9.4)	562(8.6)	
60-69 years	573(4.7)	315(5.7)	258(3.9)	
≥ 70 years	404(3.3)	186(3.3)	218(3.3)	
BMI groups < 18.5	673(5.6)	315(5.7)	358(5.5)	< 0.001
18.5-24.9	3783(31.2)	1807(32.4)	1976(30.1)	
25-29.9	3642(30.0)	1812(32.5)	1830(27.9)	
≥ 30	4028(33.2)	1637(29.4)	2391(36.5)	
Monthly Income < 4000 SR	5255(43.3)	2175(39.0)	3080(46.1)	< 0.001
4000-8000 SR	4438(36.6)	2173(39.0)	2265(34.6)	
> 8000 SR	2433(20.1)	1223(21.95)	1210(18.46)	
Smoking	1564(12.9)	1475(26.5)	89(1.4)	< 0.001
Educational level: Illiterate	2417(19.9)	554(9.94)	1863(28.42)	
Less than high school	3648(30.1)	1855(33.3)	1793(27.4)	
More than or equal high school	6061(49.1)	3162(56.8)	2899(44.2)	
Family history of: Diabetes Mellitus	6200(51.1)	2896(51.1)	3304(50.4)	0.083
Hypertension	4212(34.7)	1887(33.9)	2325(35.5)	0.066
Metabolic Syndrome Prevalence				
IDF criteria (WC + ≥ 2risk factors)	3833(31.6)	1917(34.4)	1916(29.2)	< 0.001
NCEP-ATP-III criteria (3 or more risk factors)	4828(39.8)	2507(45.0)	2321(35.4)	< 0.001

NCEP-ATP-III;, National Cholesterol Education Program and Adult Treatment Panel III, HDL; high density lipoprotein, IDF; International Diabetes Federation, LDL; low density lipoprotein, WC; waist circumference, WHR; waist-to-hip ratio

metabolic syndrome was low HDL that affected around 80% of the sample. Abdominal obesity ranged between 25% and 70%, whereas elevated blood glucose affected 25% to 60% according to the age group. Elevated triglycerides and high blood pressure were the components of metabolic syndrome that occurred least frequently.

Both male and female subjects showed an increasing prevalence of metabolic syndrome with age, although this was more pronounced according to the ATP III criteria. Men had a higher prevalence of metabolic syndrome compared to women in the younger age groups; whereas women had a higher prevalence in the age group ≥70 years. Middle-aged men and women had an almost similar prevalence of metabolic syndrome. Women in different age groups showed a high prevalence of low HDL and abdominal obesity, whereas the prevalence of elevated blood pressure, blood glucose, and triglycerides was higher among men as compared to women in 10-year age intervals, as shown in Table 2. Figure 2 shows the frequency of one or more components of metabolic syndrome, according to differences in age and sex distribution. As the number of metabolic syndrome components increase, the relative frequency is reduced, regardless of age group or sex. The frequency of three or more components of metabolic syndrome increased with age in both male and female subjects. In addition, the frequency of three or more risk factors for metabolic syndrome was found to be higher among men than women, with the exception of the > 70 age group, in which women had a higher frequency than men.

Risk factors

When the risk factors for metabolic syndrome were assessed in the current study, any age ≥ 45 years was the most important and significant risk factor in both unadjusted and multivariate models. The male gender, smoking, and increased BMI were each independently and significantly associated with an increased risk of metabolic syndrome. Higher monthly income and low educational level were found to be significant risk factors for metabolic syndrome, when the unadjusted model was used. However, high monthly income remained

significant only in the age- and sex-adjusted model, and low educational level remained independently significant only in the multivariate adjusted model. Living in an urban area was significantly associated with an increased risk of metabolic syndrome in the age- and sex- or multivariate adjusted models. Family history of DM and hypertension were also associated with an increased risk of metabolic syndrome after adjusting for age and sex, whereas only family history of hypertension remained significant in the multivariate adjusted model, as shown in Table 3.

Discussion

Saudi Arabia is known to be one of the top countries worldwide with a high prevalence of diabetes, and similarly high rate of obesity that has a direct effect on more than one third of its adult population [17]. In addition, the prevalence of other components of metabolic syndrome is reaching soaring heights in the Kingdom [14]. Therefore, with such a high prevalence of the various components of metabolic syndrome, the prevalence of metabolic syndrome in Saudi Arabia would be expected to exceed that is reported in other countries. The current study shows the prevalence of metabolic

Table 2 Prevalence of metabolic syndrome (95%CI) and its components according to age and sex strata

Age groups	Abdominal obesity	Elevated blood pressure	Elevated blood glucose	Elevated triglycerides	Low HDL cholesterol	Metabolic syndrome	
						IDF	NCEP-ATP III
Total							
18-29 years	25.3(24.1-26.5)	12.0 (11.2-12.9)	25.0(23.8-26.2)	22.0(20.85-23.11)	75.7 (74.5-76.9)	13.4(12.4-14.3)	19.6(18.5-20.7)
30-39 years	51.4(49.5-53.3)	24.7(23.0-26.3)	34.6(32.7-36.4)	38.83(37.0-40.7)	80.2(78.6-81.7)	33.8(31.96-35.6)	42.7(40.8-44.6)
40-49 years	66.3(64.3-68.3)	38.6(36.5-40.6)	46.8(44.7-48.8)	41.55(39.5-43.6)	81.4(79.8-83.0)	49.4(47.3-51.5)	57.9(55.8-59.9)
50-59 years	70.4(67.7-73.2)	53.31(50.3-56.3)	56.5(53.6-59.5)	42.4(39.4-45.3)	82.2(79.96-84.5)	56.3(53.3-49.2)	66.8(64.0-69.6)
60-69 years	69.8(66.1-73.5)	63.4(59.4-67.3)	59.9(55.9-63.9)	44.0(39.9-48.0)	79.8(76.5-83.1)	58.5(54.4-62.5)	71.0(67.3-74.7)
≥ 70 years	59.7(54.9-64.4)	66.8(62.2-71.4)	57.7(52.9-62.5)	38.4(33.6-43.1)	78.7(74.7-82.7)	50.7 (45.9-55.6)	65.8(61.2-70.5)
Men							
18-29 years	27.7(25.9-29.5)	16.5(15.0-18.0)	28.4(26.6-30.3)	28.4(26.6-30.2)	71.0(69.2-72.9)	16.4(14.9-17.9)	24.4(22.7-26.2)
30-39 years	52.4(49.6-55.1)	30.4 (27.9-32.9)	41.4(38.7-44.1)	49.61(49.9-52.4)	77.6(75.3-79.9)	39.26(36.7-41.94)	51.7(49.0-54.5)
40-49 years	63.1(60.0-66.1)	41.2(38.1-44.3)	49.2(46.0-52.3)	51.1(47.9-54.3)	77.3(74.6-80.0)	49.5(46.3-52.7)	60.3(57.2-63.4)
50-59 years	68.9(64.9-72.9)	58.2(54.0-62.4)	57.4(53.2-61.7)	49.6(45.3-53.9)	79.8(76.3-83.2)	57.25(53.0-61.5)	70.8(66.9-74.7)
60-69 years	69.2(64.1-74.3)	61.9(56.5-67.3)	58.7(53.3-64.2)	47.0(41.5-52.5)	75.2(70.5-80.0)	58.7(53.3-64.2)	71.11(66.1-76.1)
≥ 70 years	55.9(48.8-63.1)	66.7(59.9-73.4)	59.7(52.6-66.7)	43.0(35.9-50.1)	69.4(62.7-76.0)	45.2(38.0-52.3)	61.8(54.9-68.8)
Women							
18-29 years	23.3(21.7-24.8)	8.40(7.38-9.42)	22.18(20.7-23.7)	16.77(15.4-18.1)	79.53(78.1-81.0)	10.9(9.8-12.1)	15.7(14.3-17.0)
30-39 years	50.5(47.9-53.1)	19.4(17.3-21.4)	28.3(25.9-30.6)	28.9(26.5-31.3)	82.5(80.5-84.5)	28.7(26.3-31.5	34.3(31.8-36.8)
40-49 years	68.7(66.1-71.3)	36.6(34.0-39.3)	45.0(42.2-47.7)	34.5(31.9-37.1)	84.5(82.5-86.5)	49.3(46.6-52.1)	56.1(53.3-58.8)
50-59 years	71.9(68.2-75.6)	48.8(44.6-52.9)	55.7(51.6-58.8)	35.6(31.6-39.6)	84.5(81.5-87.5)	55.3(51.2-59.5)	63.0(59.0-67.0)
60-69 years	70.5(65.0-76.1)	65.1(59.3-70.9)	61.2(55.3-67.2)	40.3(34.3-46.3)	85.3(81.0-89.6)	58.1(52.1-64.2)	70.9(65.4-76.5)
≥ 70 years	62.8(56.4-69.3)	67.0(60.7-73.2)	56.0(49.4-62.6)	34.4(28.1-40.7)	86.7(82.2-91.2)	55.5(48.9-62.1)	69.27(63.15-75.39)

NCEP-ATP-III;, National Cholesterol Education Program and Adult Treatment Panel III, HDL; high density lipoprotein, IDF; International Diabetes Federation, LDL; low density lipoprotein

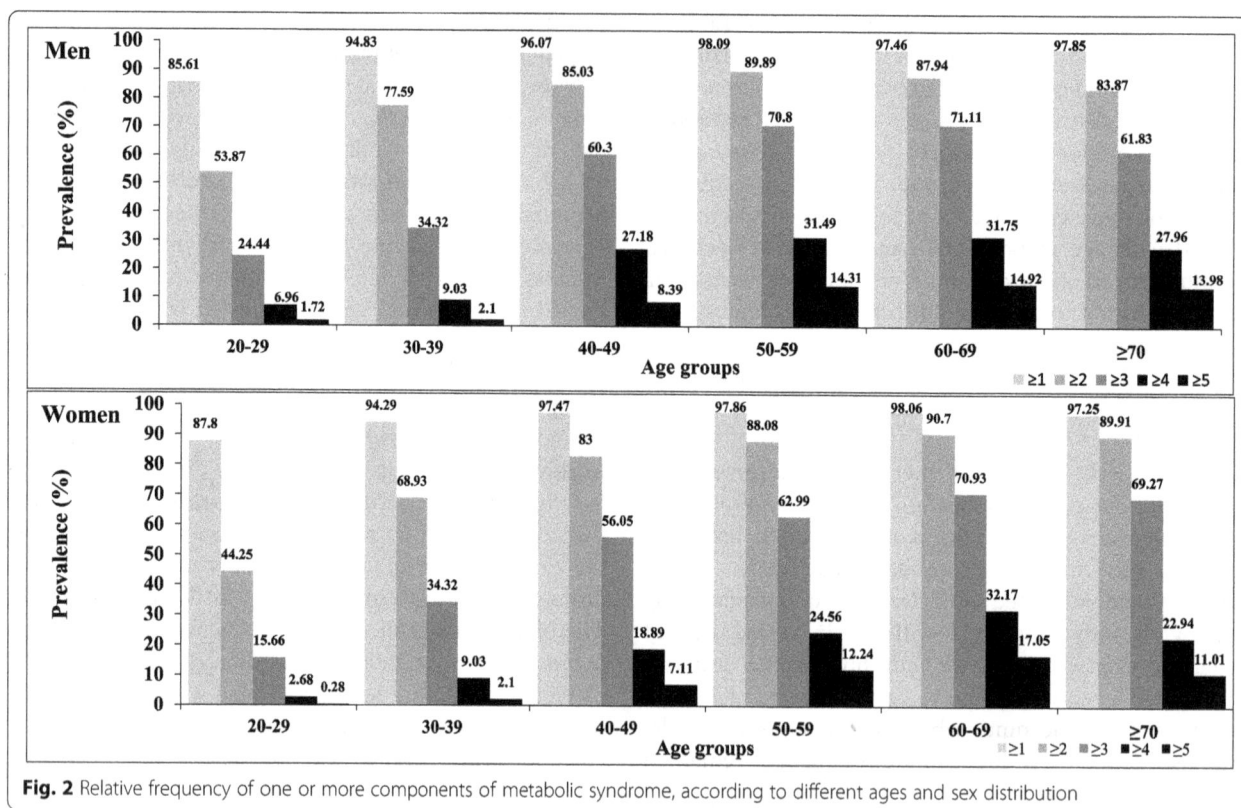

Fig. 2 Relative frequency of one or more components of metabolic syndrome, according to different ages and sex distribution

syndrome in Saudi Arabia to be 39.8% according to the ATP III criteria and 31.6% according to the IDF criteria, when local waist circumference cutoff values have been implemented [16]. Gulf countries that have passed through similar socio-economic transitions have also shown similar levels of prevalence of metabolic syndrome, in spite of the use of lower cutoff values for waist circumference in both men and women in the current study [18–20]. The prevalence of metabolic syndrome in these countries ranged from 33.7% [21] to 40.5% according to the IDF criteria [13], and from 17% [12] to 39.6% [11] according to the ATP III criteria. The prevalence of metabolic syndrome reported in other MENA countries show a comparatively lower prevalence. The prevalence in Iran was reportedly 32.1% and 33.2% in 2006, according to the IDF and ATP III criteria, respectively [22]; and that in Tunisia it was 30.0% according to the ATP III criteria [23].

These findings indicate that in terms of the prevalence of metabolic syndrome, Saudi Arabia is one of the leading MENA countries. The prevalence of metabolic syndrome among the Saudi population is also higher than that reported among ethnicities, such as the adult Spanish [24] and Australian [25] populations, in which the prevalence is reported as 31.0% for Spaniards and 30.7% for Australians, according to the ATP III and IDF

Table 3 Risk factors for metabolic syndrome odds ratio (95% CI) assessment with sex and gender and multivariate adjustment

Number of components factors	Unadjusted OR (95% CI)	Age and sex Adjusted OR (95% CI)	Multivariate OR (95% CI)
Age ≥ 45 years	4.4(4.0-4.8)	–	3.9(3.4-4.5)
Male gender	1.5(1.39-1.60)	–	2.0(1.8-2.3)
Smoking	1.6(1.4-1.8)	1.2(1.0-1.4)	1.4(1.1-1.6)
High monthly income	1.1(1.0-1.2)	1.2(1.1-1.3)	1.1(1.0-1.2)
Low educational level	1.5(1.4-1.7)	1.1(1.0-1.2)	1.3(1.1-1.5)
Urban residency	1.0(1.0-1.1)	1.2(1.0-1.2)	1.1(1.0-1.3)
Body mass index	1.6(1.1-1.2)	1.1 (1.13-1.15)	1.2(1.1-1.2)
Family history of diabetes mellitus	1.0(1.0-1.1)	1.3(1.2-1.4)	1.0(0.9-1.1)
Family history of hypertension	1.0(1.0-1.1)	1.3(1.2-1.4)	1.2(1.1-1.4)

OR; odds ratio, CI; confidence interval. Adjustement was performed for all factors listed in the table

criteria, respectively. In addition, the prevalence of metabolic syndrome in the Saudi population, according to the revised ATP III criteria, was higher than that reported in Korea and South Asia [26, 27], despite of the use of lower Asian-specific cutoff values for abdominal obesity of 90 cm and 80 cm for men and women, respectively.

The current study shows that men were more frequently affected by metabolic syndrome than women, based on both sets of criteria. These findings are inconsistent with those reported among the Caucasian ethnicity [28]. The male predominance observed in the current study could be explained by the higher frequency of diabetes, hypertension, hypertriglyceridemia, and smoking among men in Saudi society, as compared to other ethnicities [15, 29–31]. Furthermore, the waist circumference cutoff values that were used for men in the community under study were lower than those proposed by the ATP III and IDF [2, 3]. However, this was not the case for women, as the waist circumference cutoff values used for Saudi women were higher than those specified by the IDF criteria, and closer to those of the ATP III criteria [16]. Another reason behind the low prevalence of metabolic syndrome among women in Saudi society is the lower rate of smoking among Saudi women. This protects them from the negative effects of tobacco smoking on the emergence of several metabolic disorders, including the more serious insulin resistance, hyperinsulinemia, and increased waist circumference [32].

Women in this cohort, older than 70 years of age, had a higher prevalence of metabolic syndrome than men. This could be explained on one hand by the postmenopausal estrogen withdrawal effect that increases the prevalence of chronic diseases [33], and on the other hand by the poor survival observed among men with metabolic syndrome at a younger age. In addition, this study highlighted the fact that being male was a significant and independent risk factor for metabolic syndrome, until the age of 70 years.

Similar to the observations reported in the NHANES study [34], the prevalence of metabolic syndrome in the current study increased with age, reaching its peak in the sixth and the seventh decades, and decreased thereafter. This might be because age is associated with hormonal alterations, increased visceral obesity, and insulin resistance [35]. Another explanation for such age-dependent increases in the prevalence of metabolic syndrome is the parallel increase in the prevalence of the distinct components of metabolic syndrome, mainly diabetes and hypertension, with age in the Saudi population [15, 29]. In addition, the current study shows that age is a significant and independent risk factor for metabolic syndrome.

Low HDL cholesterol was the most frequent component of metabolic syndrome observed in the current study, and this finding has also been reported in other population-based studies in South Asia [26] and the Middle East [22, 36]. Low HDL cholesterol was observed more frequently in women; a finding that is consistent with most of the other studies conducted among different ethnicities [22, 36]. This observation could be explained by the higher rate of abdominal obesity observed among women in the current study, a factor that is known to lower HDL values [37]. In the present cohort, 43.4% of the participants had more than two risk factors for metabolic syndrome, a number that is higher than that observed among Omanis [38], but lower than that observed among Kuwaitis [36]. These subjects represent a high-risk group for the development of metabolic syndrome. This warrants early intervention to prevent the progression of this very expensive and even life-threatening syndrome, by adopting alternative measures that include lifestyle modifications.

Living in urban areas and a lower education level were significant risk factors for metabolic syndrome in Saudi society, a finding that is similar to those observed in other ethnicities [39–41]. This significant association is expected, because urbanization is associated with an increased prevalence of cardiovascular risk factors, such as hypertension, obesity, and dyslipidemia, as it offers economic improvement to the rural population and exposes them to additional health risks, including a poor diet and sedentary lifestyle [40, 41]. Such effects of urbanization are obvious in populations that have experienced rapid urbanization and swift lifestyle changes, such as those in Saudi Arabia and other Gulf countries [42]. The significant association between a low educational level and metabolic syndrome could be mediated by other risk factors, such as smoking and high carbohydrate intake [23].

No significant effect of a high monthly income on metabolic syndrome was noted in the current study. This finding was unexpected and differed from previous reports of other Gulf countries; however, it is in line with the inconsistency observed in the reported relationship between a high-income status and the development of metabolic syndrome [7, 20].

The current study gains its strength from the fact that it was a nationwide study with a large number of participants. Another strength of the current study was the use of a clear case definition that was based on diagnostic confirmation, using blood tests to identify diabetic and dyslipidemic cases, and country-specific waist circumference cutoff values. However, the study was limited by the fact that it was a cross-sectional study; thus, the causal relationship between metabolic syndrome and certain risk factors could not be elicited. The study was also compromised by the exclusion of physical activity and dietary assessments, both of which are important contributing factors for metabolic syndrome.

Conclusions

In conclusion, this study places Saudi Arabia as one of the countries with the highest prevalence of metabolic syndrome. Although the risk factors for metabolic syndrome in Saudi society were similar to those reported internationally, men were particularly at a greater risk of having metabolic syndrome. A high income had no effect on the prevalence of metabolic syndrome; thus, any prevention program should not consider income as a selection factor.

These findings are startling and should alert policy makers in Saudi Arabia to consider the implementation of preventive lifestyle interventions that include smoking cessation and weight control programs. Furthermore, in order to prevent metabolic syndrome, policy makers should consider the promotion of a healthy diet and physical activity in the planning of future health care strategies in Saudi Arabia.

Abbreviations

BMI: Body mass index; CHD: Coronary heart disease; CI: Confidence intervals; DBP: Diastolic blood pressure; FPG: Fasting plasma glucose; HDL: High-density lipoprotein; IDF: International Diabetes Federation; IRB: Institutional Review Board; LDL: Low-density lipoprotein; MENA: Middle East and North Africa; NCEP ATP III: National Cholesterol Education Program and Adult Treatment Panel III; NHANES: National Health and Nutrition Examination Survey; OR: Odds ratio; PHCC: Primary health care center; SAUDI-DM: Saudi Abnormal Glucose Metabolism and Diabetes Impact Study; SBP: Systolic blood pressure; SD: Standard deviation; UAE: United Arab Emirates; WHR: Waist-to-hip ratio

Acknowledgments

The authors thank the professionals of the centers that assisted in data collection and all the participating patients.

Funding

This study was funded by the University Diabetes Center at King Saud University, Ministry of Health, and the Tawuniya Company for health insurance.

Authors' contributions

KA, YA, NB, and AMY designed the study, wrote the manuscript, designed figures, interpreted data, and critically revised the article. AAA HMA, BA, FIA, KAN, KAS researched data, wrote the manuscript, and critically revised the article. All authors read and approved the final manuscript

Competing interests

The authors declare that they have no competing interests.

Author details

[1]University Diabetes Center, College of Medicine, King Saud University, PO Box 18397, Riyadh, Riyadh 11415, Saudi Arabia. [2]Nutrition Department, University Diabetes Center, King Saud University, Riyadh, Saudi Arabia. [3]Registry Department, University Diabetes Center, King Saud University, Riyadh, Saudi Arabia. [4]College of Medicine, King Saud University, Riyadh, Saudi Arabia.

References

1. Reaven GM. Role of insulin resistance in human disease. Diabetes. 1988;37: 1595–607.
2. Grundy SM, Cleeman JI, Daniels SR, Donato KA, Eckel RH, Franklin BA, et al. Diagnosis and management of the metabolic syndrome: an American Heart Association/National Heart, Lung, and Blood Institute scientific statement. Circulation. 2005;112:2735–52.
3. Alberti KGMM, Zimmet P, Shaw J. IDF epidemiology task force consensus group. The metabolic syndrome–a new worldwide definition. Lancet. 2005; 366:1059–62.
4. Grundy SM, Brewer HB Jr, Cleeman JI, Smith SC Jr, Lenfant C. National Heart, Lung, and Blood Institute; American Heart Association. Definition of metabolic syndrome: report of the National Heart, Lung, and Blood Institute/American Heart Association conference on scientific issues related to definition. Arterioscler Thromb Vasc Biol. 2004;24:e13–8.
5. Malik S, Wong ND, Franklin SS, Kamath TV, L'Italien GJ, Pio JR, et al. Impact of the metabolic syndrome on mortality from coronary heart disease, cardiovascular disease, and all causes in United States adults. Circulation. 2004;110:1245–50.
6. International Diabetes Federation: IDF Worldwide Definition of the Metabolic Syndrome. http://www.idf.org/metabolic-syndrome Accessed 13 Feb 2017.
7. Kaur J. A comprehensive review on metabolic syndrome. Cardiol Res Pract. 2014; https://doi.org/10.1155/2014/943162.
8. Ford ES. Prevalence of the metabolic syndrome defined by the international diabetes federation among adults in the U.S. Diabetes Care. 2005;28:2745–9.
9. Waterhouse DF, McLaughlin AM, Sheehan F, O'Shea D. An examination of the prevalence of IDF- and ATPIII-defined metabolic syndrome in an Irish screening population. Ir J Med Sci. 2009;178:161–6.
10. Zhao Y, Yan H, Yang R, Li Q, Dang S, Wang Y. Prevalence and determinants of metabolic syndrome among adults in a rural area of Northwest China. PLoS One. 2014;9:e91578.
11. Bouguerra R, Alberti H, Smida H, Salem LB, Rayana CB, El Atti J, et al. Waist circumference cut-off points for identification of abdominal obesity among the Tunisian adult population. Diabetes Obes Metab. 2007;9:859–68.
12. Al-Lawati JA, Mohammed AJ, Al-Hinai HQ, Jousilahti P. Prevalence of the metabolic syndrome among Omani adults. Diabetes Care. 2003;26:1781–5.
13. Malik M, Razig SA. The prevalence of the metabolic syndrome among the multiethnic population of the United Arab Emirates: a report of a national survey. Metab Syndr Relat Disord. 2008;6:177–86.
14. Al-Nozha M, Al-Khadra A, Arafah MR, Al-Maatouq MA, Khalil MZ, Khan NB, et al. Metabolic syndrome in Saudi Arabia. Saudi Med J. 2005;26:1918–25.
15. Al-Rubeaan K, Al-Manaa H, Khoja T, Ahmad N, Al-Sharqawi A, Siddiqui K, et al. The Saudi abnormal glucose metabolism and diabetes impact study (SAUDI-DM). Ann Saudi Med. 2014;34:465–75.
16. Al-Rubean K, Youssef AM, AlFarsi Y, Al-Sharqawi AH, Bawazeer N, AlOtaibi MT, et al. Anthropometric cutoff values for predicting metabolic syndrome in a Saudi community: from the SAUDI-DM study. Ann Saudi Med. 2017;37: 21–30.
17. Al-Nozha MM, Al-Mazrou YY, Al-Maatouq MA, Arafah MR, Khalil MZ, Khan NB, et al. Obesity in Saudi Arabia. Saudi Med J. 2005;26:824–9.
18. Khader Y, Bateiha A, El-Khateeb M, Al-Shaikh A, Ajlouni K. High prevalence of the metabolic syndrome among northern Jordanians. J Diabetes Complicat. 2007;21:214–9.
19. Al-Shaibani H, El-Batish M, Sorkhou I, Al-Shamali N, Al-Namash H, Habiba S, et al. Prevalence of insulin resistance syndrome in a primary health care center in Kuwait. Fam Med. 2004;36:540.
20. Mabry RM, Reeves MM, Eakin EG, Owen N. Gender differences in prevalence of the metabolic syndrome in gulf cooperation council countries: a systematic review. Diabet Med. 2010;27:593–7.
21. Bener A, Zirie M, Musallam M, Khader YS, Al-Hamaq AOAA. Prevalence of metabolic syndrome according to adult treatment panel III and international diabetes federation criteria: a population-based study. Metab Syndr Relat Disord. 2009;7:221–9.

22. Zabetian A, Hadaegh F, Azizi F. Prevalence of metabolic syndrome in Iranian adult population, concordance between the IDF with the ATPIII and the WHO definitions. Diabetes Res Clin Pract. 2007;77:251–7.

23. Belfki H, Ben Ali S, Aounallah-Skhiri H, Traissac P, Bougatef S, Maire B, et al. Prevalence and determinants of the metabolic syndrome among Tunisian adults: results of the transition and health impact in North Africa (TAHINA) project. Public Health Nutr. 2013;16:582–90.

24. Fernández-Bergés D, Cabrera de León A, Sanz H, Elosua R, Guembe MJ, Alzamora M, et al. Metabolic syndrome in Spain: prevalence and coronary risk associated with harmonized definition and WHO proposal. DARIOS study. Rev Esp Cardiol (Engl Ed). 2012;65:241–8.

25. Cameron AJ, Magliano DJ, Zimmet PZ, Welborn T, Shaw JE. The metabolic syndrome in Australia: prevalence using four definitions. Diabetes Res Clin Pract. 2007;77:471–8.

26. Aryal N, Wasti SP. The prevalence of metabolic syndrome in South Asia: a systematic review. Int J Diabetes Dev Ctries. 2016; http://doi.org/10.1007/s13410-015-0365-5.

27. Hong AR, Lim S. Clinical characteristics of metabolic syndrome in Korea, and its comparison with other Asian countries. J Diabetes Investig. 2015;6:508–15.

28. O'Neill S, O'Driscoll L. Metabolic syndrome: a closer look at the growing epidemic and its associated pathologies. Obes Rev. 2015;16:1–12.

29. Al-Nozha MM, Abdullah M, Arafah MR, Khalil MZ, Khan NB, Almazrou YY, et al. Hypertension in Saudi Arabia. Saudi Med J. 2007;28:77–84.

30. Al-Nozha MM, Arafah MR, Al-Maatouq MA, Khalil MZ, Khan NB, Al-Marzouki K, et al. Hyperlipidemia in Saudi Arabia. Saudi Med J. 2008;29:282–7.

31. Bassiony MM. Smoking in Saudi Arabia. Saudi Med J. 2009;30:876–81.

32. Sun K, Liu J, Ning G. Active smoking and risk of metabolic syndrome: a meta-analysis of prospective studies. PLoS One. 2012;7:e47791.

33. Rosano GMC, Vitale C, Marazzi G, Volterrani M. Menopause and cardiovascular disease: the evidence. Climacteric. 2007;10(1):19–24.

34. Park YW, Zhu S, Palaniappan L, Heshka S, Carnethon MR, Heymsfield SB. The metabolic syndrome: prevalence and associated risk factor findings in the US population from the third National Health and nutrition examination survey, 1988-1994. Arch Intern Med. 2003;163:427–36.

35. Boden G, Chen X, DeSantis RA, Kendrick Z. Effects of age and body fat on insulin resistance in healthy men. Diabetes Care. 1993;16:728–33.

36. Al Zenki S, Al Omirah H, Al Hooti S, Al Hamad N, Jackson RT, Rao A, et al. High prevalence of metabolic syndrome among Kuwaiti adults–a wake-up call for public health intervention. Int J Environ Res Public Health. 2012;9:1984–96.

37. Després JP, Tremblay A, Pérusse L, Leblanc C, Bouchard C. Abdominal adipose tissue and serum HDL-cholesterol: association independent from obesity and serum triglyceride concentration. Int J Obes. 1988;12:1–13.

38. Al-Lawati JA, Jousilahti P. Body mass index, waist circumference and waist-to-hip ratio cut-off points for categorisation of obesity among Omani Arabs. Public Health Nutr. 2008;11:102–8.

39. Kim MH, Kim MK, Choi BY, Shin YJ. Educational disparities in the metabolic syndrome in a rapidly changing society–the case of South Korea. Int J Epidemiol. 2005;34:1266–73.

40. Vorster HH. The emergence of cardiovascular disease during urbanisation of Africans. Public Health Nutr. 2002;5:239–43.

41. Zhu YG, Ioannidis JPA, Li H, Jones KC, Martin FL. Understanding and harnessing the health effects of rapid urbanization in China. Environ Sci Technol. 2011;45:5099–104.

42. United Nations - Population Division - Department of Economic and Social Affairs. World Urbanization Prospects 2014. https://esa.un.org/unpd/wup/. Accessed 13 Feb 2017.

9

Association of retinol binding protein 4 and transthyretin with triglyceride levels and insulin resistance in rural thais with high type 2 diabetes risk

Karunee Kwanbunjan[1*], Pornpimol Panprathip[1], Chanchira Phosat[2], Noppanath Chumpathat[3], Naruemon Wechjakwen[4], Somchai Puduang[1], Ratchada Auyyuenyong[5], Ina Henkel[6] and Florian J. Schweigert[6]

Abstract

Background: Retinol binding protein 4 (RBP4), a protein secreted by adipocytes and bound in plasma to transthyretin (TTR), has been associated with obesity, the early phase of insulin resistance, metabolic syndrome, and type 2 diabetes mellitus. The objective of this study was to elucidate the relationship between RBP4, TTR, triglyceride (TG) and type 2 diabetes risk in rural Thailand.

Methods: We measured the serum RBP4, TTR, glucose, triglyceride and insulin levels, and glucose tolerance of 167 volunteers from Sung Noen District, Nakhon Ratchasima Province, Thailand. Student's t-test, Pearson's correlation and logistic regression analysis were used to evaluate the relationships between RBP4, TTR and type 2 diabetes markers.

Results: RBP4 and TTR levels, as well as homeostatic model assessment of insulin resistance (HOMA-IR) values, were significantly elevated among subjects with high triglyceride levels ($p < 0.01$, $p < 0.05$, $p < 0.05$, respectively). Triglyceride levels correlated with RBP4 ($r = 0.34$, $p < 0.001$) and TTR ($r = 0.26$, $p < 0.01$) levels, as well as HOMA-IR values ($r = 0.16$, $p < 0.05$). After adjustment for age and gender, the risk of hypertriglyceridemia was 3.7 times greater (95% CI = 1.42–9.73, $p = 0.008$) in the highest RBP4 tertile as compared to the lowest tertile. Similarly, the highest TTR and HOMA-IR tertiles had greater risk of hypertriglyceridemia at 3.5 (95% CI = 1.30–9.20, $p = 0.01$) and 3.6 (95% CI = 1.33–9.58, $p = 0.01$) times higher than the respective lowest tertiles. The correlation between TTR and blood glucose was statistically significant ($r = 0.18$, $p < 0.05$), but not found this relationship in RBP4.

Conclusions: The associations of RBP4 and TTR with hypertriglyceridemia and insulin resistance may have important implications for the risk of heart disease and stroke.

Keywords: RBP4, TTR, HOMA-IR, Hypertriglyceridemia, Type 2 diabetes

Background

Retinol binding protein (RBP4) is an adipokine that may be linked to type 2 diabetes (T2DM), which leads to cardiovascular disease (CVD). Several studies have reported elevated plasma RBP4 in T2DM subjects with obesity [1], impaired glucose tolerance [2–4], and T2DM with nephropathy [5]. RBP4 has also been found to affect the insulin signaling cascade, leading to insulin resistance. This adipokine is also associated with CVD, a complication induced by diabetes. While it has been shown that elevated serum RBP4 levels manifest in the development of systemic insulin resistance in rats [6], evidence for an effect of RBP4 on obesity and insulin resistance in humans is controversial. Studies have reported early states of T2DM with both increased and decreased levels of RBP4 [7–10]. Transthyretin (TTR), a transport protein, carries RBP4 and the thyroid hormone, thyroxin (T4), through the blood [11].

* Correspondence: karunee.kwa@mahidol.ac.th
[1]Department of Tropical Nutrition and Food Science, Faculty of Tropical Medicine, Mahidol University, Bangkok 10400, Thailand
Full list of author information is available at the end of the article

Recently, a human study found that circulatory RBP4 and TTR is associated with glucose intolerance and obesity, and T2DM and RBP4 is associated with insulin resistance [12].

Elevated plasma triglyceride (TG) concentration is a common biochemical finding associated with insulin resistance and is a valuable clinical marker of the metabolic syndrome. Observational and meta-analytic studies have shown relationships between increased cardiovascular risk and hypertriglyceridemia [13–15]. Numerous and complex cases of dyslipidemia, hypertension, hypercoagulability, and atherosclerosis are linked with insulin resistance. The inability of insulin-resistant fat cells to store TG is very likely the initial step in the development of the dyslipidemia. Based on in-vitro studies, short-term increases in insulin levels are associated with increased TG synthesis [16].

Metabolic syndrome consists of a clustering of several metabolic risk factors in an individual and is a major component of atherogenic dislipidemia, increased blood pressure, elevated glucose, and a prothrombotic state [17]. T2DM is a major public health problem in Thailand, with over 4 million cases of diabetes reported in 2015 [18, 19]. CVD has been the leading cause of death for over a decade and diabetes is likely to be an important factor in the vascular disease burden [20–22]. The objective of the present study was to investigate whether RBP4 and TTR are associated with insulin resistance, prediabetes and triglyceride levels in rural Thais with high T2DM risk.

Methods
Subjects
This cross-sectional study involved 167 participants aged between 35 and 66 years, from Sung Noen District, Nakhon Ratchasima Province, Thailand. Subjects were randomized and free of baseline T2DM and other any chronic diseases. Those pregnant, within a 6-month lactation period, or those regularly taking any medicine or having any infections, were excluded from the study. Informed consent was obtained from the subjects after explaining the study procedures in detail. The study protocol was approved by the Ethics Committee of the Faculty of Tropical Medicine (TMEC 13–073), Mahidol University.

Anthropometric assessment
Each subject was weighed (in kilograms) and measured for height (in meters) to evaluate individual body mass index (BMI, kg/m^2). Waist circumference (WC) and hip circumference (HC) were measured and used to determine waist-to-hip ratio (WHR). A body composition monitor (model HBF-375, Omron Healthcare, Kyoto, Japan) was used to determine each subject's body composition, including percentage of body fat (BF), visceral fat (VF), and muscle.

Measurement of laboratory parameters
Blood samples were taken from the antecubital veins after a fasting period of at least 12 h, and were used to assess fasting blood glucose (FBG), glycohemoglobin (HbA$_{1c}$), fasting insulin, total cholesterol (TC), HDL-c and TG. Another blood sample was taken 2 h after a 75 g oral glucose load to determine glucose tolerance. Blood samples were centrifuged and blood serum was immediately frozen at 80 °C until analysis. FBG, HbA$_{1c}$, 2-h blood glucose (2hBG), and TG were analyzed using a Cobas 6000 analyzer (Roche Diagnostics Ltd., Basel, Switzerland). A human insulin ELISA kit (EMD Millipore, Billerica, MA, USA) was used to measure fasting insulin levels. Insulin resistance was evaluated by the homeostatic model assessment of insulin resistance (HOMA-IR) i.e. HOMA-IR = [Fasting insulin (μIU/mL) × Fasting glucose (mmol/L)] / 22.5.

TC and HDL-c were determined by enzymatic assay (Thermo Fisher Scientific Inc., Waltham, Massachusetts, USA). Levels of TC, HDL-c, and TG were then used to calculate low density lipoprotein cholesterol (LDL-c) using the Friedewald equation i.e. LDL-c = TC − (HDL-c + TG / 5). Serum RBP4 and TTR levels were assessed by non-commercial enzyme-linked immunosorbent assays using polyclonal rabbit anti-human antibodies (DakoCytomation, Hamburg, Germany), as previously described [23]. Both assays were calibrated using the standards obtained from human blood (N Protein Standard SL; Dade Behring, Marburg, Germany).

Dietary assessment
A validated semi-food frequency questionnaire (semi-FFQ) containing checklists of various food and beverages, food portion sizes, and consumption frequencies, was used to estimate dietary intake. Energy, protein, carbohydrate and fat intake were calculated using Nutri-Survey software (version 2007; SEAMEO-TROPMED RCCN, University of Indonesia).

Statistical analysis
Statistical analysis was conducted using SPSS (version 15.0; SPSS, Chicago, IL, USA), with results expressed as mean and standard deviation. A Student's t-test was performed to compare the means between the two groups. Correlations among variables were calculated using Pearson's correlation with the associations estimated using odd ratios (OR) and 95% confidence

intervals (CI) obtained from logistic regression. P values < 0.05 were considered statistically significant.

Results

Biometric and biochemical characteristics of the study groups

The study participants were divided into two groups according to TG level using a 150 mg/dl cut-off point [24]. The group with normal TG levels (TG < 150 mg/dl) contained 110 subjects, with the remaining 57 subjects positive for hypertriglyceridemia (TG ≥ 150 mg/dl). A comparison of age, BMI, WC, HC, WHR, BF, VF, and muscle between normal and high TG subjects is shown in Table 1. Normal and high TG subjects were in the same age range. Body size and composition, measured by BMI, HC, WHR, BF, and muscle, showed no significant differences between normal and high TG groups. Conversely, the central obesity indicators WC and VF were significantly elevated in the high TG group ($p < 0.05$). Likewise, the high TG group had higher diastolic blood pressure readings than the normal TG group ($p = 0.03$), though there were no significant differences between groups for systolic blood pressure, FBG, 2hBG, and HbA$_{1c}$. Regarding lipid profiles, there were no significant differences in TC, HDL-c, or LDL-c between the normal and high TG groups. The results from the semi-FFQ showed that the normal- and high TG groups had similar dietary intake patterns. The average energy intake of the normal TG group was 2404.82 kcal/day, and of the high TG group 2382.24 kcal/day, with carbohydrates constituting the highest proportion by weight (Table 2).

Increased RBP4 and TTR levels and HOMA-IR values in the high TG group

Serum RBP4 and TTR were significantly elevated in the high TG group ($p < 0.05$) (Fig. 1a, b). HOMA-IR values corresponded to the levels of RBP4 and TTR, with the high TG group showing higher HOMA-IR values than the normal TG group ($p = 0.02$) (Fig. 1c). Significant positive correlations were found between serum TG and RBP4 ($r = 0.34$, $p = 0.000$), TTR ($r = 0.26$, $p = 0.001$), and HOMA-IR ($r = 0.16$, $p = 0.039$).

The risk of hypertriglyceridemia was evaluated by multivariate analysis (Table 3). Fasting RBP4 and TTR levels were divided into tertiles, with the lowest tertile being the reference tertile. The results showed that after adjustment for age and gender, individuals with RBP4 levels in the highest tertile had 3.7 times higher risk of developing hypertriglyceridemia than those in the lowest tertile (OR $= 3.71$, 95% CI $= 1.42$–9.73). Similarly, subjects in the highest TTR and HOMA-IR tertiles had 3.5 times (OR $= 3.46$, 95% CI $= 1.30$–9.20) and 3.6 times (OR $= 3.58$, 95% CI $= 1.33$–9.58) higher risk of developing hypertriglyceridemia, respectively, than those in the lowest tertiles.

Association of RBP4, TTR, and HOMA-IR with serum glucose

Pearson correlation coefficients were used to assess the relationship between blood glucose and study parameters. Blood glucose showed a non-significant positive correlation with most of the study parameters, including WHR ($r = 0.031$), systolic ($r = 0.194$) and diastolic ($r = 0.112$) blood pressure, VF ($r = 0.036$),

Table 1 Characteristic of the study group

Variables	Normal TG group ($n = 110$)	High TG group ($n = 57$)	P-value
Gender (male/female)	32/79	15/42	0.80*
Age (year)	46.27 ± 5.92	47.26 ± 5.94	0.31
Hip circumference (cm)	92.35 ± 11.43	94.21 ± 8.34	0.28
Waist-hip ratio	0.89 ± 0.09	0.91 ± 0.06	0.30
Body fat (%)	29.86 ± 7.96	30.59 ± 6.81	0.55
Visceral fat (%)	8.70 ± 5.09	10.48 ± 5.54	0.04
Muscle (%)	26.11 ± 4.05	25.75 ± 3.62	0.57
Systolic blood pressure (mmHg)	122.75 ± 18.58	123.88 ± 20.94	0.72
Diastolic blood pressure (mmHg)	72.55 ± 10.45	76.98 ± 13.53	0.03
Fasting blood glucose (mg/dL)	94.22 ± 13.43	96.18 ± 23.55	0.49
2hBG (mg/dL)	122.67 ± 49.62	137.46 ± 70.90	0.12
HbA$_{1c}$ (%)	5.43 ± 0.67	5.54 ± 1.04	0.43
Total cholesterol (mg/dL)	200.23 ± 58.94	212.14 ± 63.17	0.23
LDL-C (mg/dL)	149.58 ± 61.17	165.63 ± 63.42	0.11
HDL-C (mg/dL)	50.65 ± 14.89	46.51 ± 15.29	0.09

Data are presented as means ±standard deviation unless otherwise specified
P-values were calculated by Student's t-test
*P-value for gender were calculated by Chi-square test

Table 2 Dietary intake of the study group

Variables	Normal group ($n = 110$)	High TG group ($n = 57$)	P-value
Energy intake per day (kcal)	2404.82 ± 681.95	2382.24 ± 815.35	0.87
Protein intake per day (g)	75.76 ± 37.85	69.78 ± 32.82	0.31
Fat intake per day (g)	65.94 ± 39.16	60.58 ± 42.80	0.42
Carbohydrate intake per day (g)	369.59 ± 119.48	377.80 ± 120.19	0.68

Data are presented as means ±standard deviation unless otherwise specified
P-values were calculated by Student's t-test

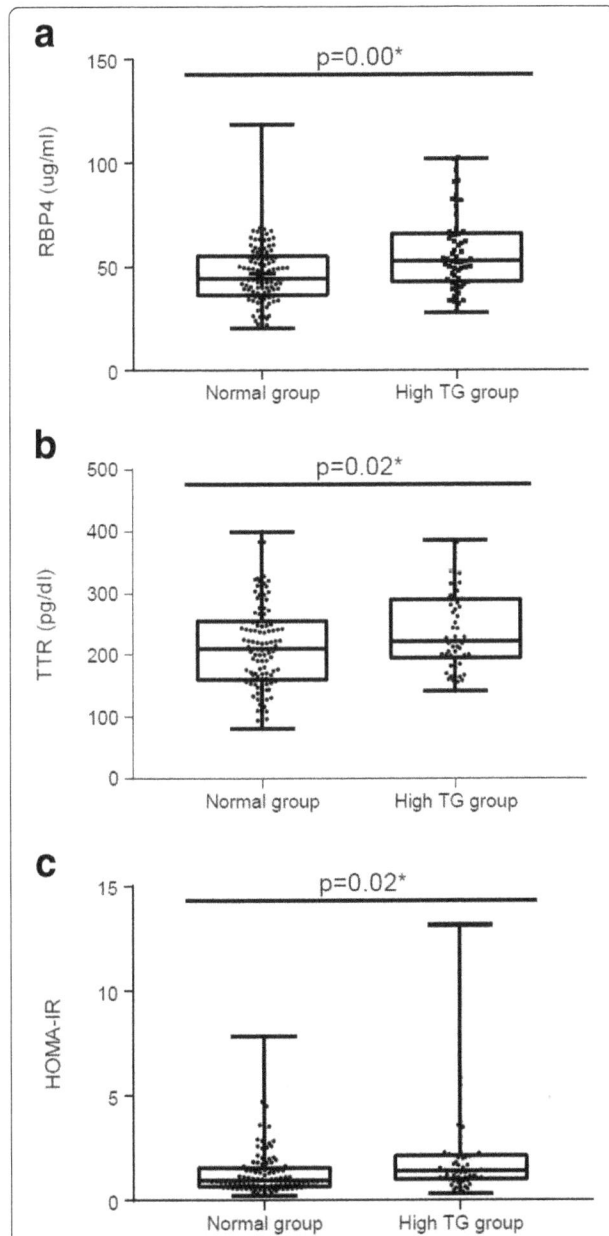

Fig. 1 Comparison of RBP 4 (**a**), TTR levels (**b**) and HOMA-IR (**c**) value between normal- and high TG groups. P-values were calculated by Student's t-test. RBP4: retinal binding protein 4, TTR: transthyretin, HOMA-IR: homeostatic model assessment of insulin resistance

muscle ($r = 0.098$), TC ($r = 0.025$), LDL-c ($r = 0.001$), and HDL-c ($r = 0.095$). To investigate T2DM risk, the study subjects were divided into two groups based on FBG, i.e. normal T2DM risk group (FBG < 100 mg/dl) and high T2DM risk group (FBG≥100 mg/dl). The high T2DM risk group showed increased TTR levels ($p = 0.02$) and HOMA-IR values ($p = 0.03$), as well as decreased RBP4 levels ($p = 0.04$) than the normal T2DM risk group (Table 4).

Correlation between RBP4, TTR, and HOMA-IR with metabolic syndrome parameters

Pearson correlation coefficients were used to assess the relationship between RBP4, TTR, and HOMA-IR, with metabolic syndrome parameters. There were many statistically significant correlations between RBP4, TTR, and HOMA-IR, with metabolic syndrome parameters including RBP4 correlated with TG ($r = 0.344$) and HDL-c ($r = 0.259$); TTR correlated with FBG ($r = 0.182$), TG (r

Table 3 Association between RBP4, TTR, HOMA-IR and risk of hypertriglyceridemia

Variables	Subjects		Odd ratio[a]	95% CI	P-value
	Control	Case			
RBP4 (µg/mL)					
≤ 39.27	33	9	1		
39.28–58.81	57	27	1.67	0.70–4.01	0.25
≥ 58.82	20	21	3.71	1.42–9.73	0.008
	110	57			
TTR (pg/mL)					
≤ 169.26	33	9	1		
169.27–272.51	55	29	2.01	0.84–4.81	0.12
≥ 272.52	22	19	3.46	1.30–9.20	0.01
	110	57			
HOMA-IR					
≤ 0.75	36	9	1		
0.76–1.80	52	29	2.23	0.92–5.39	0.08
≥ 1.81	22	19	3.58	1.33–9.58	0.01
	110	57			

[a]Odd ratios were adjusted by age and gender
95% CI and P-values were calculated by logistics regression model

Table 4 Comparison of RBP4, TTR, and HOMA-IR between normal group and T2DM risk group base on fasting blood glucose levels

Variables	FBG< 100 mg/dL ($n = 122$)	FBG ≥ 100 mg/dL ($n = 45$)	P- value
RBP 4 (µg/mL)	51.87 ± 17.41	45.95 ± 13.74	0.04
TTR (pg/mL)	215.36 ± 67.98	242.65 ± 66.49	0.02
HOMA-IR	1.36 ± 1.42	1.90 ± 1.32	0.03

Data are presented as means ±standard deviation unless otherwise specified
P-values were calculated by Student's t-test

= 0.260), and HDL-c ($r = 0.168$) was also significant; HOMA-IR correlated with FBG ($r = 0.216$), TG ($r = 0.160$), and HDL-c ($r = 0.186$). RBP4 showed a negative correlation with FBG ($r = -0.057$) and a positive correlation with HOMA-IR ($r = 0.134$), but without statistical significance. TTR was also found to be non-statistically significant with HOMA-IR ($r = -0.046$). However, the correlation between TTR and FBG was statistically significant ($r = 0.182$).

Discussion

The subjects with hypertriglyceridemia in this study presented a higher risk of metabolic syndrome due to their above normal TG levels and abdominal obesity indicator values (WC and VF). These subjects may also have increased insulin resistance, since they showed increased HOMA-IR values. Many other investigators have reported that hypertriglyceridemia is closely related to an insulin resistant state. Patients with primary hypertriglyceridemia have increased non-esterified fatty acid turnover rates and secretion by adipose tissue, supplying an excess of fatty acids to the liver for synthesis of TG. This increase suggests that patients with hypertriglyceridemia have insulin resistance at the level of the adipose tissues [25–27]. Björntorp suggests that abdominal obesity is closely linked to insulin resistance, because the mobilized TG in visceral fat creates large amounts of free fatty acid in the portal vein, which can affect liver function and lead to hypertriglyceridemia [28].

There is evidence to suggest that RBP4 and TTR play a role in the development of insulin resistance [1, 12, 29] and metabolic syndrome [30–32]. RBP4 was found to interrupt the insulin signaling cascade causing insulin resistance. In addition, relationships have been found between RBP4 and diabetes complications, such as atherosclerosis and CVD [6]. Several studies have investigated the association of RBP4 with T2DM risk, however the results are conflicting. In a cross-sectional study by Comucci et al., Brazilian subjects with T2DM showed lower RBP4 levels than the control group, though RBP4 was not related to T2DM [33]. TTR functions as a carrier for RBP4, and since hepatic secretion of TTR is affected by dietary protein and energy intake, TTR is also used as a biomarker for assessing nutritional status [34]. TTR levels were reported to be elevated in T2DM subjects and to correlate positively with TG level [30]. Pandey et al. have shown higher circulatory levels of RBP4 and TTR in T2DM subjects, as well as a significant association between T2DM and RBP4 (OR = 1.11, 95% CI: 1.01–1.21) and TTR (OR = 1.34, 95% CI: 1.17–1.55) after adjusting for confounding factors [12]. In the present study, subjects with FBG ≥100 mg/dl had significantly lower serum levels of RBP4 and higher levels of TTR than those with FBG < 100 mg/dl. Moreover, a significant correlation was found between FBG and TTR levels ($p = 0.018$), although the results for a correlation between FBG and RBP4 levels were inconclusive. Moreover, a relationship between RBP4, TTR and metabolic syndrome components was found in this study. Classified by TG level, subjects with high TG showed increased RBP4 and TTR levels, as well as increased HOMA-IR values. In addition, the risk of hypertriglyceridemia was approximately 4-fold greater in subjects with high serum RBP4 and TTR levels and HOMA-IR values. An association between increased levels of both RBP4 and TTR and an elevated risk of insulin resistance (the precursor state to T2DM) and CVD (the macrovascular complication of diabetes) has been reported in several studies [1, 2, 35]. A positive correlation has also been found between plasma RBP4 and TG levels in subjects with T2DM [7, 35, 36]. Hypertriglyceridemia has been independently associated with an elevated risk of CVD [37, 38]. However, while associations between plasma RBP4 levels, TG levels and insulin resistance have been shown in many human studies, while other studies report an insulin resistance-independent association between plasma RBP4 and TG levels [7, 9]. Nevertheless, the results of the present study suggest associations between RBP4, TTR, TG, and insulin resistance. In particular, our results indicate that TTR may play a role in the pathophysiology of diabetic hypertriglyceridemia.

Conclusions

The relationships between RBP4 and TTR levels and FBG abnormalities in this study remain ambiguous. Conversely, our results show a significant association between serum TG levels and insulin resistance. TTR was associated with prediabetes and TG level, whereas RBP4 was only associated with TG. Our findings indicated that RBP4 and TTR are related to hypertriglyceridemia and insulin resistance; therefore, these markers may involve the risk of heart disease and stroke. However, the cross-sectional nature of this study means that these associations reflect a single time point only. A cohort study is therefore required to confirm the associations of these markers with blood glucose and serum TG levels.

Abbreviations
2hBG: 2-h blood glucose; 95% CI: 95% confidence intervals; BF: Body fat; BMI: Body mass index; CVD: Cardiovascular disease; FBG: Fasting blood glucose; HbA1c: Glycated hemoglobin; HC: Hip circumference; HDL-c: High density lipoprotein cholesterol; HOMA-IR: The homeostatic model assessment of insulin resistance; LDL-c: Low density lipoprotein cholesterol; p: p-value; r: Regression coefficient; RBP4: Retinol binding protein 4; Semi-FFQ: Semi-quantitative food frequency questionnaire; T2DM: Type 2 diabetes mellitus; TC: Total cholesterol; TG: Triglyceride; TTR: Transthyretin; VF: Visceral fat; WC: Waist circumference; WHR: Waist to hip ratio

Acknowledgments
We thank the staff at Nong Waeng Promoting Hospital, Thailand and our laboratory-based colleagues from the Institute of Nutritional Science of the University of Potsdam, Germany, especially Ms. Undine Ullrich-Schaare. We also thank our subjects for their participation in our study, and Alice Tait, PhD, from Edanz Group, Mr. Robert Sine and Mr. Paul Adams from ORS, Faculty of Tropical Medicine for English editing of this manuscript.

Funding
This research was supported by Mahidol University and Katholischer Akademischer Ausländer-Dienst (KAAD).

Authors' contributions
KK, PP, CP, NC, NW, SP, RA, IH, FS designed the study. KK, PP, CP, NC, NW, SP, obtained data. KK and PP analyzed and interpreted data. KK, PP, CP, NC, NW, SP, RA, IH, FS provided advice. KK wrote the first draft. All authors read and approved the final manuscript.

Competing interests
The authors declare that they have no competing interest.

Author details
[1]Department of Tropical Nutrition and Food Science, Faculty of Tropical Medicine, Mahidol University, Bangkok 10400, Thailand. [2]Department of Nutrition, Faculty of Public Health, Mahidol University, Bangkok 10400, Thailand. [3]Faculty of Nursing, Huachiew Chalermprakiet University, Samut Prakan 10540, Thailand. [4]Faculty of Public Health, Nakhonratchasima Rajabhat University, Nakhon Ratchasima 30000, Thailand. [5]Department of Food Business and Nutrition, Faculty of Agriculture, Ubon Ratchathani Rajabhat University, Ubon Ratchathani 34000, Thailand. [6]Institute of Nutritional Science, University of Potsdam, 14558 Potsdam, Germany.

References
1. Graham TE, Yang Q, Blüher M, Hammarstedt A, Ciaraldi TP, Henry RR, et al. Retinol-binding protein 4 and insulin resistance in lean, obese, and diabetic subjects. New Engl J Med. 2006;354:2552–63.
2. Cho YM, Youn BS, Lee H, Lee N, Min SS, Kwak SH, et al. Plasma retinol-binding protein-4 concentrations are elevated in human subjects with impaired glucose tolerance and type 2 diabetes. Diabetes Care. 2006;29:2457–61.
3. Chavez AO, Coletta DK, Kamath S, Cromack DT, Monroy A, Folli F, et al. Retinol-binding protein 4 is associated with impaired glucose tolerance but not with whole body or hepatic insulin resistance in Mexican Americans. Am J Physiol Endocrinol Metab. 2009;296:E758–64.
4. Xu M, Li XY, Wang JG, Wang XJ, Huang Y, Cheng Q, et al. Retinol-binding protein 4 is associated with impaired glucose regulation and microalbuminuria in a Chinese population. Diabetologia. 2009;52:1511–9.
5. Murata M, Saito T, Otani T, Sasaki M, Ikoma A, Toyoshima H, et al. An increase in serum retinol-binding protein 4 in the type 2 diabetic subjects with nephropathy. Endocr J. 2009;56:287–94.
6. Li F, Xia K, Sheikh MS, Cheng J, Li C, Yang T. Retinol binding protein 4 promotes hyperinsulinism induced proliferation of rat aortic smooth muscle cells. Mol Med Rep. 2014;9:1634–40.
7. von Eynatten M, Lepper PM, Liu D, Lang K, Baumann M, Nawroth PP, et al. Retinol-binding protein 4 is associated with components of the metabolic syndrome, but not with insulin resistance, in men with type 2 diabetes or coronary artery disease. Diabetologia. 2007;50:1930–7.
8. Kowalska I, Straczkowski M, Adamska A, Nikolajuk A, Karczewska-Kupczewska M, Otziomek E, et al. Serum retinol binding protein 4 is related to insulin resistance and nonoxidative glucose metabolism in lean and obese women with normal glucose tolerance. J Clin Endocrinol Metab. 2008;93:2786–9.
9. Lewis JG, Shand BI, Frampton CM, Elder PA, Scott RS. Plasma retinol-binding protein is not a marker of insulin resistance in overweight subjects: a three year longitudinal study. Clin Biochem. 2008;41:1034–8.
10. Gavi S, Qurashi S, Stuart LM, Lau R, Melendez MM, Mynarcik DC, et al. Influence of age on the association of retinol-binding protein 4 with metabolic syndrome. Obesity (Silver Spring). 2008;16:893–5.
11. Zanotti G, Berni R. Plasma retinol-binding protein: structure and interactions with retinol, retinoids, and transthyretin. Vitam Horm. 2004;69:271–95.
12. Pandey GK, Balasubramanyam J, Balakumar M, Deepa M, Anjana RM, Abhijit S, et al. Altered circulating levels of retinol binding protein 4 and transthyretin in relation to insulin resistance, obesity, and glucose intolerance in Asian Indians. Endocr Pract. 2015;21:861–9.
13. Patel A, Barzi F, Jamrozik K, Lam TH, Ueshima H, Whitlock G, et al. Serum triglycerides as a risk factor for cardiovascular diseases in the Asia-Pacific region. Circulation. 2004;110:2678–86.
14. Sarwar N, Danesh J, Eiriksdottir G, Sigurdsson G, Wareham N, Bingham S, et al. Triglycerides and the risk of coronary heart disease: 10,158 incident cases among 262,525 participants in 29 western prospective studies. Circulation. 2007;115:450–8.
15. Murad MH, Hazem A, Coto-Yglesias F, Dzyubak S, Gupta S, Bancos I, et al. The association of hypertriglyceridemia with cardiovascular events and pancreatitis: a systematic review and meta-analysis. BMC Endocr Disord. 2012;12:2.
16. Henry N. Ginsberg. Insulin resistance and cardiovascular disease. J Clin Invest. 2000;106:453–8.
17. Grundy SM. Hypertriglyceridemia, atherogenic dyslipidemia, and the metabolic syndrome. Am J Cardiol. 1998;81:18B–25B.
18. International Diabetes Federation. Diabetes atlas, 7th edition. 2017. www.idf.org/diabetesatlas. Accessed 21 June 2017.
19. International Diabetes Federation. WP Region. 2017. https://www.idf.org/our-network/regions-members/western-pacific/members/115-thailand.html. Accessed 21 June 2017.
20. World Health Organization. Cardiovascular disease. 2017. http://www.who.int/cardiovascular_diseases/en/. Accessed 21 June 2017.
21. World Health Organization. Noncommunicable Diseases (NCD) Country Profiles. 2014. http://www.who.int/nmh/countries/tha_en.pdf. Accessed 21 June 2017.
22. National Institutes of Health. Metabolic Syndrome. 2017. https://www.nhlbi.nih.gov/health/health-topics/topics/ms. Accessed 21 June 2017.

23. Raila J, Henze A, Spranger J, Mohlig M, Pfeiffer AFH, Schweigert FJ. Microalbuminuria is a major determinant of elevated plasma retinol-binding protein 4 in type 2 diabetic patients. Kidney Int. 2007;72:505–11.

24. National Cholesterol Education Program (NCEP) Expert Panel on Detection, Evaluation, and Treatment of High Blood Cholesterol in Adults (Adult Treatment Panel III). Third report of the National Cholesterol Education Program (NCEP) expert panel on detection, evaluation, and treatment of high blood cholesterol in adults (adult treatment panel III) final report. Circulation. 2002;106:3143–421.

25. Grundy SM. Hypertriglyceridemia, insulin resistance, and the metabolic syndrome. Am J Cardiol. 1999;83(9B):25F–9F.

26. Steiner G. Hyperinsulinaemia and hypertriglyceridaemia. J Intern Med Suppl. 1994;736:23–6.

27. Despres JP. The insulin resistance-dyslipidemic syndrome of visceral obesity: effect on patients' risk. Obes Res. 1998;6:8S–17S.

28. Bjorntorp P. New concepts in the relationship obesity–non-insulin dependent diabetes mellitus. Eur J Med. 1992;1:37–42.

29. Saki F, Ashkani-Esfahani S, Karamizadeh Z. Investigation of the relationship between retinol binding protein 4, metabolic syndrome and insulin resistance in Iranian obese 5-17 year old children. Iran J Pediatr. 2013;23:396–402.

30. Yoshida A, Matsutani Y, Fukuchi Y, Saito K, Naito M. Analysis of the factors contributing to serum retinol binding protein and transthyretin levels in Japanese adults. J Atheroscler Thromb. 2006;13:209–15.

31. Qi Q, Yu Z, Ye X, Zhao F, Huang P, Hu FB, et al. Elevated retinol-binding protein 4 levels are associated with metabolic syndrome in Chinese people. J Clin Endocrinol Metab. 2007;92:4827–34.

32. Mostafaie N, Sebesta C, Zehetmayer S, Jungwirth S, Huber KR, Hinterberger M, et al. Circulating retinol-binding protein 4 and metabolic syndrome in the elderly. Wien Med Wochenschr. 2011;161:505–10.

33. Comucci EB, Vasques AC, Geloneze B, Calixto AR, Pareja JC, Tambascia MA. Serum levels of retinol binding protein 4 in women with different levels of adiposity and glucose tolerance. Arq Bras Endocrinol Metabol. 2014;58:709–14.

34. Ingenbleek Y, Young V. Transthyretin (prealbumin) in health and disease: nutritional implications. Annu Rev Nutr. 1994;14:495–533.

35. Takebayashi K, Suetsugu M, Wakabayashi S, Aso Y, Inukai T. Retinol binding protein-4 levels and clinical features of type 2 diabetes patients. J Clin Endocrinol Metab. 2007;92:2712–9.

36. Cabré A, Lázaro I, Girona J, Manzanares JM, Marimón F, Plana N, et al. The APOA5-1131 T>C variant enhances the association between RBP4 and hypertriglyceridemia in diabetes. Nutr Metab Cardiovasc Dis. 2010;20:243–8.

37. West KM, Ahuja MM, Bennett PH, Czyzyk A, De Acosta OM, Fuller JH, et al. The role of circulating glucose and triglyceride concentrations and their interactions with other "risk factors" as determinants of arterial disease in nine diabetic population samples from the WHO multinational study. Diabetes Care. 1983;6:361–9.

38. Fontbonne A, Eschwège E, Cambien F, Richard JL, Ducimetière P, Thibult N, et al. Hypertriglyceridaemia as a risk factor of coronary heart disease mortality in subjects with impaired glucose tolerance or diabetes. Results from the 11-year follow-up of the Paris prospective study. Diabetologia. 1989;32:300–4.

10

Patients' and caregivers' experiences of using continuous glucose monitoring to support diabetes self-management: qualitative study

J. Lawton[1*], M. Blackburn[1], J. Allen[2,3], F. Campbell[4], D. Elleri[5], L. Leelarathna[6], D. Rankin[1], M. Tauschmann[2,3], H. Thabit[6] and R. Hovorka[2,3]

Abstract

Background: Continuous glucose monitoring (CGM) enables users to view real-time interstitial glucose readings and provides information on the direction and rate of change of blood glucose levels. Users can also access historical data to inform treatment decisions. While the clinical and psychological benefits of CGM are well established, little is known about how individuals use CGM to inform diabetes self-management. We explored participants' experiences of using CGM in order to provide recommendations for supporting individuals to make optimal use of this technology.

Methods: In-depth interviews ($n = 24$) with adults, adolescents and parents who had used CGM for ≥4 weeks; data were analysed thematically.

Results: Participants found CGM an empowering tool because they could access blood glucose data effortlessly, and trend arrows enabled them to see whether blood glucose was rising or dropping and at what speed. This predicative information aided short-term lifestyle planning and enabled individuals to take action to prevent hypoglycaemia and hyperglycaemia. Having easy access to blood glucose data on a continuous basis also allowed participants to develop a better understanding of how insulin, activity and food impacted on blood glucose. This understanding was described as motivating individuals to make dietary changes and break cycles of over-treating hypoglycaemia and hyperglycaemia. Participants also described how historical CGM data provided a more nuanced picture of blood glucose control than was possible with blood glucose self-monitoring and, hence, better information to inform changes to background insulin doses and mealtime ratios. However, while participants expressed confidence making immediate adjustments to insulin and lifestyle to address impending hypoglycaemia and hypoglycaemia, most described needing and expecting health professionals to interpret historical CGM data and determine changes to background insulin doses and mealtime ratios. While alarms could reinforce a sense of hypoglycaemic safety, some individuals expressed ambivalent views, especially those who perceived alarms as signalling personal failure to achieve optimal glycaemic control.

Conclusions: CGM can be an empowering and motivational tool which enables participants to fine-tune and optimize their blood glucose control. However, individuals may benefit from psycho-social education, training and/or technological support to make optimal use of CGM data and use alarms appropriately.

Keywords: Continuous glucose monitoring, Type 1 diabetes, Qualitative, Patient experience, Caregiver experience

* Correspondence: j.lawton@ed.ac.uk
[1]Usher Institute of Population Health Sciences and Informatics, University of Edinburgh, Edinburgh, UK
Full list of author information is available at the end of the article

Background

Continuous glucose monitoring (CGM) enables users to view real-time interstitial glucose readings and provides information on the direction and rate of change of blood glucose levels. Multiple alarms can be set to alert users if blood glucose either rises or falls (or is predicted to rise or fall) beyond predefined target ranges, and individuals are able to access historical data to inform diabetes self-management decisions. CGM is associated with reductions in glycated haemoglobin (HbA1c) levels in both adults and children, especially when used frequently [1–4]. CGM has also been shown to reduce hypoglycaemia and hyperglycaemia [2, 3, 5], severe hypoglycaemia [6]; and, improve treatment satisfaction [7–9] and quality of life outcomes [10, 11].

While the clinical and psychological benefits of CGM are well established, less is known about how individuals use CGM to make informed treatment decisions and why high levels of treatment satisfaction exist. Only limited qualitative research, focusing on user and/or caregiver experiences, has been conducted. This includes work exploring barriers to using, and reasons for discontinuing, CGM in adolescent [12] and adult groups [13]; adult users' attitudes and characteristics which might help predict effective use of CGM [14]; and, how use of CGM may influence couple's diabetes management and marital relationships [15]. More recently, Pickup et al. [16] used an open-ended survey question to explore user and caregiver experiences of CGM, including benefits and drawbacks encountered. While this is the most comprehensive study in terms of scope and sampling, Pickup et al.'s design did not permit user experiences to be explored in detail; hence, they recommended further, in-depth research be undertaken [16]. In line with this recommendation, we conducted in-depth interviews with individuals (adults, adolescents and parents) who made nonadjunctive use of CGM over ≥4 weeks in the initial training phase of a closed-loop study. The aim of this interview study was to understand and explore how participants used CGM to support diabetes self-management and what they considered the main benefits and drawbacks to be. Our objectives were to aid interpretation of findings from earlier CGM studies; and, provide recommendations for supporting individuals using CGM. An additional objective was to collect data to allow comparisons to be drawn with participants' later experiences of using a closed-loop system as part of the trial; these data will be reported separately.

Methods

Participants and devices

Inclusion criteria for trial enrolment included a screening HbA1c ≥7.5% (58.5 mmol/mol) and ≤10% (86 mmol/mol) and a diabetes duration of at least 6 months [17].

Individuals were required to have used an insulin pump for at least 3 months, with good knowledge of insulin self-adjustment as judged by the investigator [17]. Individuals were ineligible for the trial if they had used CGM regularly in the previous three months.

Following trial recruitment, participants were trained to use the study insulin pump (MiniMed™ 640G pump, Medtronic, Northridge, CA, USA) and glucose sensor (Guardian™ Sensor 3, Medtronic by health care professionals who followed a common outline curriculum. Key areas covered in the training included: an insertion and initiation of sensor session, using the sensor menu of the insulin pump and sensor calibrations, use of software to analyse CGM data and use of CGM data to optimise treatment. Written guidelines for the operation and use of the CGM device were also provided in the form of the manufacturer's user manual. Alarm settings on the CGM device were initially standardized but participants were allowed to adjust these during the study period. Parents/caregivers were unable to remote access their child's CGM data.

Participants who took part in the interview study comprised: individuals aged ≥16 years; individuals aged 13–15 years and their parent(s)/caregiver(s); and, parents/caregivers of those aged ≤12 years. The decision to interview parents/caregivers of those aged ≤12 years and those aged 13–15 years was made because, in younger groups, parents take responsibility for most diabetes management tasks [18], while supporting and sharing responsibility with adolescents [19]. Interviewees were invited to take part in the qualitative study by members of the clinical team in the four participating UK sites (Cambridge, Manchester, Leeds, and Edinburgh). The clinical team informed these individuals that the qualitative research was being conducted by an independent research team and gave them reassurances of confidentiality. Recruitment and data collection continued until there was representation of different age groups in the final sample and data saturation had occurred; that is, until no new findings were identified in new data collected. The study received approval from the independent Cambridge East Research Ethics Committee (REC ref. 15/EE/0324). Participants aged ≥16 years and parents or guardians of participants aged < 16 years provided signed informed consent; written assent was obtained from minors before study-related activities.

Qualitative study design

In-depth interviews were used as the method of data collection, as these afforded the flexibility needed for participants to discuss issues they perceived as salient, including those unforeseen at the study's outset [20], while use of topic guides helped ensure the data collected remained relevant to the study aims and objectives. An inductive approach was used informed by general principles of Grounded Theory research [21]. This entailed simultaneous data collection and analysis, with findings from early interviews informing areas explored in later ones.

Data collection and analysis

Interviews were conducted by MB at a time and location of participants' choosing (mostly in their own homes) immediately before they moved into the main phase of the trial, at which point they had used CGM in real-life situations for a minimum of 4 weeks. Topic guides were developed based on literature reviews, input from clinical team members, and revised in light of emerging findings, in line with an inductive approach. Key areas explored included: previous experience of using CGM and self-monitoring of blood glucose (SMBG); understandings and expectations of CGM and impact of CGM (if any) on diabetes self-management; likes and dislikes of the technology; and views about information and training needed to support effective use of CGM. Patients aged 13–15 years old and their parents were interviewed separately. The interviews took place between July 2016 and May 2017. They typically lasted 1–2 h, were digitally recorded and transcribed in full for in-depth analysis.

Data were analysed by three experienced qualitative researchers (JL, MB and DR) using a thematic approach informed by the method of constant comparison; this entailed cross-comparison of all interviews to identify recurrent themes, before a coding framework was developed to capture these themes and contextual information needed to aid data interpretation. Nvivo, a qualitative software package, was used to facilitate data coding and retrieval and coded datasets were subjected to further analyses to allow more nuanced interpretations of the data to be developed.

Results

The sample comprised 12 participants aged 16+ years, three participants aged 13–15 years and nine parents (see Table 1). A 100% opt-in was achieved. Eighteen interviewees (including six parents of child participants) described having had prior experiences of using CGM (e.g. to manage diabetes or as part of an earlier research study).

Ease of access to continuous data

A key benefit of CGM, as all participants highlighted, was the ease with which they were able to access information about their blood glucose levels. Indeed, it was precisely because this process was so effortless that participants said they were much more aware of what their (or their child's) blood glucose levels were throughout the day than when only SMBG was used:

Table 1 Characteristics of study participants

Participants with type 1 diabetes ($n = 15$)		
Gender, female (n,%)		7(46.7)
Age at recruitment (years)		
	13–15	3
	16–20	2
	21–30	1
	31–40	6
	41–50	2
	51–60	
	60+	1
Occupation/education (n,%)		
	Professional	5(33.3)
	Semi-skilled	4(26.7)
	Retired	1(6.7)
	Higher education	2(13.3)
	Secondary school	3(20)
Self-reported diabetes duration (mean, SD, range - years)		
	≤12 years	4 ± 2.9 (2–9)
	13–17	9.25 ± 3.9 (4.5–13.75)
	18+	25 ± 11.1 (15–45)
Sensor use run-in (% over 4 weeks)		
	≤12 years	81.2 ± 13.8 (64–99)
	13–17	85.6 ± 10.8 (77–98)
	18+	89.9 ± 6.4 (77–97)
Parents of paediatric patients ($n = 9$)[a]		
Gender, female (n,%)		7(77.8)
Age at recruitment (years)		
	31–40	2
	41–50	5
	51–60	2
Occupation (n,%)		
	Professional	5(55.6)
	Semi-skilled	3(33.3)
	Unemployed/Full time Carer	1(11.1)

[a]This includes: parents who represented children aged ≤12 years ($n = 5$) and parents of children aged 13–15 ($n = 4$). In one instance, both parents of a child aged 13–15 participated in an interview

"It's so much easier with anything isn't it, where you can just glance at it. It's, you know, if to tell the time, rather than just glancing at your watch you had to sort of get something out, open it up, fiddle around with it, you wouldn't worry so much about checking the time, would you?" (Parent 6)

Indeed, many participants drew a strong contrast between their experiences of using CGM and those of SMBG with Participant 3, like others, noting the limitations arising from the latter:

"it's [SMBG] frustrating.. cause you don't know what's happening … it's like walking around with a blindfold on. And you can walk into a room every now and then and take the blindfold off for 60 seconds. And then you have to put it back on."

Predicting and managing the future

As Participant 3 went on to elaborate, SMBG was of limited benefit not only because one could not instantly and effortlessly access one's blood glucose levels, but also because it was not possible to establish "whether you're going up or down, and how fast". Indeed, a central benefit of CGM, as all participants observed, were the opportunities trend arrows presented to predict the future by virtue of being able to tell whether their blood glucose was rising or dropping and at what speed. This included Participant 1 who discussed how CGM data, when compared to SMBG results, enabled them to "make more informed decisions on what you're going to do. And probably a lot sooner" because, as they explained, "I can see ok I'm actually going up. I'm going up really quickly. Or I'm coming down, I'm coming down fast, so I need to do something about it. As opposed to just a snapshot."

As various individuals noted, CGM thus helped enable them to pre-empt and prevent hypo- and hyperglycaemia, and thereby achieve more stable blood glucose levels, because, "obviously you're ready before it happens" (Parent 2). Specifically, participants discussed how the predictive information provided by CGM prompted proactive use of corrective insulin doses or consumption of carbohydrate to prevent their (or their child's) blood glucose levels moving out of target ranges:

"if she [teenaged daughter] says: 'oh I don't feel quite right', she can glance at it and think: 'oh yeah I'm going high and I've got an arrow going straight up'. So she can then say: 'oh yeah, actually I need to actually put a bolus in'. And equally if she's got an arrow going straight down, she can say: 'actually although I'm six, I've got an arrow going straight down. So I need something [to eat] within the next 20 minutes, half an hour, otherwise I'm gonna hypo'. So that's good. You can almost stop things happening before they get to the critical point." (Parent 6)

Some individuals also discussed how the predictive information provided by CGM enabled short-term lifestyle

planning, whether this be, as Participant 2 described, by changing the timing of a meal or, in Participant 7's case, reducing the length of a walk, to avoid hypo- or hyperglycaemia:

"It's easier to do the stuff I wanna do, because I can read my pump. I can see: am I going up? Am I going down? Should I have lunch before I do this? Or can I do this before lunch kind of thing?... [using CGM] I can say: oh we'll have lunch in half an hour. Or I can- I'll just finish what I'm doing, or. So I think it's giving me more personal freedom if you like." (Participant 2)

"Yes, the arrow- well that's good for going low. Em, it's a good- great indicator to see that it's- my sugars are actually- they're dropping a little bit faster than I expected. They're maybe dropping according to the graphs, but dropping a lot faster. Em, it means I can get, if I'm out for a walk with the dog, I can think: okay. Right I need to cut the walk short, because I'm going to go low otherwise." (Participant 7)

While individuals described having received some instruction from health professionals on how to interpret and respond to the information provided by trend arrows, most emphasised that they found this information to be intuitive and easy to understand and as having prompted common-sense responses:

"they told me what the arrows mean... But I've- I've kind of taken it upon myself to interpret that into three arrows and active insulin, get something quick, and quick-acting. Em so I've kind of used what I think is my best judgement on that." (Participant 9)

Understanding the impact of lifestyle and insulin on blood glucose levels

Participants also described how having easy access to CGM data on a continuous basis had enabled them to develop a much better understanding of how insulin, food and physical activity impacted on their blood glucose levels. As several individuals noted, such information had been an informative and motivational tool which had prompted positive changes to how they had approached and managed their diabetes. This included Participant 10 who described how they had broken a pattern of over-treating hypoglycaemia after 'real time' CGM data had provided evidence and reassurance that a more restrained approached was more efficacious:

"when I'd be treating a low, before I just thought I'll just eat and eat. And, obviously the sensor showed me that when I did that I would just bounce way way back up, too high, because before, you know, I couldn't physically see [this] on my pump with the arrows .. So now I know that I just- I can't eat- I just don't need to eat as much. I don't need to panic as much."

Participant 14, likewise, described adopting a more "patient" approach to their diabetes self-management in light of information provided by CGM, one which meant they were now less likely to over-correct for hyperglycaemia:

"So when I've used the pump to correct for it [high blood glucose] and I can see [from 'real time' CGM data], well actually I probably won't need to, I can probably be a bit more patient and wait for it to catch up. And that's quite helpful because that means I am less likely to have a hypo as a result of overcorrecting."

In another pertinent example, Parent 2 noted how her 12 year old daughter has been motivated to make dietary changes after CGM data had alerted her to how consumption of high sugar foods, such as breakfast cereals, were causing her blood glucose to spike:

"she herself, off her own back, has been able to see, physically see on the line, where something has affected her blood sugar. Whereas before it will have affected it, and, you know, we treat it. But .. cause it's a visual line she can see, that eating something's gonna make her shoot up- it's kind of- I think it's struck a chord, in that she's going: 'well actually, that's not really that good'. So she's making conscious decisions in what she chooses to eat, without any kind of enforcement or- or guiding... changed the type of breakfast she has, so that she- she's been having more smoothies rather than these high sugar, carby breakfasts."

Using the past to improve the future; retrospective analysis of data
Participants also discussed how the retrospective data provided by CGM enabled them to develop insight into their blood glucose control at times when they were much less likely to undertake SMBG, principally when they were asleep. In some cases, being able to examine graphs of night-time readings offered peace of mind that in target and stable blood glucose control was being achieved. In others, such as Participant 14, retrospective review of CGM data had alerted participants to un-known problems with their blood glucose control:

"And you can see what the history's like and the trends and stuff. And I find that really, really helpful, because it's like looking back over the period you've been asleep. And you can see what your blood sugar's been doing... Sometimes you go to bed with a really normal blood sugar and you wake up and it's normal. But over the night it's just done this. And it's like: 'Wow'. Before I would have thought: 'ah pretty good control really (laughs). But there's something weird happening in the middle of the night.'" (Participant 14)

As participants also discussed, having access to graphs which captured historical data provided useful informa-tion which could be used to inform changes to basal rates and/or mealtime ratios:

"So you know, retrospectively you can look up the past couple of weeks and have a look at each day and you can see much better the patterns that come from your blood sugars and then you can adjust your insulin far more easily. ... if you can see a pattern from the CGM charts I can change those instantly, the basal patterns and the ratios far more easily.. to get better stable control." (Participant 3)

Indeed, while participants did note that it was possible to generate data for retrospective analysis using SMBG, because CGM captured data at five minute intervals, it also allowed a much more nuanced and informative pic-ture to be generated than could be captured through periodic snapshots:

"Em, but since I've had the sensor, because I've got continuous points I'm getting a nice clean graph, rather than working off five or six points a day. So I'm able to make a lot better decision, rather than having to check my sugars every 30 minutes to try to get a nice trend pattern, I'm now getting a really good set of results that I can work off." (Participant 7)

Independent and dependent adjustments
However, while participants, including Participant 7, noted the value of the retrospective information pro-vided by CGM, only a minority described having the confidence and ability to use this information to make independent adjustments to pump settings (basal rates) and/or meal time ratios. Indeed, in line with their earlier, pre-trial experiences of using insulin pumps (without CGM) where participants reported experiencing similar difficulties, the majority described both needing and expecting input and help from health professionals prior to changing basal rates and meal ratios. This was not only because participants questioned their own numeric

skills and ability to analyse CGM data, but also because deferring to health professional expertise appeared, for many, to have been a habituated, taken-for-granted practice which pre-dated their use of CGM:.

"It's quite- a quite complicated set up. So yes I have different basal rates, for different times. And we do change that. I don't change it on my own...it's not something I'd do without talking to some other clever girls.... only because I think it is so fundamental of my regime, that I would be worried about changing it without understanding 100% if it should be up or down. So it's more insecurity I think, of my own knowledge about the basal." (Participant 2)

"I see the consultant or the nurse often enough to do that with them...I wouldn't feel that comfortable messing with- the insulin ratio- your insulin to carb ratios... because the ability to look at the data is less so than in the clinic, if that makes sense." (Participant 4)

Some individuals, however, highlighted a need for education and training to make effective and independent use of historical CGM data while others, including Participant 7, pointed to the potential benefits of including pattern recognition software with future CGM devices:

"because I can see so many more variants in the line it makes me more determined to try and work out how to prevent, like monitor and check and find out why we have spikes and troughs ... I'm at the stage- where at the moment I can do one change at a time. I know it just made me more determined to wanna be able to be in more control with her, working out what settings need changing, which is why I asked (names hospital) if they could give me that training." (Parent 2)

"But it's difficult to sort of detect the trends, which is where it's nice in some software where it- it actually highlights stuff that it's noticed." (Participant 7)

Tolerating and experiencing glitches and inaccuracies

In keeping with findings from previous studies [8, 13, 14, 16] participants reported various glitches and frustrations arising from using CGM. These included difficulties inserting and/or removing the device, finding a comfortable and discrete place on the body upon which to locate it, occasional loss of signal and challenges arising from needing to calibrate their devices at regular (12 hourly) intervals, especially when they did not lead routinized lives e.g. due to shift working. Participants, however, always tempered any criticisms with positive remarks and all emphasised that the

clinical and psychological benefits of CGM outweighed any challenges encountered: "Calibration's a pain but, you know, I've just got to do it.... And sort of it's worth the effort" (Participant 4). Participants also indicated that that their tolerance of "technical hitches" (Participant 5) arose partly from their understanding that they were in a clinical trial, and their expectation that, over time, CGM technology would improve. In some cases, this expectation appeared to have resulted from earlier experiences of using CGM and observing developments in its accuracy and usability:

"and I've noticed.. as we've taken part in a lot of trials, these sensors are getting better.. the finger test and the sensor is becoming close and closer. I remember four, five years ago they were wide apart. And you thought, 'well what's the point, you know if it's going to be so widely different.' So we start seeing an improvement in the technology and how accurate the sensor's becoming." (Parent 5)

Alarms

In general, individuals pointed to clear clinical and psychological benefits to alarms alerting them to high/low blood glucose:

"It beeps when you're going high. Having that, just that- that knowledge that you've got something looking out for you, just in case you do miss it, is- is so relieving, like ridiculously good... it's just- just another level of freedom. You just- you know you're safe... yeah, just added security." (Participant 9)

Indeed, in one parent's case, the existence of the alarm was believed to have saved her young child's life:

"So, for instance a week ago, em [child's name has] never had a hypo at 11 o'clock at night, never. I heard an alarm going off and thought: what the hell was that? He'd dropped to 2.2. I wasn't due to test [child's name] until 12 o'clock and I think it was about 11 o'clock. So I would have left him another hour, before I tested him. By then, he could have died or gone into a coma." (Parent 7)

However, others noted how alarms could result in poor or interrupted sleep and/or unwelcomed distractions in the workplace or at school; with various children, including Parent 1's daughter, reportedly switching alarms off in school due to concerns about drawing attention to themselves and distracting peers:

"The thing is she can't really have the alarms at school cause the teacher is not very happy about her beeping. So, and if she does she just stops it so the kids are not looking at her because she's beeping. So it doesn't really have any kind of positive effect, the alarms during the day. So she would just switch them off. She doesn't even check why is it beeping... Just because she don't want them going off in school cause it'll draw attention to her." (Parent 1)

Others described feeling that alarms 'nagged' them: "I suppose the worst of it would be the beeping... its beeping at you to tell you the sensor's doing something, or it's going too low, or something like that, so it nags" (Participant 3). This 'nagging' was described in particularly ambivalent ways by those, such as Participant 6, who suggested that she did not want to always lead a life dominated and dictated by her diabetes:

"I kind of love it and I hate it, cause I hate the fact that it shouted at me all the time. And they're like [names health professional] 'that's what you want, so you can make sure you're ok'. I'm like: 'not at 3 o'clock in the morning, I don't care.'" (Participant 6)

For similar reasons, Participant 10 also expressed ambivalence; in this individual's case because the alarms acted as a tangible and difficult reminder not only that they had diabetes but also of their struggles to achieve optimal blood glucose control:

"It goes off a lot, it will vibrate and vibrate, and then this big alarm will go off... And it wakes me up. And it goes off in lessons. And it really frustrates me. And it's like any diabetic will know if something annoys you about your diabetes, it's more than being annoyed, it's deep anger...it's telling me I am high or it's telling me I'm low." (Participant 10)

Data lag

Others noted how, by virtue of the lag between CGM readings and actual blood glucose levels, they were sometimes exposed to information which was unhelpful:

"It alerts when I'm going low or I'm going high. So I do a sugar test: it says 13 the (CGM) reading says I'm 13.5 going up. So it'll constantly beep... saying you're 13.6, 13.7, you're going up, you're going up. And actually I'm going down. But it hasn't caught up with it yet." (Participant 13)

Indeed due to this lag and other occasional inaccuracies, some participants emphasised the importance of undertaking SMBG before addressing high/low blood glucose: "We don't rely on it. You know if she's [teenage daughter] having a hypo I'd still suggest that she tested" (Parent 6). Most participants, however, also described finding the lag relatively unproblematic because of how they actually made use of CGM data. For instance, it was noted that the small lag between actual blood glucose levels and CGM readings was unimportant when retrospective analysis of data was undertaken to spot patterns and trends which could inform changes to pump settings. In addition, when CGM data prompted participants to make more immediate changes to prevent high/low blood glucose, most noted how it was predictive information rather than actual blood glucose readings which they found most useful and informative:

"in a way... the arrows are more useful to you than the actual number because it's not about what you are right now, is it. It's about what's gonna happen while you're asleep, or while you're going for your run... or whatever it is, like in a way that's more helpful to you in terms of what's happening next." (Participant 6)

Discussion and conclusions

This qualitative study has provided an in-depth understanding of participants' experiences of, and views about, using CGM; and how, and why, CGM can be used to promote diabetes self-management. In doing so, we have offered a more detailed and nuanced perspective than is possible with quantitative/survey research. Specifically, our findings help explain why high levels of treatment satisfaction, reported in previous questionnaire studies [7–9], exist amongst CGM users. As we have shown, this is not only because CGM allows information about blood glucose to be accessed instantly and effortlessly, but also because trend arrows provide insightful information that enables diabetes to be managed in more proactive and effective ways than are possible with SMBG. Specifically, participants described using trend arrow information to pre-empt and prevent hyper- and hypoglycaemia by making proactive and appropriate use of carbohydrate consumption, corrective doses and short-term lifestyle planning. Such observations also help explain clinical research and trial findings that CGM can reduce hypo and hyperglycaemic excursions [2, 3, 5] and amplify and support findings of survey research undertaken with CGM users [22].

Participants also highlighted how CGM offered rich, informative data which enhanced knowledge of their blood glucose control at time points (e.g. night-time) when they were least likely to perform SMBG, and which could be used to adjust insulin basal rates and/or mealtime ratios to optimize or improve glycaemic control. However, while participants felt confident and able to make immediate, and what they saw as common-sense changes to lifestyle, food intake or insulin to address impending hypo- or hyperglycaemia, most described feeling much less confident and competent to undertake retrospective review of CGM data, spot patterns and trends and use these to inform independent adjustments to basal rates and mealtime ratios. While the former observation lends support to Bode and Battelino's [23] suggestion that CGM usage remains largely intuitive, the latter raises important questions about whether the clinical benefits of CGM are always fully realised. Indeed, in keeping with observations and recommendations made by others [2, 11, 24] our findings point to a need for psycho-education and training amongst those using CGM to make optimal use of this technology. Specifically, as Ritholz et al. [14] have noted, we would recommend preparation and follow-up training about retrospective data use and analysis be given to individuals using CGM, a training need which has also been identified in other patient groups using flexible intensive insulin regimens [25, 26]. To address users' education and training needs, staff training needs and workloads may also need to be taken into account [27]. The potential use of technologies, such as pattern recognition software, could also be considered [25]; indeed, such a recommendation was made by some of those who took part in this study. Another alternative may be to consider use of an individualised decision support system exploiting cloud-based technologies with or without health care professional input [28, 29].

Like others, we found that, while accounts of using CGM were overwhelmingly positive, participants encountered some difficulties and hassles using their devices [16]. These included calibration issues, equipment failure and problems inserting and/or removing the device [30]. While, in keeping with other studies, we found that disturbance caused by alarms could be a source of annoyance, especially to school-aged children [13, 30], our data reveal a richer and more complex picture. First, we have shown that, as well as causing frustration and disrupted sleep, alarms can also provide comfort and reassurance by alerting individuals to low (and high) blood glucose in a timely manner, thereby reinforcing a sense of hypoglycaemic safety [11]. Second, as our findings also suggest, some participants' ambivalence about alarms appeared to arise from a more general dislike of having diabetes and an association made between alarming and what they saw as personal failure to achieve optimal blood glucose control. This is an issue which could be explored further in psychological work, to help determine whether some individuals, especially those with sub-optimal self-management behaviours and/or a high HbA1c, would benefit from psychosocial support prior to initiation of

CGM to help maximise the benefits from alarms while preventing alarm fatigue [31]. However, on a more immediate and practical level, we would recommend that, as part of CGM training, individuals would benefit from instruction on how to switch alarms off and use different alarm profiles during different parts of the day. In addition, the snooze time of different alarms should be appropriately set to avoid repeated alarms.

While concerns about sensor inaccuracies and the lag between recorded and actual blood glucose levels have been highlighted by others [13], these were not found to be unduly problematic in the current study. While this may be due to improvements in CGM technology over time, we have also shown that participants found CGM data useful even if, because of the lag, they questioned the accuracy of readings. This was largely due to participants valuing predictive (trend arrow) information over actual readings, and also because retrospective review of data was not seen as being compromised by a small data lag. Some participants also emphasised the value of undertaking SMBG before taking action to address high/low blood glucose recorded by their sensors, a usage that may have been reinforced by the education and training they were given in the run up to the trial.

A key study strength is our use of an open-ended exploratory design which, as already indicated, offered a level and depth of insight not possible in clinical and survey research. An additional strength is the multi-centre study design and the inclusion of a diverse age range of individuals in our sample, together with parents of those aged 15 years and under. This potentially means our findings have greater generalizability than those of other qualitative studies undertaken to date, although it should be noted that there is a skew in the sample towards those aged 31–40 years. Like others, [11, 14] our sample, which was recruited from a clinical trial, was heavily skewed towards well-educated/professional individuals, some of whom who had participated in earlier studies/trials of CGM. Consequently, such individuals may have been particularly motivated and interested in diabetes self-care and had an above average understanding of CGM. In addition, some participants' earlier experiences of using CGM, and of seeing the technology improve over time, may have resulted in a form of 'therapeutic optimism' [32]. Specifically, participants may have hoped or believed that CGM technology will continue to improve, leading to overly positive and uncritical accounts. This may limit the generalizability of our findings; as may the fact that, in the currently study, only one particular CGM monitor was used and Polonsky et al.'s [11] observation that there are notable differences in usability, reliability and performance of CGM devices. In addition, we only focused on people's experiences of using CGM for a limited number of weeks and it is possible that participants might have experienced fatigue had they used CGM for longer due to frustrations arising from alarms and CGM systems prompting action as soon as blood glucose moves out of predefined ranges [33, 34]. It should also be noted that, as we only interviewed people using insulin pumps, the findings may not be generalizable to those using injection regimens. For the aforementioned reasons, we would recommend further qualitative research be undertaken with more diverse socio-economic groups, recruited out with clinical trials, who use CGM for longer periods of time and/or who use multiple daily injection regimens.

Abbreviations
CGM: Continuous glucose monitoring; DAFNE: Dose Adjustment for Normal Eating; HbA1c: Glycated haemoglobin; SMBG: Self-monitoring of blood glucose

Acknowledgments
We would like to thank all of the individuals who took part in the interview study and the health professionals who assisted with recruitment and patient care. Additional thanks goes to Josephine Hayes, University of Cambridge, who provided administrative support and was the trial study coordinator.

Funding
Artificial Pancreas research at Cambridge is supported by JDRF, National Institute for Health Research Cambridge Biomedical Research Centre, National Institute of Diabetes and Digestive and Kidney Diseases, Horizon 2020, Helmsley Trust, and Wellcome Strategic Award (100574/Z/12/Z).

Authors' contributions
JL conceived and designed the study, performed data analysis and interpretation, and drafted the manuscript. MB collected data, performed data analysis and interpretation, and contributed to drafting and revising the manuscript. DR performed data analysis and interpretation, and contributed to drafting and revising the manuscript. JA, FC, DE, LL, MT, HT and RH contributed to drafting and revising the manuscript. All authors read and approved the final manuscript.

Competing interests
RH reports having received speaker honoraria from Eli Lilly, Novo Nordisk and Astra Zeneca, serving on advisory panel for Eli Lilly and Novo Nordisk, receiving license fees from BBraun and Medtronic; having served as a consultant to BBraun; patents and patent applications. MT reports having received speaker honoraria from Novo Nordisk and Medtronic. LL reports having received speaker honoraria from Medtronic, Animas, Sanofi and Novo Nordisk, serving on advisory panel for Animas, Medtronic and Novo Nordisk. JL, DR, MB, JMA, DE and HT have no conflicts of interest to disclose.

Author details
[1]Usher Institute of Population Health Sciences and Informatics, University of Edinburgh, Edinburgh, UK. [2]Wellcome Trust-MRC Institute of Metabolic Science, University of Cambridge, Cambridge, UK. [3]Department of Paediatrics, University of Cambridge, Cambridge, UK. [4]Leeds Children's Hospital, Leeds, UK. [5]Royal Hospital for Sick Children, Edinburgh, UK. [6]Manchester Diabetes Centre, Central Manchester University Hospitals NHS Foundation Trust, Manchester Academic Health Science Centre, Manchester, UK.

References
1. Wong JC, Foster NC, Maahs DM, Raghinaru D, Bergenstal RM, Ahmann AJ, et al. Real-time continuous glucose monitoring among participants in the T1D exchange clinic registry. Diabetes Care. 2014;37:2702–9.
2. Pickup JC, Freeman SC, Sutton AJ. Glycaemic control in type 1 diabetes during real time continuous glucose monitoring compared with self monitoring of blood glucose: meta-analysis of randomised controlled trials using individual patient data. BMJ. 2011;343:d3805.
3. Battelino T, Conget I, Olsen B, Schütz-Fuhrmann I, Hommel E, Hoogma R, et al. The use and efficacy of continuous glucose monitoring in type 1 diabetes treated with insulin pump therapy: a randomised controlled trial. Diabetologia. 2012;55:3155–62.
4. Beck RW, Riddlesworth T, Ruedy K, Ahmann A, Bergenstal R, Haller S, et al. Effect of continuous glucose monitoring on glycemic control in adults with type 1 diabetes using insulin injections: the DIAMOND randomized clinical trial. JAMA. 2017;317:371–8.
5. Ly TT, Nicholas JA, Retterath A, Lim EM, Davis EA, Jones TW. Effect of sensor-augmented insulin pump therapy and automated insulin suspension vs standard insulin pump therapy on hypoglycemia in patients with type 1 diabetes: a randomized clinical trial. JAMA. 2013;310:1240–7.
6. van Beers CA, DeVries JH, Kleijer SJ, Smits MM, Geelhoed-Duijvestijn PH, Kramer MH, et al. Continuous glucose monitoring for patients with type 1 diabetes and impaired awareness of hypoglycaemia (IN CONTROL): a randomised, open-label, crossover trial. Lancet Diabetes Endocrinol. 2016;4:893–902.
7. Hommel E, Olsen B, Battelino T, Conget I, Schütz-Fuhrmann I, Hoogma R, et al. Impact of continuous glucose monitoring on quality of life, treatment satisfaction, and use of medical care resources: analyses from the SWITCH study. Acta Diabetol. 2014;51:845–51.
8. Tansey M, Laffel L, Cheng J, Beck R, Coffey J, Huang E, et al. Satisfaction with continuous glucose monitoring in adults and youths with type 1 diabetes. Diabet Med. 2011;28:1118–22.
9. Beck R, Lawrence J, Laffel L, Wysocki T, Xing D, Huang E, et al. Quality-of-life measures in children and adults with type 1 diabetes: Juvenile Diabetes Research Foundation continuous glucose monitoring randomized trial. Diabetes Care. 2010;33:2175–7.
10. Halford J, Harris C. Determining clinical and psychological benefits and barriers with continuous glucose monitoring therapy. Diabetes Technol Ther. 2010;12:201–5.
11. Polonsky WH, Hessler D. What are the quality of life-related benefits and losses associated with real-time continuous glucose monitoring? A survey of current users. Diabetes Technol Ther. 2013;15:295–301.
12. Rashotte J, Tousignant K, Richardson C, Fothergill-Bourbonnais F, Nakhla MM, Olivier P, et al. Living with sensor-augmented pump therapy in type 1 diabetes: Adolescents' and parents' search for harmony. Can J Diabetes. 2014;38:256–62.
13. Schmidt S, Duun-Henriksen AK, Nørgaard K. Psychosocial factors and adherence to continuous glucose monitoring in type 1 diabetes. J Diabetes Sci Technol. 2012;6:986–7.
14. Ritholz M, Atakov-Castillo A, Beste M, Beverly E, Leighton A, Weinger K, et al. Psychosocial factors associated with use of continuous glucose monitoring. Diabet Med. 2010;27:1060–5.
15. Ritholz M, Beste M, Edwards S, Beverly E, Atakov-Castillo A, Wolpert H. Impact of continuous glucose monitoring on diabetes management and marital relationships of adults with type 1 diabetes and their spouses: a qualitative study. Diabet Med. 2014;31:47–54.
16. Pickup JC, Ford Holloway M, Samsi K. Real-time continuous glucose monitoring in type 1 diabetes: a qualitative framework analysis of patient narratives. Diabetes Care. 2015;38:544–50.
17. Bally L, Tauschmann M, Allen JM, Hartnell S, Wilinska ME, Exall J, et al. Assessing the effectiveness of 3 months day-and-night home closed-loop control combined with pump suspend feature compared to sensor augmented pump therapy in youths and adults with sub-optimally controlled type 1 diabetes: a randomised parallel study protocol. BMJ Open. 2017;7(7):e016738.
18. Lawton J, Waugh N, Barnard K, Noyes K, Harden J, Stephen J, et al. Challenges of optimizing glycaemic control in children with type 1 diabetes: a qualitative study of parents' experiences and views. Diabet Med. 2015;32:1063–70.
19. Williams C. Doing health, doing gender: teenagers, diabetes and asthma. Soc Sci Med. 2000;50:387–96.
20. Pope C, Mays N. Reaching the parts other methods cannot reach: an introduction to qualitative methods in health and health services research. BMJ. 1995;311:42–5.

21. Glaser B, Strauss A. The discovery of grounded theory. Chicago: Aldine Publishing Co.; 1967.
22. Pettus J, Price DA, Edelman SV. How patients with type 1 diabetes translate continuous glucose monitoring data into diabetes management decisions. Endocr Pract. 2015;21:613–20.
23. Bode BW, Battelino T. Continuous glucose monitoring in 2014. Diabetes Technol Ther. 2015;17(Suppl 1):S12–20.
24. Battelino T, Liabat S, Veeze H, Castañeda J, Arrieta A, Cohen O. Routine use of continuous glucose monitoring in 10 501 people with diabetes mellitus. Diabet Med. 2015;32:1568–74.
25. Lawton J, Rankin D, Cooke D, Elliott J, Amiel S, Heller S, et al. Patients' experiences of adjusting insulin doses when implementing flexible intensive insulin therapy: a longitudinal, qualitative investigation. Diabetes Res Clin Pract. 2012;98:236–42.
26. Lawton J, Kirkham J, Rankin D, Barnard K, Cooper C, Taylor C, et al. Perceptions and experiences of using automated bolus advisors amongst people with type 1 diabetes: a longitudinal qualitative investigation. Diabetes Res Clin Pract. 2014;106:443–50.
27. James S, Perry L, Gallagher R, Lowe J. Diabetes educators: perceived experiences, supports and barriers to use of common diabetes-related technologies. J Diabetes Sci Technol. 2016;10:1115–21.
28. Reddy M, Pesl P, Xenou M, Toumazou C, Johnston D, Georgiou P, et al. Clinical safety and feasibility of the advanced bolus calculator for type 1 diabetes based on case-based reasoning: a 6-week nonrandomized single-arm pilot study. Diabetes Technol Ther. 2016;18:487–93.
29. Glooko, Inc. Remote Patient Monitoring for Diabetes Mobile and population health for patients and care teams. https://www.glooko.com. Accessed 24 May 2017.
30. Barnard KD, Wysocki T, Allen JM, Elleri D, Thabit H, Leelarathna L, et al. Closing the loop overnight at home setting: psychosocial impact for adolescents with type 1 diabetes and their parents. BMJ Open Diabetes Res Care. 2014;2:e000025.
31. Shivers JP, Mackowiak L, Anhalt H. "Turn it off!": diabetes device alarm fatigue considerations for the present and the future. J Diabetes Sci Technol. 2013;7:789–94.
32. Jansen LA. Two concepts of therapeutic optimism. J Med Ethics. 2011; 37:563–6.
33. Battelino T, Bode BW. Continuous glucose monitoring in 2013. Diabetes Technol Ther. 2014;16(Suppl 1):S11–6.
34. Anhalt H. Limitations of continuous glucose monitor usage. Diabetes Technol Ther. 2016;18:115–7.

11

Associations between ERα/β gene polymorphisms and osteoporosis susceptibility and bone mineral density in postmenopausal women: a systematic review and meta-analysis

Heping Zhu[1,2], Jiannong Jiang[1], Qiang Wang[1], Jun Zong[1], Liang Zhang[3], Tieliang Ma[4], Youjia Xu[2]* and Leiyan Zhang[1]*

Abstract

Background: Many studies have reported associations between estrogen receptor (ER) gene polymorphisms and postmenopausal osteoporosis (PMOP) risk and bone mineral density (BMD), but the results are controversial. The aim of the present meta-analysis is to verify the association between ERα and ERβ gene polymorphisms and osteoporosis susceptibility and BMD in postmenopausal women.

Methods: PubMed, EMBASE, Web of Science, the Cochrane Library and China WeiPu Library were searched. OR and WMD with 95% CI were calculated to assess the association.

Results: Overall, no significant association was observed between ERα XbaI, ERα PvuII and PMOP susceptibility in either overall, Caucasian or Asian populations. ERα G2014A was significantly associated with a decreased risk of PMOP in Caucasian populations. There was a significant association between ERβ RsaI and PMOP risk in both overall and Asian populations. Caucasian PMOP women with ERα XbaI XX and Xx genotypes had a higher LS Z value than women with xx genotype. ERα XbaI XX genotype was associated with increased FN BMD in overall and Caucasian populations, an increased FN Z value in Asians, and a decreased FN Z value in Caucasians. There was also a significant association between ERα XbaI Xx genotype and an increased FN Z value in either Asians or Caucasians. ERα PvuII PP genotype was associated with a low LS Z value in Caucasians and a low FN BMD and Z value in Asians. Pp genotype in PMOP women was significantly correlated with low LS BMD in overall populations, a low FN Z value in either overall, Caucasian or Asian populations.

Conclusion: Each ERα and ERβ gene polymorphism might have different impact on PMOP risk and BMD in various ethnicities.

Keywords: Estrogen receptor, Postmenopausal osteoporosis, Gene polymorphism, Meta-analysis

* Correspondence: xuyoujia@suda.edu.cn; 2004zhp-pp@sohu.com
[2]Department of Orthopedics, The Second Affiliated Hospital of Soochow University, Suzhou 215004, China
[1]Department of Orthopedics, The Affiliated Yixing Hospital of Jiangsu University, Yixing 214200, China
Full list of author information is available at the end of the article

Background

Postmenopausal osteoporosis (PMOP) is a common metabolic bone disorder characterized by low bone mineral density (BMD) and increased fracture risks [1–3]. It is estimated that osteoporosis affects approximately 10 million American adults, with another 34 million being at high risk due to low bone mass [4].

The pathophysiology of PMOP is considered as a disorder or negative imbalance of bone metabolism and remodeling, with bone resorption outpacing bone formation [3], suggesting that vitamin D and parathyroid hormone (PTH) and other factors related to bone resorption and formation may play a key role in the underlying mechanism and pathophysiology of PMOP [5–8]. Furthermore, genetic factors including genes and gene polymorphisms may also play an important role in the development of PMOP [9].

Estrogen is another important hormone that plays an important role in the pathogenesis of PMOP, knowing that reduced ovarian production of estrogen after menopause is a cause for the initial phase of rapid bone loss and osteoporosis in women [3]. Estrogen is known as an important regulator of bone metabolism, and estrogen deficiency is believed to be the cause of BMD loss, increased mechanical loading-induced bone remodeling, and the development of PMOP [10]. Knowing that the action of estrogen is predominantly mediated by estrogen receptor (ER), including ERα and ERβ by binding to different ligands to mediate various biological effects [3, 10], more attention has been paid to the relationship between ERs and PMOP risk and BMD in postmenopausal women [11–38]. However, the results of studies currently available about this issue are controversial.

Previous meta-analyses have been performed to assess the pooled effects of ER gene polymorphisms on BMD and fracture risk [39–41]. WANG et al. [39] showed that the ERα XbaI (rs9340799) polymorphism was associated with BMD at diverse skeletal sites, and ERα PvuII (rs2234693) PP genotype played a role in protecting the lumbar spine but on the other hand might be a risk factor for the femoral neck fracture. However, to the best of our knowledge, no meta-analysis has been performed to explore the relationships between ER gene [ERα XbaI (rs9340799), ERα PvuII (rs2234693) and ERα G2014A (rs2228480)] and ERβ gene [ERβ AluI (rs4986938) and ERβ RsaI (rs1256049)] polymorphisms and PMOP susceptibility and BMD of the lumbar spine and femoral neck in postmenopausal women. To address these issues, we performed a meta-analysis of all currently available studies relating ER gene [ERα XbaI (rs9340799), ERα PvuII (rs2234693) and ERα G2014A (rs2228480)] and ERβ gene [ERβ AluI (rs4986938) and ERβ RsaI (rs1256049)] polymorphisms with PMOP risk and BMD.

Methods

Data sources and searches

We searched PubMed, EMBASE, Web of Science, the Cochrane Library and China WeiPu Library to identify case-control studies that investigated the associations between ERα gene polymorphisms [ERα XbaI (rs9340799), ERα PvuII (rs2234693) and ERα G2014A (rs2228480)] ERβ gene polymorphisms [ERβ AluI (rs4986938) and ERβ RsaI (rs1256049)] and osteoporosis susceptibility and BMD in postmenopausal women by using the following search terms ('PMOP' OR 'Postmenopausal osteoporosis' OR 'Postmenopausal') AND ('Estrogen Receptor' OR 'ER') AND ('polymorphism' OR 'single nucleotide polymorphism' OR 'SNP' OR 'variation'). To analyze the pooled effects of ER gene polymorphisms on BMD, the following search terms were used: ('PMOP' OR 'Postmenopausal osteoporosis' OR 'Postmenopausal') AND ('Estrogen Receptor' OR 'ER') AND ('polymorphism' OR 'single nucleotide polymorphism' OR 'SNP' OR 'variation') AND ('BMD' OR 'bone mineral density'). Then, one-by-one screening was performed by two authors according to the inclusion and exclusion criteria. No language restrictions were applied. Secondary searches of eligible studies were conducted by searching the reference lists of the selected studies, reviews or comments.

Inclusion and exclusion criteria

The inclusion criteria of our meta-analysis are as follows: (1) case-control studies; (2) studies on BMD and fracture risks in postmenopausal women with PMOP due to estrogen deficiency using postmenopausal women without PMOP or healthy volunteers as control; (3) studies reporting alleles and genotypes of at least one of the ER gene polymorphisms in women with or without PMOP: ERα XbaI (rs9340799), ERα PvuII (rs2234693), ERα G2014A (rs2228480), ERβ AluI (rs4986938) and ERβ RsaI (rs1256049); (3) studies reporting the sample size, mean and standard deviation (SD) of BMD (g/cm^2) or BMD Z value in PMOP women with at least one of the ER genotypes; and (4) studies with sufficient data. The exclusion criteria were: (1) reviews or case reports without controls, and (2) studies with no availability of current data; and (3) duplicated reports.

Data extraction

Data from the eligible studies were extracted according to the inclusion and exclusion criteria by two authors, and a consensus was reached by discussion. In the study of associations between ER gene polymorphisms and PMOP risk, the following data were collected: author list, year of publication, ethnicity, sample size, alleles, genotype of each gene polymorphism and Hardy-Weinberg equilibrium (HWE). The following data were collected for analysis of differences in BMD in PMOP women with various ER genotypes: author list, year of publication, ethnicity, the number of cases and mean and SD of BMD (g/cm^2) and BMD Z value.

Data synthesis and statistical analysis

We calculated odds ratios (OR) and 95% confidence interval (CI) to evaluate the association between ER gene polymorphisms and PMOP risk (osteoporosis occurred in postmenopausal women due to estrogen deficiency as represented by low BMD and increased fracture risks). The strength of association between ER gene polymorphisms and PMOP susceptibility was evaluated by OR and 95% CI under the allele contrast model, heterozygote model, homozygote model, dominant model and recessive model. HWE was calculated in the control population to evaluate the quality of the data by using chisquare test. Regarding the associations between BMD and ER gene polymorphisms, we compared BMD (g/cm^2) and BMD Z value in PMOP women under the heterozygote and homozygote model respectively using the

weight mean difference (WMD) and 95% CI. Heterogeneity of the included studies was examined by a chi-squared-based Q statistical test and quantified by I2 metric value. If I2 value was > 50% or $P < 0.10$, ORs and WMD were pooled by the random effect model; otherwise, the fixed effect model was used. Power analysis was performed using the Power and Precision V4 software (Biostat Inc., Englewood, USA). Sensitivity analysis was performed to assess the impact of each study on the combined effect of the present meta-analysis. Besides, subgroup analysis was also performed according to the ethnicity of the study populations. Stata 12.0 software (StataCorp, College Station, TX, USA) was used and a $P < 0.05$ was considered as statistically significant.

Results

Study selection and characteristics

A total of 28 studies [11–38] were finally recruited in our meta-analysis. The study selection and inclusion process is shown in Fig. 1. Fourteen studies [11–24]

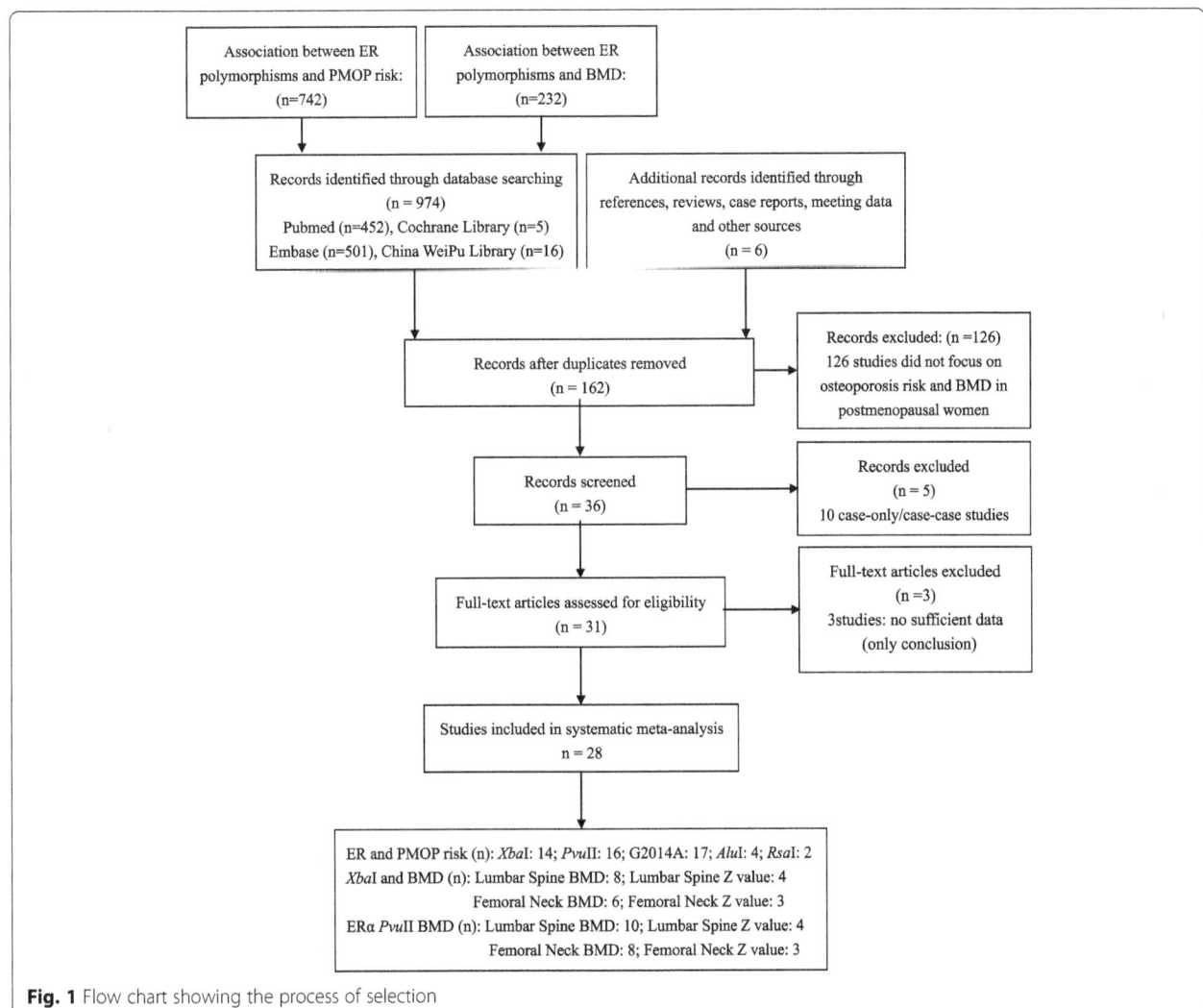

Fig. 1 Flow chart showing the process of selection

reported the association between ERα XbaI and PMOP risk, and the number of the included studies that reported the alleles and genotypes of ERα PvuII, ERα G2014A, ERβ AluI and ERβ RsaI was 16 [11–25, 32], 4 [26–29], 4 [17, 30–32] and 2 [30, 31], respectively. Ivanova et al. [20], Albagha et al. [33], Aerssens et al. [24], Kurt et al. [34], Ge et al. [36] and Pérez et al. [19] reported both the lumbar spine and femoral neck BMD (g/cm²). Jeedigunta et al. [15] and Kurabayashi et al. [35] were also recruited in the assessment of the lumbar spine BMD (g/cm²) in ERα XbaI genotypes. Ivanova et al. [20], Albagha et al. [33] and An et al. [38] reported both the lumbar spine and femoral neck Z values. Shang et al. [11] also studied the lumbar spine Z value in PMOP with ERα XbaI genotypes. Ten studies [15, 19, 20, 23, 24, 33–37] and 8 studies [19, 20, 23, 24, 33, 34, 36, 37] were recruited in the pooled analysis of differences in lumbar spine and femoral neck BMD (g/cm²) in PMOP women carrying ERα PvuII, respectively. With regard to differences in lumbar spine and femoral neck Z value in PMOP women with ERα PvuII, 4 studies [11, 20, 33, 38] and 3 studies [20, 33, 38] were included in our meta-analysis, respectively. In addition, all these studies complied with HWE. The characteristics of the included studies are shown in Tables 1, 2 and 3.

Power analysis

Before initiation of the meta-analysis, a power analysis was conducted by using the Power and Precision V4 software to verify whether the included studies could offer adequate power (> 80%). The result showed that the statistical power in our study was sufficient to detect the associations between ER gene polymorphisms and PMOP risk.

Associations between ER gene polymorphisms and PMOP risk

Overall, we did not find any significant association between ERα XbaI and ERα PvuII polymorphisms and risk of PMOP in either overall, Caucasian or Asian populations (all P > 0.05) (Table 4). ERα G2014A polymorphism played a protcetive role in developing PMOP in Caucasian populations, while no significant association was observed in overall and Asian populations (both P > 0.05). All the data are shown in Table 4 and Fig. 2.

With regard to ERβ polymorphism, ERβ AluI was significantly associated with the risk of developing PMOP in Asian postmenopausal women under the recessive model; however, we did not observe any significant association between ERβ AluI and PMOP risk in overall and Caucasian populations (both P > 0.05) (Table 4 and Fig. 3). Furthermore, we also found that there was a remarkable association between ERβ RsaI polymorphism

and decreased PMOP risk in overall and Asian populations (Table 4).

Associations between ER gene polymorphisms and BMD in PMOP women

ERa XbaI and lumbar spine bone mineral density (BMD g/cm² and BMD Z value)

In our meta-analysis, no significant difference in lumbar spine BMD (g/cm²) was observed between PMOP women with ERα XbaI XX, ERα XbaI Xx and ERα XbaI xx genotype in either overall, Caucasian or Asian populations (all P > 0.05) (Table 5). The lumbar spine BMD Z value in Caucasian PMOP women carrying ERα XbaI XX genotype was greater than that in those carrying xx genotype, while no significant difference was observed in overall and Asian populations (both P > 0.05). ERα XbaI Xx genotype was found to be significantly associated with high lumbar spine BMD Z value in either overall or Caucasian populations but not in Asian populations.

ERa XbaI and femoral neck bone mineral density (BMD g/cm² and BMD Z value)

Our pooled analyses indicated that the ERα XbaI XX genotype was significantly associated with increased femoral neck BMD in overall and Caucasian populations. In contrast, ERα XbaI XX genotype did not play a key role in femoral neck BMD in Asian populations (Table 5 and Fig. 4). Interestingly, compared with PMOP women with xx genotype, XX genotype was significantly associated with decreased femoral neck Z value in Caucasians, and increased femoral neck Z value in Asians (Table 5). However, no significant association was observed between XX genotype and the femoral neck Z value in overall populations. In addition, Caucasians and Asians carrying the ERα XbaI Xx genotype were at risk of a high femoral neck Z value, while no significant association was found in overall populations. We did not observe remarkable relationships between ERα XbaI Xx genotype and femoral neck BMD in either overall, Caucasian or Asian populations (all P > 0.05). All data are shown in Table 5.

ERa PvuII and lumbar spine bone mineral density (BMD g/cm² and BMD Z value)

With regard to ERα PvuII, the difference in the lumbar spine Z value between the PP and pp. genotypes was – 0.07 (95% CI = – 0.03 to – 0.01, P = 0.031) in Caucasian PMOP women; however, no significant difference was observed in overall and Asian populations. For the Pp versus pp. genotype, the difference in lumbar spine BMD was – 0.01 (95% CI = – 0.02 to – 0.00, P = 0.036) in overall populations, and the difference in the lumbar spine Z value was – 0.16 (95% CI = – 0.20 to – 0.12, P < 0.001) in Caucasian

Table 1 General characteristics of studies assciated with postmenopausal osteoporosis risk

Author	Year	Ethnicity	Sample Size		ERα *XbaI* Case					Control					HWE
			Case	Control	X	x	XX	Xx	xx	X	x	XX	Xx	xx	
Shang et al.	2016	Asian	198	276	338	58	146	46	6	109	443	10	89	177	0.77
Wang et al.	2015	Asian	72	72	125	19	55	15	2	132	12	62	8	2	0.21
Li et al.	2014	Asian	440	791	254	626	31	192	217	404	1178	48	308	435	0.50
Erdogan et al.	2011	Caucasian	50	30	41	59	7	27	16	28	32	6	16	8	0.70
Jeedigunta et al.	2010	Asian	247	254	253	241	60	133	54	306	202	81	144	29	0.32
Tanriover et al.	2010	Caucasian	50	50	48	52	5	38	7	54	46	12	30	8	0.14
Harsløf et al.	2010	Caucasian	228	225	134	322	19	96	113	164	286	30	104	91	0.97
Musumeci et al.	2009	Caucasian	100	200	130	70	35	60	5	155	245	13	129	58	0.26
Pérez et al.	2008	Caucasian	64	68	48	80	9	30	25	46	90	5	36	27	0.13
Ivanova et al.	2007	Caucasian	220	180	256	184	73	110	37	163	197	25	113	42	0.58
Huang et al.	2006	Asian	66	116	19	113	2	15	49	46	186	4	38	74	0.74
Nam et al.	2005	Asian	6	168	0	12	0	0	6	63	273	6	51	111	0.96
Qin et al.	2004	Asian	244	273	120	368	11	98	135	137	409	13	111	149	0.18
Aerssens et al.	2000	Caucasian	135	239	92	178	14	64	57	175	303	32	111	96	0.99

Author	Year	Ethnicity	Sample Size		ERα *PvuII* Case					Control					HWE
			Case	Control	P	p	PP	Pp	pp	P	p	PP	Pp	pp	
Shang et al.	2016	Asian	198	276	156	240	28	100	70	386	166	138	110	28	0.38
Wang et al.	2015	Asian	60	60	30	90	3	24	33	32	88	3	26	31	0.40
Li et al.	2014	Asian	440	791	368	512	65	238	137	498	1084	69	360	362	0.12
Sonoda et al.	2012	Asian	114	171	118	110	24	70	20	137	205	31	75	65	0.26
Erdogan et al.	2011	Caucasian	50	30	42	58	8	26	16	38	22	10	18	2	0.11
Jeedigunta et al.	2010	Asian	247	254	181	313	50	81	116	232	276	60	112	82	0.08
Tanriover et al.	2010	Caucasian	50	50	39	61	7	25	18	48	52	14	20	16	0.79
Harsløf et al.	2010	Caucasian	228	224	198	258	46	106	76	233	215	63	107	54	0.52
Musumeci et al.	2009	Caucasian	100	200	120	80	30	60	10	186	214	31	124	45	0.53
Pérez et al.	2008	Caucasian	64	68	56	72	11	34	19	58	78	12	34	22	0.86
Ivanova et al.	2007	Caucasian	220	180	226	214	58	110	52	148	212	21	106	53	0.37
Morón et al.	2006	Caucasian	87	175	79	95	17	45	25	171	179	45	81	49	0.33
Huang et al.	2006	Asian	66	116	79	53	23	33	10	68	164	11	46	59	0.64
Nam et al.	2005	Asian	6	168	2	10	1	0	5	130	206	25	80	63	0.96
Qin et al.	2004	Asian	244	273	193	295	40	113	91	223	323	43	137	93	0.52
Aerssens et al.	2000	Caucasian	135	239	120	150	27	66	42	219	259	47	125	67	0.41

Author	Year	Ethnicity	Sample Size		ERα G2014A Case					Control					HWE
			Case	Control	A	G	AA	GA	GG	A	G	AA	GA	GG	
Wajanavisit et al.	2015	Asian	99	113	94	104	33	28	38	179	47	72	35	6	0.53
Gómez et al.	2007	Caucasian	70	500	30	110	2	26	42	303	697	40	223	237	0.21
Ongphiphadhanakul et al.	2003	Asian	33	325	23	43	5	13	15	129	521	13	103	209	0.94
Ongphiphadhanakul et al.	2001	Asian	106	122	56	156	8	40	58	37	207	2	33	87	0.57

Table 1 General characteristics of studies assciated with postmenopausal osteoporosis risk *(Continued)*

Author	Year	Ethnicity	Sample Size		ERβ AluI										HWE
					Case					Control					
			Case	Control	A	G	AA	GA	GG	A	G	AA	GA	GG	
Shoukry et al.	2015	Caucasian	200	180	223	177	75	73	52	125	235	30	65	85	0.46
Huang et al.	2015	Asian	413	890	678	148	285	108	20	1384	396	541	302	47	0.57
Harsløf et al.	2010	Caucasian	228	224	154	302	26	102	100	186	262	35	116	73	0.32
Morón et al.	2006	Caucasian	88	177	76	100	11	54	23	146	208	34	78	65	0.23

Author	Year	Ethnicity	Sample Size		ERβ RsaI										HWE
					Case					Control					
			Case	Control	A	G	AA	GA	GG	A	G	AA	GA	GG	
Shoukry et al.	2015	Caucasian	200	180	52	348	2	48	150	37	323	1	35	144	0.47
Huang et al.	2015	Asian	413	777	329	497	63	203	147	759	795	169	421	187	0.28

populations; however, we did not find any significant difference in lumbar spine BMD in either Caucasians or Asians, and in the lumbar spine Z value in overall and Asian populations (Table 5 and Fig. 5). In addition, no significant difference in lumbar spine BMD was observed between PP and pp. genotypes ($P > 0.05$) (Table 5).

ERa PvuII and femoral neck bone mineral density (BMD g/cm² and BMD Z value)

We further found that the ERα PvuII PP genotype was associated with decreased femoral neck BMD and Z value compared with the pp. genotype in Asians, while no significant difference in femoral neck BMD and Z value was observed in either overall and Caucasian populations (both $P > 0.05$) (Table 5). Furthrmore, PMOP women carrying the Pp genotype were at risk of a low femoral neck Z value, which was found in overall, Caucasian and Asian populations. Our study showed that there was no significant difference in femoral neck BMD between PMOP women with the Pp genotype and those with the pp. genotype ($P > 0.05$). All the data are shown in Table 5.

Sensitivity analysis and publication bias

We performed a leave-one-out analysis to estimate the sensitivity of our study and found that omission of any single study did not affect the overall statistical significance, indicating that the results of our meta-analysis are stable. Therefore, we could conclude that our meta-analysis data are relatively stable and credible. To estimate the publication bias of our meta-analysis, the Begg's and Egger's test was performed (Table 4), indicating that there was minimal evidence of publication bias. The shape of funnel plot was symmetrical, which also showed no publication bias in our study (Fig. 6).

Discussion

Associations between ERα gene polymorphisms and PMOP risk

ERα XbaI and ERα PvuII are the two restriction fragment length polymorphisms of ERα gene located in Intron 1 [14]. Many studies [11–25, 32] have been performed to explore the relationships between ERα XbaI, ERα PvuII and PMOP risk; however, these studies have yielded inconsistent data [11–25, 32]. Overall, we did not observe any significant association between ERα XbaI and ERα PvuII polymorphisms and PMOP risk in either overall, Caucasian or Asian populations. In our opinion, the inadequate sample size, different ethnicities, various genotyping techniques, the presence of admixture in the population, gene-environment interactions, differences in age and measurement errors of different investigators might be important factors contributing to these controversial results. ERα XbaI and ERα PvuII have proven to play key roles in attainment and maintenance of peek bone mass during young adulthood, and it might be difficult to document their effects in a population of postmenopausal women [24]. In addition, PvuII and XbaI polymorphisms are located in a non-functional area of the ER gene [20], which might also contribute to our polled results. With regard to ERα G2014A, it is located on the exon region of chromosome 6p25.1, and may contribute via the epigenetic level for the efficiency of translation or receptor protein expression [26]. Our results showed that a significant association between ERα G2014A and PMOP risk was observed only in Caucasian populations but not in overall and Asian populations.

Associations between ERβ gene polymorphisms and PMOP risk

ERβ has been found to be more abundant than ERα in trabecular bone, and more potent than ERα in

Table 2 Characteristics of included studies of lumbar spine BMD, femoral neck BMD, lumbar spine Z value and femoral neck Z value in ERα XbaI genotypes

ERα XbaI

Author	Year	Ethnicity	Lumbar Spine BMD (g/cm²)					
			XX		Xx		xx	
			N	Mean ± SD	N	Mean ± SD	N	Mean ± SD
Ivanova et al.	2007	Caucasian	73	0.75 ± 0.17	110	0.81 ± 0.06	37	0.87 ± 0.07
Albagha et al.	2001	Caucasian	27	0.88 ± 0.03	89	0.88 ± 0.02	90	0.85 ± 0.02
Aerssens et al.	2000	Caucasian	14	0.94 ± 0.21	64	0.93 ± 0.22	57	0.88 ± 0.16
Jeedigunta et al.	2010	Asian	60	0.89 ± 0.15	133	0.86 ± 0.13	54	0.64 ± 0.16
Kurt et al.	2012	Caucasian	41	0.95 ± 0.12	94	0.92 ± 0.12	40	0.93 ± 0.10
Kurabayashi et al.	1999	Asian	1	1.18 ± 0.00	20	0.92 ± 0.04	61	0.92 ± 0.02
Ge et al.	2006	Asian	37	0.73 ± 0.08	134	0.74 ± 0.09	26	0.75 ± 0.13
Pérez et al.	2008	Caucasian	7	0.70 ± 0.02	31	0.67 ± 0.02	24	0.66 ± 0.02

ERα XbaI

Author	Year	Ethnicity	Femoral Neck BMD (g/cm²)					
			XX		Xx		xx	
			N	Mean ± SD	N	Mean ± SD	N	Mean ± SD
Ivanova et al.	2007	Caucasian	73	0.69 ± 0.08	110	0.69 ± 0.04	37	0.65 ± 0.03
Albagha et al.	2001	Caucasian	27	0.77 ± 0.03	89	0.73 ± 0.01	90	0.72 ± 0.02
Aerssens et al.	2000	Caucasian	14	0.73 ± 0.03	64	0.68 ± 0.09	57	0.70 ± 0.20
Kurt et al.	2012	Caucasian	41	0.79 ± 0.09	94	0.8 ± 0.08	40	0.83 ± 0.10
Ge et al.	2006	Asian	37	0.70 ± 0.10	134	0.68 ± 0.07	26	0.67 ± 0.07
Pérez et al.	2008	Caucasian	7	0.59 ± 0.02	36	0.58 ± 0.01	20	0.56 ± 0.02

ERα XbaI

Author	Year	Ethnicity	Lumbar Spine Z value					
			XX		Xx		xx	
			N	Mean ± SD	N	Mean ± SD	N	Mean ± SD
Shang et al.	2016	Asian	146	−1.98 ± 0.91	146	−1.65 ± 0.02	6	−0.35 ± 2.19
Ivanova et al.	2007	Caucasian	73	−2.10 ± 0.00	110	−0.6 ± 0.00	37	−01 ± 0.00
Albagha et al.	2001	Caucasian	27	−0.34 ± 0.20	89	−0.29 ± 0.11	90	−0.47 ± 0.11
An et al.	2000	Asian	10	0.48 ± 0.49	84	0.12 ± 0.85	152	−0.26 ± 0.58

ERα XbaI

Author	Year	Ethnicity	Femoral Neck Z value					
			XX		Xx		xx	
			N	Mean ± SD	N	Mean ± SD	N	Mean ± SD
Ivanova et al.	2007	Caucasian	73	−2.00 ± 0.00	110	−2.00 ± 0.00	37	−1.90 ± 0.00
Albagha et al.	2001	Caucasian	27	−2.00 ± 0.23	89	−0.42 ± 0.10	90	−0.52 ± 0.12
An et al.	2000	Asian	10	0.42 ± 0.57	84	0.11 ± 0.66	152	−0.32 ± 0.76

Table 3 Characteristics of included studies of lumbar spine BMD, femoral neck BMD, lumbar spine Z value and femoral neck Z value in ERα *PvuII* genotypes

ERα *PvuII*

Author	Year	Ethnicity	Lumbar Spine BMD (g/cm²) PP		Pp		pp	
			N	Mean ± SD	N	Mean ± SD	N	Mean ± SD
Ivanova et al.	2007	Caucasian	58	0.70 ± 0.09	110	0.71 ± 0.10	52	0.77 ± 0.06
Albagha et al.	2001	Caucasian	37	0.87 ± 0.03	102	0.86 ± 0.02	67	0.88 ± 0.02
Aerssens et al.	2000	Caucasian	27	0.93 ± 0.18	66	0.91 ± 0.22	42	0.89 ± 0.17
Jeedigunta et al.	2010	Asian	50	0.92 ± 0.18	81	0.89 ± 0.11	116	0.81 ± 0.14
Kurt et al.	2012	Caucasian	44	0.93 ± 0.13	104	0.93 ± 0.11	46	0.93 ± 0.09
Kurabayashi et al.	1999	Asian	19	0.99 ± 0.04	27	0.89 ± 0.03	36	0.91 ± 0.02
Ge et al.	2006	Asian	38	0.73 ± 0.10	93	0.74 ± 0.09	67	0.75 ± 0.10
Ge et al.	2006	Asian	38	0.73 ± 0.10	92	0.74 ± 0.09	67	0.75 ± 0.10
Qin et al.	2004	Asian	40	0.70 ± 0.01	113	0.70 ± 0.01	91	0.72 ± 0.01
Pérez et al.	2008	Caucasian	11	0.73 ± 0.03	34	0.66 ± 0.02	17	0.65 ± 0.02

ERα *PvuII*

Author	Year	Ethnicity	Femoral Neck BMD (g/cm²) PP		Pp		pp	
			N	Mean ± SD	N	Mean ± SD	N	Mean ± SD
Ivanova et al.	2007	Caucasian	58	0.52 ± 0.02	110	0.68 ± 0.01	52	0.76 ± 0.05
Albagha et al.	2001	Caucasian	37	0.75 ± 0.02	102	0.71 ± 0.01	67	0.75 ± 0.02
Aerssens et al.	2000	Caucasian	27	0.69 ± 0.06	66	0.70 ± 0.09	42	0.69 ± 0.11
Kurt et al.	2012	Caucasian	44	0.77 ± 0.08	104	0.81 ± 0.09	46	0.82 ± 0.09
Ge et al.	2006	Asian	38	0.68 ± 0.09	93	0.67 ± 0.07	67	0.69 ± 0.08
Ge et al.	2006	Asian	38	0.68 ± 0.09	92	0.67 ± 0.08	67	0.69 ± 0.08
Qin et al.	2004	Asian	40	0.57 ± 0.01	113	0.60 ± 0.01	91	0.59 ± 0.01
Pérez et al.	2008	Caucasian	9	0.59 ± 0.01	37	0.57 ± 0.01	16	0.57 ± 0.02

ERα *PvuII*

Author	Year	Ethnicity	Lumbar Spine Z value PP		Pp		pp	
			N	Mean ± SD	N	Mean ± SD	N	Mean ± SD
Shang et al.	2016	Asian	28	-1.54 ± 0.35	100	-1.67 ± 0.91	70	-2.79 ± 1.46
Ivanova et al.	2007	Caucasian	58	-2.40 ± 0.00	110	-2.10 ± 0.00	52	-1.50 ± 0.00
Albagha et al.	2001	Caucasian	37	-0.35 ± 0.16	102	-0.44 ± 0.10	67	-0.28 ± 0.14
An et al.	2000	Asian	53	-0.53 ± 0.16	128	-0.21 ± 0.99	65	0.22 ± 0.46

ERα *PvuII*

Author	Year	Ethnicity	Femoral Neck Z value PP		Pp		pp	
			N	Mean ± SD	N	Mean ± SD	N	Mean ± SD
Ivanova et al.	2007	Caucasian	58	-2.00 ± 0.00	110	-1.90 ± 0.00	52	-0.70 ± 0.00
Albagha et al.	2001	Caucasian	37	-0.29 ± 0.17	102	-0.59 ± 0.09	67	-0.28 ± 0.15
An et al.	2000	Asian	53	-0.48 ± 0.90	128	-0.19 ± 0.80	128	0.31 ± 0.49

Table 4 Results of genetic models for ERα *Xba*I, ERα *Pvu*II, ERα G2014A, ERβ *Alu*I and ERβ *Rsa*I polymorphisms and osteoporosis susceptibility in postmenopausal women

Comparison	N	Test of association			Model	Test of heterogeneity		Begg's test	Egger's test
		OR	95% CI	P value		P value	I^2 (%)	P value	P value
ERα *Xba*I									
Overall	14								
X vs. x		1.21	0.73–2.00	0.455	R	< 0.001	96.4	0.584	0.955
XX vs. xx		1.84	0.71–4.75	0.206	R	< 0.001	93.7	0.443	0.465
Xx vs. xx		1.19	0.83–1.70	0.357	R	< 0.001	80.1	0.511	0.610
Xx/XX vs. xx		1.34	0.82–2.18	0.240	R	< 0.001	90.4	0.661	0.545
XX vs. Xx/xx		1.50	0.70–3.24	0.296	R	< 0.001	93.4	0.443	0.875
Caucasian	7								
X vs. x		1.15	0.76–1.74	0.510	R	< 0.001	88.0		
XX vs. xx		1.56	0.56–4.39	0.399	R	< 0.001	88.9		
Xx vs. xx		1.13	0.76–1.67	0.540	R	0.021	59.8		
Xx/XX vs. xx		1.24	0.76–2.01	0.387	R	< 0.001	76.2		
XX vs. Xx/xx		1.30	0.56–3.03	0.536	R	< 0.001	88.2		
Asian	7								
X vs. x		1.23	0.47–3.25	0.668	R	< 0.001	98.0		
XX vs. xx		2.18	0.37–12.73	0.388	R	< 0.001	98.1		
Xx vs. xx		1.22	0.63–2.36	0.553	R	< 0.001	88.0		
Xx/XX vs. xx		1.39	0.56–3.46	0.481	R	< 0.001	94.6		
XX vs. Xx/xx		1.77	0.44–7.14	0.424	R	< 0.001	96.0		
ERα *Pvu*II									
Overall	16								
P vs. p		0.96	0.71–1.29	0.769	R	< 0.001	92.3	0.753	0.616
PP vs. pp		0.99	0.55–1.78	0.961	R	< 0.001	90.8	1.000	0.886
Pp vs. pp		1.01	0.72–1.41	0.956	R	< 0.001	82.3	0.753	0.501
PP/Pp vs. pp		0.97	0.65–1.43	0.868	R	< 0.001	88.7	0.893	0.539
PP vs. Pp/pp		0.99	0.65–1.53	0.977	R	< 0.001	87.3	0.893	0.976
Caucasian	8								
P vs. p		0.95	0.71–1.26	0.716	R	< 0.001	79.2		
PP vs. pp		0.93	0.49–1.79	0.831	R	< 0.001	81.4		
Pp vs. pp		0.98	0.73–1.31	0.877	R	0.112	40.0		
PP/Pp vs. pp		0.97	0.67–1.39	0.861	R	0.008	63.5		
PP vs. Pp/pp		0.97	0.59–1.58	0.895	R	< 0.001	78.2		
Asian	8								
P vs. p		0.97	0.57–1.66	0.919	R	< 0.001	95.6		
PP vs. pp		1.08	0.40–2.96	0.877	R	< 0.001	94.4		
Pp vs. pp		1.04	0.58–1.88	0.889	R	< 0.001	90.2		
PP/Pp vs. pp		0.98	0.50–1.95	0.962	R	< 0.001	93.8		
PP vs. Pp/pp		1.05	0.50–2.20	0.891	R	< 0.001	91.8		
ERα G2014A									
Overall	4								
A vs. G		0.89	0.32–2.51	0.825	R	< 0.001	95.1	0.308	0.237

Table 4 Results of genetic models for ERα *Xba*I, ERα *Pvu*II, ERα G2014A, ERβ *Alu*I and ERβ *Rsa*I polymorphisms and osteoporosis susceptibility in postmenopausal women *(Continued)*

Comparison	N	Test of association			Model	Test of heterogeneity		Begg's test	Egger's test
		OR	95% CI	P value		P value	I^2 (%)	P value	P value
AA vs. GG		0.88	0.08–9.19	0.912	R	< 0.001	92.9	0.734	0.419
GA vs. GG		0.76	0.28–2.03	0.581	R	< 0.001	88.1	0.734	0.530
GA/AA vs. GG		0.73	0.22–2.41	0.601	R	< 0.001	92.8	0.734	0.530
AA vs. GA/GG		1.13	0.23–5.72	0.878	R	< 0.001	88.6	0.734	0.299
Caucasian	1								
A vs. G		0.63	0.41–0.96	0.032	R	–	–		
AA vs. GG		0.28	0.07–1.21	0.089	R	–	–		
GA vs. GG		0.66	0.39–1.11	0.116	R	–	–		
GA/AA vs. GG		0.60	0.36–1.00	0.050	R	–	–		
AA vs. GA/GG		0.34	0.08–1.43	0.141	R	–	–		
Asian	3								
A vs. G		1.00	0.23–4.46	0.996	R	< 0.001	96.6		
AA vs. GG		1.28	0.05–30.10	0.878	R	< 0.001	95.2		
GA vs. GG		0.77	0.17–3.45	0.736	R	< 0.001	91.3		
GA/AA vs. GG		0.76	0.12–4.62	0.765	R	< 0.001	94.8		
AA vs. GA/GG		1.69	0.20–14.27	0.630	R	< 0.001	92.2		
ERβ *Alu*I									
Overall	4								
A vs. G		1.25	0.78–2.00	0.362	R	< 0.001	91.5	1.000	0.997
AA vs. GG		1.27	0.52–3.13	0.597	R	< 0.001	88.4	0.734	0.647
GA vs. GG		1.16	0.65–2.07	0.606	R	0.001	81.0	0.734	0.408
GA/AA vs. GG		1.29	0.66–2.53	0.459	R	< 0.001	87.8	0.734	0.612
AA vs. GA/GG		1.21	0.65–2.24	0.553	R	< 0.001	85.7	0.497	0.646
Caucasian	3								
A vs. G		1.23	0.58–2.57	0.590	R	< 0.001	94.3		
AA vs. GG		1.28	0.34–4.84	0.717	R	< 0.001	92.2		
GA vs. GG		1.30	0.60–2.78	0.504	R	0.001	86.5		
GA/AA vs. GG		1.36	0.55–3.39	0.507	R	< 0.001	91.8		
AA vs. GA/GG		1.10	0.37–3.22	0.863	R	< 0.001	90.3		
Asian	1								
A vs. G		1.31	1.06–1.62	0.012	R	–	–		
AA vs. GG		1.24	0.72–2.13	0.441	R	–	–		
GA vs. GG		0.84	0.48–1.48	0.548	R	–	–		
GA/AA vs. GG		1.10	0.64–1.87	0.739	R	–	–		
AA vs. GA/GG		1.44	1.12–1.84	0.004	R	–	–		
ERβ *Rsa*I									
Overall	2								
A vs. G		0.92	0.50–1.70	0.785	R	0.010	85.0		
AA vs. GG		0.49	0.34–0.70	< 0.001	F	0.261	20.9		
GA vs. GG		0.87	0.41–1.84	0.722	R	< 0.001	85.9		
GA/AA vs. GG		0.85	0.37–1.95	0.704	R	< 0.001	88.9		

Table 4 Results of genetic models for ERα *Xba*I, ERα *Pvu*II, ERα G2014A, ERβ *Alu*I and ERβ *Rsa*I polymorphisms and osteoporosis susceptibility in postmenopausal women (*Continued*)

Comparison	N	Test of association			Model	Test of heterogeneity		Begg's test	Egger's test
		OR	95% CI	P value		P value	I² (%)	P value	P value
AA vs. GA/GG		0.66	0.48–0.90	0.009	F	0.408	0		
Caucasian	1								
A vs. G		1.30	0.83–2.04	0.245	R	–	–		
AA vs. GG		1.92	0.17–21.41	0.596	F	–	–		
GA vs. GG		1.32	0.80–2.15	0.273	R	–	–		
GA/AA vs. GG		1.33	0.82–2.17	0.246	R	–	–		
AA vs. GA/GG		1.81	0.16–20.11	0.630	F	–	–		
Asian	1								
A vs. G		0.69	0.58–0.82	< 0.001	R	–	–		
AA vs. GG		0.47	0.33–0.68	< 0.001	F	–	–		
GA vs. GG		0.61	0.47–0.81	< 0.001	R	–	–		
GA/AA vs. GG		0.57	0.44–0.74	< 0.001	R	–	–		
AA vs. GA/GG		0.65	0.47–0.89	0.007	F	–	–		

R Random effect model
F Fixed effect model

mediating estrogen-induced repression of TNF-α expression, which is considered an important contributor to PMOP [30]. ERβ *Alu*I is one of the widely-studied ERβ gene polymorphisms, knowing that it could alter mRNA stability and protein levels, leading to reduced synthesis of ERβ [30]. In our study, ERβ *Alu*I was found to be significantly associated with increased risk of PMOP in Asian populations, while no significant relationship was observed in overall and Caucasian populations. Thus, different genetic backgrounds, environmental effects and/or their internal interactions could explain the diverse results in various ethnicities. ERβ *Rsa*I is another

important polymorphism of ERβ. Our subgroup analysis revealed a significant association between ERβ *Rsa*I and PMOP risk in overall populations, which is consistent with the studies of Shoukry et al. [30], and Huang et al. [31].

Associations between ERα *Xba*I and lumbar spine and femoral neck BMD

Our pooled results showed that there was no significant difference in lumbar spine BMD between PMOP women carrying XX, Xx and xx genotype in either overall, Caucasian or Asian populations. However, WANG et al. [39] reported that the *Xba*I

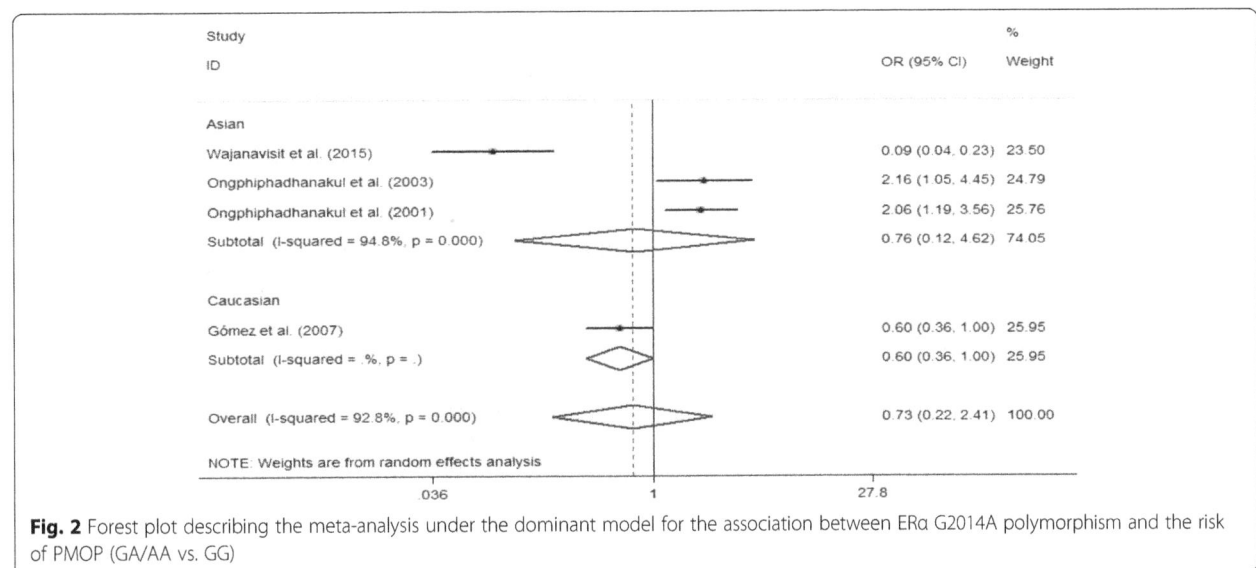

Fig. 2 Forest plot describing the meta-analysis under the dominant model for the association between ERα G2014A polymorphism and the risk of PMOP (GA/AA vs. GG)

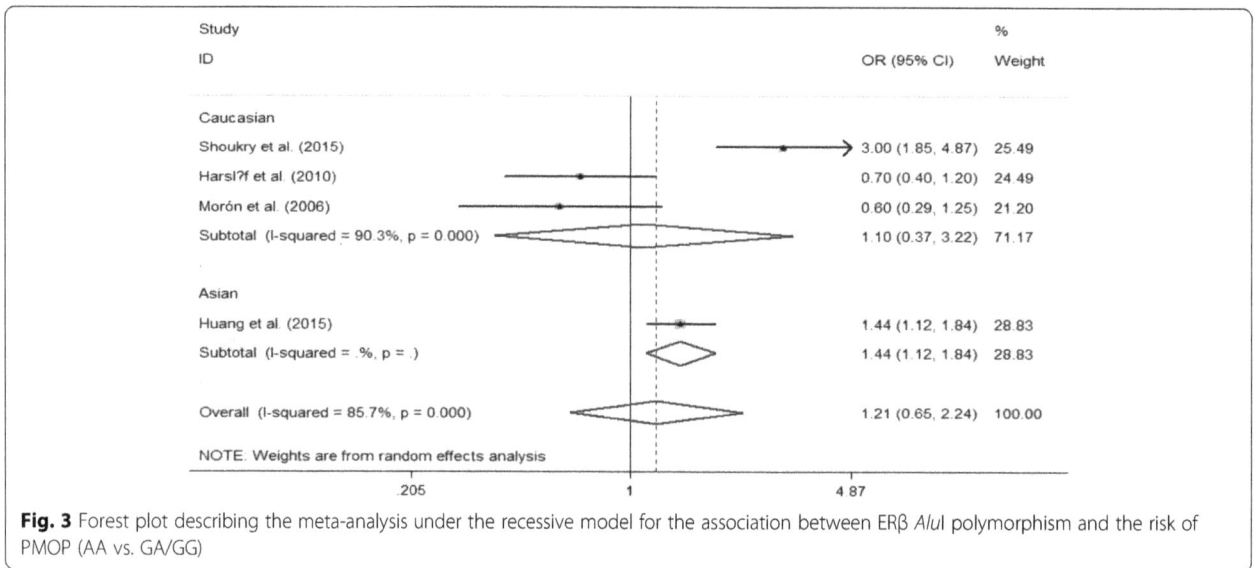

Fig. 3 Forest plot describing the meta-analysis under the recessive model for the association between ERβ *AluI* polymorphism and the risk of PMOP (AA vs. GA/GG)

polymorphism was significantly associated with BMD of the lumbar spine, and XX had a protective effect in comparison with carriers of the x alleles, which is consistent with the report of Ioannidis et al. [41]. Both WANG and Ioannidis included all types of osteoporotic patients, not only postmenopausal women, which might be the most important reason for the difference between our results and theirs. As mentioned above, ERα *Xba*I might not play a key role in attainment and maintenance of peek bone mass in postmenopausal women [24], and therefore it could be easily understood why no significant association was observed between ERα *Xba*I and lumbar spine BMD. With regard to femoral neck BMD, our study indicated that the femoral neck BMD in PMOP women with XX genotype was significantly higher than that in women with xx genotype in overall and Caucasian populations, which highlights the theory that ERα gene is involved in the pathogenesis of PMOP. No significant difference of femoral neck BMD was observed between PMOP women with Xx and xx genotype in each subgroup. Although no significant association was observed between lumbar spine BMD and ERα *Xba*I, we found that the lumbar spine Z value in both PMOP women carrying XX and those carrying Xx genotype was significantly higher than that in Caucasians carrying xx genotype. We also observed that XX genotype was associated with a low femoral neck Z value in Caucasians and high femoral neck Z value in Asians. In addition, Caucasians and Asians carrying Xx genotype were at risk of a high femoral neck Z value. However, why ERα *Xba*I plays a contradictory role in BMD and Z value at the lumar spine and femoral neck, and

the mechanisms by which it is associated with BMD and Z value remains unclear and needs further investigation.

Associations between ERα *Pvu*II and lumbar spine and femoral neck BMD

Although the molecular mechanism underlying the effect of ERα *Pvu*II on bone mass is poorly understood, it is believed that ERα *Pvu*II might play a key role in BMD as it is in linkage disequilibrium with the TA polymorphism in the ER promoter that is associated with altered gene transcription [20]. Our pooled analysis indicated that PMOP women with the Pp genotype had lower lumbar spine BMD than those with the pp. genotype. We also found that there was no significant difference in lumbar spine BMD between women with the PP genotype and those with the pp. genotype, which is consistent with the meta-analysis of Wang et al. [40]. Furthermore, we observed that the PP genotype was associated with decreased femoral neck BMD in Asians, while Pp might not play a key role in femoral neck BMD in all subgroups. Interestingly, WANG et al. [39] reported that PP play a role in protecting the lumbar spine but on the other hand it might be a risk factor for the femoral neck fracture. Wang CL [40] and WANG KJ [39] conducted their meta-analyses on osteoporotic women during menopause while our study included osteoporotic women post menopause, which might be the most important reason for the difference between our study and theirs. In addition, both PP and Pp genotypes were significantly associated with low lumbar spine Z value in Caucasians,

Table 5 Meta-analysis of differences of Lumbar Spine BMD, Femoral Neck BMD, Lumbar Spine Z value and Femoral Neck Z value between each genotype of ERα *Xba*I and ERα *Pvu*II polymorphism

ERα *Xba*I	XX vs. xx						Xx vs. xx					
	Test of differences			Model	Test of heterogeneity		Test of differences			Model	Test of heterogeneity	
	N	WMD (95% CI)	P value		P value	I^2 (%)	N	WMD (95% CI)	P value		P value	I^2 (%)
Lumbar Spine BMD (g/cm^2)												
Overall	8	0.03 (−0.02, 0.08)	0.198	R	< 0.001	94.2	8	0.02 (− 0.00, 0.05)	0.086	R	< 0.001	94.1
Caucasian	5	0.00 (−0.04, 0.04)	0.917	R	< 0.001	90.2	5	0.00 (−0.02, 0.02)	0.862	R	< 0.001	91.1
Asian	3	0.11 (−0.16, 0.38)	0.414	R	< 0.001	97.8	3	0.07 (−0.07, 0.20)	0.326	R	< 0.001	97.3
Lumbar Spine Z value												
Overall	3	0.22 (−0.40, 0.83)	0.495	R	< 0.001	88.5	3	0.24 (0.00, 0.47)	0.046	R	0.041	68.6
Caucasian	1	0.13 (0.05, 0.21)	0.001	R	–	–	1	0.18 (0.15, 0.21)	< 0.001	R	–	–
Asian	2	−0.28 (−2.58, 2.02)	0.811	R	0.009	85.2	2	−0.23 (− 1.81, 1.36)	0.780	R	0.062	71.3
Femoral Neck BMD (g/cm^2)												
Overall	6	0.03 (0.01, 0.05)	0.003	R	0.001	75.5	6	0.01 (−0.00, 0.03)	0.057	R	< 0.001	84.7
Caucasian	5	0.03 (0.01, 0.05)	0.009	R	< 0.001	80.4	5	0.01 (−0.00, 0.03)	0.094	R	< 0.001	87.7
Asian	1	0.03 (−0.01, 0.08)	0.110	R	–	–	1	0.01 (−0.02, 0.04)	0.350	R	–	–
Femoral Neck Z value												
Overall	2	−0.38 (−2.56, 1.80)	0.733	R	< 0.001	99.2	2	0.25 (−0.07, 0.58)	0.130	R	0.001	91.6
Caucasian	1	−1.48 (−1.57, −1.39)	< 0.001	R	–	–	1	0.10 (0.07, 0.13)	< 0.001	R	–	–
Asian	1	0.74 (0.37, 1.11)	< 0.001	R	–	–	1	0.43 (0.24, 0.62)	< 0.001	R	–	–
ERα *Pvu*II	PP vs. pp						Pp vs. pp					
	Test of differences			Model	Test of heterogeneity		Test of differences			Model	Test of heterogeneity	
	N	WMD (95% CI)	P value		P value	I^2 (%)	N	WMD (95% CI)	P value		P value	I^2 (%)
Lumbar Spine BMD (g/cm^2)												
Overall	10	0.02 (− 0.01, 0.04)	0.216	R	< 0.001	95.5	10	−0.01 (− 0.02, − 0.00)	0.036	R	< 0.001	84.0
Caucasian	5	0.01 (−0.04, 0.06)	0.793	R	< 0.001	95.5	5	−0.02 (− 0.03, 0.00)	0.106	R	< 0.001	84.9
Asian	5	0.03 (−0.02, 0.08)	0.288	R	< 0.001	96.2	5	−0.00 (− 0.02, 0.02)	0.912	R	< 0.001	86.4
Lumbar Spine Z value												
Overall	3	0.11 (−0.55, 0.78)	0.742	R	< 0.001	98.7	3	0.13 (−0.40, 0.67)	0.623	R	< 0.001	95.9
Caucasian	1	−0.07 (− 0.13, − 0.01)	0.031	R	–	–	1	− 0.16 (− 0.20, − 0.12)	< 0.001	R	–	–
Asian	2	0.24 (−1.72, 2.20)	0.809	R	< 0.001	99.0	2	0.34 (−1.18, 1.85)	0.665	R	< 0.001	97.9
Femoral Neck BMD (g/cm^2)												
Overall	8	−0.04 (− 0.09, 0.01)	0.135	R	< 0.001	99.3	8	−0.02 (− 0.04, 0.01)	0.132	R	< 0.001	98.2
Caucasian	5	−0.06 (− 0.16, 0.05)	0.295	R	< 0.001	99.6	5	−0.03 (− 0.05, 0.00)	0.054	R	< 0.001	95.2
Asian	3	−0.01 (− 0.02, − 0.01)	< 0.001	R	1.000	0.00	3	−0.00 (− 0.03, 0.02)	0.768	R	0.009	78.7
Femoral Neck Z value												
Overall	2	−0.39 (−1.15, 0.37)	0.315	R	< 0.001	97.0	2	−0.39 (− 0.57, − 0.20)	< 0.001	R	0.024	80.3
Caucasian	1	−0.01 (− 0.08, 0.05)	0.718	R	–	–	1	− 0.31 (− 0.35, − 0.27)	< 0.001	R	–	–
Asian	1	−0.79 (−1.05, − 0.53)	< 0.001	R	–	–	1	− 0.50 (− 0.66, − 0.34)	< 0.001	R	–	–

R Random effect model
F Fixed effect model

but not in overall and Asian populations, probably because of the different genetic backgrounds in various ethnicities and interactions between genetic and non-genetic factors. PMOP women with the PP and Pp genotypes had lower femoral neck Z value than those with the pp. genotype in overall, Caucasian and Asian populations.

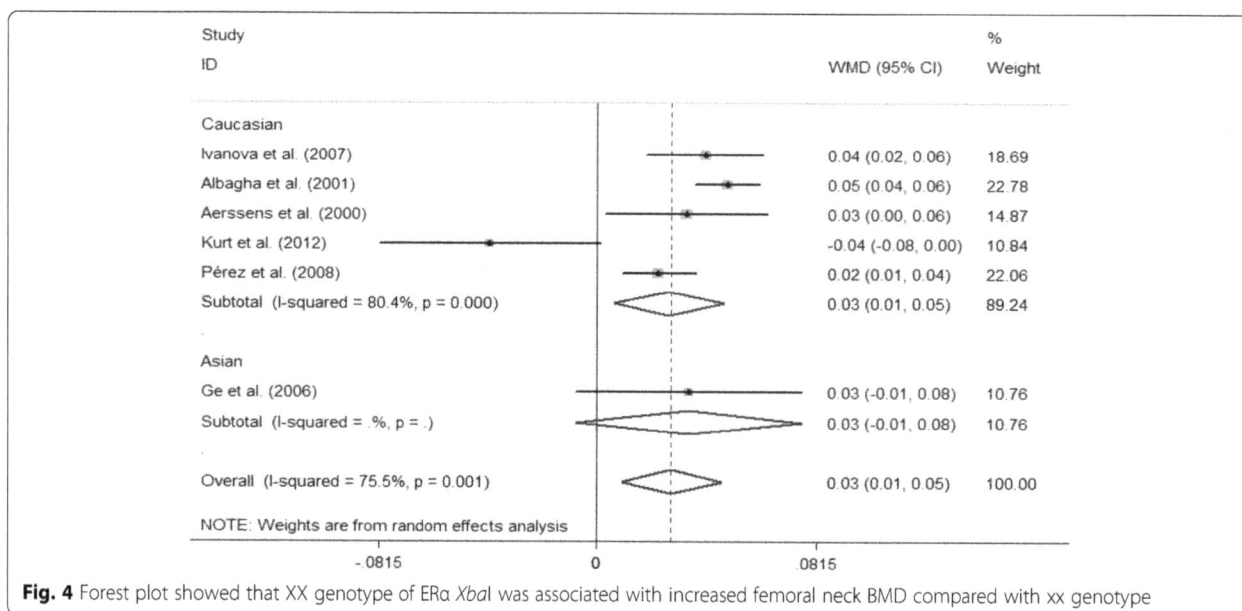

Fig. 4 Forest plot showed that XX genotype of ERα *Xba*I was associated with increased femoral neck BMD compared with xx genotype

Limitations

Although we performed a comprehensive analysis of the association between ERα, ERβ gene polymorphisms and PMOP risk and BMD in postmenopausal women, there are some limitations that should be addressed. First, high heterogeneity was observed in some of our pooled results, which might have negative impact on our conclusions. Second, PMOP is a disease whose etiology might be involved in several confounding factors, and other confounding factors such as age, years since menopause and estrogen therapy might interact with each other and play a key role in the etiology and progression of PMOP. However, no data available could be used in all recruited studies to detect the interactions between these confounding factors in PMOP patients. We should take all these confounding factors into consideration in our study rather than studying them separately, which is also a limitation of our meta-analysis. Third, we failed to perform a pooled analysis to detect whether ERα G2014A, ERβ *Alu*I and ERβ *Rsa*I were correlated with BMD in postmenopausal women as no sufficient data could be collected and analyzed. Therefore, larger-scale and better-designed studies are necessary to determine the association between ERα/β gene polymorphisms and PMOP risk and BMD in postmenopausal women.

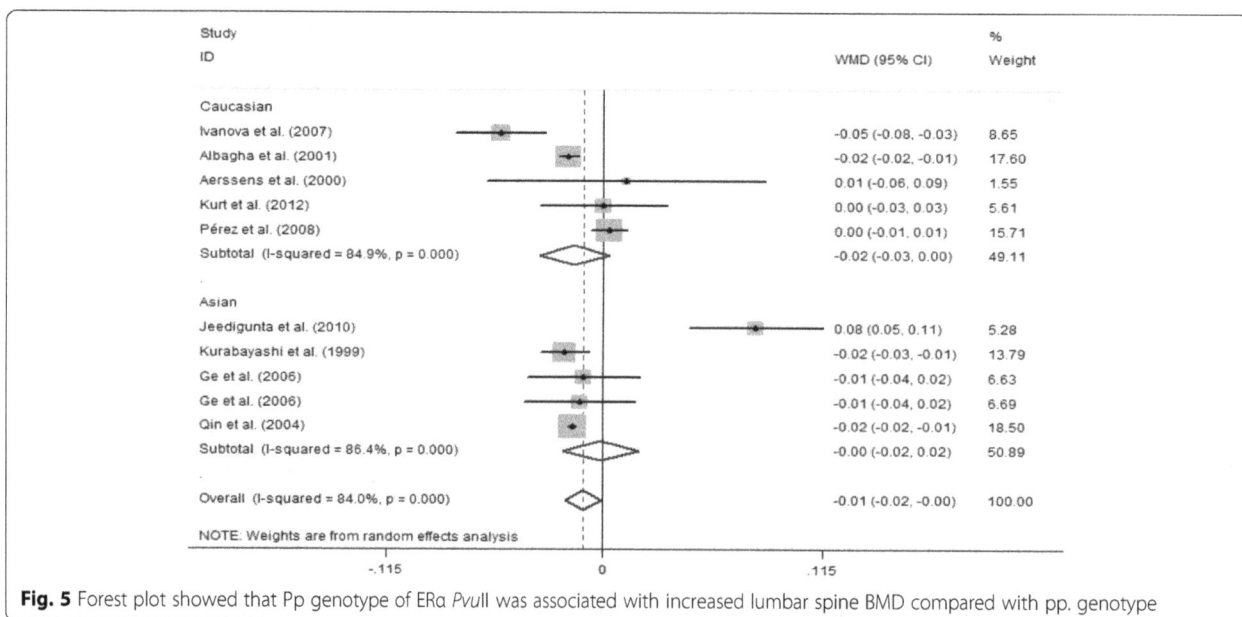

Fig. 5 Forest plot showed that Pp genotype of ERα *Pvu*II was associated with increased lumbar spine BMD compared with pp. genotype

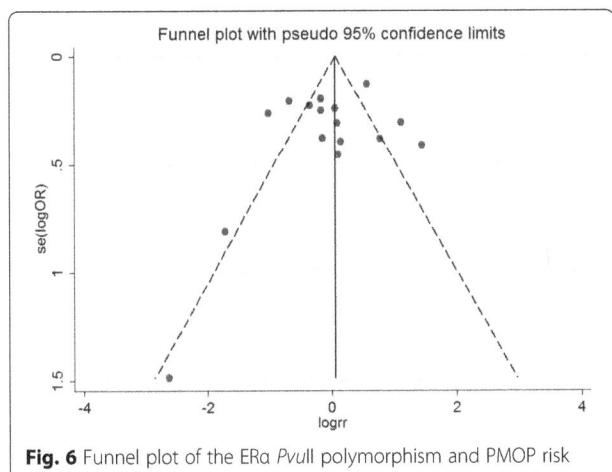

Fig. 6 Funnel plot of the ERα *PvuII* polymorphism and PMOP risk

Conclusion

ERα/β gene polymorphisms were significantly associated with PMOP risk and BMD in postmenopausal women, but each ERα/β gene polymorphism may have a distinct effect on PMOP risk and BMD in Asian and Caucasian populations.

Abbreviations

BMD: Bone mineral density; CI: Confidence interval; ER: Estrogen receptor; Lactase: LCT; OR: Odds ratios; PMOP: Postmenopausal Osteoporosis; PTH: Parathyroid Hormone; TGF-β: Transforming growth factor-β; WMD: Weight mean difference

Acknowledgements

Not applicable

Funding

No

Authors' contributions

HPZ and JNJ participated in the study design. QW and JZ made contributions to the data collection. LZ, YJX and TLM were responsible for the statistical analysis. HPZ and LYZ participated in the writting and LYZ was also responsible for the final proofing. All authors read and approved the final manuscript.

Competing interests

The authors declare that they have no competing interests.

Author details

[1]Department of Orthopedics, The Affiliated Yixing Hospital of Jiangsu University, Yixing 214200, China. [2]Department of Orthopedics, The Second Affiliated Hospital of Soochow University, Suzhou 215004, China. [3]Department of Orthopedics, Northern Jiangsu People's Hospital, Yangzhou 225001, China. [4]Central Laboratory, The Affiliated Yixing Hospital of Jiangsu University, Yixing 214200, China.

References

1. Gokosmanoglu F, Varim C, Atmaca A, Atmaca MH, Colak R. The effects of zoledronic acid treatment on depression and quality of life in women with postmenopausal osteoporosis: a clinical trial study. Journal of research in medical sciences : the official journal of Isfahan University of Medical Sciences. 2016;21:112.
2. Bandeira L, Bilezikian JP. Novel therapies for postmenopausal osteoporosis. Endocrinol Metab Clin N Am. 2017;46(1):207–19.
3. Eastell R, O'Neill TW, Hofbauer LC, Langdahl B, Reid IR, Gold DT, Cummings SR. Postmenopausal osteoporosis. Nature reviews Disease primers. 2016;2: 16069.
4. Wensel TM, Iranikhah MM, Wilborn TW. Effects of denosumab on bone mineral density and bone turnover in postmenopausal women. Pharmacotherapy. 2011;31(5):510–23.
5. Paschalis EP, Gamsjaeger S, Hassler N, Fahrleitner-Pammer A, Dobnig H, Stepan JJ, Pavo I, Eriksen EF, Klaushofer K. Vitamin D and calcium supplementation for three years in postmenopausal osteoporosis significantly alters bone mineral and organic matrix quality. Bone. 2017;95: 41–6.
6. Ebina K, Kashii M, Hirao M, Hashimoto J, Noguchi T, Koizumi K, Kitaguchi K, Matsuoka H, Iwahashi T, Tsukamoto Y, et al. Comparison of the effects of denosumab between a native vitamin D combination and an active vitamin D combination in patients with postmenopausal osteoporosis. J Bone Miner Metab. 2016;
7. Safer U, Safer VB, Demir SO, Yanikoglu I. Effects of bisphosphonates and calcium plus vitamin-D supplements on cognitive function in postmenopausal osteoporosis section sign. Endocrine, metabolic & immune disorders drug targets. 2016;16(1):56–60.
8. Gennari L, Rotatori S, Bianciardi S, Nuti R, Merlotti D. Treatment needs and current options for postmenopausal osteoporosis. Expert Opin Pharmacother. 2016;17(8):1141–52.
9. Xie W, Ji L, Zhao T, Gao P. Identification of transcriptional factors and key genes in primary osteoporosis by DNA microarray. Medical science monitor : international medical journal of experimental and clinical research. 2015;21: 1333–44.
10. Macari S, Ajay Sharma L, Wyatt A, Knowles P, Szawka RE, Garlet GP, Grattan DR, Dias GJ, Silva TA. Osteoprotective effects of estrogen in the maxillary bone depend on ERalpha. J Dent Res. 2016;95(6):689–96.
11. Shang DP, Lian HY, Fu DP, Wu J, Hou SS, Lu JM. Relationship between estrogen receptor 1 gene polymorphisms and postmenopausal osteoporosis of the spine in Chinese women. Genetics and molecular research : GMR. 2016;15(2)
12. Wang ZR. Age diference of estrogen receptor gene polymorphisms in the elderly women with hip osteoporosis. Chin. J.of Tissue Engmeenng Res. 2015;19(7):991–5.
13. Hai L, Jishen X, Bingpu C, Hailing H, Jinhua W, Jianhai C, xiaoyan F. Estrogen receptor- alpha gene Pvull, Xbal polymorphism, camellia oil and post-menopausal osteoporosis relevance in Guangxi Zhuang. Chinese. J Anat. 2014;37(5):581–4.
14. Erdogan MO, Yildiz H, Artan S, Solak M, Tascioglu F, Dundar U, Eser B, Colak E. Association of estrogen receptor alpha and collagen type I alpha 1 gene polymorphisms with bone mineral density in postmenopausal women. Osteoporosis international : a journal established as result of cooperation between the European Foundation for Osteoporosis and the National Osteoporosis Foundation of the USA. 2011;22(4):1219–25.
15. Jeedigunta Y, Bhoomi Reddy PR, Kolla VK, Munshi A, Ananthapur V, Narasimulu G, Akka J. Association of estrogen receptor alpha gene polymorphisms with BMD and their affect on estradiol levels in pre- and postmenopausal women in south Indian population from Andhra Pradesh. Clin. Chim. Acta ; Int. J. of clin. Chem. 2010;411(7–8):597–600.
16. Durusu Tanriover M, Bora Tatar G, Uluturk TD, Dayangac Erden D, Tanriover A, Kilicarslan A, Oz SG, Erdem Yurter H, Sozen T, Sain Guven G. Evaluation of the effects of vitamin D receptor and estrogen receptor 1 gene polymorphisms on bone mineral density in postmenopausal women. Clin Rheumatol. 2010;29(11):1285–93.

17. Harslof T, Husted LB, Carstens M, Stenkjaer L, Langdahl BL. Genotypes and haplotypes of the estrogen receptor genes, but not the retinoblastoma-interacting zinc finger protein 1 gene, are associated with osteoporosis. Calcif Tissue Int. 2010;87(1):25–35.

18. Musumeci M, Vadala G, Tringali G, Insirello E, Roccazzello AM, Simpore J, Musumeci S. Genetic and environmental factors in human osteoporosis from sub-Saharan to Mediterranean areas. J Bone Miner Metab. 2009;27(4):424–34.

19. Perez A, Ulla M, Garcia B, Lavezzo M, Elias E, Binci M, Rivoira M, Centeno V, Alisio A, Tolosa de Talamoni N. Genotypes and clinical aspects associated with bone mineral density in argentine postmenopausal women. J Bone Miner Metab. 2008;26(4):358–65.

20. Ivanova JT, Doukova PB, Boyanov MA, Popivanov PR. PvuII and XbaI polymorphisms of the estrogen receptor gene and bone mineral density in a Bulgarian population sample. Hormones (Athens, Greece). 2007;6(1):36–43.

21. Wang W, Fu SJ, Wang XS, Zhang YP, Wang SW, Zhong B. The relationship between ER gene polymorphisms and postmenopause osteoporosis of spine in southern Chinese women. Jurnal of Clinical Orthopsedics. 2006;9(6):562–5.

22. Nam HS, Shin MH, Kweon SS, Park KS, Sohn SJ, Rhee JA, Choi JS, Son MH. Association of estrogen receptor-alpha gene polymorphisms with bone mineral density in postmenopausal Korean women. J Bone Miner Metab. 2005;23(1):84–9.

23. Qin YJ, Zhang ZL, Huang QR, He JW, Zhou Q, Hu YQ, Li M, Liu YJ. Association of ER alpha gene PvuII and XbaI polymorphisms and related factors with osteoporosis in postmenopausal women: a case-control study. Chin J Geriatr. 2004;23(6):380–3.

24. Aerssens J, Dequeker J, Peeters J, Breemans S, Broos P, Boonen S. Polymorphisms of the VDR, ER and COLIA1 genes and osteoporotic hip fracture in elderly postmenopausal women. Osteoporosis international : a journal established as result of cooperation between the European Foundation for Osteoporosis and the National Osteoporosis Foundation of the USA. 2000;11(7):583–91.

25. Sonoda T, Takada J, Iba K, Asakura S, Yamashita T, Mori M. Interaction between ESRα polymorphisms and environmental factors in osteoporosis. J Orthop Res. 2012;30(10):1529–34.

26. Wajanavisit W, Suppachokmongkorn S, Woratanarat P, Ongphiphadhanakul B, Tawonsawatruk T. The association of bone mineral density and G2014A polymorphism in the estrogen receptor alpha gene in osteoporotic hip fracture in Thai population. Journal of the Medical Association of Thailand = Chotmaihet thangphaet. 2015;98(Suppl 8):S82–7.

27. Gomez R, Magana JJ, Cisneros B, Perez-Salazar E, Faugeron S, Veliz D, Castro C, Rubio J, Casas L, Valdes-Flores M. Association of the estrogen receptor alpha gene polymorphisms with osteoporosis in the Mexican population. Clin Genet. 2007;72(6):574–81.

28. Ongphiphadhanakul B, Chanprasertyothin S, Payattikul P, Saetung S, Rajatanavin R. The implication of assessing a polymorphism in estrogen receptor alpha gene in the risk assessment of osteoporosis using a screening tool for osteoporosis in Asians. Osteoporosis international : a journal established as result of cooperation between the European Foundation for Osteoporosis and the National Osteoporosis Foundation of the USA. 2003;14(10):863–7.

29. Ongphiphadhanakul B, Chanprasertyothin S, Payattikul P, Saetung S, Piaseu N, Chailurkit L, Rajatanavin R. Association of a G2014A transition in exon 8 of the estrogen receptor-alpha gene with postmenopausal osteoporosis. Osteoporosis international : a journal established as result of cooperation between the European Foundation for Osteoporosis and the National Osteoporosis Foundation of the USA. 2001;12(12):1015–9.

30. Shoukry A, Shalaby SM, Etewa RL, Ahmed HS, Abdelrahman HM. Association of estrogen receptor beta and estrogen-related receptor alpha gene polymorphisms with bone mineral density in postmenopausal women. Mol Cell Biochem. 2015;405(1–2):23–31.

31. Huang HL, Tan HH, Chen BP, Li H, Xie JS, Zhao QZ. Correlation of polymorphism of estrogen receptor-β and camellia oil with post-menopausal osteoporosis in Zhuang women of Guangxi. Chinese Journal of Anatomy. 2015;03:323–325,343.

32. Moron FJ, Mendoza N, Vazquez F, Molero E, Quereda F, Salinas A, Fontes J, Martinez-Astorquiza T, Sanchez-Borrego R, Ruiz A. Multilocus analysis of estrogen-related genes in Spanish postmenopausal women suggests an interactive role of ESR1, ESR2 and NRIP1 genes in the pathogenesis of osteoporosis. Bone. 2006;39(1):213–21.

33. Albagha OM, FE MG, Reid DM, Ralston SH. Estrogen receptor alpha gene polymorphisms and bone mineral density: haplotype analysis in women from the United Kingdom. Journal of bone and mineral research : the official journal of the American Society for Bone and Mineral Research. 2001;16(1):128–34.

34. Kurt O, Yilmaz-Aydogan H, Uyar M, Isbir T, Seyhan MF, Can A. Evaluation of ERalpha and VDR gene polymorphisms in relation to bone mineral density in Turkish postmenopausal women. Mol Biol Rep. 2012;39(6):6723–30.

35. Kurabayashi T, Tomita M, Matsushita H, Yahata T, Honda A, Takakuwa K, Tanaka K. Association of vitamin D and estrogen receptor gene polymorphism with the effect of hormone replacement therapy on bone mineral density in Japanese women. Am J Obstet Gynecol. 1999;180(5):1115–20.

36. Ge JR, Zhu XX, Chen K. Effect of estrogen receptor gene Px haplotype on bone mineral density in female postmenopausal osteoporosis. Chin J Geriatr. 2006;25(6):416–9.

37. Ge JR, Wang HM, Zhu XX, Chen K. Effect of PvuIIpolymorphisms of estrogen receptor gene on filtering risk factors in postmenopansal osteoporosis. Chin J Osteopors. 2006;12(1):38–40.

38. An SJ, Li E, Tong XX, Liu K, Zhao JS. Study on relationship between estrogen receptor gene polymorphism and syndrome differentiation typing of female postmenopausal osteoporosis in traditional Chinese medicine. Chinese Journal of Integrated Traditional and Western Medicine. 2000;20(12):907–10.

39. Wang KJ, Shi DQ, Sun LS, Jiang X, Lu YY, Dai J, Chen DY, Xu ZH, Jiang Q. Association of estrogen receptor alpha gene polymorphisms with bone mineral density: a meta-analysis. Chin Med J. 2012;125(14):2589–97.

40. Wang CL, Tang XY, Chen WQ, Su YX, Zhang CX, Chen YM. Association of estrogen receptor alpha gene polymorphisms with bone mineral density in Chinese women: a meta-analysis. Osteoporosis international : a journal established as result of cooperation between the European Foundation for Osteoporosis and the National Osteoporosis Foundation of the USA. 2007;18(3):295–305.

41. Ioannidis JP, Stavrou I, Trikalinos TA, Zois C, Brandi ML, Gennari L, Albagha O, Ralston SH, Tsatsoulis A. Association of polymorphisms of the estrogen receptor alpha gene with bone mineral density and fracture risk in women: a meta-analysis. Journal of bone and mineral research : the official journal of the American Society for Bone and Mineral Research. 2002;17(11):2048–60.

12

Association between thyroid hormones and the components of metabolic syndrome

Jieun Jang[1,2†], Youngsook Kim[3†], Jaeyong Shin[2,4], Sang Ah Lee[1,2], Young Choi[1,2] and Eun-Cheol Park[2,4*] (iD)

Abstract

Background: Thyroid hormones are known to have direct and indirect effects on metabolism. Individuals with metabolic syndrome, a disease that is growing in incidence at a rapid rate, are at higher risk for cardiovascular disease, diabetes, and cancer. The aim of this study was to identify whether significant correlations exist between thyroid hormone levels and components of the metabolic syndrome in the general population of Korea.

Methods: The data were collected from the sixth Korea National Health and Nutrition Examination Surveys from 2013 to 2015. A total of 1423 participants were tested for thyroid function. The analysis of variance and multiple linear regression were performed to analyze the relationship between thyroid hormone level and components of the metabolic syndrome.

Results: A positive association between free thyroxine and fasting glucose level was observed in patients with high free thyroxine levels ($\geq$1.70 ng/dL, $\beta = 15.992$, $p = < 0.0001$), when compared with patients with normal-middle free thyroxine levels. Moreover, a negative association was observed between free thyroxine and triglyceride levels in patients with normal-high free thyroxine levels ($\beta = -21.145$, $p = 0.0054$) and those with high free thyroxine levels ($\beta = -49.713$, $p = 0.0404$).

Conclusion: Free thyroxine shows a partially positive association with fasting glucose and a partially negative association with triglycerides in the Korean population. In patients with abnormal thyroid function, follow up tests for glucose levels and lipid profiling during treatment for thyroid dysfunction would be beneficial in terms of overlooking metabolic syndrome and to prevent related diseases.

Keywords: Thyroid hormone, Metabolic syndrome, Free thyroxine, FT4

Background

Metabolic syndrome, a well-known cluster of cardiovascular risk factors, is a major public health concern worldwide [1, 2]. Metabolic syndrome increases the risk for cardiovascular disease, diabetes, and even certain types of cancer [3]. According to the National Cholesterol Education Program's Adult Treatment Panel III definition, metabolic syndrome is the presence of abnormal values for at least three of the following criteria: waist circumference, serum triglycerides, high-density lipoprotein (HDL) cholesterol, blood pressure, and fasting glucose [3]. The prevalence of metabolic syndrome is increasing rapidly [4]. According to data from the National Health and Nutrition Examination Survey (NHANES) 2011–2012, about 34.7% of US adults were estimated to have metabolic syndrome [4]. Similar increasing trends have been observed in Europe and other countries [2, 5]. According to the National Cholesterol Education Program's Adult Treatment Panel III criteria, and per the World Health Organization Asia-Pacific guidelines, the prevalence of metabolic syndrome was approximately 28.2% in the general population of Korea in 2012 [6]. The mortality rate due to cardiovascular disease has increased from 35.6 to 52.4 out of 100,000 persons over 2003–2014. Thus, more focus and effort is needed to reduce the prevalence of metabolic syndrome,

* Correspondence: ECPARK@yuhs.ac

†Jieun Jang and Youngsook Kim contributed equally to this work.
Jieun Jang and Youngsook Kim are co-first authors.
²Institute of Health Services Research, Yonsei University, Seoul, Republic of Korea
⁴Department of Preventive Medicine & Institute of Health Services Research, Yonsei University College of Medicine, 50 Yonsei-ro, Seodaemun-gu, Seoul 120-752, Republic of Korea
Full list of author information is available at the end of the article

while considering the rapidly increasing frequency of mortality due to related diseases [7].

Thyroid hormones have an important role in metabolism [8]. Abnormal levels of thyroid hormones alter metabolism, and some of these changes share common pathophysiologic processes with metabolic syndrome. Therefore, thyroid dysfunction can affect metabolic syndrome. Lambadiari et al. reported that thyroid hormones are significant determinants of glucose homeostasis [9], and affect fasting glucose levels by antagonizing insulin action [9]. For instance, hyperthyroidism leads to impaired insulin secretion, which suppresses hepatic glucose production and promotes glucose uptake in the muscle [9]. Similarly, Dimitriadis et al. showed that the increased glucose levels in hyperthyroidism could be explained by an increase in endogenous glucose production via of gluconeogenesis [10]. Studies have also demonstrated an association between thyroid hormones and glucose levels. Klein et al. reviewed several studies regarding the mechanism of action of thyroid hormones on the cardiovascular system [11]. They concluded that thyroid hormones have direct and indirect impacts on the cardiovascular system. Patients with thyroid disease, especially hyperthyroidism, often demonstrated signs and symptoms of cardiovascular changes [11]. Several other studies have shown that overt hypothyroidism induces an increase in blood pressure and plasma cholesterol levels [12]. However, most of the studies that assessed the relationships between abnormal thyroid hormone levels and metabolic syndrome have been conducted in Caucasian populations [2, 13]. Therefore, the aim of this study was to assess the relationships between thyroid hormone levels and metabolic syndrome components in a nationally representative sample of South Korean adults.

Methods
Study population
This study was conducted using data from the sixth Korea National Health and Nutrition Examination Surveys (KNHANES VI, 2013–2015), a nationwide cross-sectional survey conducted by the Korean Centers for Disease Control and Prevention (Seoul, Korea) to assess the health and nutritional status of the South Korean population. The institutional review board of the Korea Centers for Disease Control and Prevention (KCDC) approved the study (IRB: 2013-07CON-03-4C, 2013-12EXP-03-5C, 2015-01-02-6C). A nationally representative sample was obtained using a stratified multistage cluster sampling design. The survey consists of a health interview, nutrition survey, and health examination. Tests for thyroid disease and metabolic syndrome components (waist circumference, triglycerides, HDL cholesterol,

blood pressure, and fasting glucose) were part of the health examination. The initial sample included 22,948 participants. The thyroid functions tests were carried out by subsampling 2400 subjects aged ≥10 years with respect to thyroid-stimulating hormone (TSH), free thyroxine (FT4), thyroid peroxidase antibody (TPOab), and urinary iodine in the sixth Korea National Health and Nutrition Examination Surveys (KNHANES VI, 2013–2015). Participants with missing thyroid function data were excluded (n = 20,591). Patients who received treatment that could interfere with the test results for thyroid hormone levels and various components of metabolic syndrome, such as radioactive iodine treatment, antithyroid drugs, thyroid hormones, other medication for thyroid disease, dyslipidemia medications, blood pressure regulators, insulin, or glucose regulators were also excluded (n = 429). The data for a total of 1423 participants without any missing variables were finally included in the analysis.

Dependent variables and variables of interest
The dependent variables were the components of metabolic syndrome. Waist circumference was measured at the narrowest spot between the lowest rib and the highest lateral border of the right iliac crest. Systolic blood pressure was measured after the participants relaxed for 5 min while sitting. Triplicate measurements of systolic blood pressure were obtained. The mean of the second and third measured value was used in the analysis. Triglycerides, HDL cholesterol, and fasting glucose levels were measured using the same Hitachi Automatic Analyzer 7600–210 (Hitachi, Tokyo, Japan).

The variable of interest in this study was thyroid hormone levels. Serum FT4, serum TSH, and TPOab levels were measured using an electro-chemiluminescence immunoassay (Cobas: Roche Diagnostics, Penzberg, Germany). Samples were sent to the central certified laboratory and analyzed. The laboratory reference ranges for FT4, TSH, and TPOab were 0.80–1.70 ng/dL, 0.50–5.0 uIU/mL, and < 34 IU/mL [14–16]. FT4 levels were divided into five categories: (1) low; under normal (< 0.80 ng/dL); (2) normal-low (< 1.17 ng/dL); (3) normal-middle (< 1.31 ng/dL); (4) normal-high (< 1.70 ng/dL); and (5) high; upper normal (≥1.70 ng/dL). TSH levels were divided as follows: low; under normal (< 0.50 uIU/mL); normal-low (< 1.80 uIU/mL), normal-middle (< 2.87 uIU/mL), normal-high (< 5.00 uIU/mL) and high; upper normal (≥5.00 uIU/mL). TPOab levels were categorized as normal (< 34 IU/mL), high with low FT4 (34 IU/mL ≤ TPOab; FT4 < 1.24 ng/dL), high with high FT4 (34 IU/mL ≤ TPOab; 1.24 ng/dL ≤ FT4). In addition, we categorized TPOab levels into normal (< 34 IU/mL), high with low

TSH (34 IU/mL ≤ TPOab; TSH < 2.25 uIU/mL), high with high TSH (34 IU/mL ≤ TPOab; 2.25 uIU/mL ≤ FT4). Considering that the TPOab titer is related to both hypothyroidism and hyperthyroidism, patients with high levels were divided into two groups using two median FT4 levels and two TSH levels.

Covariates

We adjusted for the covariates of sociodemographic factors, socioeconomic factors, health-behavior factors, and health-condition factors. Sociodemographic factors included age (19–44 years, 45–64 years, > 64 years) and gender (male and female). Socioeconomic factors included educational level (elementary school or less, middle school, high school, and college or over), marital status (married and cohabit, married but no cohabit or bereaved or divorced, and unmarried), household income level (divided into quartiles), region (urban or rural), and occupation (white collar, pink collar, blue collar, and unemployed or else). Urban areas included capitals and metropolitan cities and rural areas comprised the remaining areas. Alcohol consumption (ever or never), smoking (ever or never), and walking activity (active or inactive) were the health-behavior factors. Health-condition factors involved stress level (high, middle, low).

Statistical analysis

Statistical analysis was performed using the SAS software, version 9.4 (SAS Institute, Cary, NC, USA). All analysis incorporated weights. The mean values and standard deviations of the components of metabolic syndrome were compared using the analysis of variance. Multiple linear regression was performed to analyze the relationship between thyroid hormone level and the components of metabolic syndrome. Subgroup analysis was performed according to age and gender. A p-value < 0.05 was considered to indicate a statistically significant result.

Results

Demographic characteristics

Table 1 presents the general characteristics of the study populations. There were 683 males (48.0%) and 740 females (52.0%) included in this study. Of the 1423 participants, 870 (61.1%) were aged between 19 and 44 years, 471 participants (33.1%) were aged between 45 and 64 years, and 82 participants (5.8%) were aged over 64 years. The mean waist circumference was 31.9 ± 4.0 in. and the mean triglycerides level was 133.0 ± 120.5 mg/dL. The mean HDL cholesterol level was 52.0 ± 12.8 mg/dL, mean blood pressure 114.2 ± 15.1 mmHg, and the mean fasting glucose level 95.0 ± 16.6 mg/dL. When analyzed according to FT4 levels, waist circumference, triglycerides, and fasting glucose results were statistically significantly different ($p < 0.05$). Patients with high FT4 levels demonstrated considerably higher fasting glucose levels (High: 109.4 ± 45.2 mg/dL; Normal-middle: 93.8 ± 12.2 mg/dL).

Multiple analysis

Table 2 shows the estimates for the components of metabolic syndrome. "β" presents standardized regression coefficient and "S.E" presents standardized error of a correlation coefficient. After controlling for covariates, the results showed a positive association between FT4 and fasting glucose level in patients with high FT4 levels when compared to those with normal-middle FT4 levels (β = 15.992; p = < 0.0001). We also identified a significant negative association between FT4 levels and triglycerides in patients with normal-high (β = − 21.145, p = 0.0054) and those with high FT4 levels (β = − 49.713, p = 0.0404). In addition, a positive association was observed between TPOab and triglycerides levels in patients with high TPOab levels in the presence of low median FT4 levels (β = 36.075, p = 0.0247). Also, positive association was identified between TPOab and triglycerides levels in patients with high TPOab levels in the presence of high median TSH levels (β = 32.181, p = 0.0368).

Sensitivity analysis

Table 3 shows the subgroup analysis of the association between the components of metabolic syndrome and FT4 hormone levels according to age and gender. When stratified by age, a significant negative association between FT4 and triglycerides was observed among patients aged 19–44 years (low: β = 124.396, p = 0.0165; normal-high: β = − 25.519, p = 0.0050). This association was stronger in the 19–44-year-old age group than in the other older age groups.

Additional file 1: Table S1 presents the subgroup analysis of the association between the components of metabolic syndrome and TSH levels stratified by age and gender. Additional file 1: Table S2 shows the subgroup analysis of the association between the components of metabolic syndrome and TPOab levels with categorizing FT4 levels stratified by age and gender. In addition, Additional file 1: Table S3 shows the subgroup analysis of the association between the components of metabolic syndrome and TPOab levels with categorizing TSH levels stratified by age and gender. TSH was not significantly associated with other components of metabolic syndrome, except HDL cholesterol. Additional file 1: Table S2 shows that a positive association between TPOab and triglycerides levels is more frequently observed in male with high TPOab titers but with low FT4 levels (β = 136.104, p = 0.0062).

Table 1 General characteristics of the study population

	Waist circumference (inches)				Triglycerides (mg/dL)		HDL cholesterol (mg/dL)		Blood pressure (mmHg)		Fasting glucose (mg/dL)	
	N	%	Mean ± SD	p-value	Mean ± SD	p-value	Mean ± SD	p-value	Mean ± SD	p-value	Mean ± SD	p-value
Total	1423	100.0	31.9	4.0	133.0	120.5	52.0	12.8	114.2	15.1	95.0	16.6
Free thyroxine hormone (ng/dL)				0.0388		0.0020		0.1873		0.9267		<.0001
Low (< 0.80)	15	1.1	32.8	2.4	162.7	74.4	51.8	13.4	116.3	12.5	97.1	14.4
Normal (low tertile) (< 1.17)	424	29.8	32.1	4.1	141.3	131.9	51.8	13.1	114.6	16.0	95.9	16.8
Normal (mid tertile) (< 1.31)	488	34.3	31.8	3.9	133.9	118.3	52.1	12.2	113.9	15.6	93.8	12.2
Normal (high tertile) (< 1.70)	472	33.2	31.9	4.2	125.2	114.9	52.2	13.2	113.9	13.9	94.5	17.5
High (1.70≤)	24	1.7	31.8	4.1	102.1	53.0	48.2	7.2	116.6	11.8	109.4	45.2
Thyroid stimulating hormone (uIU/mL)				0.2965		0.9867		0.1489		0.6965		0.1958
Low (< 0.50)	30	2.1	30.8	2.9	108.4	66.1	55.9	14.5	116.3	14.2	94.9	10.9
Normal (low tertile) (< 1.80)	476	33.5	32.1	4.1	136.6	144.8	51.3	13.1	114.3	14.9	96.2	19.4
Normal (mid tertile) (< 2.87)	468	32.9	32.1	4.0	131.7	111.9	52.1	12.5	113.6	14.8	94.6	13.4
Normal (high tertile) (< 5.00)	334	23.5	31.6	4.1	132.0	104.4	52.5	12.7	114.7	16.0	94.8	18.4
High (5.00≤)	115	8.1	31.7	4.0	132.9	96.0	51.6	12.3	114.0	14.7	92.1	10.8
Thyroid peroxidase antibody (IU/mL)				0.5217		0.5189		0.4016		0.0369		0.9543
Normal (< 34)	1324	93.0	31.9	4.1	132.2	120.2	52.0	12.8	114.0	15.1	95.1	17.0
High (under low FT4) (34≤)	56	3.9	31.7	4.0	155.3	149.2	50.6	12.5	114.4	13.1	92.6	10.1
High (under high FT4) (34≤)	43	3.0	31.5	3.1	127.9	79.6	51.5	13.7	119.4	16.6	94.0	10.6
Thyroid peroxidase antibody (IU/mL)				0.9967		0.3755		0.5473		0.0827		0.5928
Normal (< 34)	1324	93.0	31.9	4.1	132.2	120.2	52.0	12.8	114.0	15.1	95.1	17.0
High (under low TSH) (34≤)	39	2.7	31.5	4.2	124.8	69.9	50.5	12.5	114.8	14.3	93.7	12.0
High (under high TSH) (34≤)	60	4.2	31.6	3.3	155.5	148.5	51.3	13.4	117.7	15.2	93.0	9.1
Age				0.4481		0.0347		0.0217		<.0001		0.0746
19–44	870	61.1	31.5	4.3	125.1	119.9	53.5	12.7	109.9	12.2	92.9	16.7
45–64	471	33.1	32.6	3.4	149.0	126.9	50.0	13.0	119.9	16.6	98.1	15.4
64<	82	5.8	32.9	3.4	125.4	69.6	47.5	9.8	126.1	16.8	98.3	19.3
Gender				<.0001		<.0001		<.0001		<.0001		<.0001
Male	683	48.0	33.7	3.8	166.2	151.9	47.7	11.1	118.4	14.2	98.0	20.1
Female	740	52.0	30.3	3.6	102.4	68.3	55.9	13.0	110.3	14.9	92.2	12.0
Education level				0.7844		0.5789		0.0002		0.0034		0.9794
Elementary school or less	119	8.4	32.8	3.1	150.5	114.0	46.3	11.0	124.4	15.0	97.6	12.0
Middle school	108	7.6	32.6	4.2	148.5	105.8	50.6	11.6	120.8	15.9	97.4	15.2

Table 1 General characteristics of the study population (Continued)

	N	%	Waist circumference (inches) Mean ± SD	p-value	Triglycerides (mg/dL) Mean ± SD	p-value	HDL cholesterol (mg/dL) Mean ± SD	p-value	Blood pressure (mmHg) Mean ± SD	p-value	Fasting glucose (mg/dL) Mean ± SD	p-value
High school	574	40.3	31.9 4.0		132.5 126.4		53.0 13.2		114.5 15.4		94.9 16.3	
College or over	622	43.7	31.6 4.2		127.4 118.2		52.3 12.7		110.8 13.3		94.1 17.8	
Marital status				<.0001		0.5017		0.0569		0.2066		<.0001
Married-cohabit	813	57.1	32.3 3.7		136.4 110.3		51.3 12.4		116.0 16.3		96.7 17.9	
Married-no co habit or bereaved or divorced	130	9.1	32.5 3.8		147.0 121.8		50.0 13.5		118.0 15.5		98.8 18.4	
Unmarried	480	33.7	31.1 4.5		123.5 135.2		53.8 12.9		110.1 11.5		91.0 12.8	
Household income level				0.0328		0.6671		0.1671		0.0484		0.4857
Quartile 1 (lowest)	346	24.3	32.5 4.3		137.7 125.9		51.3 13.0		116.5 16.3		95.2 15.3	
Quartile 2	336	23.6	31.8 3.8		124.2 100.7		52.5 13.2		113.5 14.2		94.8 18.1	
Quartile 3	386	27.1	31.9 3.8		137.2 115.6		51.0 12.4		113.9 14.5		94.3 11.8	
Quartile 4 (highest)	355	24.9	31.5 4.1		132.2 136.4		53.1 12.6		112.7 15.1		95.6 20.5	
Region				0.0163		0.0112		0.3290		0.6709		0.7321
Urban area	1043	73.3	31.7 3.9		127.4 113.4		52.3 12.6		113.6 15.1		94.6 16.4	
Rural area	380	26.7	32.5 4.3		148.5 137.1		51.1 13.2		115.9 14.9		96.0 17.2	
Occupation				0.1036		0.7295		<.0001		0.5925		0.1260
White color	445	31.3	31.9 4.1		132.0 117.5		51.7 13.2		111.4 13.5		94.9 19.3	
Pink color	209	14.7	32.0 3.9		126.2 95.8		52.9 12.5		114.1 14.1		94.6 13.6	
Blue color	315	22.1	33.0 3.6		157.2 147.9		51.4 13.3		120.1 15.9		98.6 17.6	
Unemployed or else	454	31.9	31.2 4.2		120.3 109.8		52.2 12.1		112.9 15.4		92.7 13.8	
Alcohol consumption				0.0108		0.3359		0.2579		0.8845		0.4812
Ever	85	6.0	32.1 3.7		123.2 95.3		51.5 13.9		116.0 17.3		95.5 11.2	
Never	1338	94.0	31.9 4.1		133.6 121.9		52.0 12.7		114.1 14.9		94.9 16.9	
Smoking				0.0062		0.0025		0.5679		0.6979		0.3499
Ever	603	42.4	33.5 4.1		167.2 146.6		48.8 12.8		117.5 15.0		97.2 16.3	
Never	820	57.6	30.8 3.6		107.9 88.9		54.2 12.3		111.7 14.7		93.3 16.7	
Walking activity				0.8915		0.3812		0.4642		0.0845		0.1128
Active	581	40.8	31.8 3.9		127.3 121.2		52.5 12.7		112.7 14.3		93.5 13.8	
Inactive	842	59.2	32.0 4.1		137.0 119.8		51.6 12.8		115.2 15.5		96.0 18.3	
Stress level				0.1867		0.0485		0.0567		0.1300		0.5092
High	451	31.7	31.9 4.4		141.3 145.7		51.9 12.6		112.6 14.0		95.0 18.7	
Middle	800	56.2	31.8 3.9		128.1 101.0		52.0 12.9		114.0 15.1		94.7 14.9	
Low	172	12.1	32.6 3.7		134.0 129.7		52.1 12.9		119.1 16.9		96.2 18.5	

Table 2 The estimates for the components of metabolic syndrome[a]

Variable	Waist circumference (inches)			Triglycerides (mg/dL)			HDL cholesterol (mg/dL)			Blood pressure (mmHg)			Fasting glucose (mg/dL)		
	β[a]	S.E	p-value	β[a]	S.E	p-value	β[a]	S.E	p-value	β[a]	S.E	p-value	β[a]	S.E	p-value
Free thyroxine hormone (ng/dL)															
Low (<0.80)	1.383	0.938	0.1407	38.690	30.172	0.2000	-0.267	3.109	0.9317	0.758	3.532	0.8301	2.727	4.217	0.5180
Normal (low tertile) (<1.17)	0.327	0.240	0.1731	9.957	7.705	0.1964	-0.279	0.801	0.7272	-0.712	0.905	0.4313	1.698	1.077	0.1152
Normal (mid tertile) (<1.31)	Ref.			Ref.			Ref.			Ref.			Ref.		
Normal (high tertile) (<1.70)	-0.426	0.236	0.0714	-21.145	7.591	0.0054	1.439	0.788	0.0681	-0.359	0.890	0.6869	0.268	1.061	0.8003
High (1.70≤)	-0.735	0.753	0.3292	-49.713	24.227	0.0404	-1.718	2.603	0.5095	2.068	2.836	0.4661	15.992	3.386	<.0001
Thyroid stimulating hormone (uIU/mL)															
Low (<0.50)	-1.253	0.673	0.0629	-20.614	21.742	0.3432	4.393	2.227	0.0487	2.656	2.569	0.3014	0.178	3.040	0.9533
Normal (low tertile) (<1.80)	-0.318	0.234	0.1742	0.479	7.559	0.9495	-0.558	0.783	0.4759	0.630	0.880	0.4743	1.680	1.057	0.1122
Normal (mid tertile) (<2.87)	Ref.			Ref.			Ref.			Ref.			Ref.		
Normal (high tertile) (<5.00)	-0.378	0.257	0.1414	3.591	8.297	0.6652	0.035	0.859	0.9671	1.283	0.966	0.1843	0.713	1.160	0.5392
High (5.00≤)	-0.093	0.374	0.8044	9.045	12.095	0.4547	-0.890	1.246	0.4748	0.660	1.406	0.6389	-1.511	1.691	0.3717
Thyroid peroxidase antibody (IU/mL)[b]															
Normal (<34)	Ref.			Ref.			Ref.			Ref.			Ref.		
High (under low FT4) (34≤)	0.396	0.498	0.4268	36.075	16.046	0.0247	-2.475	1.674	0.1396	-0.814	1.866	0.6626	-2.152	2.249	0.3387
High (under high FT4) (34≤)	-0.620	0.556	0.2655	-6.054	17.922	0.7356	0.118	1.862	0.9493	4.319	2.084	0.0384	-1.604	2.512	0.5232
Thyroid peroxidase antibody (IU/mL)[c]															
Normal (<34)	Ref.			Ref.			Ref.			Ref.			Ref.		
High (under low TSH) (34≤)	-0.307	0.587	0.6014	-5.248	18.895	0.7812	-1.617	1.966	0.4110	-0.493	2.198	0.8225	-1.511	2.648	0.5682
High (under high TSH) (34≤)	0.111	0.478	0.8162	32.181	15.396	0.0368	-1.130	1.608	0.4825	2.723	1.791	0.1288	-2.169	2.157	0.3149

[a]Models is adjusted by age, gender, education level, marital status, household income level, region, occupation, alcohol consumption, smoking, walking activity and stress level
[b]Considering that thyroid peroxidase antibody related to both hypothyroidism and hyperthyroidism, high groups were divided into two groups by two median of free thyroxine
[c]Considering that thyroid peroxidase antibody related to both hypothyroidism and hyperthyroidism, high groups were divided into two groups by two median of thyroid stimulating hormone

Table 3 Subgroup analysis of components of metabolic syndromes with free thyroxine hormone levels stratified by age and gender

Variables	Free thyroxine hormone levels												
	Low			Normal (low tertile)			Normal (mid tertile)	Normal (high tertile)			High		
	β^a	S.E	p-value	β^a	S.E	p-value	β^a	β^a	S.E	p-value	β^a	S.E	p-value
Waist circumference													
Age													
19~44	3.248	1.715	0.0586	0.400	0.345	0.2471	Ref.	−0.537	0.300	0.0738	−1.062	0.892	0.2343
45~64	0.745	1.113	0.5037	0.470	0.352	0.1818	Ref.	0.078	0.410	0.8495	0.394	1.668	0.8134
64<	−1.085	3.667	0.7684	−0.026	0.927	0.9777	Ref.	−1.638	1.226	0.1868	−3.990	3.705	0.2859
Gender													
Male	1.998	2.172	0.3580	0.804	0.405	0.0477	Ref.	−0.270	0.336	0.4206	−0.684	0.957	0.4749
Female	1.481	0.982	0.1322	0.070	0.284	0.8061	Ref.	−0.556	0.328	0.0909	−2.002	1.277	0.1173
Triglycerides													
Age													
19~44	124.396	51.798	0.0165	10.341	10.430	0.3217	Ref.	−25.519	9.066	0.0050	−49.843	26.938	0.0646
45~64	22.880	41.955	0.5858	14.699	13.253	0.2680	Ref.	−11.085	15.441	0.4732	−78.026	62.873	0.2153
64<	−29.035	77.925	0.7108	−6.737	19.693	0.7335	Ref.	20.424	26.056	0.4363	−21.240	78.744	0.7883
Gender													
Male	−8.759	88.150	0.9209	19.926	16.443	0.2260	Ref.	−29.603	13.619	0.0301	−56.536	38.816	0.1457
Female	59.246	19.538	0.0025	6.175	5.645	0.2744	Ref.	−8.730	6.527	0.1815	−39.210	25.395	0.1230
HDL cholesterol													
Age													
19~44	−3.987	5.399	0.4605	0.135	1.096	0.9021	Ref.	2.554	0.952	0.0075	−0.867	2.954	0.7692
45~64	0.799	4.276	0.8518	−1.313	1.360	0.3348	Ref.	−1.687	1.581	0.2868	−5.880	6.408	0.3594
64<	6.579	10.435	0.5309	1.360	2.688	0.6149	Ref.	3.663	3.507	0.3007	10.076	10.581	0.3450
Gender													
Male	−4.968	6.373	0.4360	−0.661	1.201	0.5824	Ref.	1.028	0.994	0.3017	0.343	2.981	0.9085
Female	1.003	3.743	0.7888	0.050	1.089	0.9634	Ref.	1.908	1.256	0.1292	−3.308	4.865	0.4968
Blood pressure													
Age													
19~44	9.081	5.089	0.0747	−0.032	1.029	0.9751	Ref.	0.639	0.893	0.4741	1.560	2.646	0.5556
45~64	−4.007	5.626	0.4767	−2.552	1.779	0.1522	Ref.	−3.081	2.075	0.1382	−1.728	8.439	0.8378
64<	−12.387	20.182	0.5417	5.314	5.101	0.3017	Ref.	−2.610	6.749	0.7003	22.083	20.395	0.2833
Gender													
Male	−12.655	7.995	0.1139	2.073	1.497	0.1666	Ref.	−0.438	1.239	0.7239	2.575	3.522	0.4649
Female	4.899	3.870	0.2060	−2.082	1.122	0.0638	Ref.	−0.001	1.294	0.9996	3.303	5.030	0.5116
Fasting glucose													
Age													
19~44	−3.880	7.421	0.6012	1.190	1.494	0.4261	Ref.	1.333	1.299	0.3050	17.139	3.859	<.0001
45~64	5.895	5.216	0.2591	1.833	1.648	0.2665	Ref.	−2.049	1.920	0.2865	14.249	7.817	0.0690
64<	13.834	18.440	0.4561	−0.592	4.660	0.8994	Ref.	1.248	6.166	0.8403	3.026	18.633	0.8715
Gender													
Male	0.545	11.505	0.9623	3.968	2.146	0.0649	Ref.	−0.335	1.778	0.8506	21.236	5.066	<.0001
Female	3.278	3.480	0.3466	0.346	1.006	0.7307	Ref.	1.431	1.163	0.2187	5.173	4.524	0.2532

^{a}Model is adjusted by age, gender, education level, marital status, household income level, region, occupation, alcohol consumption, smoking, walking activity and stress level

Discussion

The purpose of this study was to identify whether any associations exist between thyroid hormone levels and metabolic syndrome components. Thyroid dysfunction is well known to affect glucose and lipid metabolism; abnormal glucose level and abnormal lipid profile are important factors of metabolic syndrome [17]. In our study, we found that glucose and lipid metabolism were associated with thyroid dysfunction. A significant positive association was observed between fasting glucose and FT4 in patients with high FT4 levels. In terms of lipid metabolism, a negative association between triglycerides and FT4 was observed among people with normal-high or high FT4 levels. In addition, there was a significant positive association between TPOab and triglycerides levels in patients with high thyroid peroxidase levels and with low median FT4 levels.

Thyroid hormones regulate carbohydrate metabolism [18]. They influence the mRNA and protein expression of the glucose transporter 4, AMP-activated protein kinase, and acetyl CoA carboxylase in skeletal muscle [19]. Hyperthyroidism usually occurs when high FT4 levels leads to its increased production and absorption from glycogen, lactic acid, glycerol, and amino acids [20]. Hyperthyroidism can also increase insulin degradation. Which deteriorates blood glucose control [19, 20]. Based on these mechanisms, other studies also showed that glucose levels are high in patients with hyperthyroidism [21]. Foss et al. demonstrated that patients with hyperthyroidism had higher blood glucose levels than the euthyroid participants, indicating increased endogenous glucose production [22]. Moreover, Roubsanthisuk et al. reported that the higher glucose intolerance showed common in hyperthyroidism compare to the normal participants [23]. This could be a major cause of the increased risk for diabetes [23]. Health professionals should conduct follow-up tests of the glucose level of patients with high thyroid hormone levels. Additionally, thyroid hormone levels should be checked regularly in patients with high glucose levels.

A significant negative association between FT4 levels and triglycerides was observed in patients with high-normal or high FT4 levels. To explain this, we presumed that thyroid hormones play a key role in the regulation of enzyme activity during lipoprotein transport [12]. The influence of thyroid function on lipid metabolism involves a pathophysiological process [24]. The negative association observed between triglycerides and thyroid hormones can be explained by the increased removal rate of triglycerides from plasma due to an increase in the activity of hepatic triglyceride lipase [25, 26]. The effects of thyroid hormone on lipid metabolism are well known [26]. Because the lipid profile tends to normalize improperly under high thyroid hormone levels, the lipid profile needs to be followed up after adjusting for thyroid hormone levels [25].

There was a significant positive association between TPOab and triglycerides levels in patients with high thyroid peroxidase levels but with low median FT4 levels. In addition, a positive association was identified between TPOab and triglycerides levels in patients with high thyroid peroxidase levels in the presence of high median TSH levels. The presence of TPOab in the blood indicates a high risk for thyroid disease due to autoimmune disorders [27, 28]. In fact, abnormal TPOab levels were observed in 90% of patients with hypothyroidism and Graves' disease [27, 28]. Therefore, the positive association between TPOab and triglycerides levels in patients with high thyroid peroxidase levels but low median FT4 levels may be related to hypothyroidism.

Based on the results of the subgroup analysis, a significant negative association was observed between FT4 and triglyceride levels in patients aged 19–44 years; this association was stronger in the 19–44-year-old age group than in the other older age groups. This finding emphasizes the possibility of accumulation of risk through one's life course. Accumulation of various risks increases owing to illness, health-damaging behaviors, and adverse environmental conditions [29]. Older people may have more risk factors owing to their risk accumulation, and are more likely to have unmeasured risk factors that we could not adjust for [30]. To address this issue, future studies developed to understand the association between thyroid hormones and metabolic syndrome should incorporate a panel design.

This study had some limitations. First, the study was based on a cross-sectional survey. Causality could not be confirmed clearly and only the association could be confirmed. Second, one of the major thyroid hormones, tri-iodothyronine, was not used in the thyroid function tests. Despite the above limitations, this study also has a few strengths. First, consistent blood tests showed accurate blood TSH levels. Second, most of the previous studies were conducted in Caucasians; therefore, this issue is worth pursuing among Koreans. Finally, this study used the most recent (KNHANES 2013–2015) nationally, multistage, stratified collected data and could therefore be considered to be representative of the Korean population.

Conclusion

FT4 showed a partially positive association with fasting glucose, and a partially negative association with triglycerides in the general Korean population. Glucose level and lipid profile are metabolic syndrome components; metabolic syndrome is strongly correlated with diseases such as diabetes and cardiovascular disease that are associated with high mortality and morbidity rates. In patients with abnormal thyroid function, follow up tests for metabolic syndrome components during thyroid dysfunction could prevent overlooking metabolic syndrome and prevent related diseases.

Abbreviations
CI: Confidence interval; FT4: Free thyroxine; KNHANES: Korea National Health and Nutrition Examination Surveys; OR: Odds ratio; TPOab: Thyroid peroxidase antibody; TSH: Thyroid-stimulating hormone

Acknowledgements
We appreciate Department of Health and Human Services Centers for Disease Control and Prevention that provided meaningful data.

Authors' contributions
E.-C.P. (corresponding author) reviewed the manuscript. J.J. (cofirst author) and Y. K. (cofirst author) wrote the draft of the manuscript and analyzed the data. J. S., S. A. L. and Y. C. provided assistance for the planning, execution, execution, and analysis of the study. All authors read and approved final manuscript. The authors appreciate the administrative support provided by the Yonsei University Institute of Health Services Research. This research study was not funded by any foundation.

Competing interests
The authors declare that they have no competing interests.

Author details
[1]Department of Public Health, Graduate School, Yonsei University, Seoul, Republic of Korea. [2]Institute of Health Services Research, Yonsei University, Seoul, Republic of Korea. [3]Department of Anesthesia, Indiana University School of Medicine, Indianapolis 46202, USA. [4]Department of Preventive Medicine & Institute of Health Services Research, Yonsei University College of Medicine, 50 Yonsei-ro, Seodaemun-gu, Seoul 120-752, Republic of Korea.

References
1. Grundy SM. Obesity, metabolic syndrome, and cardiovascular disease. J. Clin. Endocrinol. Metab. 2004;89(6):2595–600.
2. Roos A, Bakker SJ, Links TP, Gans RO, Wolffenbuttel BH. Thyroid function is associated with components of the metabolic syndrome in euthyroid subjects. J. Clin. Endocrinol. Metab. 2007;92(2):491–6.
3. Ramachandran A, Snehalatha C, Satyavani K, Sivasankari S, Vijay V. Metabolic syndrome in urban Asian Indian adults—a population study using modified ATP III criteria. Diabetes Res Clin Pract. 2003;60(3):199–204.
4. Aguilar M, Bhuket T, Torres S, Liu B, Wong RJ. Prevalence of the metabolic syndrome in the United States, 2003-2012. JAMA. 2015;313(19):1973–4.
5. Vishram JK, Borglykke A, Andreasen AH, Jeppesen J, Ibsen H, Jørgensen T, Palmieri L, Giampaoli S, Donfrancesco C, Kee F. Impact of age and gender on the prevalence and prognostic importance of the metabolic syndrome and its components in Europeans. The MORGAM prospective cohort project. PLoS One. 2014;9(9):e107294.
6. Park S, Kim S-J, Lee M, Kang K-A, Hendrix E. Prevalence and associated factors of metabolic syndrome among south Korean adults. J Community Health Nurs. 2015;32(1):24–38.
7. Korea S: Cause of death statistics. Statistics Korea 2016.
8. Mullur R, Liu Y-Y, Brent GA. Thyroid hormone regulation of metabolism. Physiol Rev. 2014;94(2):355–82.
9. Lambadiari V, Mitrou P, Maratou E, Raptis AE, Tountas N, Raptis SA, Dimitriadis G. Thyroid hormones are positively associated with insulin resistance early in the development of type 2 diabetes. Endocrine. 2011;39(1):28–32.
10. Dimitriadis G, Raptis S. Thyroid hormone excess and glucose intolerance. Exp Clin Endocrinol Diabetes. 2001;109(Suppl 2):S225–39.
11. Klein I, Ojamaa K. Thyroid hormone and the cardiovascular system. N Engl J Med. 2001;344(7):501–9.
12. Duntas LH. Thyroid disease and lipids. Thyroid. 2002;12(4):287–93.
13. Ruhla S, Weickert MO, Arafat AM, Osterhoff M, Isken F, Spranger J, Schöfl C, Pfeiffer AF, Möhlig M. A high normal TSH is associated with the metabolic syndrome. Clin Endocrinol. 2010;72(5):696–701.
14. Yang M, Qu H, Deng H-C. Acute pancreatitis induced by methimazole in a patient with Graves' disease. Thyroid. 2012;22(1):94–6.
15. Davies PH, Franklyn JA, Daykin J, Sheppard MC. The significance of TSH values measured in a sensitive assay in the follow-up of hyperthyroid patients treated with radioiodine. J. Clin. Endocrinol. Metab. 1992;74(5): 1189–94.
16. Goswami R, Goel S, Tomar N, Gupta N, Lumb V, Sharma YD. Prevalence of clinical remission in patients with sporadic idiopathic hypoparathyroidism. Clin Endocrinol. 2010;72(3):328–33.
17. Rizos C, Elisaf M, Liberopoulos E. Effects of thyroid dysfunction on lipid profile. Open Cardiovasc. Med. J. 2011;5:76.
18. de Jesus G-GJ, Alvirde-Garcia U, Lopez-Carrasco G, Mendoza MEP, Mehta R, Arellano-Campos O, Choza R, Sauque L, Garay-Sevilla ME, Malacara JM. TSH and free thyroxine concentrations are associated with differing metabolic markers in euthyroid subjects. Eur J Endocrinol. 2010;163(2):273–8.
19. Crunkhorn S, Patti M-E. Links between thyroid hormone action, oxidative metabolism, and diabetes risk? Thyroid. 2008;18(2):227–37.
20. Bhattacharyya A, Wiles P. Diabetic ketoacidosis precipitated by thyrotoxicosis. Postgrad Med J. 1999;75(883):291–3.
21. Gu Y, Li H, Bao X, Zhang Q, Liu L, Meng G, Wu H, Du H, Shi H, Xia Y. The relationship between thyroid function and the prevalence of type 2 diabetes mellitus in euthyroid subjects. J. Clin. Endocrinol. Metab. 2016;jc:2016–965.
22. Foss MC, Paccola GM, Saad MJ, Pimenta WP, Piccinato CE, Iazigi N. Peripheral glucose metabolism in human hyperthyroidism. J. Clin. Endocrinol. Metab. 1990;70(4):1167–72.
23. Roubsanthisuk W, Watanakejorn P, Tunlakit M, Sriussadaporn S. Hyperthyroidism induces glucose intolerance by lowering both insulin secretion and peripheral insulin sensitivity. J. Med. Assoc. Thai. = Chotmaihet thangphaet. 2006;89(Suppl 5):S133–40.
24. Park SB, Choi HC, Joo NS. The relation of thyroid function to components of the metabolic syndrome in Korean men and women. J Korean Med Sci. 2011;26(4):540–5.
25. Pucci E, Chiovato L, Pinchera A. Thyroid and lipid metabolism. Int J Obes. 2000;24(S2):S109.
26. Tulloch B, Lewis B, Fraser TR. Triglyceride metabolism in thyroid disease. Lancet. 1973;301(7800):391–4.
27. Sultana Q, Anjum A, Fathima N, Siraj M, Ishaq M. Seropositivity to anti-thyroid peroxidase and anti-thyroglobulin autoantibodies in hypo and hyper-thyroidism: Diagnostic and epidemiological significance. IJMR. 2016; 3(4):368–72.
28. Swain M, Swain T, Mohanty BK. Autoimmune thyroid disorders—an update. Indian J Clin Biochem. 2005;20(1):9–17.
29. Kuh D, Ben-Shlomo Y, Lynch J, Hallqvist J, Power C. Life course epidemiology. J Epidemiol Community Health. 2003;57(10):778.
30. Organization WH: Life course perspectives on coronary heart disease, stroke and diabetes: key issues and implications for policy and research: summary report of a meeting of experts, 2–4 may 2001. 2001.

13

A predictive model of thyroid malignancy using clinical, biochemical and sonographic parameters for patients in a multi-center setting

Jia Liu[1,2,3], Dongmei Zheng[1,2,3,8*], Qiang Li[4], Xulei Tang[5], Zuojie Luo[6], Zhongshang Yuan[7], Ling Gao[2,3] and Jiajun Zhao[1,2,3]

Abstract

Background: Thyroid nodules are highly prevalent, but a robust, feasible method for malignancy differentiation has not yet been well documented. This study aimed to establish a practical model for thyroid nodule discrimination.

Methods: Records for 2984 patients who underwent thyroidectomy were analyzed. Clinical, laboratory, and US variables were assessed retrospectively. Multivariate logistic regression analysis was performed and a mathematical model was established for malignancy prediction.

Results: The results showed that the malignant group was younger and had smaller nodules than the benign group (43.5 ± 11.6 vs. 48.5 ± 11.5 y, $p < 0.001$; 1.96 ± 1.16 vs. 2.75 ± 1.70 cm, $p < 0.001$, respectively). The serum thyrotropin (TSH) level (median = 1.63 mIU/L, IQR (0.89–2.66) vs. 1.19 (0.59–2.10), $p < 0.001$) was higher in the malignant group than in the benign group. Patients with malignancies tested positive for anti-thyroglobulin antibody (TGAb) and anti-thyroid peroxidase antibody (TPOAb) more frequently than those with benign nodules (TGAb, 30.3% vs. 15.0%, $p < 0.001$; TPOAb, 25.6% vs. 18.0%, $p = 0.028$). The prevalence of ultrasound (US) features (irregular shape, ill-defined margin, solid structure, hypoechogenicity, microcalcifications, macrocalcifications and central intranodular flow) was significantly higher in the malignant group. Multivariate logistic regression analysis confirmed that age (OR = 0.963, 95% CI = 0.934–0.993, $p = 0.017$), TGAb (OR = 4.435, 95% CI = 1.902–10.345, $p = 0.001$), hypoechogenicity (OR = 2.830, 95% CI = 1.113–7.195, $p = 0.029$), microcalcifications (OR = 4.624, 95% CI = 2.008–10.646, $p < 0.001$), and central intranodular flow (OR = 2.155, 95% CI = 1.011–4.594, $p < 0.05$) were independent predictors of thyroid malignancy. A predictive model including four variables (age, TGAb, hypoechogenicity and microcalcification) showed an optimal discriminatory accuracy (area under the curve, AUC) of 0.808 (95% CI = 0.761–0.855). The best cut-off value for prediction was 0.52, achieving sensitivity and specificity of 84.6% and 76.3%, respectively.

Conclusion: A predictive model of malignancy that combines clinical, laboratory and sonographic characteristics would aid clinicians in avoiding unnecessary procedures and making better clinical decisions.

Keywords: Thyroid nodules, Malignancy, Predictive model

* Correspondence: dmeizheng@163.com
[1]Department of Endocrinology, Shandong Provincial Hospital Affiliated to Shandong University, Jinan, Shandong 250021, China
[2]Shandong Clinical Medical Center of Endocrinology and Metabolism, Jinan, Shandong 250021, China
Full list of author information is available at the end of the article

Background

Thyroid nodules are highly prevalent in the general adult population, with a detection rate of 19–67% during routine ultrasound examinations [1]. An epidemiological study showed that approximately 5–15% of these nodules are malignant [2]. Despite the high incidence of thyroid malignancy, most patients referred for suspected nodules have benign conditions. The overestimation of malignancy leads to the performance of unnecessary procedures and causes a burden for both society and patients. Therefore, distinguishing thyroid nodules preoperatively is required.

To date, the Thyroid Imaging Reporting and Data System (TIRADS) and American Thyroid Association guidelines are considered as the main criteria for determining malignancy and are generally followed by radiologists in practice [3]. However, these categorization systems were established based on fine needle aspiration (FNA) cytology results that included data from nodules > 1 cm. In addition, a few reports have presented serum thyrotropin (TSH) and positive thyroid autoantibodies as possible predictors of thyroid malignancy [4, 5]. However, these guidelines or studies either used FNA cytology results for their final diagnoses, which are less reliable than those confirmed via surgical inspection, or they included a relatively small number of patients. Additionally, most studies to date have focused on single risk factors, clinical, biochemical or radiological, and only a few studies have analyzed these risk factors in combination. A robust predictive model involving easily accessible clinical, laboratory and radiological risk factors may serve as a pragmatic aid in making decisions regarding malignancy differentiation.

In the present study, we reviewed a large cohort of 2984 patients in China who underwent thyroid surgery and had final pathological data available. The purpose of our study was to verify the independent risk factors of clinical, laboratory and ultrasonographic (US) features in patients with thyroid carcinomas and to establish a predictive model for determining malignancy that can be used by clinical practitioners.

Methods

Patients

We retrospectively studied the data from 3145 consecutive patients who mostly received routine neck ultrasound detections and underwent total or partial thyroid surgery between 2006 and 2009 at four tertiary hospitals in China. Patients with a previous thyroid surgery or radiation ablation and patients who were taking thyroxine or antithyroid drugs were not included. Patients with medullary thyroid cancer, anaplastic cancer or lymphoma were considered TSH-nonresponsive and were excluded. After the exclusions, 2984 patients were included in the analysis. Their clinical, laboratory, and US variables were assessed retrospectively. This study had institutional review board approval.

US imaging analysis

US examinations of the four tertiary hospitals were performed using US scanner GE LOGIQ9 (USA) equipped with a 5–12-MHz linear transducer for morphological examinations and a 4.7-MHz transducer for color Doppler evaluations. The examinations were conducted and recorded by two skilled sonographers from respective hospitals according to a standard procedure and interobservers reached agreement on the results of each US findings. The following US parameters of the nodules were recorded: (1) number of nodules, (2) nodule size, (3) echoic texture, (4) echogenicity, (5) shape, (6) margin, (7) calcification (microcalcification, macrocalcification, or egg-shell calcification) and (8) intranodular central flow.

Laboratory variables

The levels of serum TSH, free triiodothyronine (FT3) and free thyroxine (FT4) were determined using chemiluminescence analyzer Roche Cobas E601 (Switzerland) and the matched kit. These values ranged from 0.35 to 5.5 UI/ml for TSH, from 11.5 to 22.7 pmol/l for FT4 and from 3.5 to 6.5 pmol/l for FT3. If the other laboratories had different normal ranges, the values were adjusted to reflect the same normal range. Anti-thyroid peroxidase antibody (TPOAb, reference value < 60 μIU/ml) and anti-thyroglobulin antibody (TGAb, reference value < 60 IU/ml) levels were measured using immunometric assays. Thyroid antibody levels higher than the upper range were considered positive.

Pathology

FNA cytology was not generally performed and considered as a routine pre-operative assessment when the study was conducted. Postoperative histopathologic evaluations were performed by pathologists experienced in thyroid pathology. The histopathologic results of the patients operated on were grouped as either malignant or benign.

Statistical analysis

Descriptive statistics are presented as the means ± standard deviations for continuous variables and as the number of patients and percentages for categorical variables. Differences between independent groups for continuous variables were evaluated using a Student's t-test or a Mann–Whitney U-test, where applicable. Categorical data were analyzed using Pearson's chi-square test. Univariate and multivariate logistic regression analyses were performed to evaluate the association between malignancy and risk factors. Appealing receiver operating characteristic (ROC) curve analyses were performed to examine the predictive power of combinations of clinical, laboratory and sonographic features. The areas under the curves (AUCs) were derived from ROC curves. The Youden index was used to define the optimal cut-off value [6]. All statistical analyses were performed using SPSS version 17.0 (SPSS, Inc., Chicago, IL). Differences between AUCs were detected using Delong's test [7]. A *p*-value of < 0.05 was considered statistically significant.

Results
Clinical characteristics
This study cohort consisted of 541 men and 2443 women. Overall, 2460 patients were diagnosed with pathologically benign nodules, and 524 patients were diagnosed with malignant nodules. The malignancy rate in our study was 17.6%. Most of the nodules were detected incidentally in routine body check-up and totally 10.5% of the patients present clinical systems such as hoarsennes, swallowing difficulty, thyroid enlargement, with the duration of symptoms varying from 7 days to 26 years. As shown in Table 1, there was no difference in the sex ratios between the patients with benign and malignant nodules. Patients with malignant nodules were younger than those without malignant nodules (43.5 ± 11.6 years vs. 48.5 ± 11.5 years, *p* < 0.001) (Table 1).

The mean maximal diameter of malignant nodules was significantly smaller than that of benign nodules (1.96 ± 1.16 cm vs. 2.75 ± 1.70 cm, *p* < 0.001). The prevalence of solitary nodules in malignant cases was not different from that in benign cases (29.0% vs. 25.1%, *p* = 0.109).

Laboratory values
As shown in Table 2, there were no significant differences in FT3 and FT4 values between the two groups. The level of TSH (median 1.63 mIU/L, IQR (0.89–2.66) vs. 1.19 (0.59–2.10), *p* < 0.001] in the malignant group was higher than in the benign group. Subsequently, based on the cutoff values predetermined in population studies, TSH levels were divided into quintiles, including below normal (< 0.35 mIU/L), above normal (> 5.5 mIU/L), and within normal, with the latter divided into tertiles of similar size

Table 1 Clinical characteristics of 2984 subjects with thyroid nodules

	Benign (*n* = 2460)	Malignant (*n* = 524)	*P* value
Gender			
Male,%	17.7%	20.0%	0.212
Age, y, mean(SD)	48.5(11.5)	43.5(11.6)	< 0.001
Nodule size, cm, mean(SD)	2.75(1.70)	1.96(1.16)	< 0.001
Solitary nodule, %	25.1%	29.0%	0.109

Continuous variables were compared using Student's tests or Mann-Whitney U tests, and categorical variables, using X²tests. *P* < 0.05 was considered significant. Nodule size was derived from ultrasound detection

Table 2 Laboratory variables of subjects with thyroid nodules

	Benign	Malignant	P value
FT3, pmol/L, median (IQR)	4.43 (3.91–5.07)	4.44 (3.96–5.00)	0.809
FT4, pmol/L, median (IQR)	14.97 (12.84–17.42)	15.76 (13.6–18.09)	0.064
TSH, mIU/ml, median (IQR)	1.19 (0.59–2.10)	1.63 (0.89–2.66)	< 0.001
TGAb, %	15.0%	30.3%	< 0.001
TPOAb, %	18.0%	25.6%	0.028

Continuous variables were compared using Mann-Whitney U tests, and categorical variables, using X² tests. P < 0.05 was considered significant
Abbreviations: FT3 free triiodothyronine, *FT4* free thyroxine, *TSH* thyrotropin, *TGAb* anti-thyroglobulin antibody, *TPOAb* anti-thyroid peroxidase antibody

(0.35–0.99 mIU/L, 1.0–2.49 mIU/L, and 2.5–5.49 mIU/L). The prevalence of malignancy was 9.8% when TSH levels were less than 0.35 mIU/L, compared with 13.2% when TSH levels were 5.5 mIU/L or greater (*p* = 0.17). In the normal range, a high rate of malignancy was observed in patients with higher TSH levels. The prevalence of malignancy was 15.8% when TSH levels were between 1.0 and 2.49 mIU/L and 24.4% when TSH levels were between 2.50 and 5.49 mIU/L, compared with 12.6% when TSH levels were between 0.35 and 0.99 mIU/L (*p* = 0.09 and *p* < 0.001, respectively) (Fig. 1).

Patients with malignant nodules had positive TGAb and TPOAb results more frequently than did patients with benign nodules (for TGAb, 30.3% vs. 15.0%, *p* < 0.001; for TPOAb, 25.6% vs. 18.0%, *p* = 0.028).

Sonographic features
The prevalences of an irregular shape (42.7% vs. 10.7%, *p* < 0.001), an ill-defined margin (38.7% vs. 9.7%, *p* < 0.001), a solid structure (75.8% vs. 41.3% *p* < 0.001), hypoechogenicity (68.5% vs. 27.1%, *p* < 0.01), microcalcification (48.5% vs. 13%, *p* < 0.001), macrocalcification (18.5% vs. 12.5%, *p* = 0.001), and an intranodular central flow (60.3% vs. 47.1%, *p* < 0.001) were significantly higher in malignant nodules than in benign nodules (Table 3). There were no differences between the benign and malignant groups for egg-shell calcifications (*p* > 0.05).

Clinical, biochemical and sonographic characteristics of microcarcinoma
Of 524 malignant nodules, 104 nodules ≤1 cm in diameter were defined as microcarcinomas. Since microcarcinoma is considered "more silent", we analyzed clinical, biochemical and sonographic parameters separately. As shown in the Additional file 1: Table S1, we found age, positive TGAb result, hypoechogenicity, microcalcification and intranodular central flow were also associated with increased risk for malignancy in the nodules less than 1 cm in diameter.

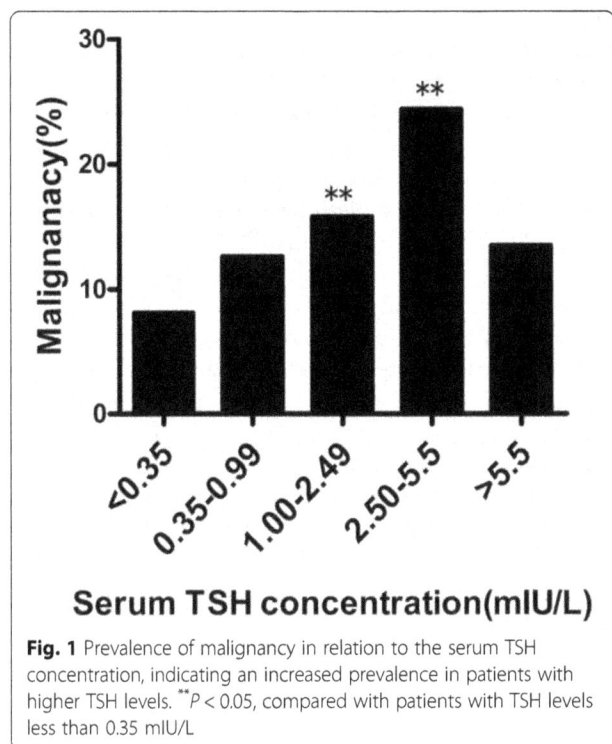

Fig. 1 Prevalence of malignancy in relation to the serum TSH concentration, indicating an increased prevalence in patients with higher TSH levels. **$P < 0.05$, compared with patients with TSH levels less than 0.35 mIU/L

Table 4 Multivariate logistic regression of risk factors for the presence of thyroid malignancy

	B	SE	OR	95%CI of OR	P value
Age	−0.038	0.016	0.963	0.934–0.993	0.017
Nodule size	−0.262	0.153	0.770	0.571–1.038	0.086
TSH	0.024	0.056	1.025	0.918–1.143	0.664
TGAb	1.490	0.432	4.435	1.902–10.345	0.001
TPOAb	−0.104	0.489	0.901	0.346–2.350	0.832
Irregular shape	1.089	0.579	2.972	0.955–9.245	0.06
Ill-defined margin	0.099	0.626	1.104	0.324–3.767	0.874
Solid structure	−0.251	0.453	0.778	0.320–1.891	0.580
Hypoechogenicity	1.040	0.476	2.830	1.113–7.195	0.029
Microcalcification	1.531	0.426	4.624	2.008–10.646	< 0.001
Macrocalcification	0.961	0.514	2.614	0.955–7.154	0.061
Central flow	0.768	0.386	2.155	1.011–4.594	0.047

Data are coefficients (B), corresponding SE, OR, 95% CI, and measure of significance (P value)
Abbreviations: CI confidence interval, *OR* odds ratio

2.830, 95% CI 1.113–7.195, $p = 0.029$; microcalcification OR 4.624, 95% CI 2.008–10.646, $p < 0.001$; central flow OR 2.155, 95% CI 1.011–4.594, $p < 0.05$, respectively).

The associations between risk factors and the presence of malignant nodules

We further explored the correlation of clinical characteristics, laboratory values and US features with the risk for malignant nodules via univariate analysis, which gave results consistent with those from the prevalence analysis (data not shown). Multivariate analysis confirmed that age had a significant negative correlation with an increased risk of thyroid malignancy (OR 0.963, 95% CI 0.934–0.993, $p = 0.017$) (Table 4). Additionally, a positive TGAb result, hypoechogenicity, microcalcification and intranodular central flow were independently associated with increased risks for malignant nodules (TGAb OR 4.435, 95% CI 1.902–10.345, $p = 0.001$; hypoechogenicity OR

Table 3 Sonographic features of subjects with thyroid nodules

	Benign	Malignant	P value
Irregular shape	10.7%	42.7%	< 0.001
Ill-defined margin	9.7%	38.7%	< 0.001
Solid structure	41.3%	75.8%	< 0.001
Hypoechogenicity	27.1%	68.5%	< 0.01
Microcalcification	13.0%	48.5%	< 0.001
Macrocalcification	12.5%	18.5%	0.001
Egg-shell calcification	1.6%	1.7%	0.797
Central flow	47.1%	60.3%	< 0.001

Categorical variables were compared using X^2 tests. $P < 0.05$ was considered significant

The performance of independent risk factors—A mathematical model to predict malignancy

To evaluate the predictive power of combinations of clinical characteristics, laboratory values and US features and to establish a mathematical model to calculate the risk for malignancy, a series of ROC curve analyses were performed, and AUCs were calculated. When the factors age, TGAb, hypoechogenicity and microcalcification were combined, the optimal AUC had a favorable value of 0.808 (0.761–0.855), indicating a diagnostic accuracy of 80.8% (Fig. 2). By combining these four independent risk factors of malignancy, we established the following formula for a predictive model:

p = (EXP(− 0.963−0.4*age + 1.108*TGAb+ 1.441*microcalcification+ 1.722*hypoechogenicity)/(1 + EXP(− 0.963− 0.4*age + 1.108*TGAb+ 1.441*microcalcification+ 1.722* hypoechogenicity)).

The best cut-off value was calculated as 0.52, with a sensitivity of 84.6% and a specificity of 76.3%.

Discussion

In this study, we verified risk factors associated with thyroid malignancy after comprehensively evaluating clinical, laboratory and sonographic variables in a population of 2984 patients who underwent thyroidectomy. Subsequently, we developed a mathematical model for cancer prediction, thereby providing a practical tool for clinicians to distinguish thyroid nodules preoperatively.

In agreement with previous studies, we identified that decreased age was one of the independent risk factors

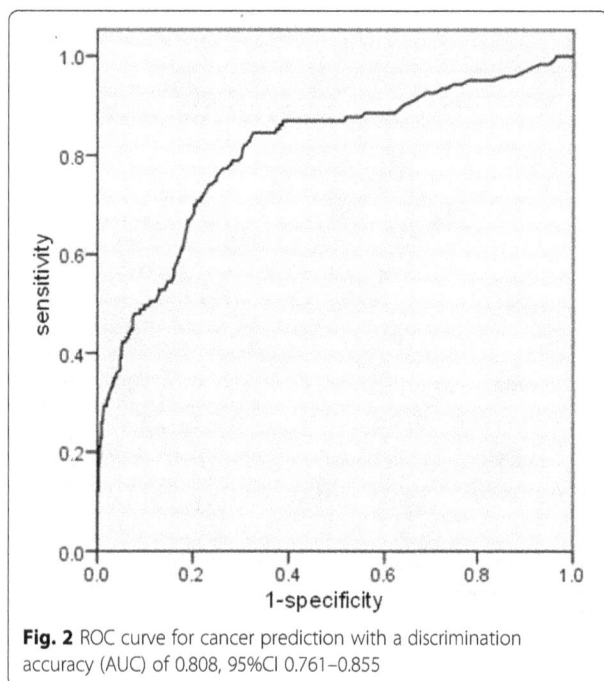

Fig. 2 ROC curve for cancer prediction with a discrimination accuracy (AUC) of 0.808, 95%CI 0.761–0.855

for thyroid cancer [8]. Malignant nodules were smaller than benign nodules (1.96 ± 1.16 cm vs. 2.75 ± 1.70 cm, $p < 0.001$). However, our multivariate logistic analysis did not confirm a predictive role of nodule size. This difference indicates that smaller nodules may not have a higher risk of malignancy because patients with larger nodules often have an increased likelihood of surgery for benign reasons, such as compressive symptoms, whereas patients with smaller nodules without any suspicious sonographic findings often select a conservative follow-up.

Higher TSH values, even within normal ranges, have been associated with a higher prevalence of thyroid malignancy in some studies [4, 5, 9, 10]. The results of our study are in agreement with those of previous studies, except for when TSH levels were higher than 5.5 mIU/l, which was not associated with a further increase in the prevalence of malignancy. This difference may be due to selection bias because we excluded patients who were taking thyroxine drugs; therefore, the number of patients with TSH levels > 5.5 mIU/L would have been quite small. However, in our study TSH lost its diagnostic value after being included in the multivariate logistic regression analysis, probably due to its weak role in predicting malignancy, which could be masked by including other co-effectors. Elevated TGAb, but not TPOAb, levels were a significant predictor of thyroid cancer, which is consistent with the findings of other reports [11–14]. Consistently, our study confirmed that the prevalence of lymphocytic thyroiditis was more frequent in malignant nodules (Additional file 2: Table S2). Additionally, our data also confirmed that patients with thyroiditis had

positive TGAb more frequently than patients without thyroiditis (63.9% vs. 13.0%, $p < 0.001$).

Numerous studies have investigated the role of US findings in the diagnosis of malignant nodules [1, 15–17]. These studies state that hypoechogenicity, microcalcification, thyroid nodules with irregular margins, and intranodular vascularity are important features in determining the risk of malignancy. However, Cappelli et al. showed that an ill-defined margin was a nonspecific finding that could be seen for both benign and malignant nodules [18]. Consistent with these previous findings, we confirmed that microcalcifications, hypoechogenicity and intranodular central flow were associated with increased risks of malignancy. Our study did not find an association between egg-shell calcification and malignancy. Peripheral-rim or eggshell calcification has generally been considered to be an indicator of a benign nodule. However, a recently published study of thyroid nodules with eggshell calcifications reported that the findings of a peripheral halo and disruption of eggshell calcifications may be useful predictors of malignancy [19, 20]. Further studies are needed to confirm this observation.

Previously, some researchers have reported several systems for maligncy assessment [21–25]. Stojadinovic et al. established a model based on the performance of electrical impedance scanning (EIS) EIS, which was not routinely scheduled in clinics [21]. Zahir et al. showed a complicated two-step predictive model which was less accesible for clinicans [22]. Koike et al. included US features alone for differentiating non-follicular neoplasms > 5 mm [23]. Maia et al. evaluated malignancy risk based on patients from a single center [24]. Banks et al. analyzed 639 patients established a diagnostic model using the variables age, nodule size and FNA cytology [25]. Different from previous reports, in this study we enrolled 2984 patients from multiple tertiary medical centers, which greatly strengthens the evidence for diagnostic evaluations. Additionally, our mathematical model is derived from a combination of easily accessible clinical, biochemical and sonographic predictors, which improves the feasibility and practical appeal, thereby helping clinicians with decision making and reducing unnecessary invasions.

In addition, we analyzed predictive variables based on postoperative pathological inspections instead of FNA cytology examinations. Although FNA is considered to be an accurate and cost-effective method for evaluating thyroid nodules with a high diagnostic sensitivity and specificity [26], there are some limitations to diagnostic FNAs. First, FNA is recommended for nodules > 1 cm at their greatest dimension with a highly or intermediately suspicious sonographic pattern and for nodules > 1.5 cm at their greatest dimension with a minimally suspicious sonographic pattern [3]. Nodules smaller than 1 cm are difficult to distinguish via FNA cytology. Second, the performance of FNA is largely affected by the experience of radiologists, and the quality of the FNA procedure may affect the results. Reflecting these limitations, a number of previous studies have analyzed risk stratification based on FNA diagnoses [4, 26, 27] and have shown that it is less reliable than postoperative pathological examinations, which were used in our study.

However, there are some limitations to this study. The US feature of a node being taller than it is wide is considered to be a reliable indicator for thyroid malignancy. Unfortunately, these data were not available for the majority of the patients; therefore, this parameter was not included in the analysis. An algorithm including this US feature might improve the diagnostic accuracy of the predictive model in our study. Although less convincing than operative confirmations, FNA cytology is a relatively effective and robust method for identifying malignancies. Unfortunately, due to limitations relating to the skill with which FNAs are performed and a lack of compliance by patients, FNAs were not routinely performed in suspicious thyroid nodules in this study. Lastly, our study is retrospective, and prospective studies in a larger patient population are required to define and verify this model of risk prediction to improve clinical management.

Conclusion

In summary, we analyzed 2984 patients who underwent thyroidectomy from multiple tertiary medical centers and established a practical model for predicting malignancies using a combination of simple and accessible clinical, biochemical and sonographic predictors. Prospective studies are required to validate this predictive model in a larger population.

Abbreviations

AUC: Area under curve; FNA: Fine needle aspiration; FT3: Free triiodothyronine; FT4: Free thyroxine; TGAb: Anti-thyroglobulin antibody; TPOAb: Anti-thyroid peroxidase antibody; TSH: Serum thyrotropin; US: Ultrasound

Acknowledgements

Not applicable.

Funding

This work was supported by grants from the National Natural Sciences Foundation of China (81100593, 81770785) and Provincial key research and development plan(2017GSF18154) to Jia Liu and was partially supported by Science and Technology Department of Shandong Province (2015GGH318016) to Dongmei Zheng.

Authors' contributions

JL conceived and designed the study, performed the data analyses and drafted the manuscript. DZ helped study design, data analysis and manuscript revision. QL,XT and ZL helped patient enrollment and data collection. ZY helped data analyses. LG and JZ participated in the design of the study and critical revision of the manuscript. All of the authors read and approved the final manuscript.

Competing interests

The authors declare that they have no competing interests.

Author details

[1]Department of Endocrinology, Shandong Provincial Hospital Affiliated to Shandong University, Jinan, Shandong 250021, China. [2]Shandong Clinical Medical Center of Endocrinology and Metabolism, Jinan, Shandong 250021, China. [3]Institute of Endocrinology and Metabolism, Shandong Academy of Clinical Medicine, Jinan, Shandong 250021, China. [4]Department of Endocrinology and Metabolism, the Second Affiliated Hospital of Harbin Medical University, Harbin, Heilongjiang 150086, China. [5]Department of Endocrinology, the First Hospital of Lanzhou University, Lanzhou, Gansu 730000, China. [6]Department of Endocrinology, the First Affiliated Hospital of Guangxi University, Nanning, Guangxi 530021, China. [7]Department of Biostatistics, School of Public Health, Shandong University, Jinan, Shandong 250021, China. [8]Department of Endocrinology and Metabolism, Shandong Provincial Hospital Affiliated to Shandong University, Jingwu Road 324, Jinan, Shandong 250021, China.

References

1. Frates MC, Benson CB, Charboneau JW, Cibas ES, Clark OH, et al. Management of thyroid nodules detected at US: Society of Radiologists in ultrasound consensus conference statement. Radiology. 2005;237:794–800.
2. Frates MC, Benson CB, Doubilet PM, Kunreuther E, Contreras M, et al. Prevalence and distribution of carcinoma in patients with solitary and multiple thyroid nodules on sonography. J Clin Endocrinol Metab. 2006;91:3411–7.
3. Haugen BR, Alexander EK, Bible KC, Doherty GM, Mandel SJ, et al. 2015 American Thyroid Association management guidelines for adult patients with thyroid nodules and differentiated thyroid cancer: the American Thyroid Association guidelines task force on thyroid nodules and differentiated thyroid cancer. Thyroid. 2016;26:1–133.
4. Boelaert K, Horacek J, Holder RL, Watkinson JC, Sheppard MC, et al. Serum thyrotropin concentration as a novel predictor of malignancy in thyroid nodules investigated by fine-needle aspiration. J Clin Endocrinol Metab. 2006;91:4295–301.
5. Polyzos SA, Kita M, Efstathiadou Z, Poulakos P, Slavakis A, et al. Serum thyrotropin concentration as a biochemical predictor of thyroid malignancy in patients presenting with thyroid nodules. J Cancer Res Clin Oncol. 2008; 134:953–60.
6. Youden WJ. Index for rating diagnostic tests. Cancer. 1950;3:32–5.
7. DeLong ER, DeLong DM, Clarke-Pearson DL. Comparing the areas under two or more correlated receiver operating characteristic curves: a nonparametric approach. Biometrics. 1988;44:837–45.
8. Baier ND, Hahn PF, Gervais DA, Samir A, Halpern EF, et al. Fine-needle aspiration biopsy of thyroid nodules: experience in a cohort of 944 patients. AJR Am J Roentgenol. 2009;193:1175–9.
9. Haymart MR, Repplinger DJ, Leverson GE, Elson DF, Sippel RS, et al. Higher serum thyroid stimulating hormone level in thyroid nodule patients is associated with greater risks of differentiated thyroid cancer and advanced tumor stage. J Clin Endocrinol Metab. 2008;93:809–14.
10. Jung KW, Park S, Kong HJ, Won YJ, Boo YK, et al. Cancer statistics in Korea: incidence, mortality and survival in 2006-2007. J Korean Med Sci. 2010;25:1113–21.
11. Kim ES, Lim DJ, Baek KH, Lee JM, Kim MK, et al. Thyroglobulin antibody is associated with increased cancer risk in thyroid nodules. Thyroid. 2010;20:885–91.
12. Chiovato L, Latrofa F, Braverman LE, Pacini F, Capezzone M, et al.

Disappearance of humoral thyroid autoimmunity after complete removal of thyroid antigens. Ann Intern Med. 2003;139:346–51.

13. Chung JK, Park YJ, Kim TY, So Y, Kim SK, et al. Clinical significance of elevated level of serum antithyroglobulin antibody in patients with differentiated thyroid cancer after thyroid ablation. Clin Endocrinol. 2002;57:215–21.

14. Sands NB, Karls S, Rivera J, Tamilia M, Hier MP, et al. Preoperative serum thyroglobulin as an adjunct to fine-needle aspiration in predicting well-differentiated thyroid cancer. J Otolaryngol Head Neck Surg. 2010;39:669–73.

15. Papini E, Guglielmi R, Bianchini A, Crescenzi A, Taccogna S, et al. Risk of malignancy in nonpalpable thyroid nodules: predictive value of ultrasound and color-Doppler features. J Clin Endocrinol Metab. 2002;87:1941–6.

16. Kim EK, Park CS, Chung WY, Oh KK, Kim DI, et al. New sonographic criteria for recommending fine-needle aspiration biopsy of nonpalpable solid nodules of the thyroid. AJR Am J Roentgenol. 2002;178:687–91.

17. Moon WJ, Jung SL, Lee JH, Na DG, Baek JH, et al. Benign and malignant thyroid nodules: US differentiation–multicenter retrospective study. Radiology. 2008;247:762–70.

18. Cappelli C, Castellano M, Pirola I, Cumetti D, Agosti B, et al. The predictive value of ultrasound findings in the management of thyroid nodules. QJM. 2007;100:29–35.

19. Kim BM, Kim MJ, Kim EK, Kwak JY, Hong SW, et al. Sonographic differentiation of thyroid nodules with eggshell calcifications. J Ultrasound Med. 2008;27:1425–30.

20. Park M, Shin JH, Han BK, Ko EY, Hwang HS, et al. Sonography of thyroid nodules with peripheral calcifications. J Clin Ultrasound. 2009;37:324–8.

21. Stojadinovic A, Peoples GE, Libutti SK, Henry LR, Eberhardt J, et al. Development of a clinical decision model for thyroid nodules. BMC Surg. 2009;9:12.

22. Taghipour Zahir S, Binesh F, Mirouliaei M, Khajeh E, Noshad S. Malignancy risk assessment in patients with thyroid nodules using classification and regression trees. J Thyroid Res. 2013;2013:983953.

23. Koike E, Noguchi S, Yamashita H, Murakami T, Ohshima A, et al. Ultrasonographic characteristics of thyroid nodules: prediction of malignancy. Arch Surg. 2001;136:334–7.

24. Maia FF, Matos PS, Silva BP, Pallone AT, Pavin EJ, et al. Role of ultrasound, clinical and scintigraphyc parameters to predict malignancy in thyroid nodule. Head Neck Oncol. 2011;3:17.

25. Banks ND, Kowalski J, Tsai HL, Somervell H, Tufano R, et al. A diagnostic predictor model for indeterminate or suspicious thyroid FNA samples. Thyroid. 2008;18:933–41.

26. American Thyroid Association Guidelines Taskforce on Thyroid N, Differentiated Thyroid C, Cooper DS, Doherty GM, Haugen BR, et al. Revised American Thyroid Association management guidelines for patients with thyroid nodules and differentiated thyroid cancer. Thyroid. 2009;19:1167–214.

27. Chang SH, Joo M, Kim H. Fine needle aspiration biopsy of thyroid nodules in children and adolescents. J Korean Med Sci. 2006;21:469–73.

14

FSH may be a useful tool to allow early diagnosis of Turner syndrome

Stela Carpini[1], Annelise Barreto Carvalho[2], Sofia Helena Valente de Lemos-Marini[1], Gil Guerra-Junior[1] and Andréa Trevas Maciel-Guerra[3*]

Abstract

Background: Ultrasensitive assays to measure pre-pubertal gonadotropins levels could help identify patients with Turner syndrome (TS) in mid-childhood, but studies in this field are scarce. The aim of this study was to analyze gonadotropins levels in girls with TS throughout childhood.

Methods: Retrospective longitudinal study conducted with 15 girls with TS diagnosed with < 5 years whose FSH and LH measures were available since then. Hormones were evaluated in newborn/mini-puberty (< 0.5 years), early childhood (0.5–5 years), mid-childhood (5–10 years) and late childhood/adolescence (> 10 years). In newborn/mini-puberty and late childhood/adolescence pre-pubertal or pubertal gonadotropins were considered normal; in early childhood and mid-childhood concentrations above the pre-pubertal range were considered abnormal.

Results: Abnormally high FSH alone was found in four of five patients in newborn/mini-puberty, 13 of 15 during early childhood and nine of 15 during mid-childhood. In the group of 12 patients in late childhood/adolescence, the three girls with spontaneous puberty had only normal levels; the remaining showed only post-menopausal concentrations. In mid-childhood one patient exhibited only pre-pubertal FSH. Conversely, most LH measurements in early and mid-childhood were normal.

Conclusion: Karyotyping of girls with short stature and high FSH levels would allow early diagnosis of Turner syndrome in a significant number of patients, particularly when resources for chromosome study of all girls with growth deficiency are limited.

Keywords: Turner syndrome, Gonadal dysgenesis, Puberty delayed, Follicle-stimulating hormone, Luteinizing hormone

Background

Even now, in the genomics era, some genetic disorders remain a challenge to diagnosis due to wide phenotypic variability and/or lack of widespread availability of genetic tests, particularly in developing countries. This is the case with Turner syndrome (TS), which has an incidence of 1:2,130 female newborns [1] and is characterized by the presence of a normal X chromosome and partial or total loss of the other sex chromosome, X or Y. Although traditionally associated with the 45,X karyotype, TS can also be due to mosaicism or structural abnormalities of sex chromosomes.

There are also strong indications that patients with a 45,X karyotype are actually mosaics (cryptic mosaicism) [2].

The clinical picture varies widely, and includes dysmorphic features of face, neck, chest and limbs. Cardiovascular and renal/collecting system anomalies may also be found, as well as autoimmune thyroid disease. Nonetheless, the most constant features are short stature and primary hypogonadism due to gonadal dysgenesis [3].

Gonadal dysgenesis in TS is the result of massive apoptosis of the oocytes during fetal life [4–6]. Though the large majority of women with TS have dysgenetic gonads, about 30% will undergo some spontaneous pubertal development, and 2–5% may achieve spontaneous pregnancy [7, 8].

A study in the 1970's revealed that plasma concentrations of follicle-stimulating hormone (FSH) and luteinizing hormone (LH) in TS patients show a biphasic pattern [9].

* Correspondence: atmg@uol.com.br
[3]Department of Medical Genetics, FCM, Unicamp, Rua Tessalia Vieira de Camargo, 126, Campinas, SP 13083-887, Brazil
Full list of author information is available at the end of the article

In that study, mean basal plasma FSH level was strikingly elevated from 2 days to 4 years; thereafter, a decline in plasma FSH to pre-pubertal levels occurred between 4 and 10 years, followed by a rise after 10 years, reaching post-menopausal levels some years later. The pattern of LH secretion was qualitatively similar to that of FSH, though the values for LH were 1/3 to 1/10 those for FSH. In that work, however, gonadotropins concentrations were determined by radioimmunoassay (RIA), which has low sensitivity.

The development of ultrasensitive immunochemilumi-nometric and immunofluorometric assays in the 1980's and 1990's demonstrated that pre-pubertal FSH and LH levels are much lower than previously thought [10]. The study of gonadotropins levels of girls with TS revealed that they remained high even at pre-pubertal age, and it was even suggested that measurement of gonadotropins could help identify prepubertal patients with primary gonadal failure [11].

However, a study of 68 girls with TS, 20 of them followed over a period of 2 years, revealed normal FSH and LH concentrations in 9 and 23.5% of patients between 0 and 5 years, respectively, and in 41 and 74% of patients between 5 and 10 years, respectively [12].

As most available data were based on transversal studies, a retrospective longitudinal one was carried out with 70 girls aged 0 to 16 years; the median ages at TS diagnosis were 5.2 years in the group of patients with a 45,X karyotype and 8.2 years in the group of patients with other chromosome constitutions. Most patients, both those with and without spontaneous pubertal development, had at least one FSH and LH value within the reference range during mid-childhood [13].

Divergences among studies about various aspects of TS phenotype are common [14]; they are due to the wide karyotypic variability of TS, including mosaicism, various structural abnormalities and different proportions of normal and abnormal cell lines. The same must apply to the extent of ovarian dysgenesis in these girls and hence to differences in the levels of gonadotropins in the pediatric age range. Thus, more data are needed to draw definite conclusions about this matter.

The aim of this work was to analyze FSH and LH levels in a sample of girls with TS who were diagnosed in early childhood (0–5 years) and followed thereafter.

Methods

A retrospective longitudinal study was conducted with patients with TS who were diagnosed since the mid-1990's with less than 5 years of age, and whose measures of FSH and LH levels were available both in early childhood and in the following years, with routine follow-up visits scheduled every 6 months. FSH and LH levels had been measured using electrochemiluminescence assays as part of their routine clinical follow-up since the time

of diagnosis; these data were obtained retrospectively from patients' files. In the absence of spontaneous puberty, only gonadotropins levels measured prior to sex hormone replacement therapy (HRT) were included.

FSH and LH levels were classified as pre-pubertal (< 3.8 mUI/mL and < 1.4 mUI/mL, respectively), post-menopausal (> 25.8 mUI/mL and > 7.7 mUI/mL, respectively) or pubertal (those within the intermediate range) according to reference values of the assays used in our service (Roche Elecsys®). Gonadotropins levels were evaluated according to age range: newborn/mini-puberty (0–0.5 years), early childhood (0.5–5 years), mid-childhood (5–10 years) and late childhood/adolescence (> 10 years). In newborn/minipuberty and in late childhood/adolescence FSH and LH levels were considered normal when they were within the prepubertal or pubertal range, while in early and mid-childhood any concentrations above the pre-pubertal ones were regarded as abnormal.

The SPSS for Windows software, version 20 (SPSS, Inc., Chicago, IL, USA) was used for data analysis. This study was carried out in accordance with the Declaration of Helsinki and the protocol was approved by the Research Ethics Committee of the State University of Campinas (931/2008; CAAE 0352.0.146.000–08). The study was exempt from written informed consent from the subjects due to its retrospective design and noninterventional nature of the study protocol.

Results

Fifteen out of 186 patients diagnosed since the mid-1990's (8%) met the inclusion criteria (Table 1). Three of them were followed only until mid-childhood and the remaining until adolescence. Mean age at diagnosis was 1.7 years, and mean age at last hormonal evaluation (that of the last visit – in prepubertal patients and those with spontaneous puberty – or the last measurement prior to initiation of HRT) was 11.4 years. The mean follow-up was 10.7 years (range: 3.0–16.5 years), and most patients had a 45,X karyotype.

Three patients had spontaneous pubertal development, one of them with a 45,X chromosome constitution in 50 cells and two with mosaicism; two had already had menarche. Six had primary hypogonadism (absence of pubertal signs and elevated gonadotropins levels) and had already initiated HRT. Three were adolescents who already had post-menopausal FSH levels but were not under HRT (patients 1, 5 and 11); the remaining had not reached adolescence at the time this study was conducted, but in one of them a post-menopausal FSH level was already detected. The number of gonadotropins measurements per patient ranged from two to 21 (median: 10) (Table 1).

Table 1 Description of the sample: age, karyotype, puberty and results of gonadotropins measurements

Patient	Age at diagnosis	Age at last hormone evaluation[a]	Karyotype	Pubertal status	Abnormal measurements/total number of measurements	
					FSH	LH
1	NB/MP	LC/A	45,X	Pre-pubertal	9/10	2/10
2	NB/MP	LC/A	45,X	Induced puberty	11/11	3/12
3	NB/MP	LC/A	45,X/46,X,+mar (SRY -)	Induced puberty	16/17	10/17
4	NB/MP	LC/A	45,X	Induced puberty	10/11	6/9
5	NB/MP	LC/A	45,X	Pre-pubertal	12/12	3/12
6	NB/MP	LC/A	45,X	Spontaneous puberty[b]	5/14	0/14
7	NB/MP	LC/A	45,X	Induced puberty	10/10	8/10
8	EC	LC/A	45,X/46,XX	Spontaneous puberty[b]	0/21	4/21
9	EC	MC	45,X	Pre-pubertal	3/3	2/3
10	EC	LC/A	45,X	Induced puberty	10/11	4/10
11	EC	LC/A	45,X	Pre-pubertal	6/6	1/6
12	EC	LC/A	45,X/46,XX	Spontaneous puberty	2/10	0/8
13	EC	MC	45,X	Pre-pubertal	2/2	1/2
14	EC	LC/A	45,X	Induced puberty	9/9	5/10
15	EC	MC	45,X/46,X,i(Xq)	Pre-pubertal	4/4	0/4

EC early childhood, *LC/A* late childhood/adolescence, *MC* midchildhood, *mo* month, *NB/MP* newborn/minipuberty, *yr*. year
[a] That of the last visit – in prepubertal patients and those with spontaneous puberty – or the last measurement prior to initiation of hormone replacement therapy
[b] Menarche already occurred

Regarding FSH, four of the five patients whose gonadotropins were measured in the first 6 months of life had abnormally high levels; none of the five girls developed spontaneous puberty. During early childhood, 13 out of 15 girls had no measurements in the normal pre-pubertal range; moreover, nine of these 13 patients had at least one measurement which was in the post-menopausal range. During mid-childhood, six of the 15 girls had at least one normal FSH concentration, but three of them also exhibited at least one post-menopausal concentration in this period; a single patient [8] exhibited only prepubertal FSH levels. Ninety-three percent of the measurements performed in early childhood and 80% of those performed in mid-childhood were abnormal. In the group of 12 patients > 10 years old, those without spontaneous pubertal development showed only post-menopausal concentrations (Fig. 1, Table 2 and Additional file 1).

Only one out of five girls had an abnormally high LH concentration detected in the first 6 months of life, and most had at least one normal measurement in early childhood and mid-childhood. Sixty-two percent of the measurements performed in early childhood and 82% of those performed in mid-childhood were in the normal pre-pubertal range. In late childhood/adolescence, five patients had at least one prepubertal or pubertal level, though two of them also had at least one post-menopausal concentration, including one of the girls with spontaneous pubertal development (patient 8); all the remaining showed only post-menopausal concentrations (Fig. 1, Table 2 and Additional file 1).

FSH levels in this sample expressed the biphasic age pattern: they were high in newborn/mini-puberty and early childhood, declined in mid-childhood, though rarely reaching the normal pre-pubertal range, and then increased again in late childhood/adolescence. In comparison, the pattern of LH, though also biphasic, revealed much higher levels in late childhood/adolescence than in newborn/mini-puberty and early childhood. In addition, in mid-childhood the decline of LH compared to the previous period was less striking than that of FSH, and prepubertal levels were often seen (Fig. 1 and Table 2).

Discussion

Gonadotropins levels in this sample expressed the same biphasic age pattern found by Conte et al. [9]; however, the use of an ultrasensitive assay in the present study revealed that, different from what was observed by those authors, the decline in plasma FSH seldom reaches pre-pubertal levels in early and mid-childhood. The significantly high mean FSH levels found in pre-pubertal TS girls in this sample were similar to those found by others [12]. Thus, our results indicate that many girls with TS could be diagnosed earlier if FSH measurements were routinely done in girls with unexplained short stature.

The results of our study differ from the other retrospective longitudinal study found in literature [13], in which most patients had at least one FSH and LH value within the reference range during mid-childhood. However, comparison between these studies is difficult. In fact,

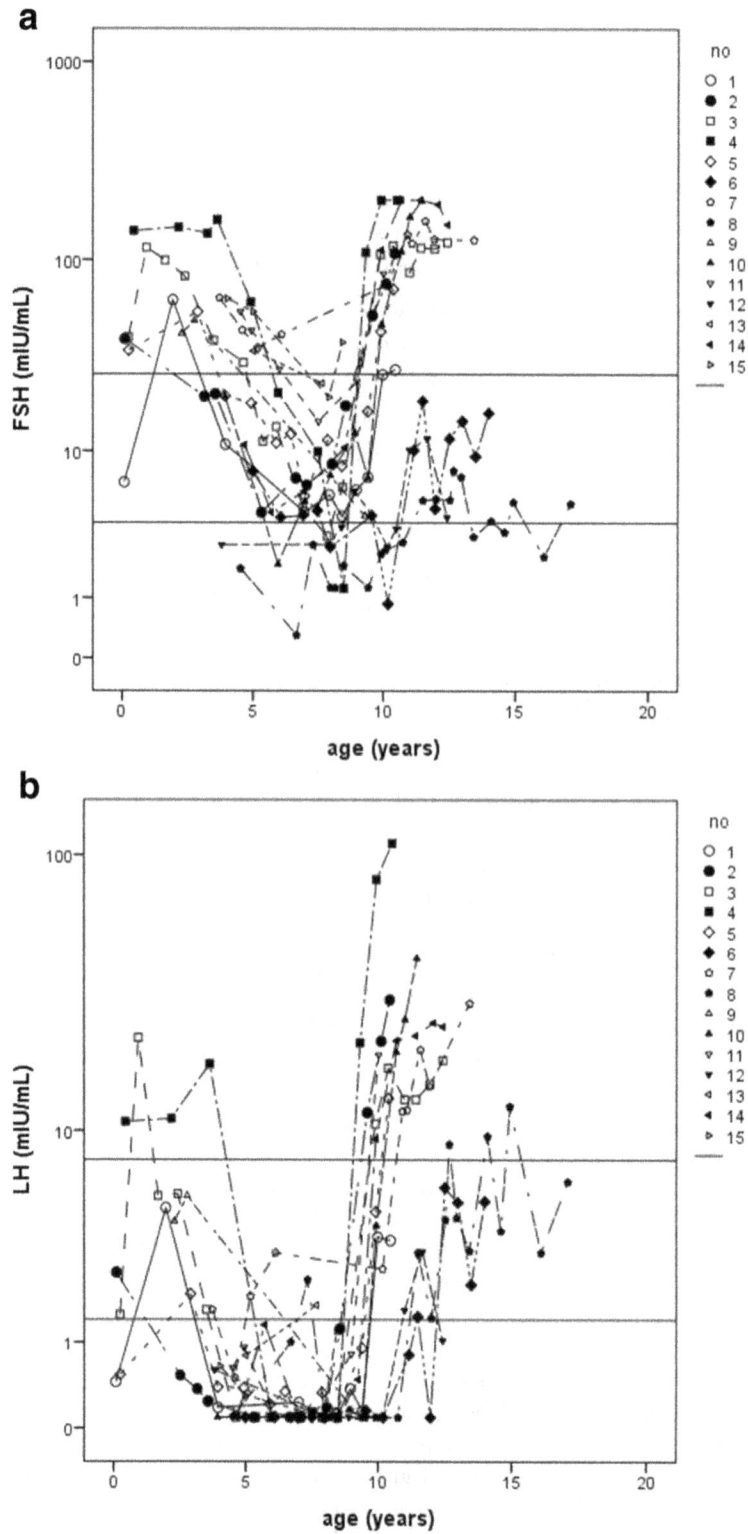

Fig. 1 Gonadotropins levels in different ages in girls with Turner syndrome. Hormone values are presented in the y-axis on a logarithmic scale. The lines on the y-axis represent the lower and upper normal limits for **a)** FSH and **b)** LH concentrations. Levels above the upper limits were considered post-menopausal and those below the lower limits were regarded as pre-pubertal

Table 2 Results of gonadotropins measurements according to age range in TS girls

| Age range (years) | N | mean | range | measurements | | | | Patients with at least one normal level for age[a] | Patients with only normal levels for age[a] | Patients with at least one abnormal level for age[a] |
				PP	P	PM	Total			
FSH										
0–0.5	5	52.05 ±51.03	6.65–140.00	0	1	4	5	1	1	4/5 (80%)
0.5–5	15	52.09 ±42.35	1.80–160.00	2	8	20	30	2	2[b]	13/15 (87%)
5–10	15	18.72 ±32.87	0.30–201.00	13	42	11	66	6	1[b]	14/15 (93%)
> 10	12	65.16 ±69.55	0.87–201.00	8	18	24	50	3	3[b]	9/12 (75%)
LH										
0–0.5	5	3.16 ±4.35	0.45–10.80	2	2	1	5	4	2	3/5 (60%)
0.5–5	15	3.07 ±5.37	0.09–22.20	18	8	3	29	13	9	6/15 (40%)
5–10	15	2.60 ±10.58	0.09–82.02	53	7	5	65	13	5	10/15 (67%)
> 10	12	12.97 ±17.36	0.09–110.00	7	17	25	49	5	3	9/12 (75%)

FSH follicle-stimulating hormone, *LH* luteinizing hormone, *N* number of patients, *P* pubertal, *PM* post-menopausal, *PP* pre-pubertal
[a] 0–0.5 years: PP or P level; 0.5–5 years and 5–10 years: PP level; > 10 years: PP or P level
[b] only patients with spontaneous pubertal development

age at diagnosis varied widely in that study (44 of the 70 girls were more than 12 years old at diagnosis) and longitudinal samples could not be obtained in all cases; in addition, length of follow-up was also variable.

A survey conducted in our university hospital in the beginning of the 1990's revealed that seven out of 38 girls with growth deficiency (18%) had TS [15]. Another study on this matter conducted with 353 subjects in China in the same decade found a very similar figure: 19% of the females had TS [16]. However, in other studies this proportion varied widely, from 4.5 to 81.7% [17–19].

Some authors have recommended routine karyotype analysis for all of these girls [20, 21], while others suggest that routine cytogenetic analysis should be restricted to those with associated congenital anomalies [19, 22], but this is still a matter of debate. In any case, karyotyping is not always available; this is particularly true in developing countries, in which the karyotype is an expensive exam and rarely offered in public health services. In addition, TS has wide phenotypic variability, and some features may not be recognized unless specifically sought [23]. As a consequence, TS may be diagnosed only in adolescence, when lack of pubertal development manifests in addition to short stature. In our institution, for instance, a recent survey revealed that mean age at diagnosis is 12 years, due to late referral by primary health services [24].

It is currently known that up to 40% of TS girls may have some degree of spontaneous pubertal development and up to 19% may have complete puberty and menses [7]; these figures may be even higher when the sample is not biased towards patients with hypogonadism [25]. Thus, some patients with residual ovarian function may have normal gonadotropins levels throughout childhood and escape diagnosis when these hormones are measured.

The majority, however, would benefit from the inclusion of FSH as an additional diagnostic tool to assess girls with unexplained growth deficiency. It has already been proposed that elevated FSH levels in childhood should prompt cytogenetic evaluation [21]. Indeed, in our sample normal measurements were uncommon both in early childhood and in mid-childhood; in addition, normal levels after 0.5 years were restricted to patients with spontaneous pubertal development. On the other hand, as most LH measurements in these age ranges were normal, its usefulness is limited.

Even though FSH measurement is not always sensitive for the diagnosis of TS in girls with unexplained short stature, this widely available and highly specific test to detect gonadal dysgenesis may lead to early diagnosis and prompt treatment in a significant number of patients by giving priority to performing their karyotype when this test is not accessible to screen all girls with growth deficiency. Even though gonadal dysgenesis is also a feature of other disorders of sex development, these conditions are usually not associated with short stature. This is the case of complete gonadal dysgenesis, either 46,XY (which may be due to mutations in *SRY* gene, among others) or 46,XX (which may be due to mutations in FSH receptor gene, among others). Thus, in some cases a normal karyotype may be found and lead to further investigations on the origin of high FSH levels.

Some of the strengths of this study are early age of diagnosis (less than 5 years in all cases), which avoids bias caused by pubertal delay as the main feature leading to clinical suspicion, and significantly long-term follow-up conducted in the same service. On the other hand, sample size is small due to definition of early age at diagnosis as an inclusion criterion.

Conclusion

In summary, follow-up of 15 girls with TS from early infancy on revealed that most FSH measurements were above the normal range for age before late childhood/adolescence. These results indicate that inclusion of this test in the guidelines for the evaluation of girls with unexplained short stature would allow early diagnosis and treatment in a significant number of patients by prioritizing their cytogenetic evaluation, particularly when resources for chromosomal studies of all girls with growth deficiency are limited.

Abbreviations

FSH: Follicular stimulating hormone; HRT: Sex hormone replacement therapy; LH: Luteinizing hormone; TS: Turner syndrome

Acknowledgements

The authors are grateful to the Main Clinical Laboratory of the University Hospital and to the Cytogenetics Laboratory of the Department of Medical Genetics of State University of Campinas (Unicamp).

Funding

This work was supported by the National Council for Scientific and Technological Development (CNPq/PIBIC).

Authors' contributions

SC contributed to the design of the work, acquisition, analysis and interpretation of data, drafting the work and final approval of the version to be published. AC contributed to acquisition of data, revising the work critically for important intellectual content and final approval of the version to be published. SL-M contributed to acquisition, analysis and interpretation of data, revising the work critically for important intellectual content and final approval of the version to be published. GG-J contributed to acquisition, analysis and interpretation of data, revising the work critically for important intellectual content and final approval of the version to be published. AM-G contributed to the design of the work, analysis and interpretation of data, drafting the work,

revising it critically for important intellectual content and final approval of the version to be published. All authors agree to be accountable for all aspects of the work in ensuring that questions related to the accuracy or integrity of any part of the work were appropriately investigated and resolved.

Competing interests

The authors declare that the research was conducted in the absence of any commercial or financial relationships that could be construed as a potential conflict of interest.

Author details

[1]Department of Pediatrics, Faculty of Medical Sciences (FCM), State University of Campinas (Unicamp), São Paulo, Brazil. [2]Post-Graduate Program in Child and Adolescent Health, FCM, Unicamp, São Paulo, Brazil. [3]Department of Medical Genetics, FCM, Unicamp, Rua Tessalia Vieira de Camargo, 126, Campinas, SP 13083-887, Brazil.

References

1. Nielsen J, Wohlert M. Chromosome abnormalities found among 34,910 newborn children: results from a 13-year incidence study in Arhus, Denmark. Hum Genet. 1991;87:81–3.
2. Fernández-García R, García-Doval S, Costoya S, Pásaro E. Analysis of sex chromosome aneuploidy in 41 patients with Turner syndrome: a study of "hidden" mosaicism. Clin Genet. 2000;58:201–8.
3. Bondy CA. Care of girls and women with Turner syndrome: a guideline of the Turner syndrome study group. J Clin Endocrinol Metab. 2007;92:10–25.
4. Modi DN, Sane S, Bhartiya D. Accelerated germ cell apoptosis in sex chromosome aneuploid fetal human gonads. Mol Hum Reprod. 2003;9:219–25.
5. Singh RP, Carr DH. The anatomy and histology of XO human embryos and fetuses. Anat Rec. 1966;155:369–83.
6. Reynaud K, Cortvrindt R, Verlinde F, De Schepper J, Bourgain C, Smitz J. Number of ovarian follicles in human fetuses with the 45,X karyotype. Fertil Steril. 2004;81:1112–9.
7. Pasquino A, Passeri F. Spontaneous pubertal development in Turner's syndrome 1. J Clin Endocrinol Metab. 1997;82:1810–3.
8. Kawagoe S, Kaneko N, Hiroi M. The pregnancy outcome of Turner syndrome: case report and review of the literature. In: Hibi I, Takano K, editors. Basic and clinical approach to Turner syndrome. Amsterdam: Elsevier Science Publishers B.V; 1993. p. 101–5.
9. Conte FA, Grumbach MM, Kaplan SL. A diphasic pattern of gonadotropin secretion in patients with the syndrome of gonadal dysgenesis. J Clin Endocrinol Metab. 1975;40:670–4.
10. Neely EK, Hintz RL, Wilson DM, Lee PA, Gautier T, Argente J, et al. Normal ranges for immunochemiluminometric gonadotropin assays. J Pediatr. 1995; 127:40–6.
11. Ropelato MG, Escobar ME, Gottlieb S, Bergadá C. Gonadotropin secretion in prepubertal normal and agonadal children evaluated by ultrasensitive time-resolved immunofluorometric assays. Horm Res. 1997;48:164–72.
12. Chrysis D, Spiliotis BE, Stene M, Cacciari E, Davenport ML. Gonadotropin secretion in girls with Turner syndrome measured by an ultrasensitive immunochemiluminometric assay. Horm Res. 2006;65:261–6.
13. Hagen CP, Main KM, Kjaergaard S, Juul A. FSH, LH, inhibin B and estradiol levels in Turner syndrome depend on age and karyotype: longitudinal study of 70 Turner girls with or without spontaneous puberty. Hum Reprod. 2010; 25:3134–41.
14. Hook EB, Warburton D. Turner syndrome revisited: review of new data supports the hypothesis that all viable 45,X cases are cryptic mosaics with a rescue cell line, implying an origin by mitotic loss. Hum Genet. 2014;133: 417–24.
15. Viguetti NL, Maciel-Guerra AT. Short stature and Turner syndrome: an association more frequent than expected. J Pediatr. 1994;70:172–4.
16. Lam WFF, Hau WLE, Lam TSS. Evaluation of referrals for genetic investigation of short stature in Hong Kong. Chin Med J. 2002;115:607–11.
17. Temtamy SA, Ghali I, Salam MA, Hussein FH, Ezz EH, Salah N. Karyotype/

phenotype correlation in females with short stature. Clin Genet. 1992;41:147–51.

18. Gicquel C, Gaston V, Cabrol S, Le Bouc Y. Assessment of Turner's syndrome by molecular analysis of the X chromosome in growth-retarded girls. J Clin Endocrinol Metab. 1998;83:1472–6.

19. Moreno-García M, Fernández-Martínez FJ, Miranda EB. Chromosomal anomalies in patients with short stature. Pediatr Int. 2005;47:546–9.

20. Sävendahl L, Davenport ML. Delayed diagnoses of Turner's syndrome: proposed guidelines for change. J Pediatr. 2000;137:455–9.

21. Saenger P, Wikland KA, Conway GS, Davenport M, Gravholt CH, Hintz R, et al. Recommendations for the diagnosis and management of Turner syndrome. J Clin Endocrinol Metab. 2001;86:3061–9.

22. Eggert P, Pankau R, Oldigs HD. How necessary is a chromosomal analysis in growth-retarded girls? Clin Genet. 1990;37:351–4.

23. Miguel-Neto J, Carvalho AB, Marques-de-Faria AP, Guerra-Júnior G, Maciel-Guerra AT. New approach to phenotypic variability and karyotype-phenotype correlation in Turner syndrome. J Pediatr Endocrinol Metab. 2016;29:475–9.

24. Carvalho AB, Guerra-Júnior G, Baptista MTM, Marques-de-Faria AP, de Lemos-Marini SHV, Maciel-Guerra AT. Turner syndrome: a pediatric diagnosis frequently made by non-pediatricians. J Pediatr. 2010;86:121–5.

25. Carpini S, Carvalho AB, Guerra-Júnior G, Baptista MTM, Lemos-Marini SHV, Maciel-Guerra AT. Spontaneous puberty in girls with early diagnosis of Turner syndrome. Arq Bras Endocrinol Metabol. 2012;56:653–7.

15

ATR-101, a selective ACAT1 inhibitor, decreases ACTH-stimulated cortisol concentrations in dogs with naturally occurring Cushing's syndrome

Daniel K. Langlois[1]*, Michele C. Fritz[1,6], William D. Schall[1], N. Bari Olivier[1], Rebecca C. Smedley[2], Paul G. Pearson[3], Marc B. Bailie[4] and Stephen W. Hunt III[5]

Abstract

Background: Cushing's syndrome in humans shares many similarities with its counterpart in dogs in terms of etiology (pituitary versus adrenal causes), clinical signs, and pathophysiologic sequelae. In both species, treatment of pituitary- and adrenal-dependent disease is met with limitations. ATR-101, a selective inhibitor of ACAT1 (acyl coenzyme A:cholesterol acyltransferase 1), is a novel small molecule therapeutic currently in clinical development for the treatment of adrenocortical carcinoma, congenital adrenal hyperplasia, and Cushing's syndrome in humans. Previous studies in healthy dogs have shown that ATR-101 treatment led to rapid, dose-dependent decreases in adrenocorticotropic hormone (ACTH) stimulated cortisol levels. The purpose of this clinical study was to investigate the effects of ATR-101 in dogs with Cushing's syndrome.

Methods: ATR-101 pharmacokinetics and activity were assessed in 10 dogs with naturally-occurring Cushing's syndrome, including 7 dogs with pituitary-dependent disease and 3 dogs with adrenal-dependent disease. ATR-101 was administered at 3 mg/kg PO once daily for one week, followed by 30 mg/kg PO once daily for one ($n = 4$) or three ($n = 6$) weeks. Clinical, biochemical, adrenal hormonal, and pharmacokinetic data were obtained weekly for study duration.

Results: ATR-101 exposure increased with increasing dose. ACTH-stimulated cortisol concentrations, the primary endpoint for the study, were significantly decreased with responders (9 of 10 dogs) experiencing a mean ± standard deviation reduction in cortisol levels of 50 ± 17% at study completion. Decreases in pre-ACTH-stimulated cortisol concentrations were observed in some dogs although overall changes in pre-ACTH cortisol concentrations were not significant. The compound was well-tolerated and no serious drug-related adverse effects were reported.

Conclusions: This study highlights the potential utility of naturally occurring canine Cushing's syndrome as a model for human disease and provides proof of concept for ATR-101 as a novel agent for the treatment of endocrine disorders like Cushing's syndrome in humans.

Keywords: Hyperadrenocorticism, Adrenocortical carcinoma, Canine models of adrenal disease

* Correspondence: langlo21@cvm.msu.edu
[1]Department of Small Animal Clinical Sciences, College of Veterinary Medicine, Michigan State University, East Lansing, MI 48824, USA
Full list of author information is available at the end of the article

Background

Hyperadrenocorticism, commonly known as Cushing's syndrome (CS), is an endocrine disorder with many similarities between dogs and humans [1]. In both species, most cases of naturally-occurring disease result from adrenocorticotropic hormone (ACTH) secreting pituitary adenomas, while remaining cases often result from cortisol-secreting adrenal tumors [2, 3]. Regardless of etiology, clinical signs are usually a result of increased circulating cortisol concentrations. Dermatologic manifestations are frequent and can include thin skin, easy bruising, hyperpigmentation, and recurrent infections [4]. The catabolic effects of cortisol often lead to muscle wasting and central obesity resulting in a classic "Cushingoid" appearance. Serious consequences such as hypertension, dyslipidemias, and thromboembolism are reported in both species [2, 5].

In addition to pathophysiologic parallels, similar treatment options exist for both species [6–8]. However, the actual treatment pursued for pituitary-dependent disease often differs as hypophysectomy and irradiation, both common therapies for humans with pituitary lesions, are infrequently performed in dogs in part due to expense and limited availability. Furthermore, depending on definition used, procedural success of dogs undergoing hypophysectomy for CS could be as low as 60% when considering post-operative mortality, treatment failures, and disease relapse [7, 9]. Direct comparative studies have not been performed, but median survival times do not appear to be substantially different in dogs undergoing hypophysectomy compared to dogs receiving medical therapy alone [9–11]. As such, most dogs with Cushing's disease are treated medically with agents that target the adrenal gland. Common therapies include trilostane, which inhibits enzymatic conversion of steroids by 3-beta-hydroxysteroid dehydrogenase, or mitotane, an adrenal cytotoxic agent [8, 12]. In veterinary medicine, the complicated dosing and side effects of mitotane have led to declining use, with a corresponding increase in trilostane treatment [13]. However, variable pharmacologic activity of trilostane has led to differing dosing recommendations with some dogs requiring up to three times daily dosing, and a small number of dogs having minimal response [14, 15]. Monitoring remains frequent, and fatal adrenal gland necrosis has been reported occasionally [15]. In humans, relapse of hypercortisolemia occurs in 15–66% of patients undergoing hypophysectomy, and persistent hypercortisolemia occurs in 14–72% of patients undergoing radiation therapy [2, 16]. Consequently, medical therapy is necessary for a subset of human patients; however, current options have limitations ranging from poor drug tolerability to variable efficacy [16].

Treatment has remained similar in dogs and humans with adrenal-dependent disease. Although adrenalectomy is curative for benign disease, management of malignant adrenocortical carcinoma (ACC) has remained challenging [17, 18]. Median survival times in dogs with detectable metastases are approximately 2–4 months despite medical or surgical intervention [18, 19]. In humans, surgical resection is palliative as the disease is often advanced at the time of diagnosis. Chemotherapeutics evaluated to date have been largely ineffective at reducing tumor burden, and controlling hypercortisolemia remains difficult [17, 20]. No drug is FDA approved for treatment of canine ACC, and the only FDA approved drug for treatment of human ACC is mitotane. However, stable disease or partial remissions only occur in approximately 30% of human patients with malignant disease, and survival times are poor [21]. Furthermore, mitotane toxicities are common and negatively affect quality of life in both humans and dogs [17, 20, 22]. Multi-agent protocols also have been used to treat human ACC; however, the median progression free survival of 5 months is discouraging [23].

Given these limitations, there is a critical need for new, targeted therapies for CS and ACC. ATR-101 (also known as PD132301–2) is a small molecule therapeutic in human clinical development for the treatment of ACC, congenital adrenal hyperplasia, and Cushing's syndrome (CS). ATR-101 is a potent (IC_{50} = 0.009 μM) and selective inhibitor of acyl coenzyme A:cholesterol acyltransferase isoform 1 (ACAT1). ACAT1 catalyzes cholesterol ester formation from cholesterol and long-chain fatty acyl-CoA [24], and in the adrenal cortex, is particularly important in creating a reservoir of substrate for steroid biosynthesis. Inhibition of this enzyme by ATR-101 at low doses results in decreases in circulating cortisol levels and other adrenal steroids in a time- and dose-dependent manner due to the lack of esterified cholesterol reservoirs. At high doses, ATR-101 leads to accumulation of free cholesterol in adrenocortical cells, ultimately leading to cellular stress and apoptosis [25–27]. As such, ATR-101 therapy could be of benefit for multiple diseases associated with adrenal steroid dysregulation [26, 27]. Recent in vivo pharmacologic studies in healthy dogs [25, 27] have provided support for development of ATR-101 in ACC and endocrine diseases such as CS and congenital adrenal hyperplasia given that ATR-101 preferentially distributes to the adrenal glands and selectively inhibits adrenal ACAT1 activity. The frequently encountered gastrointestinal and neurologic side effects of mitotane have not been observed in initial studies of ATR-101 administration to healthy dogs [27]. A recent study has suggested that ACAT1 may also be a target of mitotane [28], but other, yet to be elucidated targets, may account for some of the effects of mitotane, although this has not been thoroughly investigated [29].

Given the similarities in dogs and humans with naturally occurring CS, the dog offers a unique opportunity to perform proof of concept clinical studies for a human therapeutic. In this study, the pharmacokinetics of ATR-

101 were determined in dogs with naturally occurring CS. Furthermore, we investigated the biochemical and adrenal hormonal effects of ATR-101 administration over a 2–4 week time period. Adrenal gland histology was evaluated in dogs with adrenal-dependent disease. The results reported herein further support the ongoing development of ATR-101 as a novel agent for treatment of endocrine disorders associated with adrenal steroid dysregulation.

Methods
Compound
ATR-101 [N-[2,6-bis(1-methylethyl)phenyl]-N´-[[1-[4-(dimethylamino)phenyl]cyclopentyl]methyl]urea, hydrochloride salt (PD132301–2)] was synthesized by PharmAgra Labs, Inc. (Brevard, NC) using a modification of previously described methods [30]. The ATR-101 (Lot 313PAL23) used in these experiments had a purity of 95. 7%. ATR-101 was compounded into gelatin capsules using microcrystalline cellulose as an excipient to meet target doses (3 mg/kg and 30 mg/kg) based on individual subject weights.

Sample size calculation
A study of a continuous response variable (post-ACTH-stimulated cortisol concentrations following initial treatment) from matched pairs of study subjects was planned using previous data from dogs treated for CS at the Michigan State University Veterinary Medical Center. In order to detect a 35% decrease in post-ACTH-stimulated cortisol concentrations, 10 subjects would be needed to be able to reject the null hypothesis that this response difference is zero with probability (power) 0.8. The Type I error probability associated with this test of this null hypothesis is 0.05.

Animal study
This study was a prospectively designed proof-of-concept study to evaluate the activity of ATR-101 in dogs with CS. Dogs with both pituitary and adrenal-dependent CS were included in the study given the clinical, hormonal, and biochemical similarities [3] coupled with current veterinary practice standards in which drugs that target the adrenal glands are used for medical management of both forms of disease [12, 19]. Considering the mechanistic features of ATR-101 [27], treatment would be expected to be of benefit for naturally occurring CS independent of etiology. Client-owned dogs with clinical signs, biochemical evidence, or a recent diagnosis of CS were recruited from the local veterinary community. All dogs underwent initial evaluation at the Michigan State University Veterinary Medical Center to include a complete patient history, thorough physical examination, complete blood count, serum biochemical profile, and urinalysis. Dogs with concurrent disease that

could account for clinical signs or dogs that received any medications within the preceding 3 months that could alter endogenous cortisol production were excluded from participation. If suspicion for CS still existed following initial evaluation, an ACTH stimulation test or a low-dose dexamethasone suppression test (LDDST) were performed for confirmation [20, 31]. Dogs with confirmed CS underwent complete abdominal ultrasound evaluation and measurement of endogenous ACTH concentrations to determine if disease etiology was pituitary or adrenal in origin [20]. Dogs were classified as having pituitary-dependent disease if normal to increased endogenous ACTH concentrations (> 9 pmol/L; reference interval, 6.7–25.0 pmol/L) were detected coupled with ultrasound observation of approximately symmetric, normal to enlarged adrenal glands. Dogs were classified as having adrenal-dependent disease if decreased endogenous ACTH concentrations (< 4 pmol/L) were detected coupled with ultrasound observation of one irregularly enlarged adrenal gland and an atrophied contralateral adrenal gland. All dogs underwent ACTH stimulation testing within one week of study commencement to serve as baseline.

All dogs enrolled in the trial received ATR-101 at an initial once daily dose of 3 mg/kg PO for one week, followed immediately by a once daily dose of 30 mg/kg PO for either one week (n = 4) or 3 weeks (n = 6). The doses selected were based on previous pharmacologic and toxicologic investigations in healthy dogs [27]. The initial 4 dogs enrolled in the study received the 30 mg/kg dose for 1 week to ensure that drug was well-tolerated. Following an interim analysis in which adverse effects were not identified, the protocol was modified to extend ATR-101 treatment to assess if any additional biochemical, adrenal hormonal, or clinical effects would be observed with a longer duration of treatment. In this out-patient study, owners were instructed to administer ATR-101 capsules in the morning, preferably on an empty stomach, or with a small amount of food, if necessary for compliance. Capsules were administered by hospital technicians on study evaluation days. Dog owners recorded medication administration and any observed clinical changes or adverse effects on a standardized medication log. Weekly physical examinations and laboratory evaluations were performed in all dogs until study completion. Blood samples for laboratory evaluations were collected via peripheral venipuncture. Following study completion, owners of dogs with pituitary-dependent disease were instructed to allow a 4 week washout period before initiating standard medical therapies for CS such as trilostane. Dogs with adrenal-dependent disease underwent surgical adrenalectomy one day following study completion. All dogs remained housed with owners for the study duration.

Measurement of ATR-101 concentrations

ATR-101 concentrations were measured in serum samples collected immediately before (time 0) and 1, 2, 4 and 8 h after ATR-101 administration on days 1 ($n = 4$), 7 ($n = 10$), 14 ($n = 10$), and 28 ($n = 5$). Concentrations of ATR-101 in serum were determined by a liquid chromatography coupled with tandem mass spectrometry (LC/MS-MS) method which was developed and validated by AIT Bioscience (Indianapolis, IN) for the quantitation of ATR-101 in K_2EDTA dog plasma and has been described elsewhere [27]. This method was developed to cover the range of 1. 00–1000 ng/mL of ATR-101, using $^{13}C_4$-ATR-101 as the internal standard. Samples were analyzed on a Waters Acquity UPLC™ liquid chromatograph interfaced with a Thermo Scientific TSQ Vantage triple quadrupole mass spectrometer with electrospray ionization in the positive ion mode. ATR-101 was detected by selected reaction monitoring of the m/z $422 \rightarrow 202$ transition and its internal standard was detected by selected reaction monitoring of the m/z $426 \rightarrow 206$ transition. Raw data from the mass spectrometer was acquired and processed in Thermo Scientific Watson Laboratory Information Management System (LIMS). Peak area ratios from the calibration standard responses were regressed using a (1/ concentration^2) linear fit for ATR-101.

Pharmacokinetic analysis

Serum ATR-101 concentrations were analyzed by non-compartmental analysis (NCA) with Phoenix™ WinNonlin® Version 6.3, using an extravascular administration model. Nominal doses and sampling times were used. Prior to T_{max}, values that were below the lower limit of quantitation (BLQ) were set to 0; other BLQ concentrations were excluded from the analysis. The area under the curve from time zero to the last measurable concentration (AUC_{0-t}) was calculated using the linear up/log down method. Log/linear regression through the last three or more time points (excluding T_{max}) was used to estimate the elimination constant (λ_z). The apparent terminal phase half-life ($T_{1/2}$) and the AUC from time zero to infinity ($AUC_{0-\infty}$) were calculated using the following equations: $T_{1/2} = \ln (2)/\lambda_z$, and $AUC_{0-\infty} = AUC_{0-t} + C_{t, pred}/\lambda_z$, where $C_{t,pred}$ is the last predicted concentration based on the exponential decline (e.g., $e^{-\lambda_z \cdot t}$). If any of the following were observed, the terminal phase-dependent parameters (e.g. , λ_z, $T_{1/2}$, $AUC_{0-\infty}$, CL/F, V_z/F) following single dose administration were not reported: λ_z indicated a positive slope ($\lambda_z > 0$); T_{max} was one of the last three time points with measurable concentrations; or the linear regression coefficient or the goodness of fit (R^2) was less than 0.80. This also applied to λ_z, $T_{1/2}$, $AUC_{0-\infty}$, and V_z/F at steady state. Mean concentration graphs were prepared with Prism™ Version 7.0 (GraphPad Software, Inc., La Jolla,

CA). If less than 50% of the animals had reportable concentrations (e.g., 24 h post dose), the means were not plotted.

Measurement of routine hematologic and serum biochemical parameters

Baseline and weekly assessment of hematologic and biochemical parameters occurred for the study duration in all dogs. Blood samples obtained via peripheral venipuncture were divided equally into a K_2EDTA plasma and a serum collection tube. Plasma and serum (following clot formation) were harvested from the collection tubes immediately following centrifugation at 1200 X g for 10 min at 4 °C. Routine whole blood hematologic and serum biochemical analyses were then performed using an Advia 120 Hematology System (Siemens Healthcare, Deerfield, IL) and an Olympus AU640^e, (Olympus America Inc., Center Valley, PA), respectively. Weekly determinations of urine specific gravity were performed on voided urine samples using a standard veterinary refractometer (Reichert TS meter, 10,406, Cambridge Instruments Inc., Buffalo, NY).

Adrenal function testing

All dogs underwent baseline and weekly ACTH stimulation testing. This test consists of plasma sampling for cortisol and aldosterone concentrations immediately before and one hour post-administration of 5 µg/kg synthetic ACTH (Cortrosyn, Amphastar Pharmaceuticals Inc., Rancho Cucamonga, CA) intravenously. Although less sensitive than the LDDST for diagnosing CS, this dynamic adrenal function assessment offers the greatest specificity of available diagnostic tests, it offsets the variability in single point measurements, and it is the standard method for monitoring the efficacy of medical therapy [20, 31, 32]. Testing was performed in the morning immediately following ATR-101 administration.

Measurement of cortisol, aldosterone, and ACTH concentrations

Blood samples obtained via peripheral venipuncture were placed into K_2EDTA collection tubes, and plasma was harvested immediately after centrifugation at 1200 X g for 10 min at 4 °C. Radioimmunoassay kits previously validated and utilized for clinical diagnostics and research at the Michigan State University Diagnostic Center for Population and Animal Health were used to measure plasma concentrations of cortisol (Coat-a-Count Cortisol, Siemens Medical Solutions Diagnostics, Los Angeles, CA) [33], aldosterone (Coat-a-Count Aldosterone, Siemens Medical Solutions Diagnostics, Los Angeles, CA) [34], and ACTH (ACTH Immunoradiometric Assay, Scantibodies Laboratory, Inc., Santee, CA) [35].

Adrenal gland histology and immunohistochemistry

Following adrenalectomy, adrenal gland specimens were fixed in 10% buffered formalin for 24 h and then routinely trimmed, embedded, processed, and stained with hematoxylin and eosin for histologic evaluation. Previous established criteria were used to classify lesions as adenomas or carcinomas [36]. In addition, immunohistochemical (IHC) labeling for Melan-A and inhibin (Dako, Carpinteria, CA, USA) was performed on 5 µm serial sections of two of the three submitted adrenal gland specimens, and immunolabeling for caspase-3 (RDI/Fitzgerald, Acton, MA, USA), was performed on two of the three adrenal gland specimens [37, 38]. Immunolabeling for inhibin was performed on a Leica Bond-Max autostainer (Leica Microsystems, Buffalo Grove, IL, USA). Antigen retrieval was performed using ER1 epitope for 20 min in citric buffer solution on-line retrieval. Sections were incubated with a mouse monoclonal primary antibody (#M3609, DAKO, Carpinteria, CA, USA) against inhibin at a dilution of 1:100. A streptavidin-biotin labeling system (polymer: Refine Detection, Leica Microsystems, Buffalo Grove, IL, USA) was used for immunolabeling, and reactions were visualized with 3,3′-diaminobenzidine. Immunolabeling for Melan-A and caspase-3 was performed on an Ultra autostainer (Ventana Medical Systems, Tucson, AZ, USA). Antigen retrieval for Melan-A was performed using PT Link, citric buffer solution for 60 min, DAKO, Carpinteria, CA, USA). Antigen retrieval for caspase-3 was performed using CC1 Standard high pH for 20 min (on-line retrieval) epitope retrieval. Sections of adrenal gland were incubated for 30 min with 1 of the following 2 primary antibodies: mouse monoclonal anti-Melan-A (A103 clone Dako M7196, Carpinteria, CA, USA) at a dilution of 1:20 or rabbit polyclonal anti-caspase-3 (# 20RCR013, RDI/Fitzgerald, Acton, MA, USA) at a dilution of 1:1000. All slides were counterstained with hematoxylin. Sections of normal canine adrenal gland were used as positive controls for inhibin and Melan-A; sections of canine lymph node were used as positive controls for caspase-3.

Statistical analysis

Data were reported as means ± standard deviations (SD) given normal distribution as assessed by Kolmogorov-Smirnov testing and boxplot analysis. For analysis of pharmacokinetic parameters, C_{max}, AUC, half-life, oral clearance (CL/F), and volume of distribution (Vz/F) at different dosages were compared using a two-tailed Student's t-test. The effect of treatment over time on cortisol and aldosterone concentrations and other clinically pertinent laboratory data were evaluated using a repeated measures analysis of variance. When a significant effect for time was detected, a Dunnett's post hoc test was performed to compare individual treatment values to pre-treatment control. For the cortisol comparisons, the tests were conducted in a one-tailed fashion based

on the prediction that cortisol values would decline. All other comparisons were made in two-tailed fashion. Differences were considered significant at $P ≤ 0.05$. Statistical analyses were performed using commercially available software (GraphPad Prism™ Version 7.0, Graphpad Software Inc., La Jolla, CA; and Statistica, Dell StatSoft Inc., Austin, TX).

Results

Animal demographics

Of 15 dogs screened for potential study participation, 10 dogs with naturally occurring CS, based on adrenal function testing, were enrolled in the clinical trial (Table 1). One dog (dog 9) was withdrawn at day 24 due to complications from an unrelated prostatic carcinoma; data through day 21 from this subject were still used for analysis. Dogs were classified as having pituitary- or adrenal-dependent disease on the basis of abdominal ultrasound examination and measurement of endogenous ACTH concentration [20]. Overall, 7 dogs were classified as having pituitary-dependent disease, while 3 were classified as adrenal-dependent. In 3 dogs (dogs 1, 8, 10), CS sub-type initially was unclear. The plasma endogenous ACTH concentrations of 5.1 pmol/L, 8.8 pmol/L, and 8.7 pmol/L for dogs 1, 8, and 10, respectively, were deemed equivocal as they were near the low-end of the reference interval (6.7–25.0 pmol/L). Results of abdominal ultrasound examination were definitive in

Table 1 Demographics of the 10 dogs enrolled in the ATR-101 clinical trial

Dog	Age (yrs)	Sex	Breed	Weight	Etiology	Protocol
1	9	M/N	Boxer	36.2 kg	pituitary	2 weeks
2	12	F/S	Lab/Chow	46.0 kg	adrenal	2 weeks
3	9	M/N	Mix	24.5 kg	pituitary	2 weeks
4	8	F/S	Labrador	44.0 kg	pituitary	2 weeks
5	12	M/N	Shi Tzu	8.9 kg	pituitary	4 weeks
6	13	F/S	American Eskimo	19.1 kg	adrenal	4 weeks
7	11	F/S	Labrador	24.0 kg	pituitary	4 weeks
8	15	F/S	Pekingese/Poodle	8.2 kg	adrenal	4 weeks
9	8	M/I	Pitbull	31.0 kg	pituitary	4 weeks[a]
10	9	M/I	Siberian Husky	34.0 kg	pituitary	4 weeks

The 10 dogs were middle-aged to older dogs with an equal distribution of males and females, similar to what has been reported previously (Melián G et al., 2010). Etiology was determined based on results of abdominal ultrasound examinations and measurements of endogenous ACTH concentrations. Protocol refers to the length of treatment with ATR-101
N, neutered; S, spayed; I, intact.
[a]Dog 9 was withdrawn from the study at day 24 due to complications from an unrelated prostatic carcinoma. This dog still was utilized in the study as clinical signs (polyuria and polydipsia, polyphagia, pot-bellied appearance, alopecia, muscle wasting), laboratory test results (stress leukogram, increased alkaline phosphatase activity, hypercholesterolemia, urine specific gravity of 1.006), and pre- (226 nmol/L; reference interval, 15–115) and post-ACTH-stimulated (1272 nmol/L; reference interval, 220–550 nmol/L) cortisol concentrations provided clear and convincing evidence for CS at the time of enrollment

all three cases (bilaterally symmetric, normal to mildly enlarged adrenal glands in 2 dogs with pituitary dependent disease; one enlarged, irregular adrenal gland with atrophy of the contralateral adrenal gland in 1 dog with adrenal dependent disease), and used for definitive classification. Results of measured endogenous ACTH concentrations and abdominal ultrasound examinations were in agreement for remaining dogs.

ATR-101 pharmacokinetics

Pharmacokinetics of ATR-101 at both 3 mg/kg and 30 mg/kg are summarized in Table 2. Overall, drug exposures were greater with increased dose (Fig. 1). There appears to be saturation of extravascular clearance (CL/F) and/or a change in bioavailability between day 1 and day 7. Drug accumulation between day 1 and day 7 was observed while accumulation at day 30 was modest. Changes in apparent (extravascular) $T_{1/2}$ were observed at 30 mg/kg after 7–14 days of once daily dosing. Increases in steady state exposure (AUC_{0-24}) after repeat daily dosing at 3 and 30 mg/kg appeared dose proportional, within the observed variability, with a 8.2-fold increase in AUC_{0-24} for a 10-fold increase in dose. The corresponding increases in C_{max} were less than dose proportional with a 4.5-fold increase in C_{max} for a 10-fold increase in dosage from 3 mg/kg to 30 mg/kg. The increases AUC_{0-24} and C_{max} were significant ($P < 0.001$). Half-life and Vz/F at steady-state appeared to increase as the dosage was increased from 3 to 30 mg/kg; however, these changes were not significant ($P > 0.05$). Oral clearance did not change as the dosage was increased from 3 to 30 mg/kg ($P > 0.05$).

Effects of ATR-101 on basal and ACTH-stimulated plasma cortisol and aldosterone concentrations

The post-ACTH-stimulated cortisol concentrations (reference interval for normal dogs; 220–550 nmol/L) at days 7, 14, 21, and 28 were decreased compared to the baseline (day 0) post-ACTH-stimulated cortisol concentration ($P < 0.05$, Fig. 2a). Overall, reductions in post-ACTH-stimulated cortisol concentrations were observed in 9 of 10 dogs, including 7 of 7 dogs with pituitary-dependent CS and 2 of 3 dogs with adrenal-dependent CS. In dogs with adrenal-dependent CS, the post-ACTH-stimulated cortisol concentrations at day 14 were increased by 43.2% in one dog (dog 2) and decreased by 36.1 and 84.2% in the other two dogs as compared to baseline (day 0) concentrations. In dogs with pituitary-dependent CS, the mean ± SD percent reduction in post-ACTH-stimulated cortisol concentrations at day 14 was 49.8 ± 12.8% as compared to baseline concentrations. Post-ACTH-stimulated cortisol concentrations were not different between dogs with adrenal- or pituitary-dependent disease ($P > 0.05$). The mean baseline pre-ACTH-stimulated cortisol concentration (reference interval for normal dogs; 15–110 nmol/L) was not different than mean pre-ACTH-stimulated cortisol concentrations after treatment with ATR-101 at either dose ($P > 0.05$); however, 4 of 10 individual dogs did experience reductions. Post-ACTH-stimulated aldosterone concentrations (reference interval; 197–2103 pmol/L) were decreased following treatment with ATR-101 at days 7 and 28 ($P < 0.05$, Fig. 2b); however, no effect was observed on pre-ACTH-stimulated aldosterone concentrations ($P > 0.05$) (reference interval; 14–957 pmol/L).

Table 2 Pharmacokinetics parameters in dogs following once daily oral administration of ATR-101

Dose (mg/kg)	Day	Animal number	$T_{1/2}$ (hr)	T_{max}[a] (hr)	C_{max} (ng/mL)	AUC_{0-8} (hr*ng/mL)	AUC_{0-24} (hr*ng/mL)	$AUC_{0-\infty}$ (hr*ng/mL)	CL/F (mL/hr./kg)	V_z/F (mL/kg)
3	1	n	3	4	4	4	3	3	3	3
		Mean	2.76	1.0	445	1240	1050	1040	3440	15,600
		SD	1.04	1.0, 4.0	159	697	462	455	1960	14,500
3	7	n	4	10	10	10	7	4	7	4
		Mean	2.78	1.0	1480	4560	5790	5050	859	3600
		SD	0.196	1.0, 4.0	1100	3180	4060	3170	665	2810
30	14	n	5	10	10	10	5	5	5	5
		Mean	6.56	2.0	6790[***]	29,900	47900[***]	53,700	706	6360
		SD	4.75	1.0, 4.0	4350	15,900	20,000	24,500	252	3640
30	28	n	2	5	5	5	4	2	4	2
		Mean	9.36	1.0	9000	39,100	62,500	66,800	497	8370
		SD	NR	1.0, 4.0	3540	11,000	12,200	NR	119	NR

All values are expressed as mean ± SD. with the exception of T_{max}. Three dogs had 24 h post-dose data reported and utilized in the analysis. $AUC_{0-\infty}$ is utilized in CL/F and V_z/F calculations on day 1 while AUC_{0-24} (e.g., AUC_{0-tau}, tau = dosing period) is utilized in CL/F and V_z/F calculations at steady state (e.g., day, 7, day 14, day 28). T_{max} as well as pharmacokinetic parameters on days 1 and 28 were not evaluated statistically due to limited sample sizes. $T_{1/2}$, elimination half-life; T_{max}, time to maximum serum concentration; C_{max}, maximum serum concentration; AUC, area under the serum concentration-time curve; CL/F, apparent total serum clearance after oral administration; V_z, Apparent volume of distribution during terminal phase after oral/extravascular administration
[a]Median and range (Min, Max) are presented
[***]$P < 0.001$ versus day 7 by a two-tailed Student's t-test

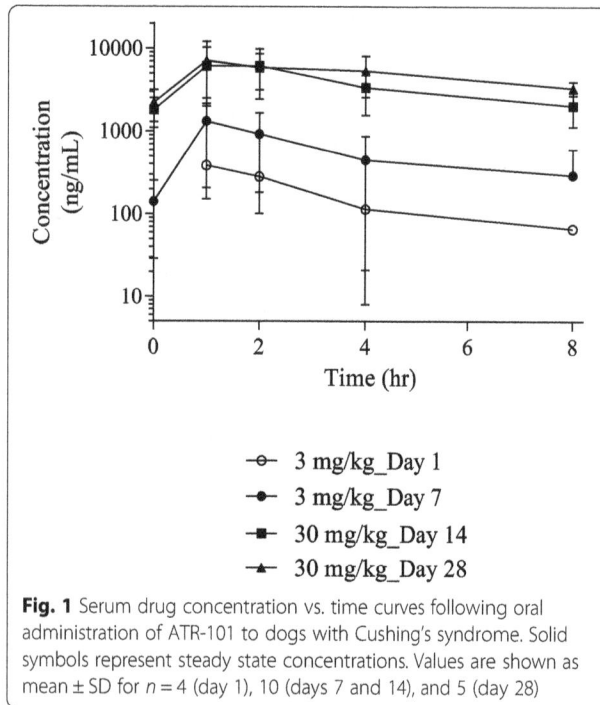

Fig. 1 Serum drug concentration vs. time curves following oral administration of ATR-101 to dogs with Cushing's syndrome. Solid symbols represent steady state concentrations. Values are shown as mean ± SD for $n = 4$ (day 1), 10 (days 7 and 14), and 5 (day 28)

Effects of ATR-101 administration on routine hematologic and serum biochemical parameters

Serum alanine aminotransferase (ALT) activity increased over time, reaching significance on day 28 ($P < 0.05$, Table 3). A similar, albeit non-significant ($P > 0.05$), trend in alkaline phosphatase (ALP) activity was observed with 8 of 10 dogs experiencing a 2 to 4 times increase in ALP activity by study completion. Mild reductions in hematocrit and serum albumin concentration also were observed ($P < 0.05$), although they remained within reference intervals throughout the study. Hematocrit rebounded on day 28, and serum albumin stabilized on day 28. Other hematologic and serum biochemical parameters, including serum sodium and potassium concentrations, did not change, and no dog in the study developed hyponatremia or hyperkalemia despite some changes in post-ACTH-stimulated aldosterone concentrations. The mean ± SD urine specific gravity of 1.016 ± 0.014 at baseline evaluation was not different from urine specific gravities of 1.018 ± 0.015 and 1.023 ± 0.019 at study completion on days 14 and 28 ($P > 0.05$).

Evaluation of clinical effects

Owners of the 10 enrolled dogs maintained daily medication logs and documented the presence or absence of potential adverse effects, including vomiting, diarrhea, anorexia, and worsening weakness (if present initially). Owners of all dogs reported that the medication was well-tolerated. Overall, out of 220 study days for the 10 dogs, 4 episodes of vomiting (dogs 6, 7, and 8) and one

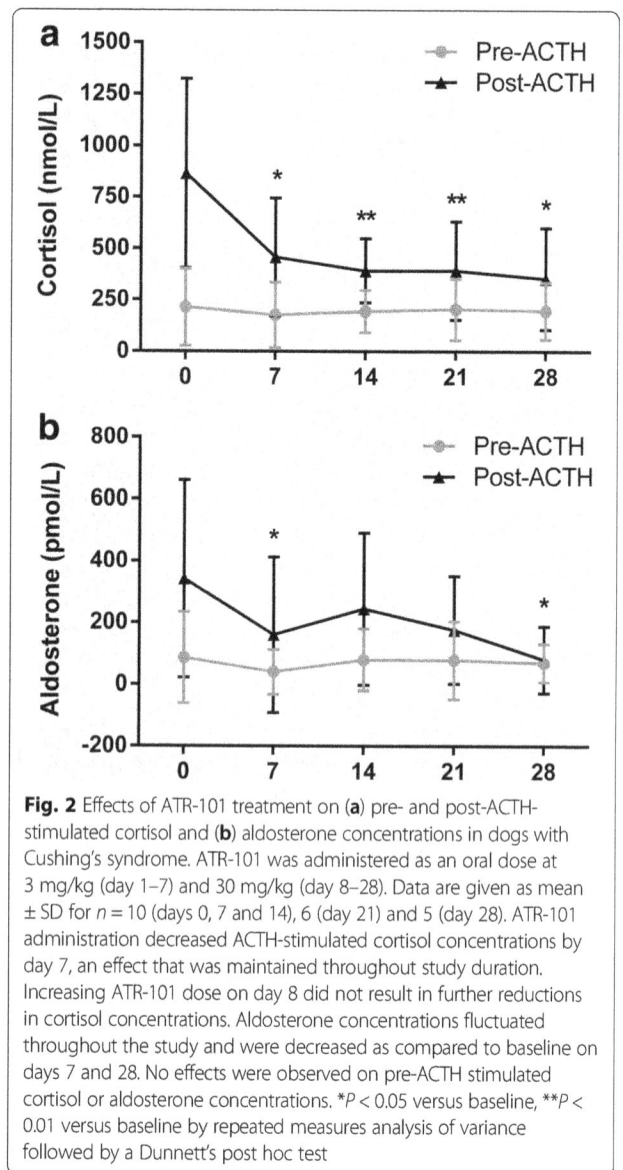

Fig. 2 Effects of ATR-101 treatment on (a) pre- and post-ACTH-stimulated cortisol and (b) aldosterone concentrations in dogs with Cushing's syndrome. ATR-101 was administered as an oral dose at 3 mg/kg (day 1–7) and 30 mg/kg (day 8–28). Data are given as mean ± SD for $n = 10$ (days 0, 7 and 14), 6 (day 21) and 5 (day 28). ATR-101 administration decreased ACTH-stimulated cortisol concentrations by day 7, an effect that was maintained throughout study duration. Increasing ATR-101 dose on day 8 did not result in further reductions in cortisol concentrations. Aldosterone concentrations fluctuated throughout the study and were decreased as compared to baseline on days 7 and 28. No effects were observed on pre-ACTH stimulated cortisol or aldosterone concentrations. *$P < 0.05$ versus baseline, **$P < 0.01$ versus baseline by repeated measures analysis of variance followed by a Dunnett's post hoc test

episode of diarrhea (dog 8) were reported. Three of 4 vomiting episodes were greater than 5 h after drug administration. Clinical signs related to CS were reported as improved in 7 dogs, unchanged in 2 dogs, and worsened in 1 dog. This included improved energy and activity level (dogs 1, 3, 6, 9 and 10), lessening polyphagia (dogs 6, 7, 9 and 10), lessening polyuria and polydipsia (dogs 7, 9, and 10), and improved dermatologic lesions (dogs 4 and 10). Dog 2 experienced worsening polyuria, polydipsia, and polyphagia and was the only dog in this study in which reductions in post-ACTH-stimulated cortisol concentrations were not observed. Dog 9, which showed clinical improvement during the first two weeks, experienced lethargy, weakness, and anorexia in the 4th week, and ATR-101 treatment was discontinued on day 24. Clinical signs persisted and the dog was euthanized

ATR-101, a selective ACAT1 inhibitor, decreases ACTH-stimulated cortisol concentrations in dogs...

141

Table 3 Results of selected serum biochemical parameters in 10 dogs with Cushing's syndrome treated with orally administered ATR-101

	Reference	Day 0	Day 7	Day 14	Day 21	Day 28
Hct	41–55 (%)	52.4 ± 5.7	50.3 ± 6.6[*]	49.0 ± 6.2[***]	44.2 ± 8.3[**]	47.6 ± 5.1
Bili	0.1– 0.4 (mg/dL)	0.19 ± 0.07	0.23 ± 0.05	0.17 ± 0.07	0.20 ± 0.00	0.14 ± 0.05
Alb	2.8– 4.0 (g/dL)	3.11 ± 0.47	3.07 ± 0.42	2.95 ± 0.43[***]	2.82 ± 0.52[**]	2.82 ± 0.48[**]
ALT	14– 102 (U/L)	136.7 ± 155.4	145.5 ± 142.4	236.7 ± 316.6	362.5 ± 331.1	445.6 ± 340.0[*]
ALP	13– 107 (U/L)	1025 ± 1633	1172 ± 1886	2121 ± 3928	4113 ± 6487	4151 ± 6555
Chol	124– 343 (mg/dL)	373.6 ± 133.8	375.1 ± 121.8	389.1 ± 147.7	340.3 ± 151.3	322.0 ± 163.4
SUN	5– 34 (mg/dL)	17.6 ± 6.2	16.7 ± 8.9	17.8 ± 6.6	20.8 ± 7.1	21.4 ± 9.0
Na	143– 149 (mmol/L)	148.5 ± 1.6	146.8 ± 1.9	146.3 ± 2.5	146.3 ± 1.4	146.4 ± 1.9
K	3.4– 5.2 (mmol/L)	4.9 ± 0.6	4.6 ± 0.5	4.6 ± 0.4	4.5 ± 0.6	4.7 ± 0.8
Cr	0.7– 2.0 (mg/dL)	0.9 ± 0.3	0.9 ± 0.3	0.9 ± 0.3	1.0 ± 0.3	1.1 ± 0.4
Glu	80– 120 (mg/dL)	99.3 ± 9.8	104.0 ± 13.4	98.4 ± 8.2	94.7 ± 8.9	94.4 ± 11.6

All value are expressed as mean ± SD for 10 dogs (days 0– 14), 6 dogs (day 21), and 5 dogs (day 28)

Hct, hematocrit; Bili, bilirubin; Alb, albumin; ALT, alanine aminotransferase; ALP, alkaline phosphatase, Chol, cholesterol; SUN, serum urea nitrogen; Na, sodium; K, potassium; Cr, creatinine, Glu, glucose

*$P < 0.05$ versus day 0; **$P < 0.01$ versus day 0; ***$P < 0.001$ versus day 0 by repeated measures analysis of variance followed by Dunnett's post hoc test

two weeks later. Based on the necropsy evaluation, which revealed numerous pulmonary metastases from a known prostatic carcinoma, the clinical signs in this dog were not thought to be related to ATR-101.

Histologic characterization of adrenal tissue in 3 dogs with cortisol secreting adrenocortical lesions

Adrenocortical lesions (Fig. 3) were confirmed in 3 dogs with adrenal dependent disease (dogs 2, 6, 8), including an adrenocortical adenoma (dog 6) and an adrenocortical carcinoma (dog 8). Moderate, multifocal necrosis, fibrosis, granulomatous inflammation, and cholesterol clefts were observed within and surrounding the neoplastic cells in dog 8, while multifocal hemorrhage and mineralization were observed within the adrenal mass in dog 6. In dog 2, histologic sections of tissue were predominantly characterized by marked necrosis, hemorrhage, fibrin accumulation, and granulating fibrosis with mild multifocal dystrophic mineralization. The extent and severity of these lesions in dog 2 precluded accurate classification as adenoma or adenocarcinoma. For dogs 6 and 8, positive immunolabeling for Melan-A (dogs 6, and 8) and inhibin (dog 8) were present in the epithelial cells, confirming adrenocortical origin. Strong nuclear immunoreactivity to caspase-3 was present in adrenocortical cells from dog 8 (80% of cells) while weaker immunolabeling was present in dog 6 (1– 2% of adrenocortical cells).

Discussion

Our results document that orally administered ATR-101 reduces post-ACTH-stimulated cortisol concentrations in dogs with naturally occurring CS. This effect was observed by day 7 of ATR-101 therapy and sustained through study conclusion on day 28. Mild reductions of

aldosterone concentrations were observed, but this effect was not thought to be clinically relevant as plasma aldosterone and serum electrolyte concentrations remained normal for the study duration. The minimal adverse effects also compare favorably with the adverse effect profiles of some currently used drugs such as mitotane. Positive hormonal (cortisol) effects were observed in all dogs with pituitary-dependent disease and 2 of 3 dogs with adrenal-dependent disease. These findings are encouraging given current limitations of medical therapy for CS in humans and the poor survival times and the difficulties in medically controlling hypercortisolemia in both humans and dogs with malignant adrenocortical lesions [16, 17, 19, 20, 39, 40]. The histologic changes in adrenal glands from dogs with adrenal-dependent disease further support previous findings in healthy dogs that ATR-101 distributes to the adrenal glands, inhibits adrenal ACAT1 activity, and induces apoptosis [25, 27]. Although this was not a blinded and controlled study, clinical improvements were reported by the majority of dog owners. In the aggregate, these results are supportive of further investigations and the ongoing development of ATR-101.

A limitation hampering human CS drug development is the paucity of disease and the failure to identify a naturally occurring model of disease. Although reported incidence varies, CS is rare in humans with an approximate annual incidence of 2 cases per million per year [41]. If CS is rare, adrenocortical carcinoma is exceedingly rare with approximately 600 new cases diagnosed in the Unites States each year [17]. In contrast, canine CS is a common endocrinologic disorder occurring at an estimated incidence of 1–2 cases per 1000 dogs per year, representing a thousand-fold greater incidence as compared to humans [42]. Despite

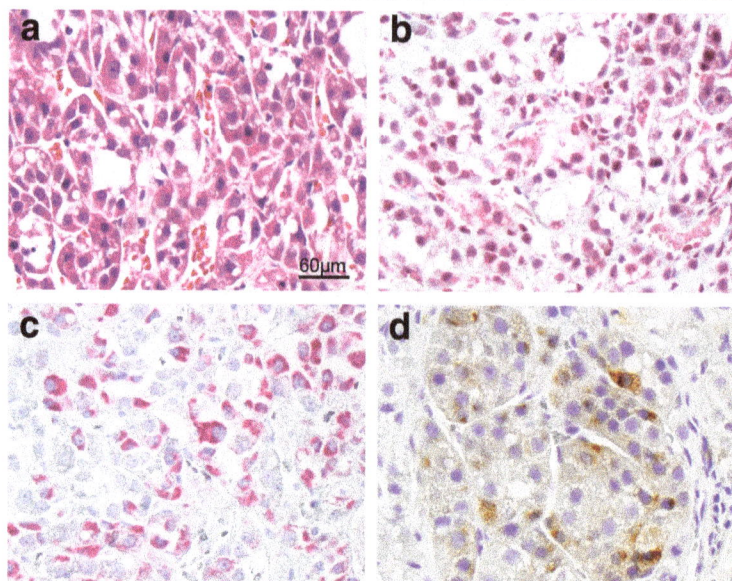

Fig. 3 Histologic approach used to evaluate adrenal tissue in dogs with adrenal-dependent Cushing's syndrome treated with ATR-101. (**a**) H&E stained adrenal tissue demonstrating proliferative neoplastic adrenocortical cells arranged in packets separated by fine fibrovascular stroma in a dog with adrenocortical carcinoma (40×, bar = 60 μm); (**b**) strong nuclear immunoreactivity for caspase-3 indicating increased cellular apoptotic activity (Vector red chromogen, 40×); positive cytoplasmic immunolabeling for Melan-A (Vector red chromogen, 40×) (**c**) and inhibin (diaminobenzidine chromogen, brown, 40×) (**d**) confirming adrenocortical origin

disparity in disease frequency, the etiology, clinical signs, and biochemical and histologic characteristics are remarkably similar between species [2, 3, 43]. Furthermore, dogs age approximately 5–7 times faster than humans, and progression of CS is also accelerated. These features make the dog appealing for both molecular studies and clinical trials. Although this potential has been recognized by others [1, 4, 43], the clinical trial reported herein is the first study using naturally occurring CS in the dog to aid in clinical proof of concept for human CS. This should establish a valuable precedent in using the dogs with naturally occurring CS for the development of human therapeutics, hopefully resulting in benefits for both species.

Although one goal in both humans and dogs is to reduce circulating cortisol concentrations and alleviate clinical signs associated with this excess, methods for monitoring medical therapy can differ [2, 16, 20, 31]. Reductions in pre-ACTH-stimulated (basal) cortisol levels were observed in 4 dogs following ATR-101 therapy, but overall changes were not significant. The exact reasons for this are unclear, but are likely related to the episodic patterns of cortisol secretion observed in dogs that are different from the circadian or diurnal patterns of cortisol secretion observed in other species [44, 45]. Cortisol levels in normal dogs can decrease below and increase above established resting intervals throughout the day. High variability in basal or non-ACTH-stimulated cortisol levels is also observed in dogs with CS [46]. Because of this, measurements of unstimulated cortisol concentrations are not of great utility in the

diagnosis or monitoring of CS in dogs [47]. While repeated 24 h urinary free cortisol determinations are routinely used for monitoring CS therapy in humans, this is impractical for most pet owners [6]. The urine cortisol to creatinine ratio, the most analogous clinical test in veterinary medicine, does not provide a consistently correct assessment of hormonal status for therapeutic monitoring of dogs with CS [20, 48, 49]. As such, the ACTH stimulation test is the current standard for monitoring medical therapy in dogs, and this was the basis for our decision to use this test for monitoring response to ATR-101 [20]. Reductions in 24 h urinary cortisol in humans and reductions in post-ACTH-stimulated cortisol concentrations in dogs do correlate with clinical improvement, and it would be logical to assume that reductions in one monitoring method would be accompanied by reductions in the other. However, one limitation of the current study is that it is unknown how well these monitoring methods correlate with each other. Given that pre-ACTH-stimulated cortisol level do not necessarily correlate to the degree of hypercortisolemia throughout the day, additional monitoring methods might prove beneficial. Although the urine cortisol to creatinine ratio is not as effective as ACTH stimulation testing for monitoring efficacy of medical therapy in dogs, values are known to decrease from baseline values following treatment with trilostane or mitotane [48, 49]. This monitoring method should be considered in future studies to enhance the translational aspect as it is most analogous to 24 h urinary free cortisol determinations utilized in humans. Other potential assessments of the degree of non-ACTH-stimulated hypercortisolism such as salivary, hair, or fecal cortisol measurements have undergone minimal investigation in dogs with CS, and their role in therapeutic monitoring is unknown [50–52]. In addition to providing another measure of efficacy, these methods might serve as a more direct correlate to the repeated 24 h urinary free cortisol measurements utilized in humans. Future studies in which dogs with naturally occurring CS are used as a human CS model should consider incorporating multiple treatment monitoring methods, including an assessment of resting hypercortisolism.

In the current study, reductions in post-ACTH-stimulated cortisol concentrations were accompanied by subjective owner-reported clinical improvements in many dogs, although complete symptom resolution was not achieved in any of the dogs. The reasons for incomplete symptom resolution are likely two-fold. First, many clinical signs, especially physical changes and dermatologic abnormalities, can take several months to resolve [20]. Second, the observed reductions in post-ACTH-stimulated cortisol concentrations were heterogeneous and not of the magnitude typically associated with resolution of clinical signs [20, 31]. The lack of further decreases in cortisol concentrations despite an increased ATR-101 dose commencing on day 8 is in contrast to a previous study of ATR-101 in healthy dogs in which dose-dependent decreases in ACTH-stimulated cortisol concentrations were observed [27]. The reasons for the heterogeneity of post-ACTH cortisol responses and the discrepancy between studies are unclear; however, it is plausible that adrenocortical ACAT1 expression could differ between normal dogs and dogs with CS, or even among individual dogs with CS [28]. Similarly, the utilization of only 2 set dosages administered at only 1 frequency in dogs with varying types and severities of CS may account for some variation. The timing of ACTH stimulation testing may also be important as the optimal time for testing in trilostane treated dogs is 4 to 6 h post-drug administration [20]. Regardless, medical therapy of CS in dogs is often individualized as variable dosages and dosing frequencies are utilized in clinical settings [14]. Extended treatment duration, higher ATR-101 dose, or more frequent dosing potentially could result in further hormonal and clinical improvement. Additional studies are needed to evaluate these hypotheses.

Clinical signs of liver disease were not observed in the current study, and biochemical parameters associated with liver function such as bilirubin, glucose, and urea nitrogen remained normal. However, the increases in liver enzyme activity are noteworthy. Dogs with CS usually have increased liver enzyme activity at diagnosis [3], but the continual increases over time despite reductions in post-ACTH-stimulated cortisol concentrations were unexpected. ACAT1 is known to be expressed in numerous tissues including Kupffer cells within the liver; however, expression of ACAT1 is markedly higher in the adrenal cortex which is likely one reason for the adrenal selective effects of ATR-101 [27, 53]. In a previous in-vitro study, ATR-101 did not induce toxic effects on hepatocytes unless the cells were pretreated with agents to block glycolysis or inhibit cytochrome P450-mediated metabolism [54]. In an unpublished toxicity study conducted by two authors of this report (MB and SH), ATR-101 administration to healthy dogs resulted in mild increases in ALP and ALT activities. Histologically, non-glycogen, non-lipid containing vacuolar hepatic change was observed which was not accompanied by necroinflammatory activity. Both abnormal enzyme activity and histologic changes resolved upon discontinuation of ATR-101. Given that ATR-101 is metabolized by the liver, the increased enzyme activity likely represents an adaptive response to hepatic drug metabolism [55], but the cause for these changes was not determined. The reported reductions in hematocrit in dogs from our study are unlikely to be of clinical significance as they remained within normal reference intervals for the study duration and rebounded by study completion. The reductions in albumin were minor and not deemed to be related to ATR-101 administration or clinically relevant as they also remained within normal reference intervals and appeared to plateau by study completion.

Conclusions

ATR-101 is well-tolerated and reduces post-ACTH-stimulated cortisol concentrations in dogs with naturally occurring CS. Given the striking similarities between CS in dogs and humans, naturally occurring canine CS appears to be a suitable model for human studies. The results reported herein further support the ongoing development of ATR-101 for treatment of disorders associated with excess adrenal steroid production in humans, such as CS, congenital adrenal hyperplasia, and ACC. Additional investigations are required to optimize dosing strategies and further evaluate the effects of prolonged drug administration on efficacy and safety.

Abbreviations
ACC: Adrenocortical carcinoma; ACTH: Adrenocorticotropic hormone; ALP: Alkaline phosphatase; ALT: Alanine aminotransferase; AUC: Area under the serum drug concentration-time curve; CS: Cushing's syndrome; LDDST: Low-dose dexamethasone suppression test

Acknowledgements
The authors thank Judy Eastman and Joe Jehl for technical assistance and pharmaceutical compounding, respectively.

Funding
This work was supported by a sponsored research agreement between Millendo Therapeutics, Inc. and Michigan State University.

Authors' contributions

DL, MF, WS, MB, and SH participated in research design. DL, MF, WS, and RS conducted the clinical experiments. DL, MF, WS, NO, PP, MB, and SH performed data analysis. DL, WS, RS, PP, MB, and SH contributed to the writing of the manuscript. All authors read and approved the final manuscript.

Competing interests

SH is an employee of Millendo Therapeutics, Inc. MB and PP are consultants to Millendo Therapeutics, Inc. Authors have no further potential conflicts of interest to report.

Author details

[1]Department of Small Animal Clinical Sciences, College of Veterinary Medicine, Michigan State University, East Lansing, MI 48824, USA. [2]Veterinary Diagnostic Laboratory, College of Veterinary Medicine, Michigan State University, East Lansing, MI 48824, USA. [3]Pearson Pharma Partners, Inc., Los Angeles, California 91362, USA. [4]Integrated Non-Clinical Development Solutions, Inc., Ann Arbor, MI 48103, USA. [5]Millendo Therapeutics, Inc., Ann Arbor, MI 48104, USA. [6]Present address: College of Human Medicine, Michigan State University, East Lansing, MI 48824, USA.

References

1. Kemppainen RJ, Peterson M. Animal models of Cushing's disease. Trends Endocrinol Metab. 1994;5:21–8.
2. Lacroix A, Feelders RA, Stratakis CA, Nieman LK. Cushing's syndrome. Lancet. 2015;386:913–27.
3. Ling GV, Stabenfeldt GH, Comer KM, Gribble DH, Schechter RD. Canine hyperadrenocorticism: pretreatment clinical and laboratory evaluation of 117 cases. J Am Vet Med Assoc 1979;174:1211-5.
4. de Bruin C, Meij BP, Kooistra HS, Hanson JM, Lamverts SW, Hofland LJ. Cushing's disease in dogs and humans. Horm Res. 2009;71(Suppl 1):140–3.
5. Nichols R. Complications and concurrent disease associated with canine hyperadrenocorticism. Vet Clin North Am Small Anim Pract. 1997;27:309–20.
6. Colao A, Boscaro M, Ferone D, Casanueva FF. Managing Cushing's disease: the state of the art. Endocrine. 2014;47:9–20.
7. Hanson JM, van't HM, Voorhout G, Teske E, Kooistra HS, Meij BP. Efficacy of transsphenoidal hypophysectomy in treatment of dogs with pituitary-dependent hyperadrenocorticism. J Vet Intern Med. 2005;19:687–94.
8. Peterson ME. Medical treatment of canine pituitary-dependent hyperadrenocorticism (Cushing's disease). Vet Clin North Am Small Anim Pract. 2001;31:1005–14.
9. van Rijn SJ, Galac S, Tryfonidou MA, Hesselink JW, Penning LC, Kooistra HS, Meij BP. The influence of pituitary size on outcome after transsphenoidal hypophysectomy in a large cohort of dogs with pituitary-dependent hypercortisolism. J Vet Intern Med. 2016;30:989–95.
10. Alenza DP, Arenas C, Lopez ML, Melian C. Long-term efficacy of trilostane administered twice daily in dogs with pituitary-dependent hyperadrenocorticism. J Am Anim Hosp Assoc. 2006;42:269–76.
11. Fracassi F, Corradini S, Floriano D, Boari A, Aste G, Pietra M, Bergamini PF, Dondi F. Prognostic factors for survival in dogs with pituitary-dependent hypercortisolism treated with trilostane. Vet Rec. 2015;176:49.
12. Neiger R, Ramsey I, O'Connor J, Hurley KJ, Mooney CT. Trilostane treatment of 78 dogs with pituitary-dependent hyperadrenocorticism. Vet Rec. 2002; 150:799–804.
13. Reine NJ. Medical management of pituitary-dependent hyperadrenocorticism: mitotane versus trilostane. Clin Tech Small Anim Pract. 2007;22:18–25.
14. Feldman EC. Evaluation of twice-daily lower-dose trilostane treatment administered orally in dogs with naturally occurring hyperadernocorticism. J Am Vet Med Assoc. 2011;238:1441–51.
15. Ramsey IK. Trilostane in dogs. Vet Clin North Am Small Anim Pract. 2010;40: 269–83.
16. Nieman LK, Biller BMK, Findling JW, Hassan Murad M, Newell-Price J, Savage MO, Tabarin A. Treatment of Cushing's syndrome: an Endocrine Society clinical practice guideline. J Clin Endocrinol Metab. 2015;100:2807–31.
17. Else T, Kim AC, Sabolch A, Raymond VM, Kandathil A, Caoili EM, Jolly S, Miller BS, Giordano TJ, Hammer GD. Adrenocortical carcinoma. Endocr Rev. 2014;35:282–326.
18. Massari F, Nicoli S, Romanelli G, Buracco P, Zini E. Adrenalectomy in dogs with adrenal gland tumors: 52 cases (2002-2008). J Am Vet Med Assoc. 2011;239:216–21.
19. Helm JR, McLauchlan G, Boden LA, Frowde PE, Collings AJ, Tebb AJ, Elwood CM, Herrtage ME, Parkin TD, Ramsey IK. A comparison of factors that influence survival in dogs with adrenal-dependent hyperadrenocorticism treated with mitotane or trilostane. J Vet Intern Med. 2011;25:251–60.
20. Melián G, Dolores Pérez-Alenza M, Peterson ME. Hyperadrenocorticism in dogs. In: Ettinger SJ, Feldman EC, editors. Textbook of Veterinary Internal Medicine, vol. Vol 2. 7th ed. St. Louis: Saunders, Inc; 2010. p. 1816–39.
21. Gonzalez RJ, Tamm EP, Ng C, Phan AT, Vassilopoulou-Sellin R, Perrier ND, Evans DB, Lee JE. Response to mitotane predicts outcome in patients with recurrent adrenal cortical carcinoma. Surgery. 2007;142:867–75.
22. Kintzer PP, Peterson ME. Mitotane treatment of 32 dogs with cortisol-secreting adrenocortical neoplasms. J Am Vet Med Assoc. 1994;205:54–61.
23. Fassnacht M, Terzolo M, Allolio B, Baudin E, Haak H, Berruti A, et al. FIRM-ACT study group. Combination chemotherapy in advanced adrenocortical carcinoma. N Engl J Med. 2012;366:2189–97.
24. Suckling KE, Stange EF. Role of acyl:CoA: cholesterol acyltransferase in cellular cholesterol metabolism. J Lipid Res. 1985;26:647–71.
25. Bailie MB, Phillips MD, Kerppola RE, Herman JE, Pearson PG, Hammer GD, Whitcomb R, Owens JC, Hunt SW III. ATR-101, a selective ACAT1 inhibitor in development for adrenocortical carcinoma, disrupts steroidogenesis and causes apoptosis in normal canine adrenals. Program of the 96th Annual Meeting of the Endocrine Society, Chicago, IL. 2014. Abstract OR14–5. https://endo.confex.com/endo/2014endo/webprogram/Paper16732.html. Accessed 06 Mar 2017.
26. Cheng Y, Kerppola RE, Kerppola TK. ATR-101 disrupts mitochondrial functions in adrenocortical carcinoma cells and in vivo. Endocr Relat Cancer. 2016;23:1–19.
27. Lapeense CR, Mann JE, Rainey WE, Crudo V, Hunt SW III, Hammer GD. ATR-101, a selective and potent inhibitor of acyl-CoA acyltransferace 1, induces apoptosis in H295R adrenocortical cells and in the adrenal cortex of dogs. Endocrinology. 2016;157:1775–88.
28. Sberia S, Leich E, Liebisch G, Sbiera I, Schirbel A, Wiemer L, Matysik S, et al. Mitotane inhibits sterol-O-acyl transferase 1 triggering lipid-mediated endoplasmic reticulum stress and apoptosis in adrenocortical carcinoma cells. Endocrinology. 2015;156:3895–908.
29. Lalli E. Mitotane revisited: a new target for an old drug. Endocrinology. 2015;156:3873–5.
30. Trivedi BK, Purchase TS, Holmes A, Augelli-Szafran CE, Essenburg AD, Hamelehle KL, Stanfield RL, Bousley RF, Krause BR. Inhibitors of acyl-CoA: cholesterol acyltransferase (ACAT). 7. Development of a series of substituted N-phenyl-N'-[(1-phenylcyclopentyl)methyl]ureas with enhanced hypocholesterolemic activity. J Med Chem. 1994;37:1652–9.
31. Gilor C, Graves TK. Interpretation of laboratory tests for canine Cushing's syndrome. Top Companion Anim Med. 2011;26:98–108.
32. van Liew CH, Greco DS, Salman MD. Comparison of the results of adrenocorticotropic hormone stimulation and low-dose dexamethasone suppression tests with necropsy findings in dogs: 81 cases (1985-1995). J Am Vet Med Assoc. 1997;211:322–5.
33. Gold AJ, Langlois DK, Refsal K. Evaluation of basal serum or plasma cortisol concentrations for the diagnosis of hypoadrenocorticism in dogs. J Vet Intern Med. 2016;30:1798–805.
34. Behrend EN, Weigand CM, Whitley EM, Refsal KR, Young DW, Kemppainen RJ. Corticosterone- and aldosterone-secreting adrenocortical tumor in a dog. J Am Vet Med Assoc. 2005;226:1662–6.
35. Fowler KM, Frank LA, Morandi F, Whittemore JC. Extended low-dose dexamethasone suppression test for diagnosis of atypical Cushing's syndrome in dogs. Domest Anim Endocrinol. 2017;60:25–30.

ATR-101, a selective ACAT1 inhibitor, decreases ACTH-stimulated cortisol concentrations in dogs...

145

36. Labelle P, Kyles AE, Farver TB, De Cock HE. Indicators of malignancy of canine adrenocortical tumors: histopathology and proliferation index. Vet Pathol. 2004;41:490–7.

37. Colgin LM, Schwahn DJ, Castillo-Alcala F, Kiupel M, Lewis AD. Pheochromocytoma in old world primates (Macaca mulatta and Chlorocebus aethiops). Vet Pathol. 2016;53:1259–63.

38. Sledge DG, Patrick DJ, Fitzgerald SD, Xie Y, Kiupel M. Differences in expression of uroplakin III, cytokeratin 7, and cyclooxygenase-2 in canine proliferative lesions of the urinary bladder. Vet Pathol. 2015;52:74–82.

39. Arenas C, Melián C, Pérez-Alenza MD. Long-term survival of dogs with adrenal-dependent hyperadrenocorticism: a comparison between mitotane and twice daily trilostane treatment. J Vet Intern Med. 2014;28:473–80.

40. Else T, Williams AR, Sabolch A, Jolly S, Miller BS, Hammer GD. Adjuvant therapies and patient and tumor characteristics associated with survival of adult patients with adrenocortical carcinoma. J Clin Endocrinol Metab. 2014;99:455–61.

41. Sharma ST, Nieman LK, Feelders RA. Cushing's syndrome: epidemiology and developments in disease management. Clin Epidemiol. 2015;7:281–93.

42. Willeberg P, Priestler WA. Epidemiological aspects of hyperadrenocorticism in dogs (canine Cushing's syndrome). J Am Anim Hosp Assoc. 1982;18:717–24.

43. Galac S. Cortisol-secreting adrenocortical tumours in dogs and their relevance for human medicine. Mol Cell Endocrinol. 2016;421:34–9.

44. Johnston SD, Mather EC. Canine plasma cortisol (hydrocortisone) measured by radioimmunoassay: clinical absence of diurnal variation and results of ACTH stimulation and dexamethasone suppression tests. Am J Vet Res. 1978;39:1766–70.

45. Kemppainen RJ, Sartin JL. Evidence for episodic but not circadian activity in plasma concentrations of adrenocorticotrophin, cortisol, and thyroxine in dogs. J Endocrinol. 1984;103:219–26.

46. Peterson ME, Orth DN, Halmi NS, Zielinski AC, Davis DR, Chavez FT, Drucker WD. Plasma immunoreactive proopiomelanocortin peptides and cortisol in normal dogs and dogs with Addison's disease and Cushing's syndrome: basal concentrations. Endocrinology. 1986;119:720–30.

47. Buckhardt WA, Boretti FS, Reusch CE, Sieber-Ruckstunl NS. Evaluation of baseline cortisol, endogenous ACTH, and cortisol/ACTH ratio to monitor trilostane treatment in dogs with pituitary-dependent hypercortisolism. J Vet Intern Med. 2013;27:919–23.

48. Angles JM, Feldman EC, Nelson RW, Feldman MS. Use of urine cortisol: creatinine ratio versus adrenocorticotropic hormone stimulation testing for monitoring mitotane treatment of pituitary-dependent hyperadrenocorticism in dogs. J Am Vet Med Assoc. 1997;211:1002–4.

49. Galac S, Buijtels JJ, Kooistra HS. Urinary corticoid: creatinine ratios in dogs with pituitary-dependent hypercortisolism during trilostane treatment. J Vet Intern Med. 2009;23:1214–9.

50. Bryan HM, Adams AG, Invik RM, Wynne-Edwards KE, Smits JE. Hair as a meaningful measure of baseline cortisol levels over time in dogs. J Am Assoc Lab Anim Sci. 2013;52:189–96.

51. Cobb ML, Iskandarani K, Chinchilli VM, Dreschel NA. A systematic review and meta-analysis of salivary cortisol measurements in domestic canines. Domest Anim Endocrinol. 2016;57:31–42.

52. Wenger-Riggenbach B, Boretti FS, Quante S, Schellenberg S, Reusch CE, Sieber-Ruckstuhl NS. Salivary cortisol concentrations in healthy dogs and dogs with hypercortisolism. J Vet Intern Med. 2010;24:551–6.

53. Lee RG, Willingham MC, Davis MA, Skinner KA, Rudel LL. Differential expression of ACAT1 and ACAT2 among cells within liver, intestine, kidney, and adrenal of nonhuman primates. J Lipid Res. 2000;41:1991–2001.

54. Vernetti LA, MacDonald JR, Pegg DG. Differential toxicity of an inhibitor of mitochondrial respiration in canine hepatocytes and adrenocortical cell cultures. Toxicol in Vitro. 1996;10:51–7.

55. Maronpot RR, Yoshizawa K, Nyska A, Harada T, Flake G, Mueller G, Singh B, Ward JM. Hepatic enzyme induction: histopathology. Toxicologic Pathol. 2010;38:776–95.

16

Design of the Growth hormone deficiency and Efficacy of Treatment (GET) score and non-interventional proof of concept study

Peter H. Kann[1*], Simona Bergmann[1], Martin Bidlingmaier[2], Christina Dimopoulou[3], Birgitte T. Pedersen[4], Günter K. Stalla[3], Matthias M. Weber[5] and Stefanie Meckes-Ferber[6]

Abstract

Background: The adverse effects of growth hormone (GH) deficiency (GHD) in adults (AGHD) on metabolism and health-related quality of life (HRQoL) can be improved with GH substitution. This investigation aimed to design a score summarising the features of GHD and evaluate its ability to measure the effect of GH substitution in AGHD.

Methods: The Growth hormone deficiency and Efficacy of Treatment (GET) score (0–100 points) assessed (weighting): HRQoL (40%), disease-related days off work (10%), bone mineral density (20%), waist circumference (10%), low-density lipoprotein cholesterol (10%) and body fat mass (10%). A prospective, non-interventional, multicentre proof-of-concept study investigated whether the score could distinguish between untreated and GH-treated patients with AGHD. A 10-point difference in GET score during a 2-year study period was expected based on pre-existing knowledge of the effect of GH substitution in AGHD.

Results: Of 106 patients eligible for analysis, 22 were untreated GHD controls (9 females, mean ± SD age 52 ± 17 years; 13 males, 57 ± 13 years) and 84 were GH-treated (31 females, age 45 ± 13 years, GH dose 0.30 ± 0.16 mg/day; 53 males, age 49 ± 15 years, GH dose 0.25 ± 0.10 mg/day). Follow-up was 706 ± 258 days in females and 653 ± 242 days in males. The GET score differed between the untreated control and treated groups with a least squares mean difference of + 10.01 ± 4.01 ($p = 0.0145$).

Conclusions: The GET score appeared to be a suitable integrative instrument to summarise the clinical features of GHD and measure the effects of GH substitution in adults. Exercise capacity and muscle strength/body muscle mass could be included in the GET score.

Keywords: Clinical study, Growth hormone, Growth hormone deficiency, Quality of life

Background

Growth hormone (GH) is a pleiotropic hormone. Whereas growth failure is the relevant symptom of childhood GH deficiency (GHD), adult GHD (AGHD) is a recognised syndrome with adverse phenotypic, metabolic and health-related quality of life (HRQoL) features [1], which improve in many patients when GH is substituted [2, 3]. For some chronic diseases with multiple clinical facets and complications (e.g., diabetes), a composite of clinical endpoints has been defined as a primary outcome measure for study purposes to evaluate the effect of therapeutic interventions [4, 5].

The objective of this project was to design and, in a second step, conduct a non-interventional proof of concept study to evaluate an instrument that allows quantification and summarising of the various facets of AGHD and the therapeutic response to GH replacement. The composite score was given the acronym "GET – Growth hormone deficiency and Efficacy of Treatment" and aimed to provide a quantitative integrative picture of parameters that, based on evidence in the literature [2, 3], are considered

* Correspondence: kannp@med.uni-marburg.de
[1]Division of Endocrinology & Diabetology, Philipp's University Marburg, D-35033 Marburg, Germany
Full list of author information is available at the end of the article

clinically, economically and socially relevant in a large population.

All the parameters chosen to be integrated into the GET score had previously been shown, according to the criteria of evidence-based medicine (EBM), to be affected by GHD and to be improved following GH substitution in AGHD. The weighting of parameters in the GET score was arbitrarily defined by the study group according to their estimated clinical relevance (experts' opinion). The parameters are all assessed in routine clinical practice and the composite score was intended to have the potential to be used for scientific purposes as well as in clinical practice. In the second step of this project, a prospective, non-interventional, multicentre proof of concept study was performed to investigate whether the GET score was able to distinguish between untreated and GH-treated patients with AGHD. Based on existing knowledge regarding the effect of GH replacement in patients with AGHD on the parameters included in the score, the difference between control and treated patients over 2 years was expected to be 10 points, and this difference was assumed to be clinically relevant (see details in Methods). If this was shown, the GET score would be considered a scientifically useful and clinically relevant instrument. In addition, the effect of GH therapy on insulin-like growth factor I (IGF-I) standard deviation score (SDS) and on the individual clinical parameters comprising the GET score was evaluated.

Methods

GET score assessment and definition

GET score items were selected according to evidence available in the literature [2, 3], and their weighting was defined arbitrarily following extensive discussion in the study group. The GET score was designed to cover a range between 0 and 100 points, composed from clinically measurable parameters. It was intended that GH-untreated patients with AGHD should be positioned approximately in the middle of the range (with a mean of ~ 50 points and a standard deviation [SD] of ~ 20 points) and that the range should allow the measurement of treatment effects. Fifty percent of the GET score points were generated from HRQoL parameters and 50% from physical measurements of somatic parameters.

The Short-Form Health Survey 36 (SF-36), one of the most commonly used generic instruments for measuring HRQoL, covers eight HRQoL elements assessing physical and psychological health [6]. Previous research has established the relationship between the EuroQol five dimensions questionnaire (EQ-5D), a generic five-item instrument providing a simple descriptive profile and a single index value for health status, and a tool used to measure HRQoL in patients with AGHD [7, 8]. An increase in the SF-36 and EQ-5D visual analogue scale (VAS) score reflects an improvement in self-perceived

health. The SF-36 and the VAS component of EQ-5D (EQ-5D-VAS) have both been used previously in patients with AGHD [7, 9]. The QoL-Assessment of GHD in Adults (QoL-AGHDA), a disease-specific, need-based measure [10], developed based on in-depth interviews with adult patients with GHD is also a recognised measure for the assessment of QoL. However, restricted licence use did not permit use of this tool in our study.

The HRQoL parameters of the GET score comprised the SF-36 score [7] (20 points) and the EQ-5D-VAS (20 points), together with the disease-related days off work (10 points).

Details on the allocation of the GET score points from SF-36 and EQ-5D-VAS are given in Additional file 1: Table S1. As the SF-36 covers eight dimensions, the arithmetic mean of the score points from each dimension was taken and included into the GET score (an example is shown in Additional file 1: Table S2). Based on data from Saller et al., [11] > 30 disease-related days off work during the previous 6 months generated a score of 0 points, and < 4 disease-related days off work generated a score of 10 points (Additional file 1: Table S1).

The somatic parameters comprised bone mineral density (BMD) (20 points), waist circumference (10 points), low-density lipoprotein cholesterol (LDL-C) (10 points), and body fat mass (10 points). Details on the allocation of the GET score points for the somatic parameters are provided in Additional file 1: Table S3.

Dual-energy X-ray absorptiometry (DXA) is the gold standard for BMD measurement [3, 12]. As patients' ages spanned more than five decades, the z-score was selected as the most suitable parameter for measuring BMD. The most pronounced effect of GH substitution on BMD is detectable at the lumbar spine [13], hence this was the measuring site for the GET score. Based on published data [14], DXA BMD lumbar spine z-score ≤ -2 was assigned a score of 0 points, and a z-score ≥ 0 was assigned a score of 20 points.

Waist circumference reflects visceral fat accumulation and is established as a key criterion for the diagnosis of metabolic syndrome and as an independent cardiovascular risk factor [15]. When including this parameter in the GET score, individual variance, risk threshold, and published data from patients with AGHD with rather small therapeutic effects had to be considered [16, 17]. Therefore, waist circumference ≥ 99 cm in females / ≥ 113 cm in males scored 0 points, and waist circumference ≤ 80 cm in females / ≤ 94 cm in males scored 10 points.

Based on the baseline values and the therapeutic effects of GH substitution on LDL-C in patients with AGHD [18, 19], LDL-C ≥ 3.98 mmol/L (154 mg/dL) scored 0 points, and ≤ 2.59 mmol/L (100 mg/dL) scored 10 points.

Using a Tanita scale, body fat mass can be assessed with body impedance analysis. Based on data from Rosenfalck et al. [20], body fat mass percentage ≥ 44.1% scored 0 points, and ≤21.5% scored 10 points.

To calculate a GET score, the first step is to calculate the overall SF-36 GET score points by taking the average of all eight SF-36 GET score points based on the transformed SF-36 domain scores (Additional file 1: Table S1). The second step is to add the GET score points for the remaining HRQoL parameters – EQ-5D-VAS and disease-related days off work (Additional file 1: Table S1). The third step is to look up the GET score points for the somatic parameters using the GET score points as shown in Additional file 1: Table S3. The addition of all components sums up to the final GET score. An example of a calculation of GET score is provided in Additional file 1: Table S4. If individual parameters are missing, the score is calculated without these parameters, but adjusted accordingly (Additional file 1: Table S5). For example, BMD has a weighting of 20%; the maximum score achievable without BMD would be 80. If a patient achieved a determined score of 67 without BMD, adjustment of the determined score would be 67/80*100, resulting in a final GET score of 83.75 (Additional file 1: Table S5). A minimum number of parameters giving a total weighting of ≥70% is required to determine the adjusted GET score, otherwise the GET score is set to missing.

Proof of concept study
Study design
GH-treatment-naïve patients with AGHD, defined according to GH Research Society criteria [3], under the care of endocrinologists, were enrolled into a prospective, observational, non-interventional, multicentre proof of concept study.

The indication and clinical decisions regarding GH replacement (Norditropin® [somatropin, recombinant human GH], Novo Nordisk A/S, Denmark) were made by the treating physician according to usual clinical practice. GH-treated patients were compared with patients in whom no treatment was initiated; the decision not to initiate GH replacement was taken jointly by the patient and the physician. The study was performed in accordance with the Declaration of Helsinki [21]. Ethical permissions were obtained from the Ethical Commission of the Chamber of Physicians of the German Federal State of Hessia. Informed consent was obtained from all study participants.

The study recruitment period was originally planned for 24 months, but extended to 36 months due to limited recruitment. Participation commenced at visit 1, when baseline data were collected and GH treatment was initiated in the treatment group. Interim follow-up visits (visits 2–4) were planned for approximately every 6 months, but occurred at varying intervals, and the participants' involvement concluded at visit 5. If the patient prematurely discontinued participation, the last interim

visit became the final visit. Duration of follow-up was calculated as days between first and last visit.

The inclusion criteria for data analysis were availability of baseline demographic data (gender, date of birth), information about GH therapy for treated patients and at least one of four follow-up visits.

The GET score was calculated, and if there were too few parameters to provide a total weighting of ≥70%, the GET score was set to missing. In the proof of concept study, IGF-I concentrations were measured mainly as a parameter for plausibility, verifying whether GH had or had not been administered. IGF-I was assessed centrally using the iSYS automated chemiluminescent IGF-I assay (Immunodiagnostic Systems Ltd., Boldon, UK). The assay employs two monoclonal antibodies and is calibrated against WHO International Standard 02/254 (National Institute for Biological Standards and Control, Hertfordshire, UK) [22].

Statistical analysis
In observational studies, clinical practice is reflected in missing values, missing visits and fewer untreated controls than treated patients, thereby providing unbalanced data; therefore, a repeated measures model was found to be the most appropriate method to analyse the available data. The study sample size was determined by the ability to recruit patients within the study period. By using the repeated measures multiple regression model for the GET score analysis, correlation of data within the individual patient were taken into account when patients were observed at several visits over time within the study period. Any overall differences between the mean GET score of the two groups in the full study period could be detected. Due to the ageing of the patients over the study period, deterioration over time could potentially occur in the parameters included in the GET score, therefore untreated controls versus treated patients were evaluated.

The model included treatment group (control and treated), visit, and the interaction term between visit and treatment as explanatory variables. Gender, age and treatment duration were also included in the model to adjust for potential differences in patient characteristics in the two groups. The overall difference in GET score between control and treated groups in the full study period was estimated by least squares means (LSM). Missing data were handled by the repeated measures model when evaluating the GET score and were considered missing completely at random. Descriptive statistics were applied for all parameters and data are presented as mean ± SD, unless otherwise stated. Statistical analysis was performed using SAS v9.4 (SAS Institute Inc., Cary, North Carolina, USA).

Results

A total of 106 patients were eligible for analysis (controls: 9 females, 13 males; GH-treated: 31 females, 53 males). Baseline characteristics for all 106 patients and mean GH starting dose for treated patients are shown in Table 1. A baseline GET score could only be calculated for 75 patients due to missing data. In the follow-up evaluation of the GET score the 75 patients were distributed as 15 control (5 females, 10 males) and 60 GH-treated (22 females, 38 males) patients.

At baseline, where all patients were in a GH-naïve stage, the overall mean ± SD GET score was estimated as 51.66 ± 20.48 score points, which was close to the intended mean baseline score of around 50 and intended SD of 20.

Baseline mean age was higher in the control versus the treated group and higher in males than females; however, the statistical model adjusted for this. Differences in age and gender did not reach a statistically significant level when included in the full repeated measures model evaluating the GET score.

Treatment (study) duration was longer for treated females (706.5 ± 258 days) versus treated males (653.6 ± 242 days). However, based on the results from the model, duration did not have a statistically significant effect on the GET score within the given study period.

GET score

Mean unadjusted GET scores by gender at baseline and follow-up visits are shown in Table 2. Mean baseline GET scores were close to 50 in all groups (female controls: 51.14 ± 21.62; treated females: 47.02 ± 22.29; male controls: 49.78 ± 19.01; treated males: 54.92 ± 19.84).

Fig. 1 shows the estimated GET scores for each group at every visit based on the repeated measures model.

The analysis showed that GH treatment had an overall clinically relevant and statistically significant effect on the GET score of the expected magnitude, with a LSM difference of + 10.01 ± 4.01 (p = 0.0145) between the control and treated groups based on the full follow-up period in the study.

Changes in individual items contributing to the GET score

HRQoL Improvements in HRQoL, as assessed with the SF-36, were observed in the GH-treated group for physical functioning (female + 4.64 ± 24.14 [n = 14]; male + 0.96 ± 14.42 [n = 26]), emotional role functioning (female + 5.36 ± 25.66 [n = 14]; male + 1.92 ± 30.49 [n = 26]) and physical role functioning (female + 12.05 ± 26.00 [n = 14]; male + 1.39 ± 20.17 [n = 27]); and in the female treated group only there were improvements in their general health perception (+ 10.93 ± 23.43 [n = 14]) and vitality (+ 9.82 ± 19.41 [n = 14]).

Using the EQ-5D-VAS, HRQoL was numerically higher at baseline in female controls (n = 6) (77.67 ± 25.32) versus treated females (n = 31) (58.71 ± 21.08), but numerically lower in male controls (n = 11) (56.36 ± 19.38) than treated males (n = 47) (65.15 ± 19.29). During the study period, mean EQ-5D-VAS score increased in GH-treated patients (mean change + 10.00 ± 11.73 females [n = 13]; + 6.38 ± 17.20 males [n = 26]). However, the score decreased substantially in female controls (n = 2) (mean change − 27.50 ± 3.54) and increased slightly in male controls (n = 6) (+ 4.33 ± 14.32). HRQoL assessed by the SF-36 was more variable than when assessed by the EQ-5D-VAS.

Disease-related days off work The number of disease-related days off work during the previous 6 months varied throughout the study. There was a decrease at each

Table 1 Baseline demographics and characteristics of the included AGHD patients

Measurement	Female control group		Female treated group		Male control group		Male treated group	
	N	Mean ± SD	N	Mean ± SD	N	Mean ± SD	N	Mean ± SD
Age (years)	9	51.60 ± 16.76	31	44.86 ± 13.05	13	57.16 ± 12.88	53	48.73 ± 14.69
GH starting dose (mg/day)	9	0.00 ± 0.00	31	0.23 ± 0.13	13	0.00 ± 0.00	53	0.20 ± 0.09
IGF-I SDS	9	−1.13 ± 2.09	26	−1.40 ± 1.44	12	−1.58 ± 1.17	44	−1.28 ± 1.72
Diagnosis at baseline	9		31		13		53	
Acquired GHD (trauma)	1		1		0		1	
Acquired GHD (pituitary tumour)	4		9		7		25	
Acquired GHD (surgery/irradiation)	1		14		5		10	
Acquired GHD (other)	2		4		0		6	
Idiopathic GHD	1		0		0		5	
Hypopituitarism/pituitary abnormality	0		3		1		5	
Craniopharyngioma	0		0		0		1	

AGHD adults with growth hormone deficiency, *GET* Growth hormone deficiency and Efficacy of Treatment, *GH* growth hormone, *GHD* GH deficiency, *IGF-I* insulin-like growth factor 1, *N* number of participants eligible for analysis, *SD* standard deviation, *SDS* standard deviation score

Table 2 Mean[a] GET score at baseline and follow-up visits by gender for GH-treated patients and controls

Visit	GET score							
	Female control group		Female treated group		Male control group		Male treated group	
	N	Mean ± SD	N	Mean ± SD	N	Mean ± SD	N	Mean ± SD
1 (baseline)	5	51.14 ± 21.62	22	47.02 ± 22.29	10	49.78 ± 19.01	38	54.92 ± 19.84
2	5	48.84 ± 13.26	19	51.45 ± 13.07	10	47.02 ± 13.76	33	57.68 ± 16.47
3	4	53.49 ± 10.96	19	52.48 ± 16.09	9	43.22 ± 18.31	32	60.97 ± 14.92
4	3	43.65 ± 24.66	12	47.60 ± 14.70	9	40.58 ± 11.79	24	58.57 ± 13.91
5	3	49.84 ± 23.29	11	47.59 ± 14.11	6	49.19 ± 17.32	29	56.03 ± 14.67

[a]Note the data presented are crude mean values and based on a variable number of patients
GH growth hormone,*GET* Growth hormone deficiency and Efficacy of Treatment, *N* number of participants in whom GET score was calculated, *SD* standard deviation

visit for GH-treated female patients, and the change from baseline was − 30.00 ± 63.44 days by visit 5 ($n = 5$). There was no discernible pattern in the number of disease-related days off in the male treated group; number of days off was 8.21 ± 44.04 days below baseline at visit 5 ($n = 19$).

Bone mineral density At baseline BMD assessed by DXA z-score was − 0.54 ± 1.42 in female controls ($n = 5$), − 0.20 ± 1.30 in male controls ($n = 9$), − 0.23 ± 1.06 in treated females ($n = 9$) and − 0.68 ± 1.86 in treated males ($n = 20$). There were small fluctuations throughout the study, with minimal change from baseline by visit 5: female controls ($n = 2$): + 0.05 ± 0.21; male controls ($n = 3$): + 0.27 ± 0.45; treated females ($n = 4$): + 0.18 ± 0.59; treated males ($n = 9$): + 0.49 ± 0.45. However, the small number of patients who underwent DXA analysis made these data difficult to interpret.

Waist circumference During the study, waist circumference (cm) increased in controls (females [$n = 6$] + 2.67 ± 5.28; males [$n = 5$] + 3.86 ± 4.84) and decreased in

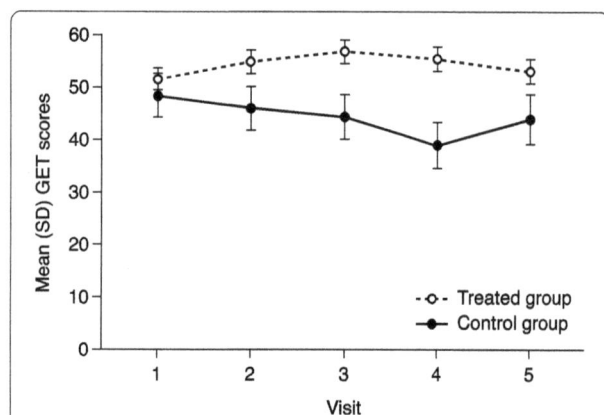

Fig. 1 Estimated difference in the GET score between control and GH-treated groups during follow-up visits (EAS)EAS, effectiveness analysis set; GET, Growth hormone deficiency and Efficacy of Treatment; GH, growth hormone.

GH-treated patients (change from baseline [cm]: female [$n = 7$] −2.86 ± 5.15; males [$n = 20$] −1.23 ± 7.55).

LDL-C During the study, LDL-C increased slightly from baseline for female controls ($n = 9$) and all male patients ($n = 12$) (female controls + 0.40 ± 0.82 mmol/L [$n = 5$]; male controls + 0.04 ± 0.72 mmol/L [$n = 7$]; treated males + 0.01 ± 0.63 mmol/L [$n = 23$]) and decreased slightly for treated females (− 0.22 ± 0.68 mmol/L [$n = 13$]).

Body fat mass Baseline body fat mass (%) was higher in females (controls: 32.98 ± 6.22 [$n = 5$]; treated: 36.81 ± 6.86 [$n = 24$]) than males (controls: 27.69 ± 8.68 [$n = 11$]; treated: 26.02 ± 6.55 [$n = 47$]). Absence of treatment was associated with an increase in body fat (mean change from baseline: female: + 0.85% ± 1.06% [$n = 11$]; male + 3.46% ± 3.07% [$n = 47$]), whereas GH treatment was associated with a decrease (mean change from baseline: female: − 2.29% ± 4.14% [$n = 15$]; male: − 1.93% ± 4.52% [$n = 27$]).

IGF-I SDS The increase in GET score was accompanied by an increase in IGF-I SDS in the GH-treated groups. Mean IGF-I SDS was below zero (− 1.13 to − 1.58) for all groups at baseline. At visit 2, change from baseline for treated females was + 1.37 ± 1.14 ($n = 23$), and for treated males was + 1.42 ± 1.21 ($n = 39$) (Fig. 2). The increased level of IGF-I SDS in the treated groups was maintained throughout the study. IGF-I SDS did not substantially change for the control group, remaining below zero at every visit.

Discussion

This study aimed to design and evaluate an experimental score that integrates the different features of AGHD and demonstrates the pleiotropic therapeutic effects of GH substitution in patients with AGHD. The GET score, which was designed based on evidence in the literature [2, 3], weights items according to their clinical relevance as considered by the study group. Importantly, the GET

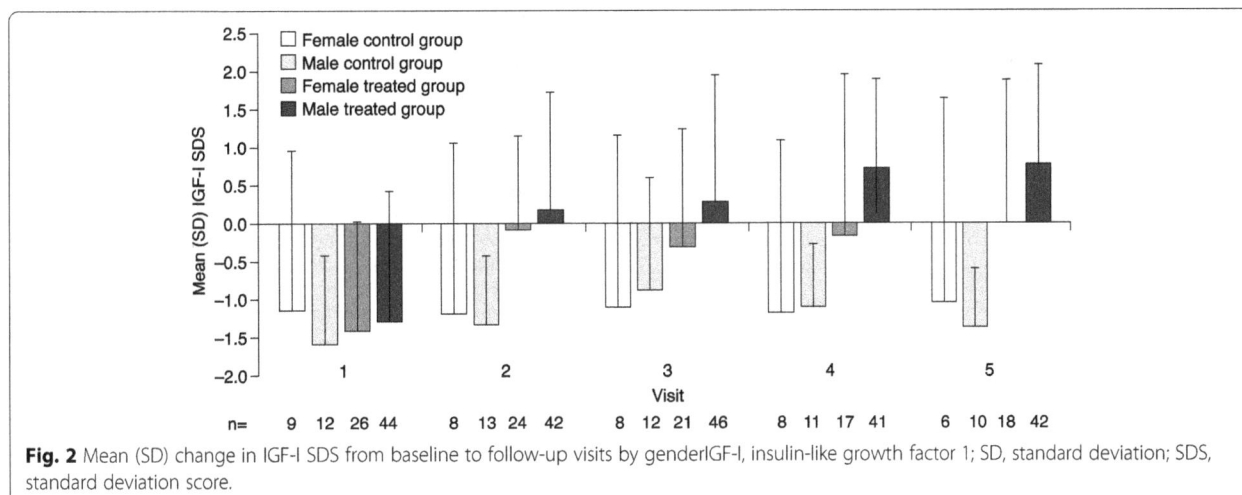

Fig. 2 Mean (SD) change in IGF-I SDS from baseline to follow-up visits by gender|IGF-I, insulin-like growth factor 1; SD, standard deviation; SDS, standard deviation score.

score can potentially be applied and calculated by physicians in everyday clinical practice.

However, our non-interventional study has shown that in a considerable proportion of patients the GET score at baseline could not be calculated due to missing data. This was surprising since the score was designed so that a GET score could be calculated with a total weighting of variables of only 70%, to account for potential missing data in a real world setting. The mean baseline GET score in GH-untreated patients was ~ 50, with a variation equivalent to ~ 20 points (SD). The contribution for each individual item to the observed GET scores was appropriately spread across the score range (i.e., 0–10 or 0–20, depending on the weighting) and mean scores were positioned, as expected, around the midpoint of the scale, indicating that the predefined score calculation was suitable. The descriptive statistics of the GET score in a GH treatment naïve situation at baseline yielded results within the expected range, indicating that the assumptions made when designing the score were appropriate.

In our proof of concept study, the GET score was evaluated and used to estimate the combined pleiotropic effects of GH by calculating the overall difference in GET score in the full follow-up period between the untreated versus treated group. This required the use of a repeated measures model to account for correlation of data within the individual patient, to handle missing and thus variable numbers of observations, and to detect any overall differences between mean GET scores of the two groups in the full study period. Due to the longitudinal nature of the study, interpretation of the study should be based on the overall difference between the two groups, as estimated by the model and shown in Fig. 1.

Based on the full follow-up period of the study, the GET score was statistically significantly different overall between untreated and GH-treated patients in the expected range of ~ 10 points, representing a clinically relevant

difference in HRQoL and/or somatic parameters. This difference was largely driven by the deterioration in GET score over time in the untreated group. The difference reached the magnitude expected, confirming that the assumptions made when designing the score were appropriate. This allows us to state that the GET score may be a suitable instrument to quantify the effects of GH treatment in patients with AGHD in an integrative way.

The GET score includes clinically relevant parameters, weighted according to potential impact on the individual patient. Patients with AGHD have reported the negative impact of their condition on many aspects of daily life [23], and the importance of HRQoL is recognised in clinical practice guidelines [24, 25]. Hence, the HRQoL parameters provide the highest overall contribution to the GET score (40%). Although the sample size of this study is limited, the results are consistent with available literature showing that GH substitution can positively influence HRQoL [26, 27].

BMD contributed significantly to the GET score (weighted 20%); however, unfortunately only a small number of patients in this study underwent DXA analysis, making interpretation of the data difficult. Many patients lacked BMD data because data collection was based on routine clinical practice and not a study protocol. During this study, BMD assessed by DXA z-score did not change significantly. Davidson et al. [28] demonstrated that clinically significant changes in BMD are observed after treatment duration of at least 18–24 months. This limitation could be addressed by studying a larger cohort over a longer period.

IGF-I serum levels are used for GH dose titration [24, 25] and provide an indication of the efficacy of GH therapy and patients' adherence with treatment. In this study, IGF-I SDS increased from baseline to near zero by visit 2 following GH treatment initiation; this level was maintained or increased throughout the study in the treated groups.

The main limitation of this proof-of-concept study was the observational, non-interventional design, which lacked the methodological rigour of a randomised controlled trial. The control group had a low number of patients and there were also differences between groups; it is likely that, as the decision for treatment was based on physician opinion, the two groups (control and treated) were not homogeneous, with differences in co-morbidities and use of concomitant medication. Treatment adherence was not evaluated in the treatment group, which may have affected the results.

As with many observational studies, missing data were a challenge, and incomplete data sets had to be handled by an appropriate statistical approach. The set of parameters chosen for the GET score was based on published evidence; however, in contrast to the published recommendations [3] these parameters do not seem to be routinely assessed when GH-treatment is warranted in AGHD. The small number of BMD examinations was unexpected for the study group. Potentially, the study duration was too short for BMD follow-up examinations. The fact that a baseline GET score could only be calculated in 75/106 patients is a concern regarding the ability of the GET score to be used in everyday clinical practice. The process of calculating the GET score, particularly the points for SF-36, is laborious, thus limiting the use in routine clinical practice. Nevertheless, an individual comparison of GET scores at baseline and after a period of GH treatment might be of clinical relevance for the assessment of individual clinical response to GHT.

Conclusions

The newly developed GET score appeared to be a suitable instrument to summarise the features of AGHD and evaluate the pleiotropic response to GH substitution therapy in an integrated way. We suggest the GET score as a tool for clinical studies rather than for routine clinical practice. A further study in a larger cohort and over a longer period of time could overcome some of the shortcomings seen in this project.

Additional file

Additional file 1: Table S1. GET score point allocation for HRQoL parameters (which comprise 50 of the total of 100 points of the GET score). Table S2 Example of a calculation of SF-36 GET score component points. Table S3 GET score point allocation for somatic parameters (which comprise 50 of the total of 100 points of the GET score).Table S4 Example of calculation of GET score including SF-36 subtotal and addition to other components of the score. GET score calculation. Table S5 Example of calculation of an adjusted GET score due to a missing value (DOCX 39 kb)

Abbreviations

AGHD: Adults with growth hormone deficiency; BMD: Bone mineral density; DXA: Dual-energy X-ray absorptiometry; EBM: Evidence-based medicine; EQ-5D: EuroQol five dimensions questionnaire; EQ-5D-VAS: VAS component of EQ-5D; GET score: Growth hormone deficiency and Efficacy of Treatment score; GH: Growth hormone; GHD: Growth hormone deficiency;

HRQoL: Health-related quality of life; IGF-I: Insulin-like growth factor I; LDL-C: Low-density lipoprotein cholesterol; LSM: Least squares means; SD: Standard deviation; SDS: Standard deviation score; SF-36: Short-Form Health Survey 36; VAS: Visual analogue scale

Acknowledgements
The authors thank the representatives of a total of 28 centres for endocrinology in Germany that contributed patients' data to the non-interventional clinical study. The authors also thank Stefan Kipper (Novo Nordisk Pharma GmbH, Mainz, Germany) for his invaluable contribution to this project, Judith L. Jacobsen (Statcon, Denmark) for perfect technical and statistical support, and Lise Højbjerre (Novo Nordisk A/S, Denmark) for review of the manuscript. Medical writing and submission support were provided by Grace Townshend and Richard McDonald of Watermeadow Medical, funded by Novo Nordisk Pharma GmbH, Mainz, Germany.

Funding
This study was sponsored by Novo Nordisk Pharma GmbH, Mainz, Germany. NCT number: NCT00934063.

Authors' contributions
PHK contributed to research design, acquisition of data, analysis/interpretation of data, revised the manuscript critically, and approved the final version. SB contributed to acquisition of data, analysis/interpretation of data, revised the manuscript critically, and approved the final version. MB contributed to acquisition of data, analysis/interpretation of data, revised the manuscript critically, and approved the final version. CD contributed to acquisition of data, analysis/interpretation of data, revised the manuscript critically, and approved the final version. BTP contributed to analysis/interpretation of data, revised the manuscript critically, and approved the final version. GKS contributed to research design, acquisition of data, analysis/interpretation of data, revised the manuscript critically, and approved the final version. MMW contributed to research design, acquisition of data, analysis/interpretation of data, revised the manuscript critically, and approved the final version. SMF contributed to analysis/interpretation of data, revised the manuscript critically, and approved the final version.

Competing interests
PHK has received research funding, honoraria for lectures and is a member of scientific boards for Novo Nordisk and Pfizer. MB has received research support, consultancy fees and/or speakers honoraria from Novo Nordisk, Pfizer, Sandoz, Novartis, IPSEN, OPKO and Genexine. BTP is an employee of Novo Nordisk A/S, Denmark. GKS has received speaker fees from Novo Nordisk and study investigator sponsored by Novo Nordisk. MMW is member of the NordiNet® ISC Board Novo Nordisk. SM-F is an employee and stockholder of Novo Nordisk Pharma GmbH, Germany. SB and CD have no conflicts of interest to declare.

Author details
¹Division of Endocrinology & Diabetology, Philipp's University Marburg, D-35033 Marburg, Germany. ²Endocrine Laboratory, Medizinische Klinik und Poliklinik IV, Ludwig-Maximilians University, 80336 Munich, Germany. ³Neuroendocrinology, Max-Planck-Institute for Psychiatry, 80804 Munich, Germany. ⁴Epidemiology, Novo Nordisk A/S, 2860 Søborg, Denmark. ⁵Endocrinology & Metabolism, Johannes Gutenberg University Hospital, 55131 Mainz, Germany. ⁶Clinical, Medical & Regulatory Department, Novo Nordisk Pharma GmbH, 55127 Mainz, Germany.

References

1. Carroll PV, Christ ER, Bengtsson BA. Growth hormone research society scientific committee. Growth hormone deficiency in adulthood and the effects of growth hormone replacement: a review. J Clin Endocrinol Metab. 1998;83:382–95.

2. Fassbender WJ, Brabant G, Buchfelder M, et al. Treatment of proven growth hormone deficiency in adults with recombinant human growth hormone according to evidence-based criteria. Dtsch Med Wochenschr. 2005;130: 2589–95.

3. Ho KK. 2007 GH deficiency consensus workshop participants. Consensus guidelines for the diagnosis and treatment of adults with GH deficiency II: a statement of the GH research society in association with the European Society for Pediatric Endocrinology, Lawson Wilkins society, European Society of Endocrinology, Japan Endocrine Society, and Endocrine Society of Australia. Eur J Endocrinol. 2007;157:695–700.

4. Gerstein HC, Miller ME, Byington RP, et al. Effects of intensive glucose lowering in type 2 diabetes. N Engl J Med. 2008;358:2545–59.

5. Patel A, MacMahon S, Chalmers J, et al. Intensive blood glucose control and vascular outcomes in patients with type 2 diabetes. N Engl J Med. 2008;358: 2560–72.

6. Ware JE Jr. SF-36 health survey update. 2007. http://www.sf-36.org/tools/SF36.shtml. Accessed July 2017.

7. Koltowska-Haggstrom M, Jonsson B, Isacson D, et al. Using EQ-5D to derive general population-based utilities for the quality of life assessment of growth hormone deficiency in adults (QoL-AGHDA). Value Health. 2007;10:73–81.

8. Busschbach JJ, Wolffenbuttel BH, Annemans L, et al. Deriving reference values and utilities for the QoL-AGHDA in adult GHD. Eur J Health Econ. 2011;12:243–52.

9. Valassi E, Brick DJ, Johnson JC, et al. Effect of growth hormone replacement therapy on the quality of life in women with growth hormone deficiency who have a history of acromegaly versus other disorders. Endocr Pract. 2012;18:209–18.

10. McKenna SP, Doward LC, Alonso J, et al. The QoL-AGHDA: an instrument for the assessment of quality of life in adults with growth hormone deficiency. Qual Life Res. 1999;8:373–83.

11. Saller B, Mattsson AF, Kann PH, et al. Healthcare utilization, quality of life and patient-reported outcomes during two years of GH replacement therapy in GH-deficient adults – comparison between Sweden, The Netherlands and Germany. Eur J Endocrinol. 2006;154:843–50.

12. Rosenfeld RG, Cohen P, Robison LL, et al. Long-term surveillance of growth hormone therapy. J Clin Endocrinol Metab. 2012;97:68–72.

13. Kann P, Piepkorn B, Schehler B, et al. Effect of long-term treatment with GH on bone metabolism, bone mineral density and bone elasticity in GH-deficient adults. Clin Endocrinol. 1998;48:561–8.

14. Kann PH. Clinical effects of growth hormone on bone: a review. Aging Male. 2004;7:290–6.

15. Alberti KG, Zimmet P, Shaw J. The metabolic syndrome – a new worldwide definition. Lancet. 2005;366:1059–62.

16. Zhu S, Heymsfield SB, Toyoshima H, et al. Race-ethnicity-specific waist circumference cutoffs for identifying cardiovascular disease risk factors. Am J Clin Nutr. 2005;81:409–15.

17. Franco C, Johannsson G, Bengtsson BA, et al. Baseline characteristics and effects of growth hormone therapy over two years in younger and elderly adults with adult onset GH deficiency. J Clin Endocrinol Metab. 2006;91:4408–14.

18. Abs R, Feldt-Rasmussen U, Mattsson AF, et al. Determinants of cardiovascular risk in 2589 hypopituitary GH-deficient adults – a KIMS database analysis. Eur J Endocrinol. 2006;155:79–90.

19. van der Klaauw AA, Romijn JA, Biermasz NR, et al. Sustained effects of recombinant GH replacement after 7 years of treatment in adults with GH deficiency. Eur J Endocrinol. 2006;155:701–8.

20. Rosenfalck AM, Maghsoudi S, Fisker S, et al. The effect of 30 months of low-dose replacement therapy with recombinant human growth hormone (rhGH) on insulin and C-peptide kinetics, insulin secretion, insulin sensitivity, glucose effectiveness, and body composition in GH-deficient adults. J Clin Endocrinol Metab. 2000;85:4173–81.

21. Divall SA, Radovick S. Growth hormone and treatment controversy; long term safety of rGH. Curr Pediatr Rep. 2013;1:128–32.

22. Bidlingmaier M, Friedrich N, Emeny RT, et al. Reference intervals for insulin-like growth factor-1 (IGF-I) from birth to senescence: results from a multicenter study using a new automated chemiluminescence IGF-I immunoassay conforming to recent international recommendations. J Clin Endocrinol Metab. 2014;99:1712–21.

23. Brod M, Pohlman B, Hojbjerre L, et al. Impact of adult growth hormone deficiency on daily functioning and well-being. BMC Res Notes. 2014;7:813.

24. ClinicalTrials.gov. A Prospective Observational Study of Effect of Somatropin on Growth Hormone Deficient Adults (HypoCCS). 2016. https://clinicaltrials.gov/ct2/show/NCT01088399. Accessed July 2017.

25. Cook DM, Yuen KC, Biller BM, et al. American Association of Clinical Endocrinologists medical guidelines for clinical practice for growth hormone use in growth hormone-deficient adults and transition patients – 2009 update. Endocr Pract. 2009;15(Suppl 2):1–29.

26. Degerblad M, Almkvist O, Grunditz R, et al. Physical and psychological capabilities during substitution therapy with recombinant growth hormone in adults with growth hormone deficiency. Acta Endocrinol. 1990;123:185–93.

27. Hull KL, Growth HS. Hormone therapy and quality of life: possibilities, pitfalls and mechanisms. J Endocrinol. 2003;179:311–33.

28. Davidson P, Milne R, Chase D, et al. Growth hormone replacement in adults and bone mineral density: a systematic review and meta-analysis. Clin Endocrinol. 2004;60:92–8.

17

Case Report: Identification of an HNF1B p.Arg527Gln mutation in a Maltese patient with atypical early onset diabetes and diabetic nephropathy

Nikolai Paul Pace[1*], Johann Craus[2], Alex Felice[1] and Josanne Vassallo[3]

Abstract

Background: The diagnosis of atypical non-autoimmune forms of diabetes mellitus, such as maturity onset diabetes of the young (MODY) presents several challenges, in view of the extensive clinical and genetic heterogeneity of the disease. In this report we describe a case of atypical non autoimmune diabetes associated with a damaging HNF1β mutation. This is distinguished by a number of uncharacteristic clinical features, including early-onset obesity, the absence of renal cysts and diabetic nephropathy. HNF1β-MODY (MODY5) is an uncommon form of monogenic diabetes that is often complicated by a wide array of congenital morphological anomalies of the urinary tract, including renal cysts. This report expands on the clinical phenotypes that have been described in the context of HNF1β mutations, and is relevant as only isolated cases of diabetic nephropathy in the setting of MODY5 have been reported.

Case presentation: An obese Maltese female with non-autoimmune diabetes, microalbuminuria, glomerular hyperfiltration, fatty liver and no renal cysts was studied by whole exome sequencing to investigate potential genes responsible for the proband's phenotype. A rare missense mutation at a highly conserved site in exon 8 of HNF1β was identified (c.1580G > A, NM_000458.3, p.Arg527Gln), with multiple in-silico predictions consistent with pathogenicity. This mutation has not been previously characterised. Additionally, several common susceptibility variants associated with early-onset obesity, polygenic type 2 diabetes and nephropathy were identified in the proband that could impose additional effects on the phenotype, its severity or its clinical course.

Conclusion: This report highlights several atypical features in a proband with atypical diabetes associated with an HNF1β missense mutation. It also reinforces the concept that monogenic causes of diabetes could be significant contributors to disease burden in obese individuals with atypical diabetes.

Keywords: MODY 5, Diabetic nephropathy, Obesity, HNF1β, Atypical diabetes

Background

The diagnosis of atypical non-autoimmune diabetes presents several challenges. These forms of diabetes are best exemplified by maturity onset diabetes of the young (MODY). MODY is a rare group of genetically heterogenous conditions characterised by beta cell dysfunction and defects in insulin secretion. Systematic screening of European and North American paediatric populations has identified a prevalence range of 1.2 to 4.2% [1–3]. Population-specific differences in the prevalence of MODY have also been reported [4, 5].

A wide array of phenotypic heterogeneity is observed in subjects with different mutations in the various genes implicated in the pathogenesis of monogenic diabetes, as this disease can mimic either type 1 or type 2 diabetes mellitus. Correctly making the diagnosis of MODY is essential in view of the therapeutic and prognostic implications. Furthermore, the autosomal dominant pattern

* Correspondence: nikolai.p.pace@um.edu.mt
[1]Centre for Molecular Medicine and Biobanking, University of Malta, Msida, Malta
Full list of author information is available at the end of the article

of inheritance mandates genetic counselling and family follow-up. The increasing availability of whole exome or targeted capture followed by high throughput sequencing facilitates the molecular diagnosis of monogenic diabetes, particularly in cases where the clinical phenotype is atypical or complicated by clinical features that are not routinely associated with MODY. Increasingly, next generation sequencing followed by interpretation using publicly-available aggregate exome variant datasets offers an unrivalled scope for the discovery and annotation of novel variants.

Identifying patients with monogenic diabetes requires an index of clinical suspicion of the disease followed by molecular diagnosis to confirm the underlying genetic defect. Guidelines issued by the International Society for Paediatric and Adolescent Diabetes (ISPAD) are available to advise clinicians, and genetic diagnosis is available in many healthcare systems [6] . Despite these guidelines, studies have shown that genetic testing for MODY is under requested and clinical prediction models have been developed to aid the identification of likely candidates for molecular genetic testing [7, 8].

In this report, we describe a rare damaging missense mutation in HNF1β that was identified in a proband with early-onset atypical diabetes with no morphological renal tract anomalies. The proband had glomerular hyperfiltration and early stage diabetic nephropathy, which is unusual in the setting of MODY5. Because of the unusual features of nephropathy in the absence of renal cysts and obesity, we performed whole exome sequencing of the proband.

Methods
Patient
This study was approved by the ethics institutional review board of the University of Malta (IRB 71/2013). Written informed consent was obtained from the proband. The mother had demised and the proband's brother and father were not available for genetic analysis at the time of the study.

Sample preparation and whole exome sequencing
Genomic DNA was extracted from a peripheral blood sample taken from the proband using a QIAamp DNA extraction kit (Qiagen, Hilden, Germany), and checked for purity and integrity using agarose gel electrophoresis and UV spectrophotometry. Sample preparation and exon enrichment for next generation sequencing was performed using a SureSelectXT All Exon V5 kit (Agilent Technologies, Santa Clara, CA). 3 µg of DNA was processed according to manufacturer's instructions. Paired end sequencing was carried out on an Illumina HiSeq 2500 sequencer (Illumina, Inc., San Diego, CA, USA).

Exome sequencing alignment, variant calling and mutation detection
Image analysis was performed with the default parameters of Illumina RTA pipeline, and base calling was carried out using CASAVA. The sequence reads were mapped and aligned to the Human Reference Genome (UCSC hg19, NCBI build 37) using the Burrows-Wheeler transformation algorithm, and duplicated reads were removed using Picard [9, 10]. FastQC was used to check the quality of sequence data [11]. Calling of SNPs and InDels was done using GATK Unified Genotyper, which uses a Bayesian genotype likelihood model to report alleles and Phred-scaled confidence values [12]. Variants (SNVs and indels) were called with SAMTools, with reference to public databases including dbSNP and 1000Genomes and gnomAD [13]. Analysis was performed with preference to variants located in genes implicated in atypical non-autoimmune forms of diabetes and early-onset obesity. The prioritized candidate gene list was obtained by reviewing publications in PubMed and OMIM. Analysis focused on non-synonymous coding variants, frameshift indels, and variants affecting splice sites, as these are most likely to be pathogenic. Non-exonic and synonymous variants were excluded from further analysis. Missense variants were evaluated for functional impact using a variety of in-silico prediction tools including SIFT [14], Polyphen2 [15], MelaLR [16], MetaSVN [16], fathmm-MKL [17], DANN [18], CADD [19], MutationTaster [20], Mutation Assesser [21] and LRT [22].

Sanger sequencing
Sanger sequencing using standard PCR amplification procedures was carried out to confirm the selected candidate variants of interest in the proband and in 300 unrelated controls of Maltese ethnicity. A 242 base pair region in exon 8 of HNF1β was amplified using the following forward primer (GGG CTC TGT ACC TGT GTC TT) and reverse primer (CCA TGG CCT TAT CAC ACC CT) with an annealing temperature of 54 degrees.

Case presentation
Clinical features
The proband is a 25 year old Caucasian female born from nonconsanguineous parents of Maltese ethnicity. She developed obesity in early childhood, with a body weight at the 97th centile at the age of 9 years. She was diagnosed with diabetes mellitus at age 11 following her presentation with osmotic symptoms of hyperglycaemia. No diabetic ketoacidosis at diagnosis was present, and both glutamic acid decarboxylase and islet cell antibodies were negative. She was initially treated by diet and lifestyle changes, and eventually started on metformin during childhood.

The proband became pregnant at age 21 years, and she delivered a healthy but macrosomic male infant by Caesarean section at 35 weeks of gestation weighing 5.18 kg. Her glycaemic control deteriorated significantly during pregnancy and was managed by combination treatment of isophane and soluble insulin. Significant weight gain also developed during pregnancy, with a BMI up to 37 kg/m². Pre-proliferative diabetic retinopathy was also present in the proband.

Since pregnancy the proband developed persistent and significant microalbuminuria (urine microalbumin > 400 mg/L), leading to macroalbuminuria (albumin-creatinine ratio > 3000 mg/g) and glomerular hyperfiltration (eGFR > 170mls/min/1.73m²) with normal creatinine levels. Urinalysis and urine microscopy showed no significant findings. Ultra-sonographic examination of the abdomen revealed normal size and echotexture in both kidneys, without any signs of obstructive uropathy, and normal cortical thickness and preservation of cortico-medullary differentiation. No evidence of autoimmune nephropathy or glomerulonephritis was present, with normal ANA, ANCA, C3, C4, rheumatoid factor IgM, uric acid, C-reactive protein and serum immunoglobulin levels. The proband also developed deranged liver function tests, with moderately elevated gamma glutamyl transferase and alanine transaminase levels. A viral hepatitis screen was negative, and hepatomegaly with no focal lesions and changes of a fatty liver were also evident on abdominal ultrasound.

As an adult, she is presently overweight (BMI 28 kg/m²) and glycaemic control is achieved by a combination of oral hypoglycaemic agents including metformin 1 g tds, gliclazide 80 mg tds and vildagliptin 50 mg daily. The proband however shows poor glycaemic control on combination oral treatment, with HbA1c values around 10%. Her fasting C-peptide concentration at the time of referral for genetic analysis was 1.4 ng/mL, indicating endogenous insulin production. Her HOMA-IR at the time was 2.8 (fasting insulin 5.7 mIU/L, fasting blood glucose 11.05 mmol/l). A repeat fasting C-peptide decreased to 1.1 ng/mL within 1 year. In addition, the proband was started on an angiotensin-converting enzyme inhibitor (perindopril, 8 mg/day) for reno-protection in view of the proteinuria and gradual increase in blood pressure that developed in the post pregnancy period. Her blood pressure control is generally well controlled on perindopril.

The proband's mother had developed diabetes at age 23, and was treated with oral hypoglycaemic agents and eventually insulin. The father developed type 2 diabetes aged 68 years, and the proband's brother developed diabetes aged 36 years. In addition, three maternal aunts also had a history of diabetes mellitus. An overview of the pedigree is shown in Fig. 1.

In view of the above clinical picture, an initial diagnosis of early-onset type 2 diabetes complicated by fatty liver and diabetic nephropathy was made. The case was subsequently revised when the proband was offered and consented to genetic analysis for monogenic diabetes. In keeping with the strong family history of early-onset diabetes and the absence of ketoacidosis, the monogenic diabetes probability calculator showed a high probability of MODY (> 75.5% positive predictive value) [8]. Whole exome sequencing was the analytical method of choice, given the possibility of a primary genetic defect underlying the associated obesity, which is an unusual feature of monogenic diabetes.

Mutation detection

A summary of the mapped sequencing data is shown in Table 1. WES yielded a total of 118,986 variants, of which 19,598 were classified as silent mutations, 16,869 as missense variants and 128 as nonsense mutations. Variants were filtered according to their frequency, location, functional consequences and clinical phenotype as outlined in the methods section.

No nonsense, frameshift, in-frame indels and variants affecting splicing sites were detected in the proband in any of the common MODY genes. A heterozygous missense mutation with predicted damaging effects in HNF1β was identified in the proband - chromosome 17, position 36,059,155, c.1580G > A, NM_000458.3, p. Arg527Gln, exon 8. In-silico analysis of pathogenicity using various bioinformatic approaches are shown in Table 2. Clearly, multiple lines of computational evidence provide support for a deleterious effect of this mutation. Evolutionary conservation analysis also shows that the p.Arg527Gln mutation occurs at a highly-conserved position within the protein sequence, and that this residue is highly conserved across multiple species. The mutation was confirmed by Sanger sequencing in the proband (Fig. 2). In addition, the mutation was not detected by Sanger sequencing in 300 DNA samples of Maltese ethnicity. In the Genome Aggregation database (gnomAD), which reports summary data from large-scale exome and genome sequencing projects, the HNF1β p.Arg527Gln mutation has a very low frequency (3/246266, frequency = 0.00001218). This mutation lies in the C-terminal transactivation domain of the protein, and is predicted to be likely pathogenic based on the above criteria.

In addition to mutations in known genes implicated in monogenic diabetes, we also screened sequence data for the presence of genomic variants that have been associated in the literature with other phenotypes present in the proband, primarily obesity and nephropathy. A summary of the relevant findings is shown in Table 3.

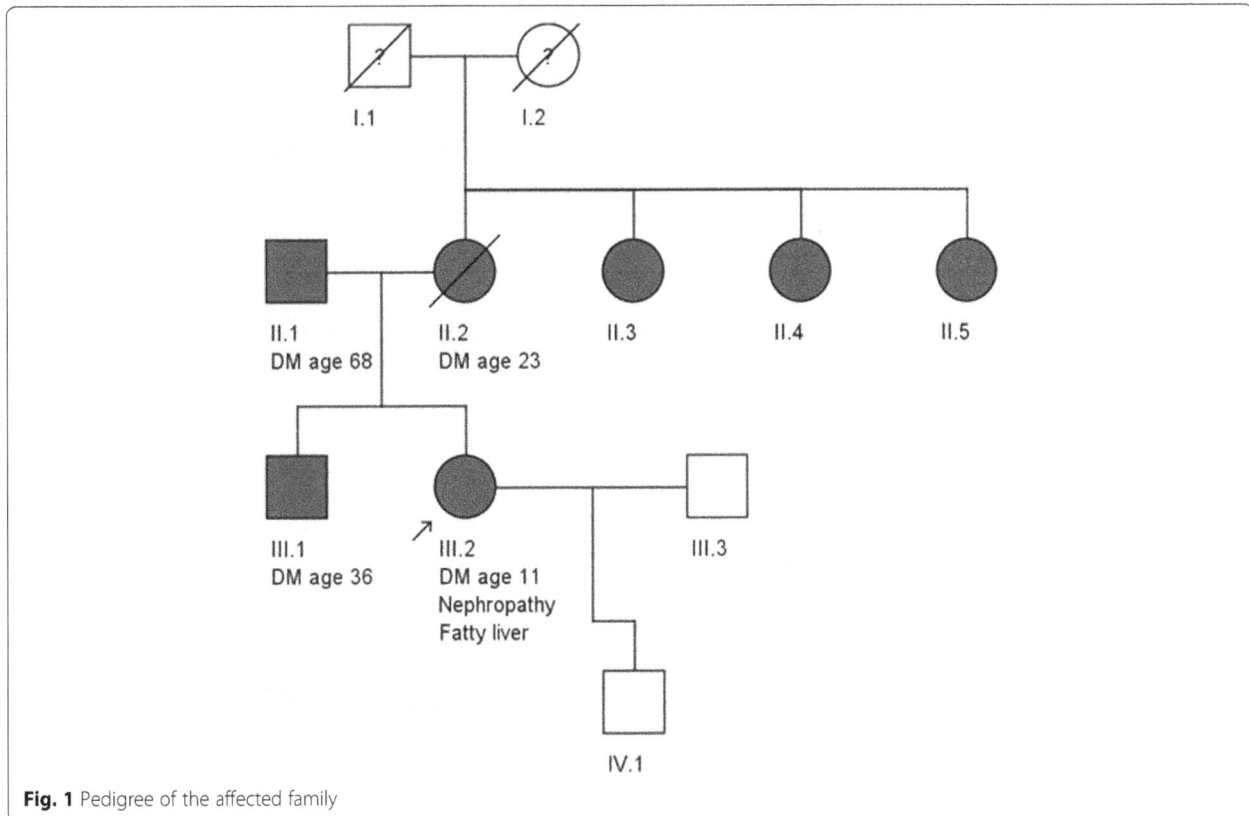

Fig. 1 Pedigree of the affected family

Discussion

In the present report, whole exome sequencing revealed a rare missense mutation in HNF1β that shows high conservation scores and has in silico predictions in favour of pathogenicity. This mutation is located in the C-terminal transactivation domain of HNF1β, is absent from controls and is present at an extremely low frequency in the Exome Aggregation Consortium dataset. Furthermore, the proband's uncharacteristic clinical phenotype and family history is suggestive of atypical or monogenic diabetes, although further evaluation of the mutation is required to provide a conclusive diagnosis of MODY5 in this case. Multiple prediction algorithms demonstrate a deleterious effect of this mutation on the

Table 1 Whole exome sequencing detail of coverage and number of read

Number of reads in raw sequence	55,723,934
Number of reads after de-duplication	96.63%
Number of mapped reads	99.53%
Number of mapped reads to targeted regions of the genome	79.11%
Average depth	66.72%
Coverage 10×	98.67%
Coverage 20×	93.93%
Coverage 50×	58.10%

gene. Missense mutations in HNF1β are commonly associated with both monogenic diabetes and kidney disease, and a number of in-vitro functional studies have demonstrated that missense mutations in HNF1β lead to impaired DNA-binding and reduced transactivation potential [23–25]. In view of these criteria, the mutation can be classified as likely pathogenic according to the established guidelines from the American College of Medical Genetics and Genomics and the Association for Molecular Pathology (ACMG/AMP) (criteria PP2, PP2, PP4, PM1, PM2) [26].

To date, around 230 mutations in HNF1β have been described [27]. This gene belongs to the homeodomain-containing family of transcription factors and is involved in the organogenesis of the kidneys, urinary tract, liver and pancreas. HNF1β functions as a homo- or hetero-dimer with a structurally related transcription factor HNF1α [28]. Mutations in HNF1α are responsible for the commonest type of monogenic diabetes (MODY3), characterised by progressive glucose intolerance due to an insulin secretory defect [7]. In contrast, mutations in HNF1β are associated with a wide array of clinical phenotypes that can include renal disease, and which are distinguished by the absence of clear genotype-phenotype associations. Primarily, heterozygous mutations in HNF1β cause a complex Renal cysts and Diabetes syndrome (RCAD) characterised by early onset diabetes (MODY5),

Table 2 In-silico predictors of pathogenicity and evolutionary conservation analysis for the HNF1βmutation described in the text

In-silico prediction of pathogenicity for HNF1β c.1580G > A (p.Arg527Gln)		
Tool	Prediction	Score
MutationTaster	Disease causing	
MutationAssessor	Medium	2.48
FATHMM-MKL	Damaging	0.9625
MetaSVM	Damaging	0.9934
MetaIR	Damaging	0.9388
LRT	Deleterious	0
PolyPhen-2 - HumVar	Probably damaging	0.998
SIFT	Damaging	0.038
DAMN score	0.9996	
CADD scaled score		35
Evolutionary conservation analysis for HNF1β c.1580G > A (p.Arg527Gln)		
Genomic Evolutionary Rate Profiling (GERP)		5.63
PhyloP20way - mammalian		0.935
SiPhy29way - mammalian		0.9297

liver dysfunction and pancreatic hypoplasia. The extent and severity of renal disease varies extensively in HNF1β mutations, ranging from congenital anomalies of the kidney and urinary tract (CAKUT), cystic kidneys to hyperuricaemia [29–31]. HNF1β mutations have been associated with isolated renal disease in the absence of diabetes and conversely, HNF1β deletions with young-onset diabetes but no kidney disease have also been described [32, 33]. Compared to other MODY genes, a high rate of de-novo mutations in HNF1β has been reported in the literature [29]. The variable expressivity of HNF1β mutations also extends to the type and age of onset of renal disease, which ranges from intrauterine life to middle age [34]. A recent multicentre retrospective co-hort study of patients with HNF1β mutations showed that stage 3–4 chronic kidney disease was present in 44% of cases, and end-stage renal disease in 21% of cases [35].

The diabetic phenotype associated with HNF1β mutations is also equally heterogenous, with severity of glycaemia ranging from impaired glucose tolerance to diabetes requiring insulin therapy. The mean age of diagnosis of diabetes is 26 years, with a range of 10–61 years [36]. HNF1β mutations

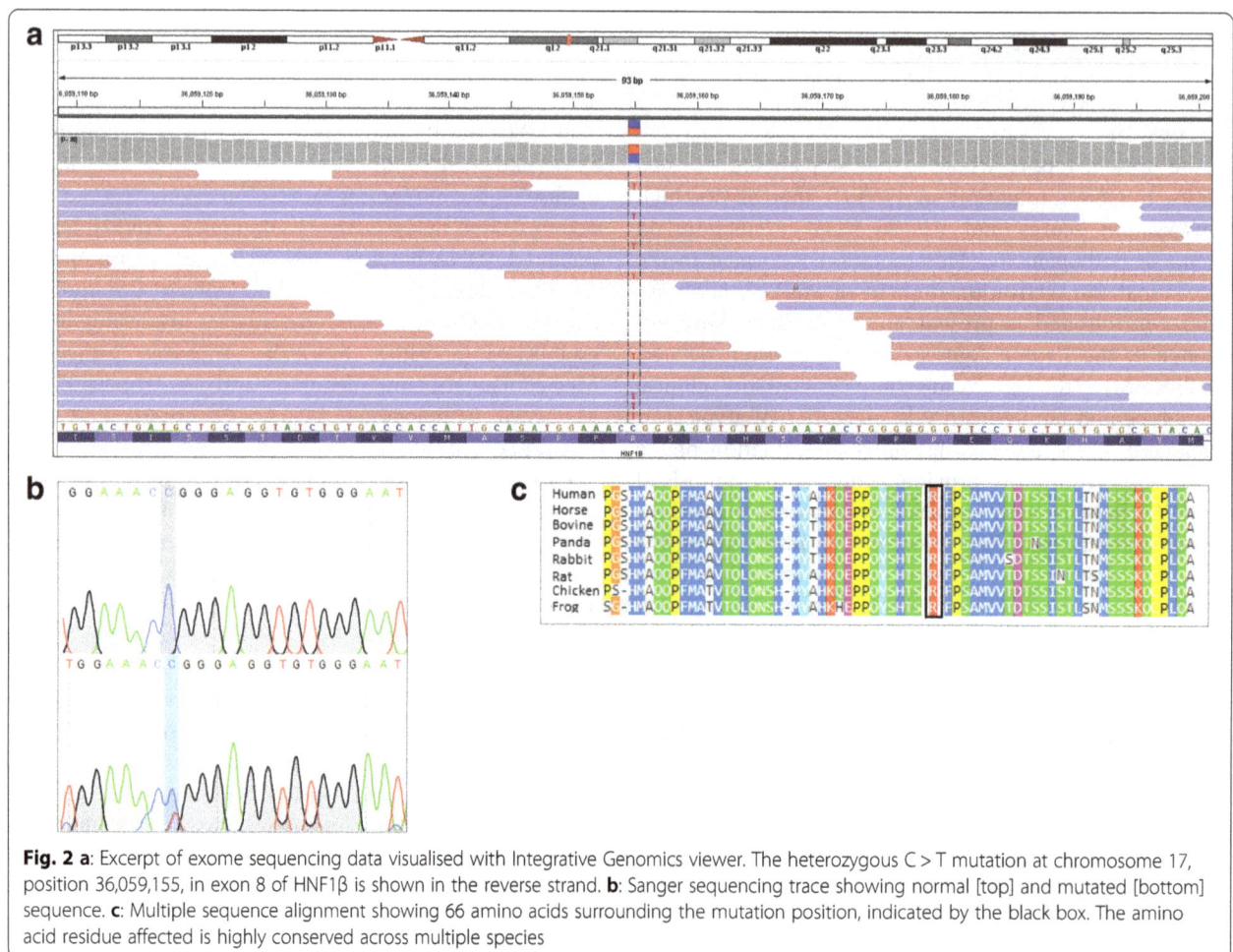

Fig. 2 a: Excerpt of exome sequencing data visualised with Integrative Genomics viewer. The heterozygous C > T mutation at chromosome 17, position 36,059,155, in exon 8 of HNF1β is shown in the reverse strand. **b**: Sanger sequencing trace showing normal [top] and mutated [bottom] sequence. **c**: Multiple sequence alignment showing 66 amino acids surrounding the mutation position, indicated by the black box. The amino acid residue affected is highly conserved across multiple species

Table 3 List of genomic variants and their respective minor allele frequency (1000 Genomes, TSI dataset) that have been identified in the proband

Chromosome	Position	dbSNP	Variant	Type	Gene	Effect	MAF	Clinical significance
chr3	10,331,457	rs696217	G/T	Missense	GHRL	p.Leu60Met	0.07	Risk factor for metabolic syndrome and childhood obesity
chr6	132,172,368	rs1044498	A/C	Missense	ENPP1	p.Lys173Gln	0.13	Susceptibility to Insulin resistance
chr4	6,292,915	rs10010131	A/G	Intronic	WFS1		0.36	Type 2 diabetes risk
chr6	149,721,690	rs237025	G/A	Missense	SUMO4	p.Val55Met	0.45	Type 2 diabetes risk, diabetic nephropathy
chr13	110,435,231	rs1805097	C/T	Missense	IRS2	p.Gly1057Asp	0.33	Type 2 diabetes risk
chr11	17,409,572	rs5219	T/C	Missense	KCNJ11	p.Lys23Glu	0.29	Type 2 diabetes risk
chr6	160,113,872	rs4880	A/G	Missense	SOD2	p.Val16Ala	0.47	Diabetic nephropathy
chr2	25,141,538	rs11676272	A/G	Missense	ADCY3	p.Ser107Pro	0.42	Childhood obesity

The variants in this table have been associated with obesity, type 2 diabetes and nephropathy in different studies

lead to beta cell dysfunction and reduced insulin secretion, which may be associated with pancreatic hypoplasia [37].

The exact cause of albuminuria and hyperfiltration in our proband is difficult to ascertain, as no evidence of renal cystic disease or of CAKUT was present on imaging. While renal cystic disease is a major manifestation of HNF1β mutations (65% of cases), considerable variation in renal phenotype exists. Similarly, studies have also shown that when renal biopsies are performed there is heterogeneity in the histological diagnosis [36]. Despite the presence of diabetes, the renal dysfunction found in carriers of HNF1β mutations is thought to be caused by renal development abnormalities rather than diabetic renal disease [38]. However, the proband also had microvascular complications of diabetes and poor glycaemic control, making associated diabetic nephropathy highly probable. A recent case report has described histologically-proven diabetic kidney disease (DKD) with glomerular sclerosis, severe diffuse mesangial cell proliferation, matrix expansion and arteriole hyalinosis in a 30 year old female with MODY 5 and macroalbuminuria caused by a missense mutation in exon 4 of HNF1β [39]. While glomerular hyperfiltration associated with early onset DM is a powerful risk factor for the development of progressive diabetic nephropathy, it is more likely attributed to glomerular DKD in our proband. Interestingly, another case report has described end-stage renal failure secondary to probable DKD in a patient with HNF1β mutation and RCAD syndrome [40].

We also examined exome data, focusing on susceptibility genes for early onset obesity, diabetic kidney disease and type 2 diabetes mellitus. Several common susceptibility variants were detected. Presumably, the additive effects of common risk variants contributes to the presentation, clinical course and progression of diabetes in the proband.

This report is significant for a number of reasons. Primarily, it expands on the mutational spectrum and wide array of clinical phenotypes associated with the HNF1β

gene. In the era of personalised medicine, it is increasingly important to place the clinical phenotype into a gene-specific context that would enable clinicians to determine both immediate and future clinical implications to both the patient and family members. Secondly, it adds to the few clinical reports that highlight the presence of early-stage diabetic nephropathy with hyperfiltration due to probable glomerular DKD in the absence of renal cysts or renal morphological abnormalities in MODY5. Furthermore, it is important to emphasise that clinicians should maintain a high index of suspicion for monogenic diabetes in young onset non-autoimmune disease, and should consider referral for HNF1β mutation analysis in the presence of renal cysts with or without diabetes. The presence of obesity from a young age in the proband is also significant, in view of the fact that the initial diagnosis was of early-onset type 2 diabetes rather than monogenic diabetes. The report also reinforces the need for increased research on the molecular epidemiology of monogenic diabetes in the Maltese islands. As yet, the prevalence of MODY in Malta is not determined. It is likely to show significant differences from studies carried out in northern European populations, in part due to strong founder effects that have been reported on the island [41]. Of note, the same missense mutation in HNF1β has also been detected in an unrelated Maltese female referred for monogenic diabetes screening. The second case involves a 30 year old female with diabetes since age 13, a family history of paternally-transmitted early-onset diabetes, a BMI of 26.32 kg/m^2, no history of diabetic ketoacidosis and treatment with long-acting insulin. Similarly, no renal cysts or structural renal tract anomalies were identified but investigation showed microalbuminuria from longstanding diabetes. The identification of the same missense mutation in two unrelated Maltese probands both with early-onset diabetes strongly suggests a possible genetic founder effect for this mutation. The authors are presently expanding genetic epidemiology studies to further investigate this.

Conclusion

In conclusion, this report has described a rare missense mutation in exon 8 of HNF1β with multiple in-silico predictions consistent with pathogenicity. The proband had childhood onset atypical diabetes complicated by obesity and early stage diabetic nephropathy in the absence of renal cysts. The broad phenotypic variability of both diabetic and renal disease probably accounts for underdiagnoses of HNF1β mutations in clinical practice. The authors also emphasise that clinicians should be vigilant for the possibility of monogenic diabetes even in obese patients with a strong family history and a high probability on MODY risk calculators. This is particularly relevant in specific populations such as in the Maltese islands, where the population carries high prevalence rates for both obesity and diabetes, and the genetic epidemiology of the disease is as yet uncharacterised.

Abbreviations
CAKUT: Congenital anomalies of the kidney and urinary tract; DKD: Diabetic kidney disease; HNF: Hepatocyte nuclear factor; MODY: Maturity onset diabetes of the young; RCAD: Renal cysts and diabetes; SNP: Single nucleotide polymorphism

Acknowledgements
We thank the proband for her collaboration in this study.

Funding
This work was supported by institutional funds of the University of Malta.

Authors' contributions
NPP and JC: Data acquisition, sequencing, analysis and clinical interpretation of data, drafting of the manuscript. JV and AF: study concept and design, analysis and interpretation of data, drafting and critical revision of the manuscript. All the authors read and approved the final manuscript.

Competing interests
The authors declare that they have no competing interests.

Author details
[1]Centre for Molecular Medicine and Biobanking, University of Malta, Msida, Malta. [2]Department of Obstetrics and Gynaecology, University of Malta, Msida, Malta. [3]Department of Medicine, University of Malta, Msida, Malta.

References

1. Fendler W, Borowiec M, Baranowska-Jazwiecka A, Szadkowska A, Skala-Zamorowska E, Deja G, et al. Prevalence of monogenic diabetes amongst polish children after a nationwide genetic screening campaign. Diabetologia. 2012;55:2631–5.
2. Pihoker C, Gilliam LK, Ellard S, Dabelea D, Davis C, Dolan LM, et al. Prevalence, characteristics and clinical diagnosis of maturity onset diabetes of the young due to mutations in HNF1A, HNF4A, and Glucokinase: results from the SEARCH for diabetes in youth. J Clin Endocrinol Metab. 2013;98:4055–62.
3. Shepherd M, Shields B, Hammersley S, Hudson M, McDonald TJ, Colclough K, et al. Systematic population screening, using biomarkers and genetic testing, identifies 2.5% of the UK pediatric diabetes population with monogenic diabetes. Diabetes Care. 2016;39:1879–88.
4. Misra S, Shields B, Colclough K, Johnston DG, Oliver NS, Ellard S, et al. South Asian individuals with diabetes who are referred for MODY testing in the UK have a lower mutation pick-up rate than white European people. Diabetologia. 2016;59:2262–5.
5. Kanthimathi S, Jahnavi S, Balamurugan K, Ranjani H, Sonya J, Goswami S, et al. Glucokinase gene mutations (MODY 2) in Asian Indians. Diabetes Technol Ther. 2014;16:180–5.
6. Rubio-Cabezas O, Hattersley AT, Njølstad PR, Mlynarski W, Ellard S, White N, et al. ISPAD clinical practice consensus guidelines 2014. The diagnosis and management of monogenic diabetes in children and adolescents. Pediatr Diabetes. 2014;15(Suppl 20):47–64.
7. Shields BM, Hicks S, Shepherd MH, Colclough K, Hattersley AT, Ellard S. Maturity-onset diabetes of the young (MODY): how many cases are we missing? Diabetologia. 2010;53:2504–8.
8. Shields BM, McDonald TJ, Ellard S, Campbell MJ, Hyde C, Hattersley AT. The development and validation of a clinical prediction model to determine the probability of MODY in patients with young-onset diabetes. Diabetologia. 2012;55:1265–72.
9. Li H, Durbin R. Fast and accurate short read alignment with burrows-wheeler transform. Bioinformatics. 2009;25:1754–60.
10. Picard. http://broadinstitute.github.io/picard. Accessed 7 May 2018.
11. Cock PJA, Fields CJ, Goto N, Heuer ML, Rice PM. The sanger FASTQ file format for sequences with quality scores, and the Solexa/Illumina FASTQ variants. Nucleic Acids Res. 2010;38:1767–71.
12. McKenna A, Hanna M, Banks E, Sivachenko A, Cibulskis K, Kernytsky A, et al. The genome analysis toolkit: a MapReduce framework for analyzing next-generation DNA sequencing data. Genome Res. 2010;20:1297–303.
13. Li H, Handsaker B, Wysoker A, Fennell T, Ruan J, Homer N, et al. The sequence alignment/map format and SAMtools. Bioinformatics. 2009;25:2078–9.
14. Kumar P, Henikoff S, Ng PC. Predicting the effects of coding non-synonymous variants on protein function using the SIFT algorithm. Nat Protoc. 2009;4:1073–81.
15. Adzhubei IA, Schmidt S, Peshkin L, Ramensky VE, Gerasimova A, Bork P, et al. A method and server for predicting damaging missense mutations. Nat Methods. 2010;7:248–9.
16. Dong C, Wei P, Jian X, Gibbs R, Boerwinkle E, Wang K, et al. Comparison and integration of deleteriousness prediction methods for nonsynonymous SNVs in whole exome sequencing studies. Hum Mol Genet. 2015;24:2125–37.
17. Shihab HA, Rogers MF, Gough J, Mort M, Cooper DN, Day INM, et al. An integrative approach to predicting the functional effects of non-coding and coding sequence variation. Bioinformatics. 2015;31:1536–43.
18. Quang D, Chen Y, Xie X. DANN: a deep learning approach for annotating the pathogenicity of genetic variants. Bioinformatics. 2015;31:761–3.
19. Kircher M, Witten DM, Jain P, O'Roak BJ, Cooper GM, Shendure J. A general framework for estimating the relative pathogenicity of human genetic variants. Nat Genet. 2014;46:310–5.
20. Schwarz JM, Cooper DN, Schuelke M, Seelow D. MutationTaster2: mutation prediction for the deep-sequencing age. Nat Methods. 2014;11:361–2.
21. Reva B, Antipin Y, Sander C. Determinants of protein function revealed by combinatorial entropy optimization. Genome Biol. 2007;8:R232.
22. Chun S, Fay JC. Identification of deleterious mutations within three human genomes. Genome Res. 2009;19:1553–61.
23. Kim EK, Lee JS, Cheong HI, Chung SS, Kwak SH, Park KS. Identification and functional characterization of P159L mutation in HNF1B in a family with maturity-onset diabetes of the young 5 (MODY5). Genomics Inform. 2014;12:240–6.

24. Barbacci E, Chalkiadaki A, Masdeu C, Haumaitre C, Lokmane L, Loirat C, et al. HNF1beta/TCF2 mutations impair transactivation potential through altered co-regulator recruitment. Hum Mol Genet. 2004;13:3139–49.

25. Raaijmakers A, Corveleyn A, Devriendt K, Tienoven V, Pieter T, Allegaert K, et al. Criteria for HNF1B analysis in patients with congenital abnormalities of kidney and urinary tract. Nephrol Dial Transplant. 2015;30:835–42.

26. Richards S, Aziz N, Bale S, Bick D, Das S, Gastier-Foster J, et al. Standards and guidelines for the interpretation of sequence variants: a joint consensus recommendation of the American College of Medical Genetics and Genomics and the Association for Molecular Pathology. Genet med off J am Coll. Med Genet. 2015;17:405–24.

27. Stenson PD, Mort M, Ball EV, Evans K, Hayden M, Heywood S, et al. The human gene mutation database: towards a comprehensive repository of inherited mutation data for medical research, genetic diagnosis and next-generation sequencing studies. Hum Genet. 2017;136:665–77.

28. Mendel DB, Hansen LP, Graves MK, Conley PB, Crabtree GR. HNF-1 alpha and HNF-1 beta (vHNF-1) share dimerization and homeo domains, but not activation domains, and form heterodimers in vitro. Genes Dev. 1991;5:1042–56.

29. Bellanné-Chantelot C, Chauveau D, Gautier J-F, Dubois-Laforgue D, Clauin S, Beaufils S, et al. Clinical spectrum associated with hepatocyte nuclear factor-1beta mutations. Ann Intern Med. 2004;140:510–7.

30. Raile K, Klopocki E, Holder M, Wessel T, Galler A, Deiss D, et al. Expanded clinical spectrum in hepatocyte nuclear factor 1b-maturity-onset diabetes of the young. J Clin Endocrinol Metab. 2009;94:2658–64.

31. Bockenhauer D, Jaureguiberry G. HNF1B-associated clinical phenotypes: the kidney and beyond. Pediatr Nephrol. 2016;31:707–14.

32. Weber S, Moriniere V, Knüppel T, Charbit M, Dusek J, Ghiggeri GM, et al. Prevalence of mutations in renal developmental genes in children with renal hypodysplasia: results of the ESCAPE study. J Am Soc Nephrol. 2006;17:2864–70.

33. Edghill EL, Stals K, Oram RA, Shepherd MH, Hattersley AT, Ellard S. HNF1B deletions in patients with young-onset diabetes but no known renal disease. Diabet Med J Br Diabet Assoc. 2013;30:114–7.

34. Heidet L, Decramer S, Pawtowski A, Morinière V, Bandin F, Knebelmann B, et al. Spectrum of HNF1B mutations in a large cohort of patients who harbor renal diseases. Clin J Am Soc Nephrol. 2010;5:1079–90.

35. Dubois-Laforgue D, Cornu E, Saint-Martin C, Coste J, Bellanné-Chantelot C, Timsit J, et al. Diabetes, associated clinical Spectrum, long-term prognosis and genotype/phenotype correlations in 201 adult patients with hepatocyte nuclear factor 1 B (HNF1B) molecular defects. Diabetes Care. 2017;40:1436–43

36. Bingham C, Hattersley AT. Renal cysts and diabetes syndrome resulting from mutations in hepatocyte nuclear factor-1β. Nephrol Dial Transplant. 2004;19:2703–8.

37. Gautier J, Bellanne-chantelot C, Dubois-laforgue D, Wilhelm J, Boitard C, Clauin S, et al. Multi-organ damage in Mody5 related to mutations of the hepatocyte nuclear factor-1βgene. Diabetes. 2002;51 https://insights.ovid.com/diabetes/diab/2002/06/002/multi-organ-damage-mody5-related-mutations/1049/00003439. Accessed 9 May 2018.

38. Magee GM, Bilous RW, Cardwell CR, Hunter SJ, Kee F, Fogarty DG. Is hyperfiltration associated with the future risk of developing diabetic nephropathy? A meta-analysis. Diabetologia. 2009;52:691–7.

39. Wang Y, Zhao Y, Zhang J, Yang Y, Liu F. A case of a novel mutation in HNF1β-related maturity-onset diabetes of the young type 5 with diabetic kidney disease complication in a Chinese family. J Diabetes Complicat. 2017;31:1243–6.

40. Hegde P, Meldon A, Lamen L, Sharma D, Kalathil D. An interesting unfolding of the diagnosis of hepatocyte nuclear factor-1 beta (HNF1β) monogenic diabetes. Pract Diabetes. 2017;34:320–322a.

41. Farrugia R, Scerri CA, Montalto SA, Parascandolo R, Neville BGR, Felice AE. Molecular genetics of tetrahydrobiopterin (BH4) deficiency in the Maltese population. Mol Genet Metab. 2007;90:277–83.

18

Predictors of vascular complications among type 2 diabetes mellitus patients at University of Gondar Referral Hospital: a retrospective follow-up study

Haileab Fekadu Wolde[1*], Asrat Atsedeweyen[1], Addisu Jember[1], Tadesse Awoke[1], Malede Mequanent[1], Adino Tesfahun Tsegaye[1] and Shitaye Alemu[2]

Abstract

Background: Type 2 Diabetes Mellitus is a serious metabolic disease that is often associated with vascular complications. There are 1.9 million people living with Diabetes in Ethiopia; diabetes mellitus is found to be the ninth leading cause of death related to its complications. Although the rate of vascular complications continues to rise, there is limited information about the problem. This study aimed to estimate the incidence and predictors of vascular complications among type 2 diabetes mellitus patients at University of Gondar Referral Hospital.

Methods: Institution based retrospective follow-up study was conducted at University of Gondar Referral Hospital with 341 newly diagnosed type 2 DM patients from September 2005 to March 2017 and the data were collected by reviewing their records. Schoenfeld residuals test and interaction of each covariate with time were used to check proportional hazard assumption. The best model was selected by using Akaike Information Criteria (AIC). Hazards ratio (HR) with its respective 95% confidence interval were reported to show strength of association.

Result: The selected patients were followed retrospectively for a median follow up time of 81.50 months (Inter quartile range (IQR) = 67.2–103.3). The mean age (± Standard deviation (SD)) of patients at baseline was 51.7(SD: ±11.5 years) and 57.48% were females. The incidence rate of vascular complications was 40.6 cases/ 1000 person years of observation. The significant predictors for vascular complications where found to be male sex (Adjusted hazard ratio (AHR) = 0.50, 95% CI: 0.27, 0.94), having hypertension at baseline(AHR = 3.99, 95% CI: 1.87, 8.56), positive protein urea at base line (AHR = 1.69, 95% CI: 1.03, 2.78), high density lipoprotein cholesterol(HDL-C) level ≥ 40 mg per deciliter (mg/dl) (AHR = 0.43, 95% CI: 0.24, 0.77), low density lipoprotein cholesterol(LDL-C) level > 100 mg/dl (AHR = 3.05, 95% CI: 1.47, 6.35) and triglyceride > 150 mg/dl (AHR = 2.74, 95% CI: 1.28, 5.84).

Conclusion: The incidence of vascular complications among type 2 diabetes patients remains a significant public health problem. Hypertension at baseline, LDL-C > 100 mg/dl, triglyceride > 150 mg/dl, HDL-C ≥ 40 mg/dl and male sex were significant predictors of vascular complication. In the light of these findings targeted interventions should be given to diabetes patients with hypertension comorbidity and dyslipidemia at follow up clinics.

Keywords: Incidence, Predictor, Type 2 diabetes

* Correspondence: haileabfekadu@gmail.com
[1]Department of Epidemiology and Biostatistics, Institute of Public Health, College of Medicine and Health Sciences, University of Gondar, Gondar, Ethiopia
Full list of author information is available at the end of the article

Background

Diabetes mellitus(DM) is a chronic metabolic disorder characterized by chronic hyperglycemia [1]. Globally, the prevalence of DM is 8.5% and it is estimated that one in 10 adults will have DM in the world by 2035 [2]. Sub Saharan African countries are expected to experience the fastest increase in the number of people living with type 2 DM in the next two decades worldwide [3]. Ethiopia is the third most populous country in the African continent with 1.9 million people living with DM [4].

The seriousness of DM is largely a result of its associated vascular complications, which can be disabling and even fatal. Vascular complications caused by type 2 DM include neuropathy, nephropathy, retinopathy, coronary heart diseases(CHD), peripheral arterial diseases (PAD) and stroke [5].

In Africa, the age standardized mortality rate due to DM and its complications is estimated to be 111.3 per 100,000 population [2]. The estimated prevalence of diabetic nephropathy is 6–16% in Sub Saharan Africa [6] and 6.1% in Ethiopia [7].In addition,the prevalence of retinopathy ranges from 31.4–41.1% in Ethiopia [8]. Type 2 DM is rapidly increasing non-communicable disease and is a major public health challenge in developing countries like Ethiopia [9] with consequences of chronicity and pre-mature death due to its vascular complications [10, 11]. In Ethiopia there were 44,655 deaths between 2012 and 2013 among people aged 20–79 years due to DM and its associated vascular complications. It was the ninth leading cause of death in Ethiopia with 22 per 1000 deaths [3, 4, 12].

There are factors which can affect the rate of vascular complications among type 2 DM patients. Among socio demographic variables females experienced higher rates of vascular complication when compared to males as the studies done in Ethiopia and India [13, 14] but not in other studies [15, 16]. Individuals who were hypertensive at the start of treatment have a positive association with the risk of vascular complications [15–19]. Patients with higher level of LDL-C and lower levels of HDL-C were at increased risk of developing vascular complications [20–22]. Higher levels of cholesterol and triglyceride were also positively associated with the risk of vascular complications [15].

Ethiopia is facing a double burden problem because type 2 DM is currently increasing due to different factors such as aging, urbanization, and an increasing prevalence of obesity. Even though the rate type 2 DM and its associated vascular complications are rising, current updated information about the problem is limited. The available literatures indicated that there were discrepancies in findings for some variables, like sex. Therefore, it is imperative to conduct a study which assesses the association between incidence of vascular complications against socio-demographic, clinical and physiologic factors using a parametric survival model.

Identifying factors which influence the rate of vascular complications would provide information for health professionals, policy makers and other governmental and non-governmental organizations to maximize efforts on prevention and risk minimization of vascular complications and deaths due to the complications in the country as well as in the study area. Thus this study aimed to determine the incidence and predictors of vascular complications among type 2 DM patients in University of Gondar Referral Hospital, Ethiopia.

Methods

Study design and period

Institution based retrospective follow up study was conducted among type 2 DM patients at University of Gondar Referral Hospital. Newly diagnosed type 2 DM patients who were enrolled between September 2005 and August 2012 were followed up to March 2017.

Study area and population

University of Gondar Referral Hospital is located in the North Gondar administrative zone, Amhara National Regional State, which is about 750 k meters (KM).

Northwest of Addis Ababa. The University of Gondar Referral Hospital is a teaching hospital which serves more than five million people in the North Gondar zone and its neighboring zones. Around 24,552 patients have chronic disease follow-up per year and among these 8880 are DM patients..Among all type 2 DM patients who are newly diagnosed between September 2005 and August 2012, newly diagnosed patients (364) who were free from any of the vascular complications at the start of treatment were selected randomly and included to the study. Patients with missing key predictor variables at baseline such as: HDL-C, LDL-C, triglyceride and hypertension status were excluded from the study.

Data collection procedures and data quality control

The study used secondary data; a data extraction check list was prepared to collect the data. Type 2 DM patients who were newly diagnosed between September 2005 and August 2012 were included. However patients who had any vascular complications mentioned at the start of the study and patients who were missing the key variables were excluded from the study. The reviewed records were identified by their medical registration or card number. The primary outcome was having any of the vascular complications such as: retinopathy, nephropathy, neuropathy, stroke, peripheral arterial dieses and coronary heart disease. These complications were determined based on the clinical decision of the physician. Diabetic retinopathy was defined by both direct and indirect ophthalmoscopy assessments done by retinal specialists confirmed by fundus photography. Neuropathy was defined by history of numbness, paraesthesia, tingling sensation confirmed by touch sensation by 10 g monofilament, vibration sense by biothesiometer and ankle reflex. Nephropathy was defined as worsening of blood pressure control, swelling of feet ankle, hands or eyes, increased need to urinate, protein in the urine with a confirmation by tests like blood test, urine test, renal function test and imaging test. Stroke is defined as patients with sudden difficulty in speech and comprehension, sudden paralysis or numbness of the face, arm or leg, sudden trouble with walking and confirmation imaging with computerized tomography (CT) scan or magnetic resonance imaging (MRI). PAD was defined by history of intermittent claudication, coldness in the lower extremities (especially when compared with the other side), weak or absent peripheral pulses in the lower extremities and confirmation via Doppler ultrasound. CHD was diagnosed by symptoms of angina, shortness of breath, a crushing sensation in the chest, pain in the shoulder or arm and sweating. Additionally CHD was confirmed by electrocardiogram (ECG) or echocardiogram [23, 24]. The patients who were included in the study were assessed for all of these vascular complications in every follow up they had in the hospital. All baseline characteristics at the start of treatment were assessed from the patient's registration document. The first characteristic assessed was the socio demographic component; this included age, sex and residence. The second characteristic assessed was the clinical component; this included hypertension comorbidity which was defined as a history of antihypertensive drug use or SBP ≥ 140 mmHg or DBP ≥ 90 mmHg [25], type of treatment, family history of DM, and body mass index (BMI). The third characteristic assessed was the physiologic component; this included HDL-C, LDL-C, triglyceride and total cholesterol which were categorized as high and low based on guidelines from the National Cholesterol Education Program (NCEP-III) and World Health Organization (WHO) [26, 27]. This also included creatinine, fasting blood sugar, systolic blood pressure(SBP), diastolic blood pressure(DBP) and protein urea which was defined as positive if the urine albumin concentration is between 30 mg(mg)/24 h and 300 mg/ 24 h and negative if it is < 30 mg/24 h. All of these characteristics of the patients were collected from their registration document. The data was collected by two health officers who had experience working in DM follow-up clinics. To control the data quality, training was given to the data collectors and their supervisor. The data extraction checklist was pre-tested for consistency of understanding the review tools and completeness of data items. The necessary adjustments were made on the final data extraction format and the filled formats were checked daily by the supervisor.

Data management and analysis strategy

The data was entered in to EPI info version 7.0 and transferred to STATA version 14.1 for analysis. Descriptive statistics were used to describe the percentage and frequency of the patients in reference to all covariates. Person-time at risk was measured starting from the time of initiation of treatment until each patient ended the follow-up. The survival experience of the patients was assessed using Kaplan-Meier survivor function. The log rank test was used to compare the survival experiences among the different groups of subjects. Schoenfeld residuals test (both global and scaled), interaction of each covariate with time and graphical methods were used to check the Cox Proportional Hazard (PH) assumption. Cox PH and three parametric models (Exponential, Weibull and Gompertz) models were fitted to identify the risk factors. The best model was selected by using Akaike information criteria (AIC), Bayesian information criteria (BIC) and log likelihood criteria. Goodness of fit of the model was assessed by using cox-snell residual technique. Variables having p - value less than 0.05 in the multivariable model were considered significantly associated with the dependent variable. Hazard ratio (HR) with its 95% confidence interval were computed to show the strength of association.

Result

Baseline characteristics of study participants

Out of the total of 341 newly diagnosed type 2 DM patients, 196 (57.48%) were females. The mean (SD) age for patients at the start of treatment was 51.7 (SD ± 11.5) years. The majority of the patients 273(80.06%) were urban dwellers. About 228(66.86%) of the patients had family history of DM and more than half of the patients 183(53.67%) had hypertension at the start of type 2 DM treatment. Almost half of the study participants 169(49.56%) had normal weight whereas 45(13.2%) were obese. About 230(67.45%) were on oral hypoglycemic agents. The majority of the patients 271(79.47%) had positive protein urea at base line. About 234(68.62%) of the patients had HDL-C level above 40 mg/dl and more than half of the patients 186(54.55%) had LDL-C level less than 100 mg/dl. More than half of type 2 DM patients included in the study 178(52.2%) had triglyceride level ≤ 150 mg/dl. The median value for creatinine and FBS was found to be 0.78 mg/dl (IQR = 0.65–0.88) and 77 mg/dl (IQR = 121–178) respectively. The mean (±SD) for SBP and DBP of the patients was 126.9(±15.8) and 78.9 (±10.1) respectively (Table 1).

Vascular complications from type 2 DM

Study subjects were followed for a median (IQR) follow up period of 81.5 months (IQR = 67.2–103.3) after initiation of treatment for a total of 2391.067 person years.

Table 1 Socio-demographic, clinical and physiologic characteristics of type 2 DM patients on anti diabetic treatment at university of Gondar referral hospital, September, 2005 – March 2017

Variable	No Vascular complication ($n = 244$)	Any one of vascular complications ($n = 97$)	Total ($n = 341$)
Sex			
Female n(%)	128(52.5)	68(70.1)	196(57.5)
Male n(%)	116(47.5)	29(29.9)	145(42.5)
Residence			
Rural n(%)	54(22.1)	14(14.4)	68(19.9)
Urban n(%)	190(77.9)	83(85.6)	273(80.1)
Occupation			
Unemployed n(%)	92(37.7)	57(58.8)	149(43.7)
Government n(%)	71(29.1)	17(17.5)	88(25.8)
NGO n(%)	16(6.6)	4(4.1)	20(5.9)
Private n(%)	65(26.6)	19(19.6)	84(24.6)
Age(year)[a]	50.1 ± 11.7	55.9 ± 9.9	51.7 ± 11.5
Family history			
Yes n(%)	178(73.0)	50(51.5)	228(66.9)
No n(%)	66(27.0)	47(48.5)	113(33.1)
Hypertension			
No n(%)	148(60.7)	10(10.3)	158(46.3)
Yes n(%)	96(39.3)	87(89.7)	183(53.7)
BMI (kg/m^2)			
< 18.5 n(%)	24(9.8)	5(5.2)	29(8.5)
18.5–24.99 n(%)	137(56.2)	32(33.0)	169(49.6)
25–29.99 n(%)	62(25.4)	36(37.1)	98(28.7)
≥ 30 n(%)	21(8.6)	24(24.7)	45(13.2)
Treatment			
OHA n(%)	163(66.8)	67(69.1)	230(67.4)
Insulin n(%)	48(19.7)	16(16.5)	64(18.8)
OHA + Insulin n(%)	33(13.5)	14(14.4)	47(13.8)
Protein urea			
Negative n(%)	217(89.0)	54(55.7)	271(79.5)
Positive n(%)	27(11)	43(44.3)	70(20.5)
HDL-C(mg/dl)			
< 40 n(%)	36(14.8)	71(73.2)	107(31.4)
≥ 40 n(%)	208(85.2)	26(26.8)	234(68.6)
LDL-C(mg/dl)			
≤ 100 n(%)	174(71.3)	12(12.4)	186(54.5)
> 100 n(%)	70(28.7)	85(87.6)	155(45.5)
Triglyceride(mg/dl)			
≤ 150 n(%)	165(67.6)	13(13.4)	178(52.2)
> 150 n(%)	79(32.4)	84(86.6)	163(47.8)
Cholesterol(mg/dl)			
≤ 200 n(%)	184(75.4)	27(27.8)	211(61.9)
> 200 n(%)	60(24.6)	70(72.2)	130(38.1)
FBS (mg/dl)[b]	136(117.5–165.5)	200(152–249)	146(121–198)

Table 1 Socio-demographic, clinical and physiologic characteristics of type 2 DM patients on anti diabetic treatment at university of Gondar referral hospital, September, 2005 – March 2017 *(Continued)*

Variable	No Vascular complication ($n = 244$)	Any one of vascular complications ($n = 97$)	Total ($n = 341$)
Creatinine(mg/dl)[b]	0.76(0.63–0.84)	0.83(0.68–1.13)	0.78(0.65–0.88)
SBP(mm Hg)[a]	122.9 ± 14.0	137.0 ± 15.8	126.9 ± 15.8
DBP(mm Hg)[a]	76.7 ± 9.3	84.5 ± 10.0	78.9 ± 10.1

[a]Expressed as mean ± SD and [b]median inter quartile range. *BMI* body mass index, *DBP* diastolic blood pressure, *FBS* fasting blood sugar, *HDL-C* high density lipoprotein cholesterol, *LDL-C* low density lipoprotein cholesterol, *SBP* systolic blood pressure

During this time period the incidence of vascular complications was found to be 40.6 cases (95% CI: 33.2, 49.5) per 1000 person year observation. From this the incidence of retinopathy was 18.4 (95% CI: 8.8, 38.6), nephropathy was 14.4(95% CI: 9.8, 21.4), neuropathy was 18.9(95%CI: 13.7, 25.9), stroke was 17.0(95%CI: 8.5, 33.9), CHD was 16.7(95%CI: 8.7, 32.1) and PAD was 15.1(95%CI: 7.9, 29.0) cases per 100 person year of observation.

The cumulative probability of developing vascular complications among type 2 DM patients who were free from any of the complications at the start of treatment was 0.0423 at month 40, 0.1653 at month 70, 0.3726 at month 100, 0.5587 at month 120 and 0.8617 at month 140 during the follow up period (Fig. 1).

Predictors of vascular complication among type 2 DM patients

After multivariable analysis using the Gompertz Cox-Regression: covariates like sex, hypertension status at baseline, protein urea at baseline, HDL-C level, LDL-C, triglyceride level were found to be independent predictors for vascular complications among type 2 DM patients (Table 2). The risk of developing vascular complications is

decreased by 50% among male type 2 DM patients than female patients. Positive protein urea at the start of treatment increased the risk of vascular complications by 69% as compared to negative protein urea. The risk of vascular complications for patients who have hypertension at baseline was 3.99 times higher than that of patients who have no hypertension. HDL-C level ≥ 40 mg/dl at the start of anti-diabetic treatment decreased the risk of developing vascular complications by 57% as compared to HDL-C < 40 mg/dl. The risk of vascular complications was 3.05 times higher among patients with baseline LDL-C > 100 mg/dl as compared to LDL-C ≤ 100 mg/dl. Triglyceride level > 150 mg/dl at the start of anti-diabetic treatment increased the risk of vascular complications by 2.74 times as compared to LDL-C ≤ 150 mg/dl.

Discussion

This study mainly investigated the incidence and predictors of vascular complications among type 2 DM patients at University of Gondar Referral Hospital, Ethiopia. This study assessed socio-demographic, clinical and physiologic characteristics of the patients based on the records taken from their medical follow up chart. As a result, factors such as male sex, history of hypertension at baseline, positive protein urea, HDL-C level ≥ 40 mg/dl, LDL-C level > 100 mg/dl and triglyceride > 150 mg/dl were found to be significantly associated with vascular complications.

The cumulative incidence of vascular complications during the study period after a median follow up time of 6.8 years were 28%. This result was slightly less than the study done in Taiwan [28] which showed the incidence to be 30.7% after a median follow up time of 5 years. In our study the incidence rate of vascular complications was 40.6 cases per 1000 person year observation. From this the incidence of coronary heart disease (CHD) and stroke was found to be 16.7 and 17.0 cases per 100 person year observation, respectively. This is lower than a study done in India [29] which showed the incidence rates to be 216 and 115 cases per 1000 person year observation, respectively. In our study the incidence rate of retinopathy was 18.4 cases per 100 person year observation, which is lower than another study done in Kenya [30] which showed the incidence to be 224.7 cases per

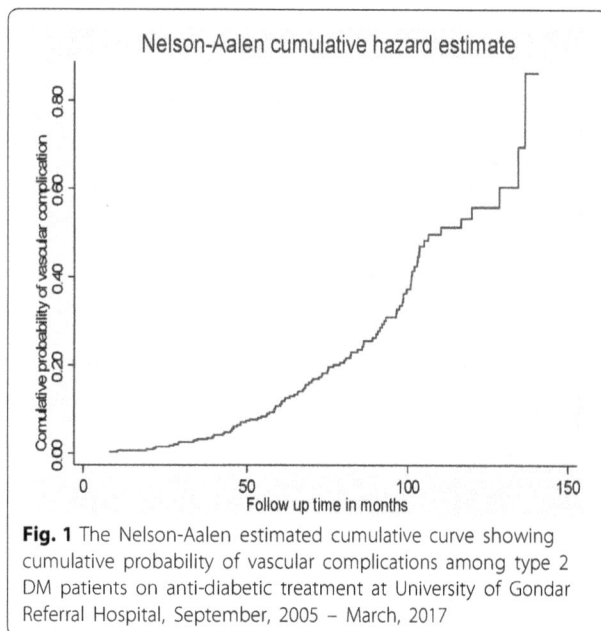

Fig. 1 The Nelson-Aalen estimated cumulative curve showing cumulative probability of vascular complications among type 2 DM patients on anti-diabetic treatment at University of Gondar Referral Hospital, September, 2005 – March, 2017

Table 2 Multivariable analysis using the Gompertz Cox-Regression model for predictor's vascular complication among type 2 DM patients in university of Gondar referral hospital September, 2005 – March 2017

Variable	Crud HR (95% CI)	Adjusted HR (95% CI)
Age(year)	1.04(1.03, 1.06)	1.02 (0.99, 1.04)
Sex		
Female	1	1
Male	0.47(0.31, 0.73)	0.50(0.27, 0.94)*
Residence		
Rural	1	1
Urban	1.47(0.84, 2.60)	0.51(0.25, 1.02)
Occupation		
Unemployed	1	1
Government	0.80(0.41,1.57)	0.796(0.41, 1.56)
NGO	0.38(0.14,1.05)	0.85 (0.27, 2.70)
Private	0.52(0.31,0.88)	0.83 (0.39, 1.74)
Family history		
Yes	1	1
NO	2.17(1.45, 3.23)	1.25 (0.78, 2.01)
Treatment Type		
OHA	1	1
Insulin	0.79(0.45, 1.36)	0.50(0.28, 1.01)
Insulin + OHA	0.87(0.46, 1.67)	0.91(0.48, 1.72)
BMI kg/m^2		
18.5–24.99	1	1
< 18.5	0.82(0.32, 2.10)	1.07(0.34, 3.27)
25–29.9	2.04(1.27, 3.29)	0.66(0.37, 1.16)
≥ 30	4.22(2.47, 7.21)	0.84(0.44, 1.61)
Hypertension		
No	1	1
Yes	10.57(5.48, 20.38)	3.99(1.87, 8.56)***
SBP(mm Hg)	1.03(1.0, 1.04)	0.995(0.97, 1.01)
DBP(mm Hg)	1.07(1.05, 1.09)	1.02(0.99, 1.05)
HDL-C(mg/dl)		
< 40	1	1
≥ 40	0.12(0.07, 0.18)	0.43(0.24, 0.77)**
LDL-C(mg/dl)		
≤ 100	1	1
> 100	13.12(7.14,24.10)	3.05(1.47, 6.35)**
Cholesterol (mg/dl)		
≤ 200	1	1
> 200	4.67(2.99, 7.28)	0.76(0.43, 1.36)
Triglyceride(mg/dl)		
≤ 150	1	1
> 150	8.08(4.50, 14.49)	2.74(1.28, 5.84)**
FBS(mg/dl)	1.008(1.006,1.010)	1.00(0.999,1.005)

Table 2 Multivariable analysis using the Gompertz Cox-Regression model for predictor's vascular complication among type 2 DM patients in university of Gondar referral hospital September, 2005 – March 2017 *(Continued)*

Variable	Crud HR (95% CI)	Adjusted HR (95% CI)
Creatinine(mg/dl)	1.003(0.995,1.010)	100(0.995, 1.009)
Protein urea		
Negative	1	1
Positive	4.14(2.77, 6.19)	1.69(1.03, 2.78)*

*** expressed as p-value< 0.001, **p-value< 0.01, *p-value< 0.05. *BMI* body mass index, *DBP* diastolic blood pressure, *FBS* fasting blood sugar, *HDL-C* high density lipoprotein cholesterol, *LDL-C* low density lipoprotein cholesterol, *SBP* systolic blood pressure

1000 person year observation. This could be due to the difference in median follow-up time used by the studies. Because the study in India used longer duration of follow-up (13 years). In addition, it could be due to the age difference of the study participants in which the study in Kenya mainly used patients who were above the age of 50 years. Moreover, the difference could be due to the difference in diagnostic methods used by the studies. In contrast to this, the incidence of retinopathy (18.4), nephropathy(14.4), neuropathy(18.9) and PAD(15.1) cases per 100 person year observation were found to be higher than incidence of retinopathy, nephropathy, neuropathy and PAD to be 78, 58, 13.9, 2, cases per 1000 person year observation in India [31]. This could be due to having a short follow up time (5.7 years) used in the India study.

In this study male type 2 DM patients accounted only 29.9% of the events and were found to have lower risk of developing vascular complications than female patients. This is in line with studies done in Ethiopia [14], India [13] and a met analysis [32] which showed female patients to have higher risk to develop vascular complications. This could be due to the hormonal differences. Because female patients encounter hormonal imbalances and decreased estrogen levels at menopause and at the same time, they lose the vasodilatory and anti-inflammatory activity of estrogen which would lead to endothelial dysfunction [33]. Another reason could be due to sex specific factors like polycystic ovarian syndrome, preeclampsia and gestational DM [34]. Another possible reason may be that women do not engage in as much physical activities as men do; physical activity contributes to improved insulin sensitivity as well as to decreased blood glucose levels and body weight [35]. In contrast to our results other retrospective follow up studies done in Iran [15] and Japan [16] showed males to be at a higher risk of developing vascular complications. Therefore, further research is needed to determine if this sex difference contributes to better outcomes in men with diabetes.

This study's findings indicated that type 2 DM patients who have history of hypertension at base line had an increased risk of developing vascular complications. This result is consistent with other studies done in Iran [15], Japan [16], India [17], and Ireland [36] which showed that a history of hypertension puts the patients at a higher risk for macro and micro vascular complications. Other studies in Cameroon and Morocco investigated the association between hypertension and specific complications; in this regard type 2 DM patients with hypertension were at increased risk of nephropathy and cardio vascular events [18, 19]. The possible reason could be the effect of hypertension on endothelial cell structure and function that leads to enhanced growth and vasoconstriction; these changes to the endothelium have a key role in the development of arthrosclerosis and glomerulosclerosis which ultimately predisposes patients to vascular complications [37].

In this study, elevated triglyceride level > 150 mg/dl and LDL-C level > 100 mg/dl were found to increase the risk of vascular complications; however an HDL-C level ≥ 40 mg/dl was associated with a decreased risk of vascular complications. This result was in accordance with other studies done in India [20], Singapore [22], Zimbabwe [38] and multi-centered study involving 28 countries from Asia, Africa, Europe and South America [21]. These four studies showed that patients with higher levels of LDL- C to have higher risk to develop vascular complications but patients with the higher levels of HDL-C have a decreased risk. Our result are also consistent with another study in India which showed increased levels of triglycerides to increase the risk of developing vascular complications like stroke and CHD [29]. This could be due to their function since the function of HDL-C is to transport fats (lipids) away from the arterial wall and in to the liver. This eventually reduces risk of accumulation fats and arthroscleroses within the arterial wall and it protects the inner wall of the arteries from damage thereby reducing the risk of CHD, stroke and other vascular diseases [39]. The reverse is true for LDL-C because it transports fates (lipids) to the arteries which in turn produce arthrosclerosis in the arteries of which increases the risk of vascular complications [40]. Excess level triglycerides above the normal range (> 150 mg/dl) also produces plaque in the arteries so it increases the risk of vascular complications. Furthermore, this retrospective follow up study found that patients with positive protein urea have an increased risk of having vascular complications which might be due to the fact that protein urea is an early sign of kidney damage. For this reason, patients with a positive protein urea are at an increased risk of vascular complications like nephropathy in the long run [41].

The clinical importance of this study was to provide information for health professionals and patients about factors that are associated with the risk of vascular complications, as well as, to improve the efforts on prevention. The public health importance of this study is to prevent economic loss associated with these diseases and its complications.

The limitation of this study was the use of secondary data collected retrospectively which results in incompleteness. This study assumed that all the vascular complications are caused by diabetes mellitus and considered vascular complication as a composite outcome for stroke, coronary heart disease, peripheral arterial disease, retinopathy, nephropathy, and neuropathy. This may over estimate the rate of vascular complication.

Conclusion

In this retrospective follow up study, findings showed that the incidence of vascular complications among type 2 DM patients at University of Gondar Referral Hospital remains a significant public health problem. Hypertension at baseline, LDL-C > 100 mg/dl, triglyceride > 150 mg/dl, HDL-C ≥ 40 mg/dl and male sex were significant predictors of vascular complications among type 2 DM patients. In light of these findings, health professionals in the DM follow up clinics should give targeted intervention for type 2 DM patients with hypertension comorbidity, dyslipidemia and positive protein urea. Patients with hypertension comorbidity should strictly control their hypertension like that of the DM.

Abbreviations

AHR: Adjusted hazard ratio; AIC: Akaike's information criteria; BIC: Bayesian information criteria; BP: Blood pressure; CHD: Coronary heart diseases; CHR: Crude hazard ratio; CKD: Chronic kidney diseases; CT: Computerized tomography (CT); CVD: Cardiovascular diseases; DBP: Diastolic blood pressure; DM: Diabetes mellitus; ECG: Electrocardiogram; FBS: Fasting blood sugar; HDL-C: High density lipoprotein cholesterol; HR: Hazard Raito; HTN: Hypertension; IQR: Inter quartile range; LDL-C: Low density lipoprotein cholesterol; NCEP: National cholesterol education program; PAD: Peripheral arterial disease; PH: Proportional hazard; WHO: World health organization

Acknowledgments

We would like to thank University of Gondar Referral Hospital administrative bodies and card room workers for their cooperation and permission to conduct the study. We are also thankful to the data collectors who participated in the study for their commitment.

Funding

We are thankful for University of Gondar for the financial support to conduct the study.

Authors' contributions

HF, AA and AJ were conception and design, acquisition of data, or analysis and interpretation of data. TA, MM, AT and SA drafting the article or revising contents. All authors read and approved the final version of the manuscript.

Competing interests

The authors declare that they have no competing interests.

Author details

[1]Department of Epidemiology and Biostatistics, Institute of Public Health, College of Medicine and Health Sciences, University of Gondar, Gondar, Ethiopia. [2]Department of Internal Medicine, School of Medicine, College of Medicine and Health Sciences, University of Gondar, Gondar, Ethiopia.

References

1. WHO, Definition, diagnosis and classification of diabetes mellitus and its complications. 1999.
2. WHO, Global report on diabetes. 2016.
3. IDF, International diabeties federation. Diabetes Atlas 7th edition. Brusseles; 2015.
4. IDF, report of non-commncaiable disease. 2015.
5. Ahmed KA, Muni S, Ismail IS. Type 2 diabetes and vascular complications: a pathophysiologic view. Biomed Res. 2010;21(2):147–55.
6. Naicker S. Burden of end-stage renal disease in sub-Saharan Africa. Clin Nephrol. 2010;74:S13–6.
7. Yirsaw B. Chronic kidney disease in sub-Saharan Africa: hypothesis for research demand. Ann Afr Med. 2012;11(2):119.
8. Ejigu A. Brief communication: patterns of chronic complications of diabetic patients in Menelik II hospital, Ethiopia. Ethiop J Health Dev. 2000;14(1):113–6.
9. Abebe SM, et al. Increasing trends of diabetes mellitus and body weight: a ten year observation at Gondar university teaching referral hospital, Northwest Ethiopia. PLoS One. 2013;8(3):e60081.
10. Berry J, Keebler ME, McGuire DK. Diabetes mellitus and cardiovascular disease. Herz. 2004;29(5):456–62.
11. Grundy SM, et al. Diabetes and cardiovascular disease. Circulation. 1999; 100(10):1134–46.
12. IDF, DF report of non-commncaiable disease. 5th edition 2012;Atlas, Brussels: IDF.
13. Raman R, et al. Prevalence and risk factors for diabetic microvascular complications in newly diagnosed type 2 diabetes mellitus. Sankara Nethralaya diabetic retinopathy epidemiology and molecular genetic study (SN-DREAMS, report 27). J Diabetes Complicat. 2012;26(2):123–8.
14. Muluneh LBaEK. Correlates of time to microvascular complications among diabetes mellitus patients usingparametric and non-parametric approaches: a case study of Ayder referral hospital, Ethiopia. Ethiop J Sci Technol. 2017; 10(1):65–80.
15. Sadeghpour S, et al. Predictors of all-cause and cardiovascular-specific mortality in type 2 diabetes: a competing risk modeling of an Iranian population. Adv Biomed Res. 2016;5(1):82.
16. Tanaka S, et al. Predicting macro-and microvascular complications in type 2 diabetes. Diabetes Care. 2013;36(5):1193–9.
17. Agrawal R, et al. Prevalence of micro and macrovascular complications and their risk factors in type-2 diabetes mellitus. JAPI. 2014;62:505.
18. Bentata Y, et al. Diabetic kidney disease and vascular comorbidities in patients with type 2 diabetes mellitus in a developing country. Saudi J Kidney Dis Transpl. 2015;26(5):1035–43.
19. Choukem SP, et al. Comparison of different blood pressure indices for the prediction of prevalent diabetic nephropathy in a sub-Saharan African population with type 2 diabetes. Pan Afr Med J. 2012;11:67.
20. Agrawal RP, et al. Prevalence of micro and macrovascular complications and their risk factors in type-2 diabetes mellitus. J Assoc Physicians India. 2014; 62(6):504–8.
21. Litwak L, et al. Prevalence of diabetes complications in people with type 2 diabetes mellitus and its association with baseline characteristics in the multinational a 1 chieve study. Diabetol Metab Syndr. 2013;5(1):57.
22. Lekshmi Narayanan RM, et al. Peripheral arterial disease in community-based patients with diabetes in Singapore: results from a primary healthcare study. Ann Acad Med Singap. 2010;39(7):525–7.
23. Marathe PH, Gao HX, Close KL. American Diabetes Association standards of medical care in diabetes 2017. J Diabetes. 2017;9(4):320–4.
24. Longo D, et al. Harrison's principles of internal medicine: volumes 1 and 2. New York: McGraw-Hill; 2012.
25. Parati G, et al. European Society of Hypertension practice guidelines for ambulatory blood pressure monitoring. J Hypertens. 2014;32(7):1359–66.
26. Marchesini G, et al. WHO and ATPIII proposals for the definition of the metabolic syndrome in patients with type 2 diabetes. Diabet Med. 2004; 21(4):383.
27. Expert Panel on Detection, E. Executive summary of the Third Report of the National Cholesterol Education Program (NCEP) expert panel on detection, evaluation, and treatment of high blood cholesterol in adults (Adult Treatment Panel III). JAMA. 2001;285(19):2486.
28. Cheng LJ, et al. A competing risk analysis of sequential complication development in Asian type 2 diabetes mellitus patients. Sci Rep. 2015;5:15687.
29. Abu-lebdeh HS, Nguyen TT. Predictors of Macrovascular Disease in Patients WithType 2 Diabetes Mellitus. Mayo Foundation for Medical Education and Research. 2001;76:707–12.
30. Bastawrous A, et al. The incidence of diabetes mellitus and diabetic retinopathy in a population-based cohort study of people age 50 years and over in Nakuru, Kenya. BMC Endocr Disord. 2017;17(1):19.
31. Amutha A, et al. Incidence of complications in young-onset diabetes: comparing type 2 with type 1 (the young diab study). Diabetes Res Clin Pract. 2017;123:1–8.
32. Collaboration, E.R.F. Diabetes mellitus, fasting blood glucose concentration, and risk of vascular disease: a collaborative meta-analysis of 102 prospective studies. Lancet. 2010;375(9733):2215–22.
33. Maric-Bilkan C. Sex differences in micro-and macro-vascular complications of diabetes mellitus. Clin Sci. 2017;131(9):833–46.
34. Carpenter MW. Gestational diabetes, pregnancy hypertension, and late vascular disease. Diabetes Care. 2007;30(Supplement 2):S246–50.
35. ADA. Standards of medical care in diabetes. Diabetes Care. 2008;31:S12–54.
36. Tracey ML, et al. Risk factors for macro-and microvascular complications among older adults with diagnosed type 2 diabetes: findings from the Irish longitudinal study on ageing. J Diabetes Res. 2016;2016:5975903.
37. Hsueh WA, Anderson PW. Hypertension, the endothelial cell, and the vascular complications of diabetes mellitus. Hypertension. 1992;20(2): 253–63.
38. Tapera, S., Prevalence and Risk Factors for Diabetes Chronic Complications in Harare, Zimbabwe, 2014. 2014, University of Zimbabwe.
39. Link JJ, Rohatgi A, de Lemos JA. HDL cholesterol: physiology, pathophysiology, and management. Curr Probl Cardiol. 2007;32(5):268–314.
40. Trialists CT. The effects of lowering LDL cholesterol with statin therapy in people at low risk of vascular disease: meta-analysis of individual data from 27 randomised trials. Lancet. 2012;380(9841):581–90.
41. Carroll MF. Proteinuria in Adults: A Diagnositc Approach. Am Fam Physician. 2000;62(6):1333–40.

General health status in Iranian diabetic patients assessed by short-form-36 questionnaire: a systematic review and meta-analysis

Masoud Behzadifar[1*] , Rahim Sohrabi[2], Roghayeh Mohammadibakhsh[3], Morteza Salemi[4], Sharare Taheri Moghadam[3], Masood Taheri Mirghaedm[3], Meysam Behzadifar[5], Hamid Reza Baradaran[6] and Nicola Luigi Bragazzi[7]

Abstract

Background: Diabetes mellitus is one of the most prevalent diseases worldwide. Diabetes is a chronic disease associated with micro- and macro-vascular complications and deterioration in general health status. Therefore, the aim of this study was to estimate general health status among Iranian diabetic patients through a systematic review and meta-analysis of study utilizing the Short-Form-36 questionnaire.

Methods: Searching the EMBASE, PubMed, ISI/Web of Sciences (WOS), MEDLINE via Ovid, PsycoINFO, as well as Iranian databases (MagIran, Iranmedex, and SID) from January 2000 to December 2017. The methodological quality of the studies was evaluated using the "A Cochrane Risk of Bias Assessment Tool: for Non-Randomized Studies of Interventions" (ACROBAT-NRSI). Random-effect model was used and the means were reported with their 95% confidence interval (CI). To evaluate the heterogeneity between studies, I^2 test was used. Egger's regression test was used to assess the publication bias.

Results: Fourteen studies were retained in the final analysis. The mean general health status using SF-36 in diabetic patients of Iran was 51.9 (95% CI: 48.64 to 53.54). The mean physical component summary was 52.92 [95% CI: 49.46–56.38], while the mean mental component summary was 51.02 [95% CI: 46.87–55.16].

Conclusion: The findings of this study showed that general health status in Iranian diabetic patients is low. Health policymakers should work to improve the health status in these patients and take appropriate interventions.

Keywords: General health status, Diabetes, Short-Form-36 questionnaire, Iran, Meta-analysis

Background

Diabetes mellitus is one of the most prevalent diseases worldwide, imposing a relevant epidemiological and clinical burden, both in terms of deaths and morbidities. The prevalence of diabetes is increasing both in developed and developing countries, and has doubled over the past three decades, with almost 80% of diabetic patients living in less developed countries [1, 2]. Population aging, lifestyle changes, lack of mobility, and many other factors characterizing modern life have contributed to such an increase [3]. In 2014, the prevalence of diabetes in people aged greater than 18 years in the world was about 8.5%. It is anticipated that diabetes will be the seventh cause of death by 2030, and, despite all efforts to control the disease, it still

* Correspondence: masoudbehzadifar@gmail.com
[1]Social Determinants of Health Research Center, Lorestan University of Medical Sciences, Khorramabad, Iran
Full list of author information is available at the end of the article

remains one of the major public health challenges [4]. The number of people with diabetes is expected to rise up to about 592 million by 2035 [5]. The prevalence of diabetes in the Middle East and North Africa is about 10.9%. In these areas, about 35 million people are affected by diabetes, with Iran having the highest prevalence (9.94%) among the countries of the Middle East [6].

Such concerns necessitate adequate health policies in order to control and prevent diabetes [7]. This disorder represents a chronic disease associated with micro- and macro-vascular complications, which dramatically impact on general health status [8]. Studies have shown that such complications can affect physical, mental and social life of people, modifying and interfering with their usual every day functioning [9]. Hence, treatments of diabetes are usually evaluated based on their effect on health status [10], which, as a key factor in effectiveness studies, refers, indeed, to the mental, physical and social status of the patient [11]. Considering the general health status among diabetic patients can provide care givers with a better understanding of patients' conditions, indicating which health

provisions are necessary for a proper management of the disease [12].

To assess general health status among diabetes patients, a variety of questionnaires have been developed that can measure different dimensions of the patients' life. The Short-Form 36 (SF-36) questionnaire is one of the most commonly used instruments [13]. It includes 36 questions distributed across eight domains (namely, vitality, physical function, body pain, health perception, physical role, emotional role, social role and mental health) [14, 15].

Various studies have been conducted to assess Iranian diabetic population's quality of life. Such information can be helpful for measuring the severity of complications and designing and implementing appropriate healthcare policies. In 2013, a review study was conducted in Iran on health status in diabetic patients. In this study, the assessment of health status of diabetics was based on all questionnaires used in Iran. Authors suggested that a meta-analysis study could better provide information about health status in diabetic patients [16]. Therefore, the aim of this study was to estimate

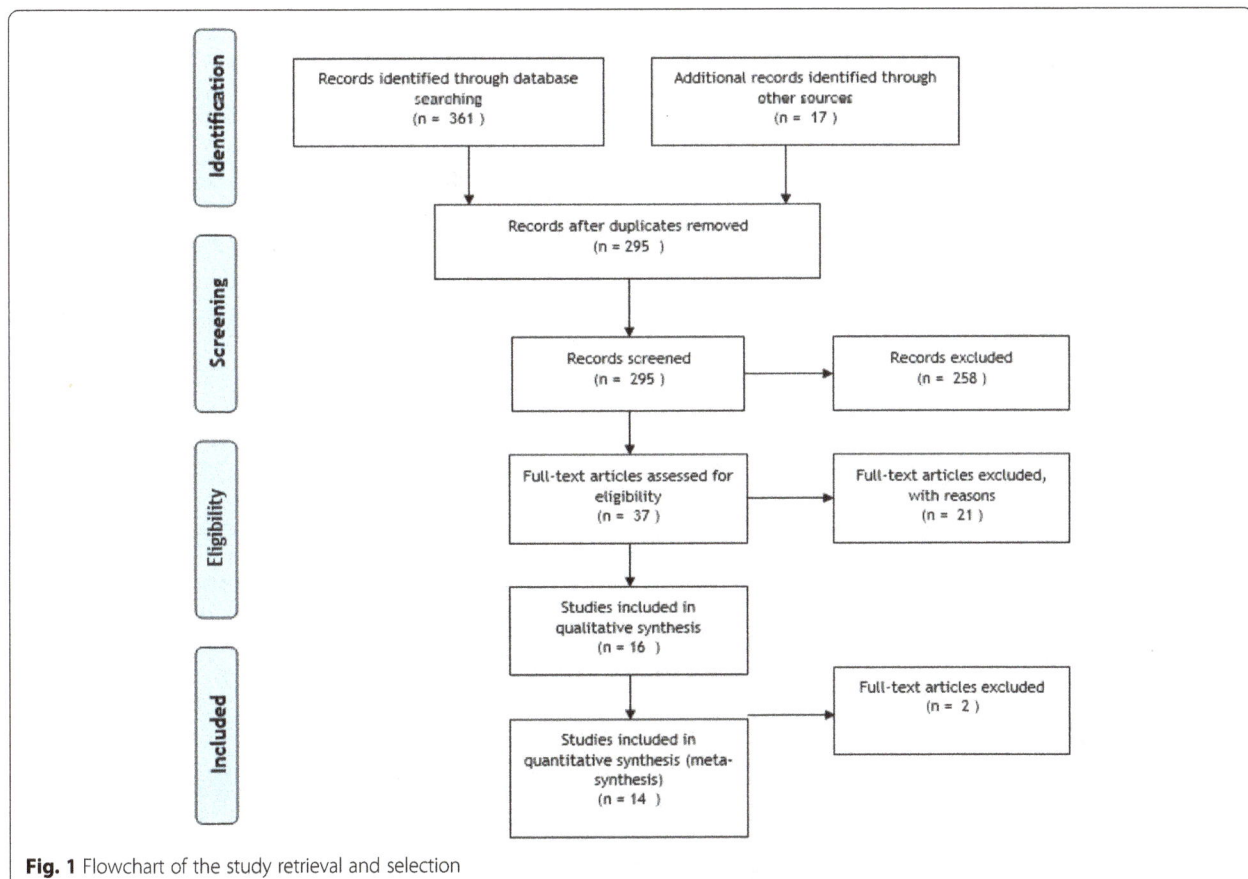

Fig. 1 Flowchart of the study retrieval and selection

Table 1 The main characteristics of the included studies about general health status in Iranian patients with diabetes

First author	Year of publication	Mean score of general health status	Sample size	Female	Male	Age (Mean ± SD)	Type of diabetes	Design of study	Duration of diabetes (Year ± SD)	Married (%)	Setting (City)	Setting (Province)
Borzou	2011	55.53	165	111	54	NA	Type 2	Cross-Sectional	NA	NA	Hamedan	Hamedan
Khaledi	2011	45.23	198	166	32	NA	Type 2	Cross-Sectional	1–5	80.8	Sannadaj	Kurdistan
Saadatjoo	2012	28.52	100	54	46	42.82 ± 16.57	Type 2	Case-Control	NA	82	Birjand	South Khorasan
Timareh	2012	52.97	350	204	146	52.91 ± 11.7	Both type	Cross-Sectional	NA	86.9	Kermanshah	Kermanshah
Sadabadi	2013	44.72	60	NA	NA	NA	Type 2	Case-Control	NA	NA	Tabriz	East Azerbaijan
Darvishpoor Kakhki	2013	46.2	131	79	52	NA	Type 2	Case-Control	NA	80.2	Tehran	Tehran
Hadi	2013	54.11	300	222	78	50.98	Both type	Cross-Sectional	NA	84	Shiraz	Fars
Darvishpoor Kakhki	2013	52.11	140	NA	NA	47.3 ± 12.7	Both type	Cross-Sectional	8.83 ± 6.10	NA	Tehran	Tehran
Mohammadshahi	2015	51.81	110	51	59	53.4 ± 8.12	Type 2	Cross-Sectional	NA	NA	Ahvaz	Khuzestan
Kashfi	2015	61.33	124	89	35	59.65 ± 12.3	Type 2	Case-Control	7.68 ± 6.93	83.9	Larestan	Fars
Borhaninejad	2016	46.48	120	69	51	71.32 ± 5.13	Type 2	Cross-Sectional	NA	73.4	Kerman	Kerman
Hajian-Tailaki	2016	56.27	747	372	375	68 ± 7.6 in male and 67.7 ± 7.9 in female	Type 2	Cross-Sectional	NA	NA	Babol	Mazandaran
Mazloomy Mahmood Abad	2017	59.27	100	59	41	51.92 ± 11.53	Type 2	Cross-Sectional	NA	94	Sirjan	Kerman
Gholami	2017	51.11	1847	1289	558	59.65 ± 12.3	Type 2	Cross-Sectional	NA	19.9	Nishabur	Razavi Khorasan

Table 2 Risk of Bias Assessment of included studies based on the ACROBAT-NRSI instrument

Study	Domains of bias						
	Bias due to confounding	Bias in selection of participants	Bias in measurement of interventions	Bias due to departures from intended interventions	Bias due to missing data	Bias in measurement of outcomes	Bias in selection of reported results
Borzou	Moderate risk	Low risk	Low risk	Low risk	Low risk	Low risk	Low risk
Khaledi	Low risk	Low risk	Low risk	Moderate risk	Low risk	Low risk	Moderate risk
Saadatjoo	Serious risk	Low risk	Serious risk	Moderate risk	Serious risk	Moderate risk	Serious risk
Timareh	Serious risk	Moderate risk	Low risk	Moderate risk	Moderate risk	Low risk	Moderate risk
Sadabadi	Moderate risk	Low risk	Moderate risk	Serious risk	Moderate risk	Moderate risk	Low risk
Darvishpoor Kakhki	Serious risk	Low risk	Low risk	Moderate risk	Low risk	Moderate risk	Low risk
Hadi	Low risk	Low risk	Moderate risk	Low risk	Low risk	Low risk	Low risk
Darvishpoor Kakhki	Moderate risk	Low risk	Low risk	Low risk	Low risk	Moderate risk	Low risk
Mohammadshahi	Low risk	Moderate risk	Low risk	Low risk	Low risk	Moderate risk	Low risk
Kashfi	Low risk	Low risk	Low risk	Low risk	Low risk	Low risk	Moderate risk
Borhaninejad	Moderate risk	Low risk	Moderate risk	Moderate risk	Low risk	Low risk	Low risk
Hajian-Tailaki	Low risk	Low risk	Low risk	Moderate risk	Moderate risk	Low risk	Low risk
Mazloomy Mahmood Abad	Low risk	Moderate risk	Low risk	Low risk	Low risk	Low risk	Low risk
Gholami	Moderate risk	Low risk	Low risk	Moderate risk	Low risk	Low risk	Low risk

	Bias due to confounding	Bias in selection of participants	Bias in measurement of interventions	Bias due to departures from intended interventions	Bias due to missing data	Bias in measurement of outcomes	Bias in selection of reported results
Borhaninejad,2016	?	+	?	?	+	+	+
Borzou, 2011	?	+	+	+	+	+	+
Darvishpoor Kakhki,2013	−	+	+	?	+	?	+
Darvishpoor Kakhki 2013	?	+	+	+	+	?	+
Gholami,2017	?	+	+	?	+	+	+
Hadi, 2013	+	+	?	+	+	+	+
Hajian-Tailaki,2016	+	+	+	?	?	+	+
Kashfi,2015	+	+	+	+	+	+	?
Khaledi, 2011	+	+	+	?	+	+	?
Mazloomy Mahmood Abad,2017	+	?	+	+	+	+	+
Mohammadshahi,2015	+	?	+	+	+	?	+
Saadatjoo, 2012	−	+	−	?	−	?	−
Sadabadi,2013	?	+	?	−	?	?	+
Timareh,2012	−	?	+	?	?	+	?

Bias due to confounding
Bias in selection of participants
Bias in measurement of interventions
Bias due to departures from intended interventions
Bias due to missing data
Bias in measurement of outcomes
Bias in selection of reported results

0% 25% 50% 75% 100%

■ Low risk of bias   ■ Unclear risk of bias   ■ High risk of bias

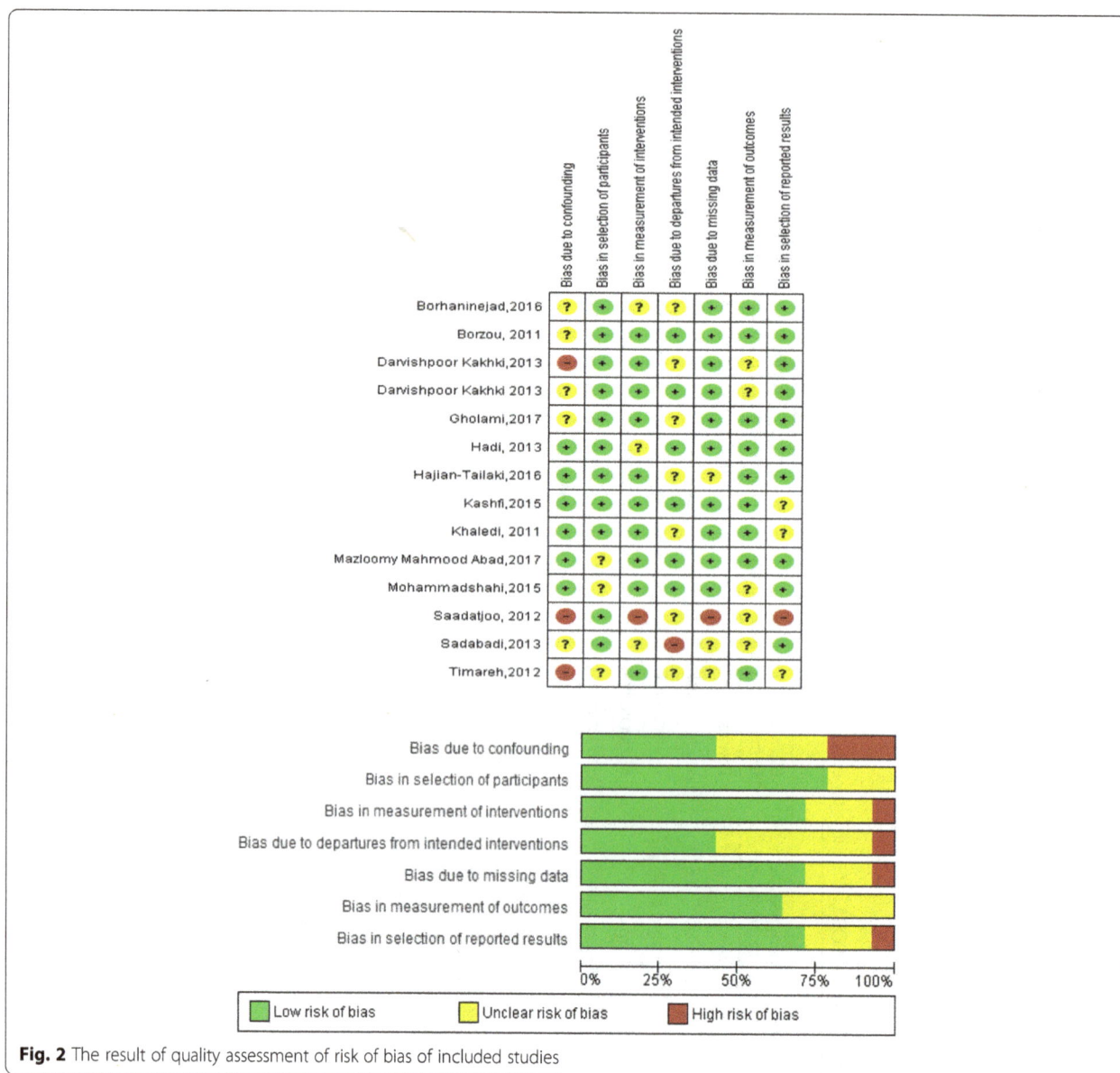

Fig. 2 The result of quality assessment of risk of bias of included studies

general health status among Iranian diabetic patients through a systematic review and meta-analysis of studies utilizing a specific instrument, namely the SF-36 questionnaire.

Methods
Literature search
The current study has been performed according to the "The Meta-analysis of Observational Studies in Epidemiology" (MOOSE) guidelines [17]. (Additional file 1).

Two authors independently searched different scholarly electronic databases: namely, EMBASE, PubMed, ISI/Web of Sciences (WOS), MEDLINE via Ovid, PsycoINFO, as well as Iranian databases (MagIran, Iranmedex, and SID). These databases were systematically searched from January 2000 to December 2017 using the following search strategies: ("general health status") AND ("Short form 36" OR "SF-36" OR "SF-36 health survey questionnaire" OR "Short form-36 health survey questionnaire") AND ("Diabetes" OR "Diabetic") AND "Iran". Studies were searched both in English and Persian (no language filter applied). Reference lists of each included study were also scanned and hand-searched for possible related studies.

Inclusion/ criteria
Studies with the following criteria were included if: i) utilizing the SF-36 questionnaire for investigating general health status among Iranian populations, ii) reporting an average score for the eight domains of the questionnaire, iii) reporting both Physical Component Summary (PCS) and Mental Components Summary

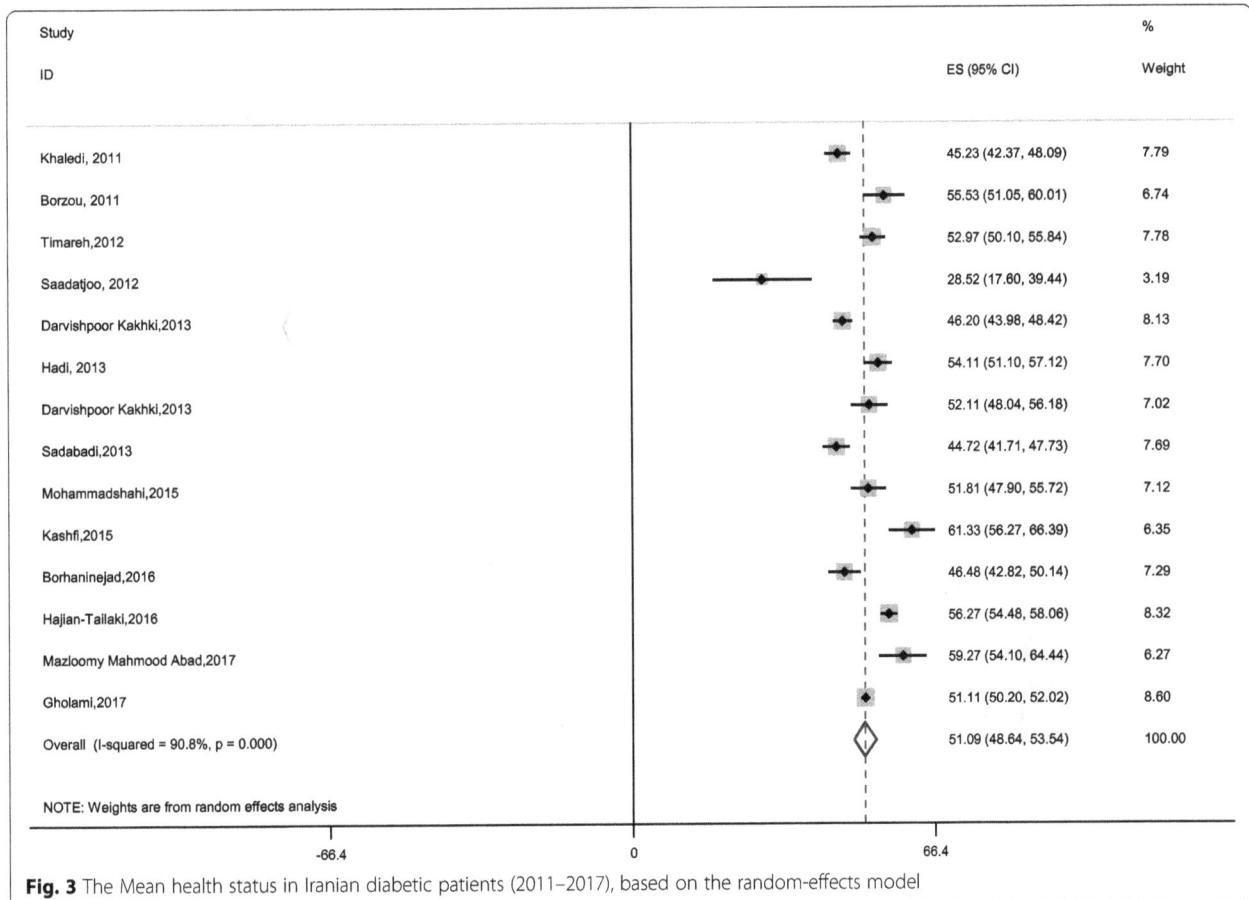

Fig. 3 The Mean health status in Iranian diabetic patients (2011–2017), based on the random-effects model

(MCS) indicators, and iv) reporting means with standard errors (SE) or standard deviations (SD). Both cross-sectional or case-control studies were considered.

Exclusion criteria

Studies were excluded if: i) designed as reviews, letters to the editor, editorials, expert opinions, commentaries, clinical trials, case-reports, case-series, or

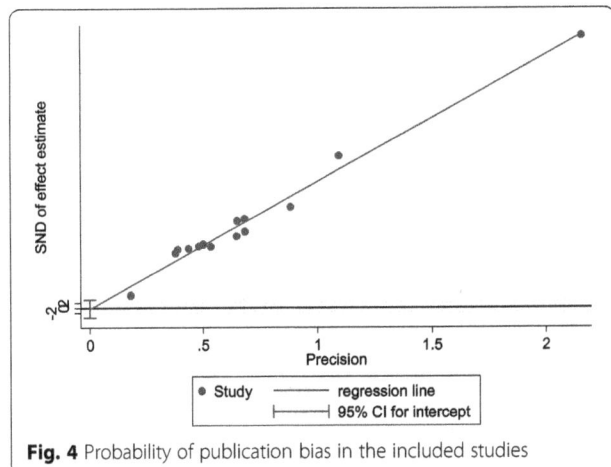

Fig. 4 Probability of publication bias in the included studies

ii) not reporting quantitative details of the SF-36 questionnaire.

Quality assessment

The methodological quality of the studies was evaluated using the "A Cochrane Risk of Bias Assessment Tool: for Non-Randomized Studies of Interventions" (ACROBAT-NRSI) [18].

Data extraction

Two authors (MB and NLB) extracted the data from the studies, and if there was a controversy between them, another author (AA) resolved the issue. The name of first authors of the studies, the year of publication, the place where the studies were conducted, the number of participants, the duration of diabetes, the design, and the mean scores of SF-36 domains were extracted.

Statistical analysis

The pooled value of the mean of overall scores, as well the scores of the eight domains of the questionnaire and the PCS and MCS scores were calculated as the mean and SE. Random-effect model was used and the means were reported with their 95% confidence interval (CI).

Table 3 The results of subgroup analysis

Variables	Number of studies	Number of participants	Mean score of general health status (95% CI)	I^2	P-value
Design of studies					
Cross-sectional	10	4077	52.32 (50.02–54.62)	86.8%	0.001
Case-control	4	415	46.47 (38.87–54.08)	93.3%	0.001
Sample size					
≤120	6	614	49.58 (43.11–56.05)	92%	0.001
> 120	8	3878	51.60 (48.95–54.24)	90.7%	0.001
Type of diabetes					
Type 2	11	3702	50.46 (47.43–53.49)	92.46%	0.001
Both type (type 1 and 2)	3	790	53.22 (51.37–55.07)	0%	0.001

To evaluate the heterogeneity among studies, I^2 test was used [19]. For evaluating the potential sources of heterogeneity, subgroup analyses based on the study design, sample size and type of diabetes (type 1 and type 2 diabetes) were conducted. Sensitivity analysis was performed to ensure that the results were stable. This analysis was also performed based on the year of publication. Egger's regression test was used to assess the publication bias [20].

Finally, case-control studies were pooled together, computing the standardized mean difference (SMD).

Figures with a *p*-value < 0.05 were considered statistically significant. All data were analyzed using Stata 12.0 software (Stata Corp LP, College Station, TX).

Results

After the initial electronic database search, 378 studies were found. Eighty-three duplicate studies were deleted. The titles of the retrieved studies were reviewed and 258 studies were excluded due to lack of relevance to the topic. Then, the title and abstract of 37 remaining studies were reviewed by two authors independently and 21 studies were excluded with reason. Finally, the full texts of the remaining 16 studies were examined and, based on the inclusion/exclusion criteria, 14 studies were retained in the final analysis [21–34]. Figure 1 summarizes the stages of the retrieval and selection of the studies.

The included studies were conducted between 2011 and 2017. The total number of participants in the studies was 4492, ranging from 60 to 1847 people. The study designs varied across studies and were cross-sectional for 10 studies and case-control for 4 studies). Table 1

shows the main characteristics of the studies retained in the present systematic review and meta-analysis.

The quality assessment of the risk of bias of the included studies is shown in Table 2 and Fig. 2.

The mean general health status using SF-36 based on the random-effect model in diabetic patients of Iran was 51.9 (95% CI: 48.64 to 53.54). The lowest health status was observed in the study of Saadatjoo with a score of 28.52 and the highest in Kashifi's study, with a value of 61.33. Figure 3 shows the overall general health status among the included studies.

Using the Egger's test, no publication bias could be detected (*p* = 0.859, see Fig. 4).

To investigate the possible sources of heterogeneity between studies, subgroup analysis was conducted based on study design, sample size and study quality. Table 3 shows the results of subgroup analysis.

For further evaluation of sources of heterogeneity, the results of meta-regression were analyzed based on the year of publication and the sample size of studies, as presented in Table 4. The results showed that the quality of life of diabetic patients has increased on a yearly basis

Table 4 The results of meta-regression

Variables	Coefficient	S.E.	t	P-value	Lower 95%	Upper 95%
Year	1.36	1.07	1.27	0.22	−0.99	3.73
Sample size	−0.00	0.00	−0.22	0.82	−0.01	0.00

Table 5 The health status based on the 8 domains of the SF-36 questionnaire

Variables	Mean (95% CI)	Heterogeneity		P-value of publication bias
		I^2	P-value	
Physical function	61.62 (55.70–67.53)	98.6%	0.001	0.78
Role physical	49.96 (44.50–55.41)	95.6%	0.001	0.83
Body pain	52.26 (48.47–56.04)	95.8%	0.001	0.57
General health	47.34 (44.15–50.53)	96.5%	0.001	0.01
Vitality	46.99 (43.28–50.69)	97.4%	0.001	0.64
Social function	57.86 (46.87–68.85)	99.7%	0.001	0.15
Role emotional	50.38 (45.29–55.47)	97.4%	0.001	0.28
Mental health	47.79 (40.06–55.52)	99.6%	0.001	0.32

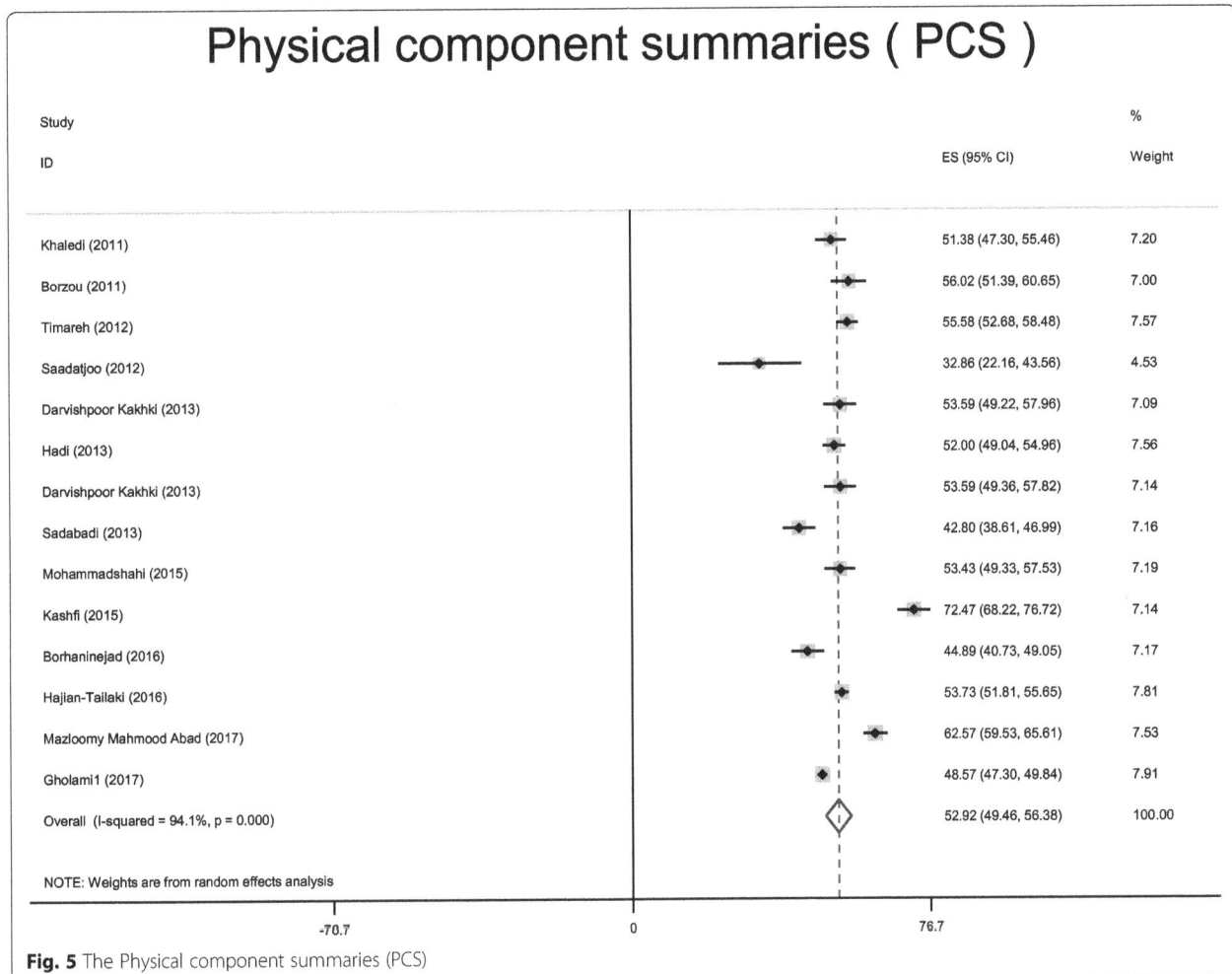

Fig. 5 The Physical component summaries (PCS)

and has decreased based on the sample size. However, none of the results were statistically significant.

The results based on the eight domains of the SF-36 questionnaire are presented in Table 5. The mean scores of PCS and MCS are shown in Figs. 5 and 6. The mean of PCS was 52.92 [95% CI: 49.46–56.38], while the mean of MCS was 51.02 [95% CI: 46.87–55.16].

Finally, case-control studies were pooled together (Fig. 7). The general health status of diabetic patients compared to healthy controls was lower with a SMD of −0.84 [95% CI: -1.83 to 0.51] and compared to the group of patients with tuberculosis with a SMD of 0.44 [95% CI: 0.21- 0.67].

Discussion

In the 14 studies included in this systematic review and meta-analysis, numerous complications and co-morbidities were reported in people with diabetes. Health policy- and decision-makers should pay attention to the implications of the reduced general health status in diabetic patients in Iran. Various studies have, indeed, shown that health status is an independent prognostic

predictor of survival and hospitalization rate in patients with peripheral arterial and renal patients, and of mortality in patients with coronary heart disease [35–38].

General health status is decreased in diabetic patients [39], when compared to the health status of general population, which, in a recent study, reported an average score of 67.69 ± 14.78 [40]. Healthcare providers should be aware of the patients' perspective and their perceived health. Preventing further diabetes complications and providing better conditions for patients' lives is fundamental. Physical and mental interventions can improve the health status of diabetic patients and avoid, or at least delay, further deterioration [41].

Our findings showed that the dimensions of physical and social function had the highest score whereas the lowest score was related to vitality and general health. The results of our study are consistent with the study done in Brazil [42], whereas other studies reported higher values [43–45]. The level of access to health services, the economic and social conditions of people, the physical and mental conditions of individuals can, at least partially, explain these differences [46, 47]. Some

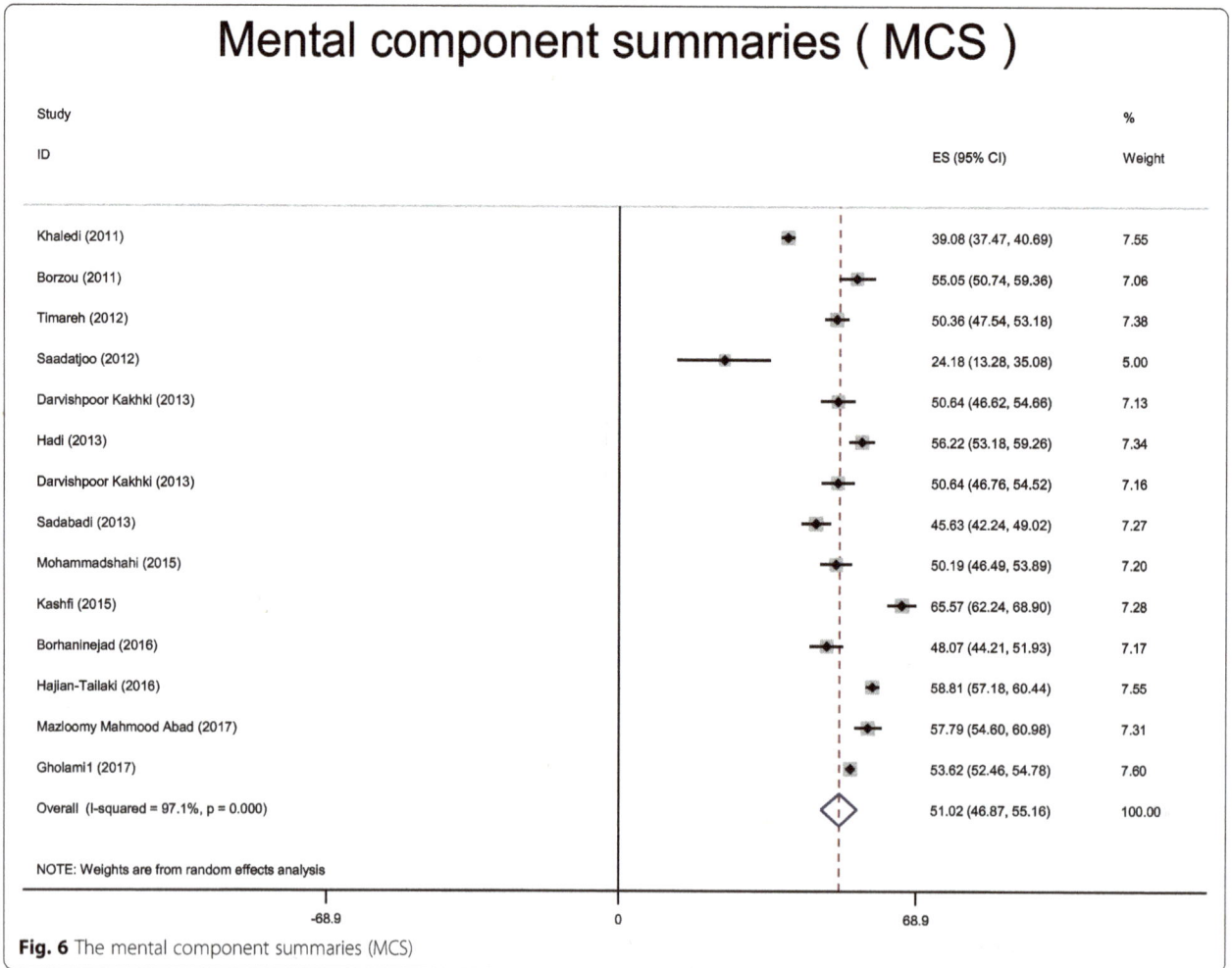

Fig. 6 The mental component summaries (MCS)

studies point to the existence of health inequalities in that people with a higher socioeconomic status have more incentive and energy to change their livelihood and are more involved in their own health care processes [48]. An important cross-sectional survey of 13 national samples from Asia, Australia, Europe and North America of 5104 patients with diabetes from the multinational study of Diabetes Attitudes, Wishes and Needs (DAWN) has shown that the reported levels of well-being, self-management, and diabetes control correlate with

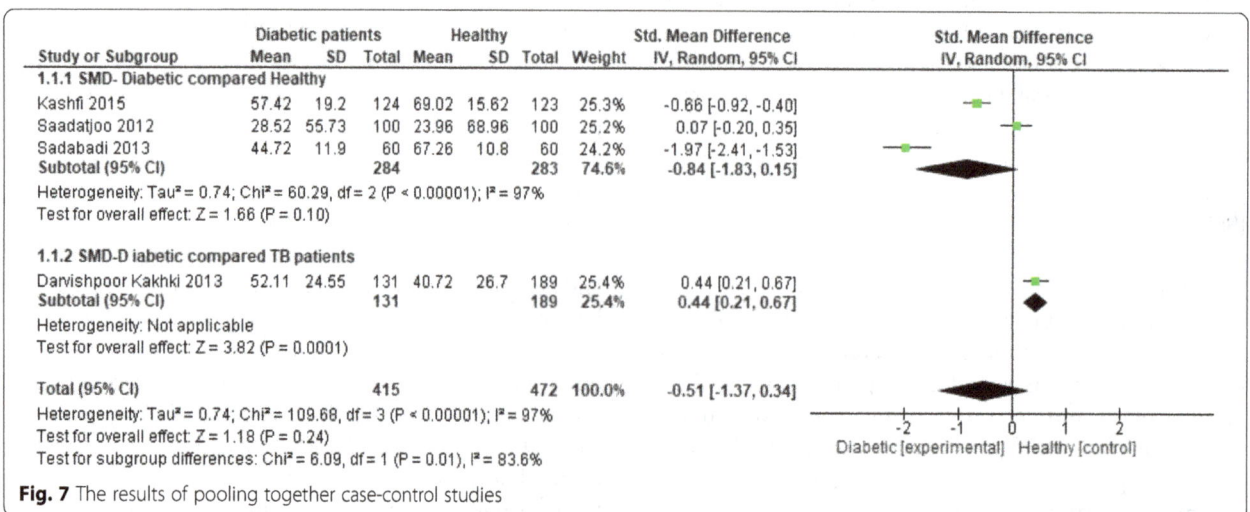

Fig. 7 The results of pooling together case-control studies

country, respondent demographic and disease character-istics, as well as with healthcare features [49]. These findings have been replicated by a follow-up study [50].

The findings of the present study indicate that diabetes dramatically affects vitality and general health domains; hence these areas should be given more attention when treating diabetic patients. In our study, MCS was less than PCS, which was consistent with the results of the Al-Shehri study [51]. Various studies have been con-ducted to show that mental disorders such as depression in patients with diabetes can be remarkably observed. In a review, results showed that depression in diabetic pa-tients had a negative effect on the treatment process and increased complications of the disease [52].

It seems that the chronic and severe nature of diabetes mellitus in the long run leads to a decrease in the gen-eral health status [53]. It should be noted that the core of the concept of reported/perceived health status is a feeling/perception of one's own health and, in fact, other aspects of the health status form a sense of health that is low in patients with diabetes. Affecting the emotional as-pects impacts on energy and vitality of patients with dia-betes. Other studies have also shown a decrease in vitality, with an increase of fatigue, depression, anxiety and stress problems, among patients with diabetes. Therefore, diabetes has a long-term negative effect on the health of patients. The decrease in the health status in patients with diabetes has also been replicated in other studies [54].

These observations can be confirmed if we compare health status of Iranian subjects with diabetes with the health status of people with chronic-degenerative disor-ders, such as rheumatoid arthritis with an average score of 52.47 [55], or cardiovascular disorders with a mean of 53.19 [56], among others. Similarly, low scores have been found for asthma [57] or chronic kidney disease [58]. Scores even lower (40.43 ± 12.7) were reported for indi-viduals with drug addiction [59].

In meta-analysis studies, taking into account potential sources of heterogeneity is crucial [60]. To investigate this aspect, we performed subgroup-analysis based on each SF-36 scale domain. The results of meta-regression were also studied for further evaluation of heterogeneity sources, which showed an increased average health sta-tus of diabetic patients based on the year of publication, even though not statistically significant. In recent years the status of services provided to diabetics is on the rise, but it seems that many of the services provided to them are not of sufficient standards, and the quality of care for these patients should be monitored more closely by healthcare providers in Iran.

However, this study has some limitations that should be properly mentioned. First, the primary studies missed to give some complementary information about patients, such as sex, other illnesses/co-morbidities, education level and income. Second, a high level of heterogeneity was observed, which can be attributed to methodological differences. Third, the health status in diabetic patients has not been studied in many Iranian provinces, which can challenge the generalizability of our estimation to all Iranian diabetic population.

Conclusion

The findings of this study showed that general health status in Iranian diabetic patients is low. Health policy- and decision-makers should work to improve the health status in these patients and take appropriate interven-tions. Therefore, it is recommended to look at important factors such as patients' attitudes in changing and im-proving their lifestyle. A combination of both clinical and non-clinical interventions should be targeted at in-creasing the standard of living of these patients.

Abbreviations

ACROBAT-NRSI: A Cochrane Risk of Bias Assessment Tool: for Non-Randomized Studies of Interventions; BP: Bodily pain; CI: Confidence intervals; ERF: Emotional role functioning; GHP: General health perceptions; MCS: Mental Component Summary; MeSH: Medical Subject Headings; MH: Mental health; PCS: Physical Component Summary; PF: Physical functioning; PRF: Physical role functioning; PROs: Patient-reported outcomes; SF-36: The Short-Form 36; SID: Scientific Information Database; SMD: Standardized Mean Difference; SRF: Social role functioning; VT: Vitality; WOS: Web of Science

Funding

This research received no specific grant from any funding agency in the public, commercial, or not-for-profit sectors.

Authors' contributions

MaB and RS designed the study. MeB, STM and RM searched databases, data extracted and study selection. MaB and MS performed data analysis. MaB, NLB, MS and MTM interpreted the results. MaB wrote the manuscript. RM, STM, and HRB been involved in drafting the manuscript or revising it critically for important intellectual content. NLB, MTM, and HRB carried out a final revision and grammar editing. All authors read and approved the final manuscript.

Competing interests

The authors declare that they have no competing interests.

Author details

[1]Social Determinants of Health Research Center, Lorestan University of Medical Sciences, Khorramabad, Iran. [2]Iranian Social Security Organization, Zanjan Province Health Administration, Zanjan, Iran. [3]Department of Health Services Management, School of Health Management and Information Sciences, Iran University of Medical Sciences, Tehran, Iran. [4]Social Determinants in Health Promotion Research Center, Hormozgan University of Medical Sciences, Bandar Abbas, Iran. [5]Health Management and Economics Research Center, Iran University of Medical Sciences, Tehran, Iran. [6]Endocrine Research Center Institute of Endocrinology and Metabolism, Iran University of Medical Sciences, Tehran, Iran. [7]School of Public Health, Department of Health Sciences (DISSAL), University of Genoa, Genoa, Italy.

References

1. Zimmet P, Alberti KG, Magliano DJ, Bennett PH. Diabetes mellitus statistics on prevalence and mortality: facts and fallacies. Nat Rev Endocrinol. 2016; 12(10):616–22.

2. NCD Risk Factor Collaboration (NCD-RisC). Worldwide trends in diabetes since 1980: a pooled analysis of 751 population-based studies with 4.4 million participants. Lancet. 2016;387(10027):1513–30.

3. Speight J, Reaney MD, Barnard KD. Not all roads lead to Rome-a review of quality of life measurement in adults with diabetes. Diabet Med. 2009;26(4):315–27.

4. Mathers CD, Loncar D. Projections of global mortality and burden of disease from 2002 to 2030. PLoS Med. 2006;3(11):e442.

5. Guariguata L, Whiting DR, Hambleton I, Beagley J, Linnenkamp U, Shaw JE. Global estimates of diabetes prevalence for 2013 and projections for 2035. Diabetes Res Clin Pract. 2014;103(2):137–49.

6. Javanbakht M, Mashayekhi A, Baradaran HR, Haghdoost A, Afshin A. Projection of diabetes population size and associated economic burden through 2030 in Iran: evidence from micro-simulation Markov model and Bayesian meta-analysis. PLoS One. 2015;10(7):e0132505.

7. Wild S, Roglic G, Green A, Sicree R, King H. Global prevalence of diabetes: estimates for the year 2000 and projections for 2030. Diabetes Care. 2004; 27(5):1047–53.

8. Papadopoulos AA, Kontodimopoulos N, Frydas A, Ikonomakis E, Niakas D. Predictors of health-related quality of life in type II diabetic patients in Greece. BMC Public Health. 2007;7:186.

9. Colberg SR, Sigal RJ, Fernhall B, Regensteiner JG, Blissmer BJ, Rubin RR, et al. Exercise and type 2 diabetes: the American College of Sports Medicine and the American Diabetes Association: joint position statement. Diabetes Care. 2010;33(12):e147–67.

10. Gusmai Lde F, Novato Tde S, Nogueira Lde S. The influence of quality of life in treatment adherence of diabetic patients: a systematic review. Rev Esc Enferm USP. 2015;49(5):839–46.

11. American Diabetes Association. Standards of medical care in diabetes-2016 abridged for primary care providers. Clin Diabetes. 2016;34(1):3–21.

12. International Diabetes Federation Guideline Development Group. Global guideline for type 2 diabetes. Diabetes Res Clin Pract. 2014;104(1):1–52.

13. Ware JE Jr, Sherbourne CD. The MOS 36-item short-form health survey (SF-36). I Conceptual framework and item selection. Med Care. 1992;30(6):473–83.

14. Al Hayek AA, Robert AA, Al Saeed A, Alzaid AA, Al Sabaan FS. Factors associated with health-related quality of life among Saudi patients with type 2 diabetes mellitus: a cross-sectional survey. Diabetes Metab J. 2014; 38(3):220–9.

15. Lyons RA, Perry HM, Littlepage BN. Evidence for the validity of the short-form 36 questionnaire (SF-36) in an elderly population. Age Ageing. 1994; 23(3):182–4.

16. Kiadaliri AA, Najafi B, Mirmalek-Sani M. Quality of life in people with diabetes: a systematic review of studies in Iran. J Diabetes Metab Disord. 2013;12:54.

17. Stroup DF, Berlin JA, Morton SC, Olkin I, Williamson GD, Rennie D, et al. Meta-analysis of observational studies in epidemiology: a proposal for reporting. Meta-analysis of observational studies in epidemiology (MOOSE) group. JAMA. 2000;283(15):2008–12.

18. Sterne JA, Hernán MA, Reeves BC, Savović J, Berkman ND, Viswanathan M, et al. ROBINS-I: a tool for assessing risk of bias in non-randomised studies of interventions. BMJ. 2016;355:i4919.

19. Higgins JP, Thompson SG, Deeks JJ, Altman DG. Measuring inconsistency in meta-analyses. BMJ. 2003;327(7414):557–60.

20. Egger M, Davey Smith G, Schneider M, Minder C. Bias in meta-analysis detected by a simple, graphical test. BMJ. 1997;315(7109):629–34.

21. Borzou SR, Salavati M, Safari M, Hadadinejad S, Zandieh M, Torkaman B. Quality of life in type II diabetic patients referred to Sina hospital, Hamadan. ZJRMS. 2011;13(4):43–6.

22. Khaledi S, Moridi G, Gharibi F. Survey of eight dimensions quality of life for patients with diabetes type II, referred to Sanandaj diabetes center in 2009. J Fasa Univ Med Sci. 2011;1(1):29–37.

23. Saadatjoo S, Rezvanee M, Tabyee S, Oudi D. Life quality comparison in type 2 diabetic patients and none diabetic persons. Mod Care J. 2012;9(1):24–31.

24. Timareh M, Rhimi M, Abbasi P, Rezaei M, Hyaidarpoor S. Quality of life in diabetic patients referred to the Diabete research center in Kermanshah. J Kermanshah Univ Med Sci. 2012;16(1):63–9.

25. Darvishpoor Kakhki A, Abed Saeedi J, Masjedi MR, Askari H. Comparison of life quality of diabetic patients with TB patients. J Knowledge Health. 2013; 8(2):71–5.

26. Darvishpoor Kakhki A, Abed saeedi Z. Health-related quality of life of diabetic patients in Tehran. Int J Endocrinol Metab. 2013;11(4):e7945.

27. Hadi N, Ghahramani S, Montazeri A. Health related quality of life in both types of diabetes in Shiraz, Iran. Shiraz E-Med J. 2013;14(2):112–22.

28. Hatamloo Sadabadi M, Babapour KJ. Comparison of Quality of Life and Coping Strategies in Diabetic and Non Diabetic People. JSSU. 2013; 20(5):581–92.

29. Kashfi SM, Nasri A, Dehghan A, Yazdankhah M. Comparison of quality of life of patients with type II diabetes referring to diabetes Association of Larestan with healthy people in 2013. J Neyshabur Univ Med Sci. 2015;3(2):32–8.

30. Mohammadshahi M, Shirani F, Elahi S, Ghasemi S, Alayi Shahni M, Haidari F. Evaluation of relationship between dietary patterns and quality of life in patients with type 2 diabetes. Daneshvarmed. 2015; 22(114):1–12.

31. Borhaninejad V, Kazazi L, Haghi M, Chehrehnegar N. Quality of life and its related factors among elderly with diabetes. Salmand. 2016;11(1):162–73.

32. Hajian-Tilaki K, Heidari B, Hajian-Tilaki A. Solitary and combined negative influences of diabetes, obesity and hypertension on health-related quality of life of elderly individuals: a population-based cross-sectional study. Diabetes Metab Syndr. 2016;10(2 Suppl 1):S37–42.

33. Gholami A, Khazaee-Pool M, Rezaee N, Amirkalali B, Abbasi Ghahremanlo A, Moradpour F, et al. Household food insecurity is associated with health-related quality of life in rural type 2 diabetic patients. Arch Iran Med. 2017; 20(6):350–5.

34. Mazloomy S, Rezaeian M, Naghibzadeh Tahami A, Sadeghi R. Association between Health–Related Quality of Life and Glycemic Control in Type 2 Diabetics of Sirjan City in 2015. JRUMS. 2017;16(1):73–82.

35. Issa SM, Hoeks SE, Scholte op Reimer WJ, Van Gestel YR, Lenzen MJ, Verhagen HJ, et al. Health-related quality of life predicts long-term survival in patients with peripheral artery disease. Vasc Med. 2010;15(3): 163–9.

36. Lopes AA, Bragg-Gresham JL, Satayathum S, McCullough K, Pifer T, Goodkin DA, et al. Health-related quality of life and associated outcomes among hemodialysis patients of different ethnicities in the United States: the Dialysis outcomes and practice patterns study (DOPPS). Am J Kidney Dis. 2003;41(3):605–15.

37. Mommersteeg PM, Denollet J, Spertus JA, Pedersen SS. Health status as a risk factor in cardiovascular disease: a systematic review of current evidence. Am Heart J. 2009;157(2):208–18.

38. Parkerson GR Jr, Gutman RA. Health-related quality of life predictors of survival and hospital utilization. Health Care Financ Rev. 2000;21(3): 171–84.

39. Schram MT, Baan CA, Pouwer F. Depression and quality of life in patients with diabetes: a systematic review from the European depression in diabetes (EDID) research consortium. Curr Diabetes Rev. 2009;5(2):112–9.

40. Ghafari R, Rafiei M, Taheri Nejad MR. Assessment of health related quality of life by SF-36 version 2 in general population of Qom city. AMUJ. 2014; 16(11):63–72.

41. Baptista LC, Dias G, Souza NR, Veríssimo MT, Martins RA. Effects of long-term multicomponent exercise on health-related quality of life in older adults with type 2 diabetes: evidence from a cohort study. Qual Life Res. 2017; 26(8):2117–27.

42. Nunes-Silva JG, Nunes VS, Schwartz RP, Mlss Trecco S, Evazian D, Correa-Giannella ML, et al. Impact of type 1 diabetes mellitus and celiac disease on nutrition and quality of life. Nutr Diabetes. 2014;7(1):e239.

43. Hervás A, Zabaleta A, De Miguel G, Beldarráin O, Díez J. Health related quality of life in patients with diabetes mellitus type 2. An Sist Sanit Navar. 2007;30(1):45–52.

44. Lindsay G, Inverarity K, McDowell JR. Quality of life in people with type 2 diabetes in relation to deprivation, gender, and age in a new community-based model of care. Nurs Res Pract. 2011;2011:613589.

45. Vázquez VC, González LM, Ruiz EM, Isidoro JM, Ordóñez MS, García CS. Assessment of health outcomes in the type 2 diabetes process. Aten Primaria. 2011;43(3):127–33.

46. Eljedi A, Mikolajczyk RT, Kraemer A, Laaser U. Health-related quality of life in diabetic patients and controls without diabetes in refugee camps in the Gaza strip: a cross-sectional study. BMC Public Health. 2006;6:268.

47. Wubben DP, Porterfield D. Health-related quality of life among North Carolina adults with diabetes mellitus. N C Med J. 2005;66(3):179–85.

48. De Vogli R, Gimeno D, Kivimaki M. Socioeconomic inequalities in health in 22 European countries. N Engl J Med. 2008;359(12):1290.

49. Rubin RR, Peyrot M, Siminerio LM. Health care and patient-reported outcomes: results of the cross-national diabetes attitudes, wishes and needs (DAWN) study. Diabetes Care. 2006;29(6):1249–55.

50. Snoek FJ, Kersch NY, Eldrup E, Harman-Boehm I, Hermanns N, Kokoszka A, et al. Monitoring of individual needs in diabetes (MIND)-2: follow-up data from the cross-national diabetes attitudes, wishes, and needs (DAWN) MIND study. Diabetes Care. 2012;35(11):2128–32.

51. Al-Shehri AH, Taha AZ, Bahnassy AA, Salah M. Health-related quality of life in type 2 diabetic patients. Ann Saudi Med. 2008;28(5):352–60.

52. Ali S, Stone M, Skinner TC, Robertson N, Davies M, Khunti K. The association between depression and health-related quality of life in people with type 2 diabetes: a systematic literature review. Diabetes Metab Res Rev. 2010;26(2):75–89.

53. King IM. Quality of life and goal attainment. Nurs Sci Q. 1994;7(1):29–32.

54. Svenningsson I, Marklund B, Attvall S, Gedda B. Type 2 diabetes: perceptions of quality of life and attitudes towards diabetes from a gender perspective. Scand J Caring Sci. 2011;25(4):688–95.

55. Karimi S, Yarmohammadian MH, Shokri A, Mottaghi P, Qolipour K, Kordi A, et al. Predictors and effective factors on quality of life among Iranian patients with rheumatoid arthritis. Mater Sociomed. 2013;25(3):158–62.

56. Yaghoubi A, Tabrizi JS, Mirinazhad MM, Azami S, Naghavi-Behzad M, Ghojazadeh M. Quality of life in cardiovascular patients in Iran and factors affecting it: a systematic review. J Cardiovasc Thorac Res. 2012;4(4):95–101.

57. Kia NS, Malek F, Ghods E, Fathi M. Health-related quality of life of patients with asthma: a cross-sectional study in Semnan, Islamic Republic of Iran. East Mediterr Health J. 2017;23(7):500–6.

58. Ghiasi B, Sarokhani D, Dehkordi AH, Sayehmiri K, Heidari MH. Quality of life of patients with chronic kidney disease in Iran: systematic review and meta-analysis. Indian J Palliat Care. 2018;24(1):104–11.

59. Heidari M, Ghodusi M. Relationship of assess self-esteem and locus of control with quality of life during treatment stages in patients referring to drug addiction rehabilitation centers. Mater Sociomed. 2016;28(4):263–7.

60. Petitti DB. Approaches to heterogeneity in meta-analysis. Stat Med. 2001; 20(23):3625–33.

20

Islet transplantation improved penile tissue fibrosis in a rat model of type 1 diabetes

Zhigang Wu[1†], Hongwei Wang[2†], Fubiao Ni[2], Xuan Jiang[4], Ziqiang Xu[3], Chengyang Liu[5], Yong Cai[3], Hongxing Fu[4], Jiao Luo[2], Wenwei Chen[6], Bicheng Chen[2*] and Zhixian Yu[6*]

Abstract

Background: Glycaemic control is one of the most effective strategies for the treatment of diabetes-related erectile dysfunction (DMED). Compared to conventional anti-diabetic drugs and insulin, islet transplantation is more effective in the treatment of diabetic complications. The aim of this study was to investigate the efficacy of islet transplantation for reversing advanced-stage DMED in rats and to observe its influence on corpus cavernosum fibrosis.

Methods: Wistar rats were intraperitoneally injected with streptozotocin to establish a diabetes model. After 12 weeks, the rats were divided into 4 groups: diabetic, insulin, islet transplantation, and normal control. Following supplementation, the changes in blood glucose and weight were determined sequentially. Penile erectile function was evaluated by apomorphine experiments in the fourth week, and the penile corpus cavernosum was also collected for assessment by Masson staining, immunohistochemistry and Western blot to observe the spongy tissue and the related cellular changes at the molecular level.

Results: Islet transplantation significantly ameliorated penile erectile function in advanced-stage diabetic rats. The ratio of corpus cavernosum smooth muscle cells to fibroblasts and the expression level of α-SMA in the islet transplantation group were significantly higher than those in the diabetic and insulin groups. In addition, the expression levels of TGF-β1, p-Samd2, and connective tissue growth factor (CTGF) in the islet transplantation and insulin groups were much lower than those in the diabetic group, while those in the islet transplantation group were significantly lower than those in the insulin group.

Conclusions: Our findings strongly suggest that islet transplantation can promote the regeneration of smooth muscle cells and ameliorate corpus cavernosum fibrosis to restore its normal structure in advanced-stage diabetic rats. The possible mechanism of ameliorating corpus cavernosum fibrosis by islet transplantation may be associated with improvement of the hyperglycaemic status in diabetic rats, thereby inhibiting the TGF-β1/Samd2/CTGF pathway.

Keywords: Diabetes mellitus, Erectile dysfunction, α-SMA, TGF-β1

Background

Clinically, diabetes mellitus is one of the most common causes of erectile dysfunction (ED) [1]. The incidence of ED in patients with diabetes is 4 times that in non-diabetic patients. Approximately 50–75% of male diabetic patients have ED, and the condition usually occurs during the early stage of diabetes [2]. Long-term hyperglycaemia not only causes corpus cavernosum blood vessel, nerve and endothelial dysfunction but also leads to penile tissue fibrosis, which damages the structure of the corpus cavernosum and decreases erectile function [3, 4]. Phosphodiesterase type 5 (PDE5) inhibitors are currently one of the most important practical treatment choices for ED; PDE5 inhibitors up-regulate the NO-cGMP pathway to improve vascular endothelial function and promote penile erection [5, 6]. However, patients with diabetes-related ED (DMED) often respond poorly to PDE5 inhibitors, potentially due to apoptosis of cavernosum smooth muscle cells (SMCs) and proliferation of cavernosum fibrous tissue [7]. Among a variety of profibrotic factors, transforming growth factor-β1

* Correspondence: chenbicheng1974@163.com; yuzhixian1979@163.com
†Zhigang Wu and Hongwei Wang contributed equally to this work.
²Hepatobiliary and pancreatic surgery laboratory, The First Affiliated Hospital of Wenzhou Medical University, Wenzhou 325000, Zhejiang Province, China
⁶Department of Urology, the First Affiliated Hospital of Wenzhou Medical University, Wenzhou 325000, Zhejiang Province, China
Full list of author information is available at the end of the article

(TGF-β1) has been regarded as the fibrogenic cytokine most closely related to cavernosum fibrosis [8].

In the early stages, strict glycaemic control is an effective strategy for inhibiting the progression of DMED [9]. Kwon et al. reported that erectile function in diabetic rats can be recovered to near normal levels by tightly controlling blood sugar levels in the early stage of diabetes [10]. However, in other stages, insulin treatment or drug therapy cannot achieve satisfactory results [11]. In addition, maintaining strict glycaemic control in every diabetic patient is almost impossible in clinical practice.

Pancreatic transplantation and islet cell transplantation are currently the most effective methods for clinical treatment of various chronic complications that are associated with diabetes [12]. Compared to pancreatic transplantation, islet transplantation is a simpler operation with a lower risk of morbidity. In addition, recipients can obtain additional donor islet cells through repeated surgeries, to fully restore blood glucose levels in diabetic patients to normal levels [13, 14]. Recent studies have shown that pancreas or islet transplantation can ameliorate and even reverse diabetic complications, including nephropathy, retinopathy and neuropathy in the early stage [15–17]. However, the effect of islet transplantation on DMED has not been reported.

In the present study, we further investigated the significance of the recovery of penile structure and function in advanced-stage DMED rats treated with islet transplantation. We also discussed the associations between the TGF-β1/Smad2 pathway and corpus cavernosum fibrosis.

Methods
Animal model and groups
A total of 42 male Wistar rats weighing 200–220 g were provided by the Experimental Animal Center of Wenzhou Medical University. All rats were housed with a 12-h light/dark cycle at 24 °C ± 1 °C and fed ad libitum for 1 week before starting the study. All animal experiments were approved by the Zhejiang Management Committee for Medical Laboratory Animal Sciences. Diabetic rat models were generated by a single intraperitoneal injection of streptozotocin (50 mg/kg of body weight) in sodium citrate buffer (pH 4.5) after an overnight fast. Plasma glucose concentrations were measured in a drop of tail vein blood using an Accu-Chek glucometer (Roche Diagnostics, Indianapolis, IN). Seven days later, a non-fasted blood glucose concentration ≥ 16.67 mmol/l for 3 days indicated the successful establishment of the rat experimental diabetic model. Twelve weeks after the induction of diabetes, rats were randomly divided into four different groups: diabetes-related erectile dysfunction group (ED group, $n = 6$), these rats were left untreated and studied 4 weeks later; islet transplantation group (IT group, $n = 6$), these rats underwent

islet transplantation under the left kidney capsule and were studied 4 weeks later; insulin treatment group (INS group, $n = 6$), these rats were given insulin (WanBang Pharmaceuticals, JiangSu, China) by subcutaneous injection at 9 a.m. and 9 p.m. every day for 4 weeks (3 U per injection); and a normal control group (control group, $n = 6$).

Islet transplantation
Islets were isolated from rat pancreases using a procedure previously described by our laboratory [18]. Islets from three donor rats were supplied for each recipient. The same procedure was followed for each rat. Briefly, rats were anaesthetized by intraperitoneal injection of chloral hydrate. Then, a laparotomy was performed to expose the pancreas. The location at which the common bile duct meets the intestine was determined and ligated, and 8 ml of collagenase V (0.8 mg/ml, dissolved in Hank's solution) was injected into the common bile duct by retrograde intubation. When the pancreas was fully inflated, it was separated from the surrounding tissues with forceps, transferred into a 50-ml centrifuge tube and digested for 10–15 min at 37 ± 0.5 °C. After digestion, the tissue was washed with Hank's solution three times. Then, the islets were purified by density gradient solutions (Histopaque-1119 and Histopaque-1077) and centrifuged at 2000 rpm for 5 min. The supernatant was poured into a new centrifuge tube and transferred to a black glass culture dish for manual selection. The final purified islets were cultured in RPMI-1640 (Gibco, Carlsbad, CA, USA) containing 10% foetal bovine serum (FBS) (Gibco, Invitrogen, Inc., USA) at 37 °C in 5% CO_2. The purified islets were adjusted to appropriate concentrations in the culture medium and transferred to a small culture dish with a 2-mm lattice for counting under a microscope. According to Lembert and others, the cell clusters were counted, and the diameters were measured with a microscope eyepiece scale. The total islet equivalents (IEQs) were calculated according to the IEQ calculation formula. A single aliquot of 100 freshly isolated islets was aspirated into a 200-μl pipette tip and transferred to a small culture dish. Propidium iodide (PI) and fluorescein diacetate (FDA) were added to evaluate islet activity by FDA-PI staining under an inverted fluorescence microscope. The activity ratio of 100 islet cell clusters was determined to estimate the total number of purified islets. From the final purified islets, approximately 800–1000 IEQs were aspirated into a 1-ml syringe connected to P-50 polyethylene tubing, and the islets were transferred to the head end of the kidney. The recipient rat was anaesthetized by intraperitoneal injection of chloral hydrate; the left flank was shaved, and the kidney was exposed through a small lumbar incision. Capsulotomy of the kidney was performed on the caudal outer surface, and the tip of the polyethylene tubing was inserted and advanced gently under the kidney capsule. The surface of the kidney was kept moist with saline during the procedure. The islets in

the tubing were pushed out slowly and carefully, and the tube was removed when the islets were transferred into the capsule. Then, the kidney was gently replaced into the peritoneum, haemostasis was performed by compression with a cotton swab, and the incision was sutured layer by layer.

Evaluation of erectile function

According to the method reported by Heaton [19], rats in each group were placed in the observation cage after feeding. The room lights were dimmed to a level that allowed observation, and the interior environment was kept quiet, allowing the rats to adapt to the environment for 10 min. Then, apomorphine (APO) was injected in the relaxed neck skin of the rat (150 µg/kg, APO dissolved in 1 mg/kg of vitamin C and physiological saline, with the volume adjusted to 5 ml/kg); each rat was recorded with a video camera during the first 30 min after injection, and the number of penile erections was observed and recorded. Penile erection was indicated by the appearance of the glans penis at the end of the penis. Each rat in each group was tested six times, and the percentage of all rats in the group with erectile function was recorded as the erectile rate.

Histological and immunohistochemical examinations

Rat cavernosum was dissected and fixed with 4% formalin. The tissue in the paraffin block was sliced to a thickness of 5 µm for immunohistochemical staining. To detect the ratio of rat cavernosum muscle to collagen, cavernosum tissue sections were stained with Masson's trichrome stain. For immunohistochemical staining, the slides were incubated overnight with antibodies against caspase-3(CST, 1:200), α-SMA (Abcam, 1:200). The tissue was then incubated with goat anti-rabbit antibody, visualized with diaminobenzidine (DAB, brown colour, ZSGB-BIO, Beijing, China) and analysed with Image-Pro Plus 6.0.

Western blot analysis

The proteins were extracted from the corpus cavernosum and quantified by BCA protein assay (Beyotime, Shanghai, China). The protein extract was electrophoresed on sodium dodecyl sulphatepolyacrylamide gel andtransferred to a polyvinylidene fluoride film, which was blocked with 5% skimmed milk at room temperature for 1 hour. The membrane was incubated overnight at 4 °C with a primary antibody: TGF-β1 (CST, 1:1000), p-Smad2 (Abcam, 1:500), Smad2 (Abcam, 1:500) and CTGF (CST, 1:1000) and then incubated with horseradish peroxidase-conjugated secondary antibody at room temperature for 2 hours. Finally, an electrochemical luminescence system (Amersham, Arlington Heights, IL, USA) was used for visualization.

Statistical analysis

All statistical data are expressed as the mean ± standard deviation. The differences among groups were analysed using one-way ANOVA; a value of $P < 0.05$ was considered statistically significant. GraphPad Prism 5.0 was used for the statistical analyses.

Results

Evaluation of islet activityand islet cells under the renal capsule

As shown in Fig. 1a, islet activity was evaluated by FDA-PI staining with an aliquot of islets before transplantation, and the results revealed a high level of islet activity. Transplanted islet cells under the renal capsule showed high activity by immunohistochemical examination for insulin 4 weeks after transplantation (Fig. 1b).

General characteristics of diabetic rats

Diabetic rats treated with insulin or islet transplantation showed a significant decrease in blood glucose levels and increase in body weight compared to rats that were not treated. Islet transplantation treatment significantly improved the blood glucose level and body weight compared to insulin treatment (Fig. 1c and d).

Islet transplantation restored erectile function

After injection with APO, the erectile response in diabetic rats was significantly lower than that in control rats. The erectile response was significantly improved in the islet transplantation and insulin groups compared to the diabetic group after subcutaneous injection of APO, but the effect of islet transplantation treatment was greater than that of insulin treatment (Fig. 2).

Islet transplantation up-regulated the smooth muscle/collagen ratio and α-SMA protein expression in the corpus cavernosum

Compared to the control group, the smooth muscle/collagen ratio and expression level of α-SMA were significantly decreased in untreated diabetic rats. Insulin treatment significantly improved these parameters compared to no treatment among diabetic rats, but the effect of islet transplantation treatment was better than that of insulin or no treatment. No significant difference was observed in these parameters between the islet transplantation and control groups (Fig. 3a and b).

Islet transplantation reduced diabetes-induced apoptosis in the corpus cavernosum

Compared to the control group, the number of capase-3-positive cells in the diabetic group was significantly increased. No significant difference was observed in the number of caspase-3-positive cells between the islet transplantation and control groups. Insulin also significantly improved this parameter, but the effect was less than that of islet transplantation (Fig. 3c).

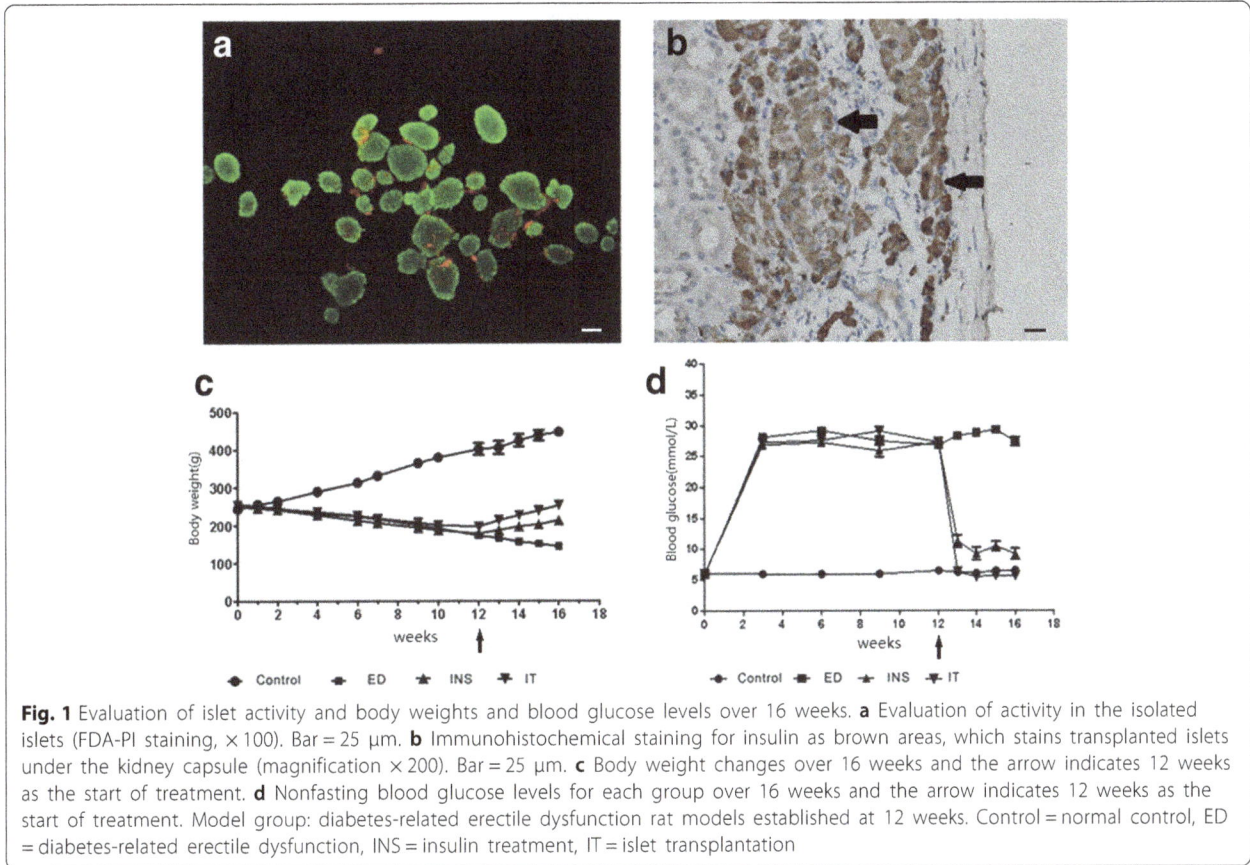

Fig. 1 Evaluation of islet activity and body weights and blood glucose levels over 16 weeks. **a** Evaluation of activity in the isolated islets (FDA-PI staining, × 100). Bar = 25 μm. **b** Immunohistochemical staining for insulin as brown areas, which stains transplanted islets under the kidney capsule (magnification × 200). Bar = 25 μm. **c** Body weight changes over 16 weeks and the arrow indicates 12 weeks as the start of treatment. **d** Nonfasting blood glucose levels for each group over 16 weeks and the arrow indicates 12 weeks as the start of treatment. Model group: diabetes-related erectile dysfunction rat models established at 12 weeks. Control = normal control, ED = diabetes-related erectile dysfunction, INS = insulin treatment, IT = islet transplantation

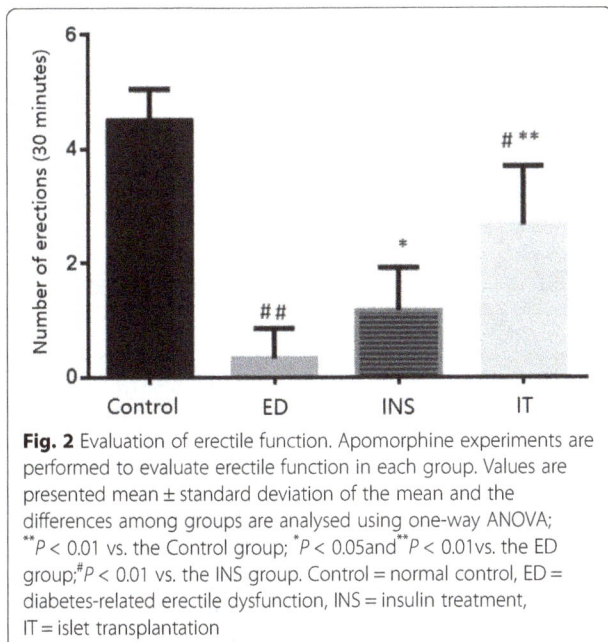

Fig. 2 Evaluation of erectile function. Apomorphine experiments are performed to evaluate erectile function in each group. Values are presented mean ± standard deviation of the mean and the differences among groups are analysed using one-way ANOVA; $^{**}P < 0.01$ vs. the Control group; $^{*}P < 0.05$ and $^{**}P < 0.01$ vs. the ED group; $^{#}P < 0.01$ vs. the INS group. Control = normal control, ED = diabetes-related erectile dysfunction, INS = insulin treatment, IT = islet transplantation

Islet transplantation inhibited diabetes-induced activation of the TGF-β1 signalling pathway

As shown in Fig. 4, the expression levels of TGF-β1, p-Smad2 and CTGF after treatment with islet transplantation and insulin were significantly decreased compared tono treatment in the diabetic rats. However, treatment with islet transplantation suppressed these parameters more significantly than treatment with insulin; no statistically significant difference was found between the islet transplantation and control groups.

Discussion

Long-term maintenance of stable and normal blood glucose levels is a key strategy for the treatment of diabetic ED. Over the past few decades, several studies have shown that pancreas or islet transplantation is an effective method to control blood glucose. Our study was designed to investigate the efficacy of islet transplantation for reversing advanced-stage DMED in rats and to establish whether this treatment is superior to insulin therapy for treating DMED in rats.

In this study, we confirmed that islet transplantation treatment significantly restored erectile function and penile structure in advanced-stage DMED rats. However, the therapeutic effect of insulin was unsatisfactory for recovering

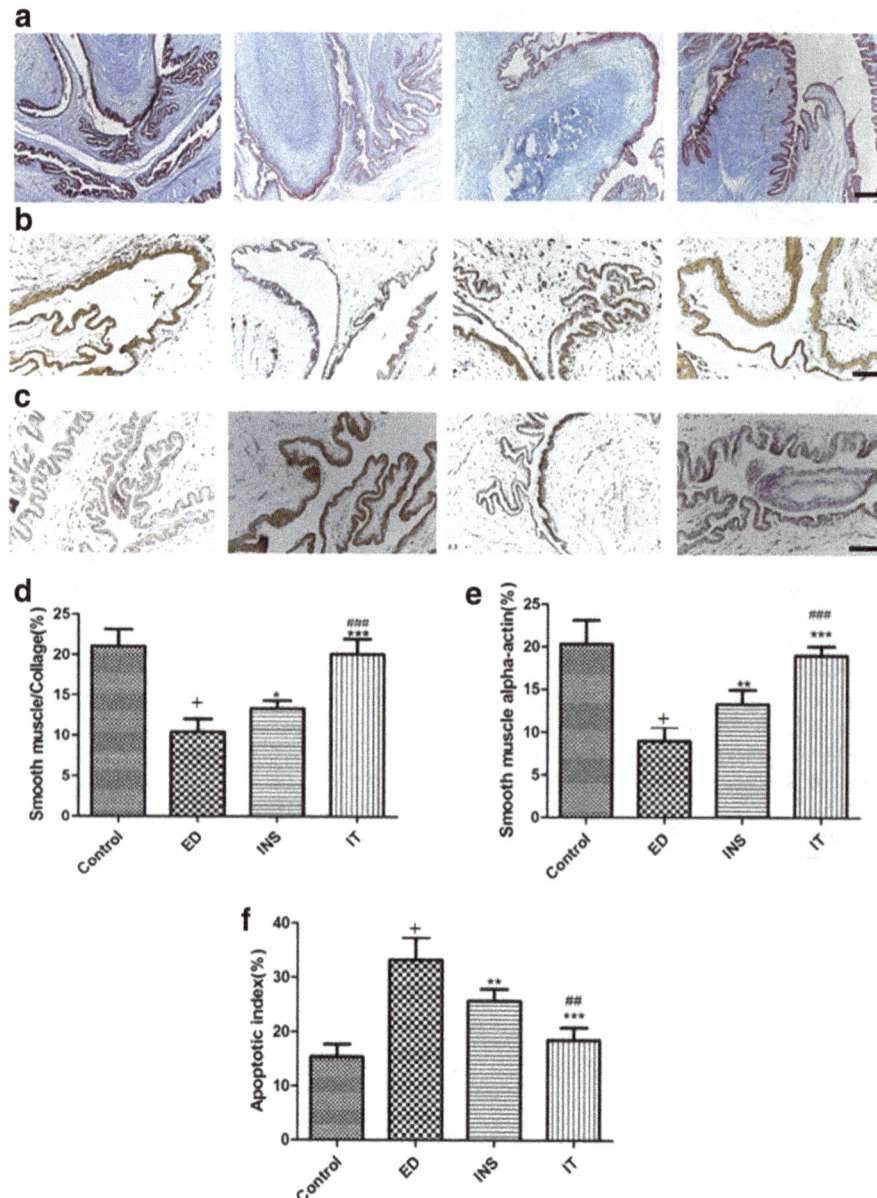

Fig. 3 Masson's trichrome staining and immunohistochemical staining. **a** Penis samples are prepared for the detection of corpus cavernosum tissue fibrosis using Masson's trichrome staining (magnification × 100). The smooth muscle components appeared red colour. The collagen components appear blue colour. Bar = 25 μm. **b** Immunohistochemical staining for α-SMA as brown areas, which stains smooth muscle cell(SMC) in the corpus cavernosum (magnification × 200). Bar = 50 μm. **c** Immunohistochemical staining for caspase-3 as brown areas, which stains SMCs apoptosis in the corpus cavernosum(magnification × 200). Bar = 50 μm. **d** Semiquantitative image analysis of muscle/collagen ratio in corpus cavernosum tissues was performed using GraphPad Prism 5.0 soft. **e** Semiquantitative image analysis of α-SMA expression in corpus cavernosum. **f** Apoptotic index presented as the ratio of apoptotic SMCs (expression of caspase-3) to the total SMCs in corpus cavernosum. Values are presented mean ± standard deviation of the mean and the differences among groups are analysed using one-way ANOVA; $+P < 0.001$ vs. the Control group; $*P < 0.05$, $**P < 0.01$, and $***P < 0.001$ vs. the ED group; ## $P < 0.01$ and ### $P < 0.001$ vs. the INS group. Control = normal control, ED = diabetes-related erectile dysfunction, INS = insulin treatment, IT = islet transplantation

erectile function and penile structure. Furthermore, the present study showed that the detailed mechanisms of islet transplantation were SMC regeneration and structural integrity recovery in penile corpus cavernosum via inhibition of the TGF-β1/Smad2/CTGF pathway.

Although oral PDE5 inhibitors are highly efficacious and safe modalities for ED, patients with DMED frequently respond poorly to these drugs [20]. Strict glycaemic control is still a basic treatment of DMED. Moreover, the effect of glycaemic control is significantly affected by the degree of

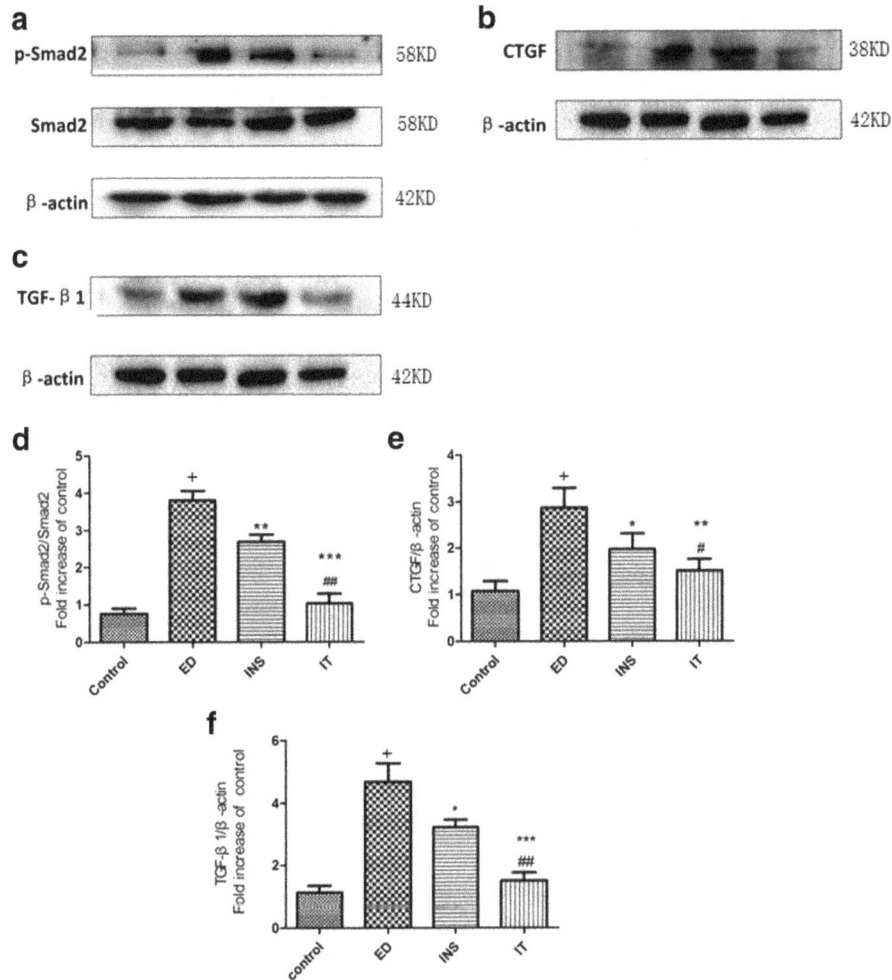

Fig. 4 Western blot analysis. **a** Western blot analysis showing the protein expression levels of P-Smad2 and Smad2 in rat corpus cavernosum tissues. **b** The expression of CTGF is measured by Western blot in rat corpus cavernosum tissues. **c** The expression of TGF-β1 is measured by Western blot in rat corpus cavernosum tissues. **d** Data are presented as the relative density of phospho-Smad2 compared with that of total Smad2. **e-f** β-actin is used as loading control and data are presented as the relative density of CTGF and TGF-β1 compared with that of β-actin. Values are presented mean ± standard deviation of the mean and the differences among groups are analysed using one-way ANOVA; $^+P < 0.001$ vs. the Control group; $^*P < 0.05$ and $^{**}P < 0.01$ vs. the ED group; $^#P < 0.05$ and $^{##}P < 0.01$ vs. the INS group. Control = normal control, ED = diabetes-related erectile dysfunction, INS = insulin treatment, IT = islet transplantation

morbidity and treatment. A previous study showed that early treatment with insulin can reverse early erectile functional changes [9]. In contrast, another study reported that the degree of glycaemic control is likely to be more important than the timing of the initiation of glycaemic control for treating DMED [11]. Clinically, various types of insulin preparations are the most widely used measures of blood sugar control. To date, however, the application of insulin to diabetic patients for strict glycaemic control is limited because patients must manage the risk of hypoglycaemic shock. Furthermore, insulin therapy cannot significantly improve diabetes-related complications in patients with advanced diabetes mellitus. No recovery of penile cavernosum was observed when insulin treatment started later than 12 weeks after inducing diabetes mellitus in rats [21]. Islet

transplantation is the most effective technique for restoring normal blood glucose levels. Yajun Ruan et al. used an APO experiment to detect penile erectile function in 12-week diabetic rats and found that the APO test was negative and used it as DMED. In addition, FENG ZHOU et al. also demonstrated that 12 weeks were sufficient to cause penile erectile dysfunction in diabetic rats [22, 23]. Therefore, in our study, the advanced-stage DMED rat model was established at 12 weeks after inducing diabetes mellitus. Insulin or islet transplantation was administered continuously in the rat model for 4 weeks. Throughout the experiment, islet transplantation could maintain the blood glucose levels of DMED rats in the normal range. However, insulin treatment was not able to maintain stable blood glucose levels. Furthermore, SMCs in the cavernosum account for 40–52% of cells and maintain penile contractility [24]. Chronic hyperglycaemia induces the loss of SMCs and leads to fibrous-muscular changes in penile tissue [25, 26]. Our studies have shown that penile erectile function is improved in advance-stage diabetic rats treated with insulin compared to rats in the DM group; however, the loss of SMCs and the increase in fibrous tissue in the corpus cavernosum were more notable in the insulin group than in the control group. In our study, penile tissues from the islet transplantation group exhibited significantly higher smooth muscle/collagen ratios and higher α-SMA expression levels in the corpus cavernosum than the insulin and DM groups. α-SMA, a typical isoform found in SMCs, is used to evaluate smooth muscle content in the corpus cavernosum [27]. Our study also confirmed that SMC apoptosis was significantly lower in the islet transplantation group than in the insulin and DM groups. Our results suggest that the cavernous structure in the islet transplantation group was similar to the normal structure of the penile sponge. Insulin treatment could delay only fibrosis of the corpus cavernosum, but islet transplantation could promote SMC regeneration, improve the penile cavernosum structure, and ultimately restore erectile function in advanced-stage DMED rats.

Expression of TGF-β1 and its downstream effectors in penile tissues was significantly increased in diabetic rats. TGF-β1 regulates fibrotic effects via activating receptor-associated Smad2 and Smad3, which translocate to the nucleus and modulate the transcription of TGF-β1 responsive genes [28]. TGF-β1 may decrease the elasticity and compliance of the penis by changing the collagen types and increasing collagen synthesis [29]. Evidence indicates that TGF-β1 signalling promotes SMC apoptosis and inhibits the regenerative capacity of SMCs in the penis [30]. CTGF, which is regulated by TGF-β1, is a vital profibrotic molecule in the tissue. Overexpression of CTGF induces fibroblast proliferation, migration, and adhesionextracellular matrix overexpression, and SMC apoptosis. Researchers have also shown that up-regulation of the TGF-β1/Smad2/CTGF pathway might play a key role in fibrosis induction in the penile tissue of diabetic rats [31]. Our studies confirmed that the TGF-β1/Smad2 and p-Smad2/CTGF pathways in the corpus cavernosum were significantly activated in advanced-stage DMED rats. Maintaining adequate blood glucose levels is the most effective measure to inhibit the TGF-β1 signalling pathway in diabetic rats. In this study, we performed immunohistochemistry and Western blotting to determine whether islet transplantation can significantly suppress the expression levels of TGF-β1, p-Smad2 and CTGF in advanced-stage DMED rats compared to those in the other groups. These results are consistent with our previous studies in which islet transplantation could decrease the expression levels of fibrotic factors including TGF-β1 and CTGF, in early diabetic nephropathy. This result may provide a better explanation for the molecular mechanism of islet transplantation in recovering erectile function and the penile cavernosum structure.

There were some limitations in the present study. First, diabetic autonomic neuropathy and endothelial dysfunction are also involved in DMED. Thus, additional studies are required to determine whether islet transplantation plays a positive role in endothelial function recovery and neural regeneration. Second, islet transplantation can also regulate C-peptide secretion. Moreover, combined treatment with C-peptide and insulin had a significant effect on diabetic neuropathy compared to insulin injection alone [32]. Thus, the relationship between C-peptide and DMED should be investigated. In addition, islet cells can also secrete some non-classical islet peptides, such as GLP-1, GIP, xenin, oxytocin secreted by pancreatic islet α cells, and PYY, NPY secreted by islet PP cells, and Urocontin3 secreted by islet β cells. These hormones can regulate the function of pancreatic β-cells and the secretion of insulin, and have great potential in the treatment of diabetic facets [33]. Among them, GLP-1 stimulates insulin secretion, inhibits glucagon secretion, reduces food intake, reduces appetite, delays gastric emptying, reduces body weight, and protects βcells from apoptosis. The American Diabetes Association (ADA) and the European Association for Diabetes Study (EASD), recommend GLP1 agonists as adjunctive agents for metformin when monotherapy fails to meet therapeutic goals. Weihao Wang et al.'s meta-analysis also demonstrated that combination therapy with GLP-1 and insulin can achieve ideal therapeutic effects on glycemic control, weight loss, and insulin dose reduction in patients with type 1 diabetes [34]. Therefore, islet transplantation may improve the effect of fibrosis in penile tissue of diabetic rats by secreting these hormones, which is worthy of further study. Finally, our data demonstrated that islet transplantation improves penile tissue fibrosis 12 weeks after diabetes induction. However, the effects of islet transplantation should be investigated for longer-term DMED.

Conclusions

This was the first study to demonstrate that islet transplantation could promote penile SMC regeneration and restore penile erectile function in advanced-stage DMED rats by inhibiting the TGF-β1/Smad2/CTGF pathway.

Abbreviations

APO: Apomorphine; CTGF: Connective tissue growth factor; DMED: Diabetes mellitus erectile dysfunction; ED: Erectile dysfunction; FDA: Fluorescein diacetate; IEQ: Total islet equivalents; PDE5: Phosphodiesterase type 5; PI: Propidium iodide; SMCs: Smooth muscle cells; STZ: Streptozotocin; TGF-β1: Transforming growthfactor beta 1; α-SMA: Alpha 2 smooth muscle actin

Funding

This project was supported by grants from the National Natural Science Foundation of China (No.81572087), Natural Science Foundation of Zhejiang province (LY17H100005), and Health and Family Planning Commission of Zhejiang Province (2015KYB240).

Authors' contributions

YZX and CBC conceived the study and takes responsibility for the integrity of the data. WZG and WHW co-write the manuscript. WHW and XJ conducted animal study. NFB and XZQ performed evaluation of erectile examinations. LJ and CWW performed histological and immunohistochemical examinations. CY and FHX performed Western blotting. LCY interpreted acquired data. All authors read and approved the final manuscript.

Competing interests

The authors declare that they have no competing interests.

Author details

[1]Department of Andrology, The First Affiliated Hospital of Wenzhou Medical University, Wenzhou 325000, Zhejiang Province, China. [2]Hepatobiliary and pancreatic surgery laboratory, The First Affiliated Hospital of Wenzhou Medical University, Wenzhou 325000, Zhejiang Province, China. [3]Department of Transplantation, The First Affiliated Hospital of Wenzhou Medical University, Wenzhou 325000, Zhejiang Province, China. [4]School of Pharmacy, Wenzhou Medical University, Wenzhou 325000, Zhejiang Province, China. [5]Department of Surgery, Perelman School of Medicine at the University of Pennsylvania, Philadelphia, PA 19104-5160, USA. [6]Department of Urology, the First Affiliated Hospital of Wenzhou Medical University, Wenzhou 325000, Zhejiang Province, China.

References

1. Zhang X, Yang B, Li N, Li H. Prevalence and risk factors for erectile dysfunction in Chinese adult males. J Sex Med. 2017;14:1201–8.
2. Hatzimouratidis K, Hatzichristou D. How to treat erectile dysfunction in men with diabetes: from pathophysiology to treatment. Curr Diab Rep. 2014;14:545–54.
3. Malavige LS, Levy JC. Erectile dysfunction in diabetes mellitus. J Sex Med. 2009;6:1232–47.
4. Lue TF. Erectile dysfunction. N Engl J Med. 2000;342:1802–13.
5. Vickers MA, Satyanarayana R. Phosphodiesterase type 5 inhibitors for the treatment of erectile dysfunction in patients with diabetes mellitus. Int J Impot Res. 2002;14:466–71.
6. Angulo J, Gonzalez-Corrochano R, Cuevas P, Fernandez A, La Fuente JM, Rolo F, Allona A, De Tejada IS. Diabetes exacerbates the functional deficiency of NO/cGMP pathway associated with erectile dysfunction in human Corpus Cavernosum and penile arteries. J Sex Med. 2010;7:758–68.
7. Gonzalez-Cadavid NF. Mechanisms of penile fibrosis. J Sex Med. 2009;6:353–62.
8. Verrecchia F, Mauviel A. Control of connective tissue gene expression by TGF beta: role of Smad proteins in fibrosis. Curr Rheumatol Rep. 2002;4:143–9.
9. Cho SY, Chai JS, Lee SH, Park K, Paick JS, Kim SW. Investigation of the effects of the level of glycemic control on erectile function and pathophysiological mechanisms in diabetic rat. J Sex Med. 2012;9:1550–8.
10. Kwon O, Cho SY, Paick JS, Kim SW. Effects of the start time of glycemic control on erectile function in streptozotocin-induced diabetic rats. Int J Impot Res. 2017;29:23–29.
11. Choi WS, Kwon OS, Cho SY, Paick JS, Kim SW. Effect of chronic administration of PDE5 combined with glycemic control on erectile function in streptozotocin-induced diabetic rats. J Sex Med. 2015;12:600–10.
12. Lundberg J, Stone-Elander S, Zhang XM, Korsgren O, Jonsson S, Holmin S. Endovascular method for transplantation of insulin-producing cells to the pancreas parenchyma in swine. Am J Transplant. 2014;14:694–700.
13. Sutherland DER. Current status of beta-cell replacement therapy (pancreas and islet transplantation) for treatment of diabetes mellitus. Transplant Proc. 2003;35:1625–7.
14. Pepper AR, Pawlick R, Gala-Lopez B, Macgillivary A, Mazzuca DM, White DJG, Toleikis PM, Shapiro AMJ, Diabetes I. Reversed in a murine model by marginal mass syngeneic islet transplantation using a subcutaneous cell pouch device. Transplantation. 2015;99:2294–300.
15. He YQ, Xu ZQ, Zhou MS, Wu MM, Chen XH, Wang SL, Qiu KY, Cai Y, Fu HX, Chen BC, Zhou MT. Reversal of early diabetic nephropathy by islet transplantation under the kidney capsule in a rat model. J Diab Res. 2016;2016:e4157313.
16. Usuelli V, La Rocca E. Novel therapeutic approaches for diabetic nephropathy and retinopathy. Pharmacol Res. 2015;98:39–44.
17. Fensom B, Harris C, Thompson SE, Al Mehthel M, Thompson DM. Islet cell transplantation improves nerve conduction velocity in type 1 diabetes compared with intensive medical therapy over six years. Diabetes Res Clin Pract. 2016;122:101–5.
18. Zmuda EJ, Powell CA, Hai T. A method for murine islet isolation and subcapsular kidney transplantation. J Vis Exp. 2011;50
19. Heaton JP, Varrin S, Morales A. The characterization of a bioassay of erectile function in a rat model. J Urol. 1991;145:1099–102.
20. Carson CC, Burnett AL, Levine LA, Nehra A. The efficacy of sildenafil citrate (Viagra) in clinical populations: an update. Urology. 2002;60:12–27.
21. Cellek S, Foxwell NA, Moncada S. Two phases of nitrergic neuropathy in streptozotocin-induced diabetic rats. Diabetes. 2003;52:2353–62.
22. Ruan Y, Li M, Wang T, Yang J, Rao K, Wang S, Yang W, Liu J, Ye Z. Taurine supplementation improves erectile function in rats with Streptozotocin-induced type 1 diabetes via amelioration of penile fibrosis and endothelial dysfunction. J Sex Med. 2016;13:78–85.
23. Zhou F, Xin H, Liu T, Li GY, Gao ZZ, Liu J, Li WR, Cui WS, Bai GY, Park NC, Xin ZC. Effects of icariside II on improving erectile function in rats with streptozotocin-induced diabetes. J Androl. 2012;33:32–44.
24. Wei AY, He SH, Zhao JF, liu Y, Liu Y, Hu YW, Zhang T, Wu ZY. Characterization of corpus cavernosum smooth muscle cell phenotype in diabetic rats with erectile dysfunction. Int J Impot Res. 2012;24:196–201.
25. Sattar AA, Wespes E, Schulman CC. Computerized measurement of penile elastic fibres in potent and impotent men. Eur Urol. 1994;25:142–4.
26. Gray MA, Wang CC, Sacks MS, Yoshimura N, Chancellor MB, Nagatomi J. Time-dependent alterations of select genes in streptozotocin-induced diabetic rat bladder. Urology. 2008;71:1214–9.
27. Mostafa ME, Senbel AM, Mostafa T. Effect of chronic low-dose Tadalafil on penile cavernous tissues in diabetic rats. Urology. 2013;81:1253–9.
28. Massague J, Chen YG. Controlling TGF-beta signaling. Genes Dev. 2000;14:627–44.
29. Yamagishi S, Inagaki Y, Okamoto T, Amano S, Koga K, Takeuchi M. Advanced glycation end products inhibit de novo protein synthesis and induce TGF beta overexpression in proximal tubular cells. Kidney Int. 2003;63:464–73.
30. Zhang LW, Piao SG, Choi MJ, Shin HY, Jin HR, Kim WJ, Song SU, Han JY, Park SH, Mamura M, Kim SJ, Ryu JK, Suh JK. Role of increased penile expression of transforming growth factor-beta 1 and activation of the smadsignaling pathway in erectile dysfunction in streptozotocin-induced diabetic rats. J Sex Med. 2008;5:2318–29.
31. Zhou F, Li GY, Gao ZZ, Liu J, Liu T, Li WR, Cui WS, Bai GY, Xin ZC. The TGF-beta1/Smad/CTGF pathway and corpus cavernosum fibrous-muscular alterations in rats with streptozotocin-induced diabetes. J Androl. 2012;33:651–9.
32. Johansson BL, Borg K, Fernqvist-Forbes E, Kernell A, Odergren T, Wahren J. Beneficial effects of C-peptide on incipient nephropathy and neuropathy in patients with type 1 diabetes mellitus. Diabet Med. 2000;17:181–9.
33. Khan D, Moffet CR, Flatt PR, Kelly C. Role of islet peptides in beta cell regulation and type 2 diabetes therapy. Peptides. 2018;100:212–8.
34. Li R, Li Y, Y W, Zhao Y, Chen H, Yuan Y, K X, Zhang H, Y L, Wang J, Li X, Jia X, Xiao J. Heparin-Poloxamer thermosensitive hydrogel loaded with bFGF and NGF enhances peripheral nerve regeneration in diabetic rats. Biomaterials. 2018;168:24–37.

21

A qualitative process evaluation of a diabetes navigation program embedded in an endocrine specialty center in rural Appalachian Ohio

Elizabeth A. Beverly[1,2]* ⓘ, Jane Hamel-Lambert[3,4], Laura L. Jensen[1], Sue Meeks[5] and Anne Rubin[6]

Abstract

Background: Diabetes in the United States has reached epidemic proportions and the people of Appalachia have been disproportionately affected by this disease. Strategies that complement standard diabetes care are critically important to mitigate the risk of complications, reduce health expenditures, and improve the quality of life of patients living in rural Appalachia. The purpose of this study was to conduct a qualitative process evaluation of a patient navigation program for diabetes after its first year of implementation.

Methods: The process evaluation assessed how the Diabetes Navigation Program was delivered as well as how it was experienced by the navigators, providers, health administrators, and office staff at an endocrine specialty center in rural Appalachian Ohio. We employed total population sampling to conduct in-depth, face-to-face interviews with all providers, health administrators, staff, and navigators at a Diabetes Endocrine Center. Interviews were transcribed, coded, and analyzed via content and thematic analyses using NVivo 11 software.

Results: Seventeen individuals (providers $n = 5$, health administrators $n = 4$, office staff members $n = 3$, and navigators n = 5) participated in in-depth, face-to-face interviews (age = 44.7 ± 11.6 years, 82.4% female, 94.1% white, 13.3 ± 9.6 years work experience). Fidelity of implementation: The navigation team carried out most of the activities denoted in the Work Plan, therefore the program was implemented somewhat successfully. Qualitative analysis revealed three themes: 1) The navigator addresses sources of health disparities: All participants described the role of the diabetes navigator as someone who is knowledgeable about diabetes and able to identify and address health disparities. 2) The navigators are the eyes in the community and the patients' homes: Navigators offered providers and clinic staff a rare glimpse into the personal lives of patients, which led to the identification of unrecognized barriers. 3) Difficulties with cross-system integration of services: Differences in the organizational culture and vision of the specialty center and navigation office contributed to systemic barriers.

Conclusions: Overall, this process evaluation highlights the importance of coordinating providers, health administrators, medical office staff, and navigators to address barriers to diabetes care. Forthcoming research is needed to document the clinical effectiveness and sustainability of the Diabetes Navigation Program in rural Appalachia.

Keywords: Diabetes, Patient navigation, Qualitative research, Process evaluation, Nursing

* Correspondence: beverle1@ohio.edu
[1]Department of Family Medicine, Ohio University Heritage College of Osteopathic Medicine, Athens, OH 45701, USA
[2]The Diabetes Institute, Ohio University, Athens, OH 45701, USA
Full list of author information is available at the end of the article

Background

Diabetes in the United States (US) has reached epidemic proportions and the people of Appalachia have been disproportionately affected by this disease. Appalachia is a 205,000-square-mile region that encompasses 420 counties in 13 states from New York to Mississippi and includes 32 counties of Ohio [1]. The Appalachian Region is 42% rural, compared to 20% of the US as a whole, and predominantly white (94.6%) [1]. The people in this region battle a poverty rate 1.5 times that of the US average, and suffer from higher unemployment, lower educational achievement, generally poorer health, and lower access to health care [1–3]. In rural southeastern Ohio, diabetes rates far exceed both the national (19.9% vs. 9.4%) [4, 5] and state prevalence (11.0%) [6]. Here, diabetes patients are more likely to have a delayed diagnosis, limited access to health care, lower health literacy, and lower empowerment [7, 8]. Moreover, the Appalachian counties located in southeastern Ohio are designated as economically "distressed," with nearly a third of residents living below the poverty line [1]. For these reasons, patients are more likely to suffer from macrovascular (i.e., cardiovascular disease) and microvascular complications (i.e., retinopathy, nephropathy, neuropathy), adult-onset blindness, lower limb amputation, food insecurity, and depression [8–11]. Thus, strategies that complement standard diabetes care are critically important to mitigate the risk of complications, reduce health expenditures, and improve the quality of life of patients living in rural Appalachian Ohio.

To address these health disparities in the region, we designed the Diabetes Navigation Program. We selected the Patient Navigation model based on empirical evidence demonstrating reduced barriers and improved outcomes for cancer care in marginalized populations [12–14]. Internationally, navigation programs have been developed to address barriers to timely and effective care in underserved populations [15–27]. Patient navigators are trained personnel, with or without a healthcare background, who engage patients on an individual basis to determine barriers to accessing care or following treatment recommendations, and provide information and services relevant to overcoming modifiable barriers, improving access to care, and facilitating self-management [28]. Patient navigators can be nurses, social workers, community health workers, and peers. Navigation addresses targeted barriers via the provision of services that may include assistance with insurance coverage [29], addressing financial barriers [30], removal of medical system barriers [30], disease-specific education [31, 32], health system education [31, 33, 34], care coordination [31], referral to community resources [32], and emotional support. Whether utilizing nurse navigators, social workers, community health workers, or peers, the evidence suggests that

navigator services have broad implications for a variety of healthcare issues, including early screening and treatment for chronic disease, improved clinical outcomes, increased clinic attendance, and reduced hospital admissions and readmissions [15–27]. For the Diabetes Navigation Program, we employed nurse navigators given the importance of understanding the complexities of diabetes and its management.

Diabetes navigation programs have shown reductions in A1C levels [35–42], reduced hypoglycemia [43], increased medical visits to providers [23, 43], reduced hospitalization/emergency department utilization [37, 43, 44], increased diabetes knowledge [36, 38], and increased diabetes self-efficacy [35, 38, 42]. Further, diabetes navigation programs are feasible with high rates of satisfaction and relatively low costs per person [45, 46]. However, to our knowledge, no patient navigation programs have employed registered nurses to address the complexities of diabetes management. Therefore, our Diabetes Navigation Program is the first of its kind to coordinate registered nurse navigators and providers to navigate diabetes patients through and around barriers in the healthcare system to reduce health disparities and ensure timely treatment. Thus, if successful, the implementation of Diabetes Navigation Program may be a promising model to address sources of health disparities in a rural, underserved setting.

As a first step in assessing the feasibility and effectiveness of the Diabetes Navigation Program, we conducted a qualitative process evaluation to assess how the program was delivered as well as how it was experienced by the navigators, providers, health administrators, and office staff of an endocrine specialty center in rural Appalachian Ohio. Process evaluations allow researchers and providers to gain insight into the best practices of the program in order to ensure its effectiveness and sustainability over time [47]. Thus, to support the advancement of the Diabetes Navigation Program, we conducted this evaluation to learn about its successes and challenges after its first year of implementation.

Method

Context – A detailed description of the diabetes navigation program

The Diabetes Navigation Program was a feasibility study designed to produce a set of findings to help determine whether an intervention should be recommended for efficacy testing of nurse navigation for diabetes [46]. The goal of the Diabetes Navigation Program was to improve health outcomes and lower health care expenditures for individuals with diabetes. We aimed to achieve these goals by expanding access to care and enhancing care coordination via nurse navigators. Our Diabetes Navigation Program shared the principles of Harold P. Freeman's model of patient navigation, with an intent to promote timely movement of patients through the frag-mented healthcare system and eliminate barriers to dia-betes care. The nurse navigators addressed the financial, communication, structural, emotional, and sociocultural barriers that prevent or delay timely care. For example, navigators explained diagnostic reports to patients, served as a consistent point of connection, accessed in-surance benefits by filling out paperwork and making phone calls, referred patients to legal services at a civil legal aid firm, referred patients to mental health pro-viders and specialty providers, increased food stamps by filling out paperwork, delivered emergency food boxes, found permanent or temporary housing by contacting Housing and Urban Development agencies, contacted Home Energy Assistance Program programs, provided diabetes education, reduced hospital bills through Hospital Care Assurance Programs, distributed diabetes medication at no or reduced cost, obtained transporta-tion services through public insurance programs, attended medical visits, and offered emotional support. By removing barriers to everyday living, such as having electricity for a refrigerator to store insulin, navigation helps patients with diabetes focus on their diabetes and participate in healthcare decisions. The nurse navigators did not provide any clinical care to patients, rather strictly navigation services.

The target population for the Diabetes Navigation Pro-gram included individuals with type 1, type 2, and gesta-tional diabetes receiving diabetes care from the Diabetes Endocrine Center. The Diabetes Navigation Program serves patients in Athens, Hocking, Meigs, Morgan, Perry, and Washington counties in Ohio. Diabetes rates are significantly higher in each of these counties) [5], compared to the United States prevalence [48]. Recent county health rankings show that the southeastern Appalachian region of Ohio ranks in the bottom half of poorest health outcomes [49]. Further, these counties are designated as health professional shortage areas (HPSA), with no diabetes specialists or hospitals in Perry or Morgan counties [50]. Approximately 46,000 diabetes patients live in these six counties.

The Diabetes Endocrine Center is recognized as the region's major diabetes management and patient care facility as well as an ever-expanding comprehensive clinical research facility for obesity, diabetes, and other metabolic diseases. Care at the center is team-based and patient-centered. The physicians work in concert with nurse practitioners, pharmacists, clinical psychologists, certified diabetes educators, dietitians, and clinical re-search nurses. All of these units are housed in the same facility for the ease of access for the patient. This pro-vides an integrated interprofessional clinical experience and a rich learning environment for future health care professionals. During Year 1 of the Diabetes Navigation

Program, the clinic treated 2124 patients for a total of 5866 visits. Providers at the Diabetes Endocrine Center referred patients with A1C levels $> 7.0\%$ with one or more health disparities to the Diabetes Navigators.

Program leadership

The Principal Investigator (EAB) of the Diabetes Naviga-tion Program was responsible for oversight of all pro-grammatic activity and fiscal responsibilities, including contracting, budget monitoring, implementation of pro-posed activities to accomplish stated objectives and goals, completing strategic planning, and conducting the systematic evaluation of the program to assess the process and outcomes. A nurse manager (SM), who has been doing family navigation for over 20 years in the region, hired and trained all of the navigators. A job description for a full-time equivalent (FTE 1.0) nurse navigator supported by external grant funding was writ-ten and posted online via the University website. Regis-tered nurses from Appalachian Ohio were given priority. Four other nurse navigators were currently employed by the University in the Family Navigation Program in the Community Clinic at the University's medical school building. These navigators included a navigator nurse manager (SM), two nurse navigators (FTE 1.0) specializ-ing in high risk pregnancies, and a part-time diabetes navigator (FTE 0.5) specializing in children and type 1 diabetes. The external grant funded the full-time dia-betes nurse navigator (FTE 1.0) and 0.1 FTE of the navigation nurse manager. The nurse manager then su-pervised the navigators to ensure that the principals and standards of services were consistent with the Patient Navigation Model [13]. Training of the newly hired dia-betes nurse navigator followed an apprentice-based model, which included shadowing the three navigators and working closely with the navigation nurse manager. In addition, the five navigators worked in close proximity at the University in an office suite and could problem-solve challenges collectively. No formal curriculum or training was utilized to train the nurse navigator.

Program recruitment

The navigation leadership team (EAB, JHL, SM, AR) met with local diabetes providers to tell them about the Diabetes Navigation Program and the services that were provided at no cost to the patient. They encouraged the five providers (three physicians, one nurse practitioner, one certified diabetes educator) from the Diabetes Endocrine Center to refer patients who were struggling with glycemic control and diabetes self-management. In addition, they encouraged providers to refer patients with barriers, such as housing issues, transportation, food insecurity, no or lack of insurance coverage, to the program. Providers were instructed to make the referral based on whether or not he/she felt that the patient was reaching individualized diabetes targets as well as to address specific health disparities. Providers asked the patient for permission to provide the referral and the patient signed a release of protected health information form. All pertinent medical information (e.g., A1C, blood pressure, lipid profiles, body mass index, diabetes complications) was sent to the Diabetes Navigation Program with the referral. Initially, providers were instructed to send all referrals from via facsimile (fax) machine. We planned to gain access during Year 1 to the Electronic Health Record (EHR) system from the Diabetes Endocrine Center to improve workflow and communication. If a patient contacted the Diabetes Navigation Program as a self-referral, we obtained permission from the primary care provider for the referral and had the patient sign the release of protected health information form so that we could obtain the necessary medical information.

All five providers from the Diabetes Endocrine Center referred patients to the Diabetes Navigation Program. From October 2015 to October 2016, a total of 39 diabetes patients (mean age = 58.5 ± 16.9, diabetes duration = 12.5 ± 9.0, A1C = 8.9 ± 2.3% or 11.6 ± 1.1 mmol/l, BMI + 36.5 ± 9.1) received navigation services from the Diabetes Navigation Program during its first year of implementation. The patients' most common barriers to diabetes care included finances (84.6%, $n = 33$), food insecurity (76.9%, $n = 30$), mental health issues (71.8%, $n = 28$), vision problems (53.8%, $n = 21$), transportation (41.0%, $n = 16$), lack of social support (38.5%, $n = 15$), housing (30.8%, n = 12), legal issues (30.8%, n = 12), literacy (15.4%, $n = 6$), and domestic violence (10.8%, $n = 4$). Length of involvement ranged from 1 day to 12 months. No minimum or maximum number of touch points (in-person meetings or phone calls – we did not document email or text message exchanges as visits) with the patients was set for the program; all interactions were based on patient need. The range in visits for Year 1 was 2 to 73 (mean = 14.7 ± 10.8). Navigators met with the patients at their homes, public spaces (e.g., libraries, restaurants), physician offices, and the navigators' offices. At the initial visit, the navigator conducted an intake lasting approximately 2 h (e.g., similar to a complete health history in nursing), which included an authorization of protected health information, a personal history, list of family and social contacts, identification of current barriers to diabetes care, diabetes health history, past medical history, medication list, depression screening (Patient Health Questionnaire 9 [51]), diabetes distress (Problem Areas in Diabetes 5 [52]), diabetes self-care (Self-Care Inventory-Revised [53]), and a diabetes care plan checklist (i.e., reinforcing diabetes education, reviewing scheduled medical appointments,

addressing diabetes self-care plan, setting individualized diabetes self-care goals). Follow-up visits were scheduled based on individual needs and urgency of issues. Navigation goals were tailored to each individual patient. Services continued until the goals or needs were met; if a goal or need could not be met, the patient was informed why this was not possible (e.g., unable to stop a house foreclosure). Our program did not have a formal termination of services protocol at the start of the program; we planned to develop a protocol over time that it was informed by patient preferences.

Process evaluation

A qualitative process evaluation was conducted to achieve a deep understanding of the experiences and views of the Diabetes Navigation Program from the perspective of the providers. Our research questions were as follows: 1) Was the Diabetes Navigation Program implemented as designed? 2) What was the role of the diabetes navigator? 3) What were the early successes of the program? 4) What were the ongoing challenges of the program? From October 2016 to December 2016, we interviewed providers, health administrators, and office staff members from the Diabetes Endocrine Center in addition to the diabetes navigators about the successes and challenges of the Diabetes Navigation Program in its first year of implementation. Inclusion criteria for the process evaluation included direct or indirect contact with the Diabetes Navigation Program. We recruited participants via email. The Ohio University Institutional Review Board approved the study (reference IRB protocol number 16 N23). All participants provided written informed consent prior to participation and received compensation for their time.

Sample

The required sample size in qualitative research relies on the quality of the of the information obtained per sampling rather than the number [54]. The logic of qualitative sampling rests not on generalizability or representativeness, but on the notion of saturation, that is, the point at which no new information is obtained. Therefore, sample size is not a criterion for evaluating the rigor of the sampling strategy but, rather, for evaluating the adequacy and the comprehensiveness of the findings [55]. We employed total population sampling, a type of purposive sampling, where the entire population is included in the sample because they have a particular set of characteristics (e.g., specific experience with the Diabetes Navigation Program) [55]. Therefore, we interviewed all of the providers at the Diabetes Endocrine Center who made referrals to the navigators, the office staff who assisted with the referral process and medical chart documentation, the administrators who oversaw the practice, and the navigators. We made the decisions to interview all five navigators, including the three navigators not funded by the external grant, because they assisted with patients who were pregnant ($n = 2$) and patients who had type 1 diabetes ($n = 4$) during Year 1 of the program.

Data collection

The multidisciplinary research team devised and field-tested a semi-structured interview guide with two individuals (see Table 1). An experienced qualitative researcher (EAB) conducted all interviews, asking participants broad, open-ended questions about the role of the diabetes navigator, experiences with the diabetes navigation, barriers to implementation, and early successes with the program. The interviewer used directive probes to elicit additional information and clarify questions. Interviews were conducted at the Diabetes Endocrine Center and University conference rooms, and lasted 20–90 min. All interviews were digitally audio-recorded and transcribed verbatim. The researchers performed quality checks of the transcribed files while listening to the interview recordings to validate the transcriptions. Participants' names and identifiers were removed to protect patient confidentiality.

Additionally, a reflexive journal (written by the interviewer) was maintained during data collection. The purpose of the reflexive journal was to record the interviewer's thoughts, beliefs, and experiences during the research process. The personal notes were used to evaluate the investigator's response to specific interviews. The

Table 1 Interview Guide Questions

1. In your own words, what is diabetes navigation?

2. What qualities make a good diabetes navigator?

3. How might diabetes navigation help patients struggling with their diabetes management?

Probe: Please provide examples of diabetes navigation successes.

4. Please describe your experience with diabetes navigation at the Diabetes Endocrine Center?

Probe: How does diabetes navigation help providers in the Diabetes Endocrine Center?

Probe: How does diabetes navigation not help providers in the Diabetes Endocrine Center?

6. What barriers have you experienced with diabetes navigation?

7. What is needed to improve the diabetes navigation program at the Diabetes Endocrine Center?

Probe: What is the diabetes navigation program doing well?

Probe: What is the diabetes navigation program not doing well?

Probe: How do you propose we improve the diabetes navigation program?

8. Do you have any other comments or suggestions about the diabetes navigation program?

value of the reflexive journal was to reduce personal bias and maintain objectivity [56]. In addition, memoing was incorporated to record ideas and insights regarding the data. Memoing is a form of data coding completed during data collection. Memos were written to connect notations with shared meaning. Such reflections helped the interviewer recognize the need for additional interviewing of the participants [57]. Salient information from the reflexive journal and memoing was integrated into the data analysis.

Data analysis

The multidisciplinary research team consisted of a diabetes behavioral specialist and qualitative methodologist, a clinical psychologist, a public health professional, a registered nurse, and a medical legal provider. Two researchers (EAB, LLJ) analyzed the data using standard qualitative techniques [58]. Specifically, the researchers performed content analysis by independently marking and categorizing key words, phrases, and texts to identify codes to describe the overarching themes [59]. Transcripts were coded and then reviewed to resolve discrepancies. This process continued until saturation was reached; that is, until no new codes emerged. After all transcripts were coded and reviewed, one member of the research team (LLJ) entered the coded transcripts in NVivo 11 software (QSR International, Victoria, Australia) to organize the data to support thematic analysis.

Rigor

To support credibility (validity), we conducted member checks with five participants to confirm participant corroboration [60, 61]. To support transferability (external validity), we described in detail specifics of the Diabetes Navigation Program, our research questions, and the evaluation methodology so that the findings are comparable to other programs [61]. To support dependability (reliability) of the data, an external researcher not involved in the data collection or analysis performed a data audit by reviewing the findings to achieve researcher corroboration [61]. Finally, to support confirmability (objectivity), we tracked the decision-making process using an audit trail [62, 63]. The audit trail is a detailed description of the research steps conducted from the development of the project to the presentation of findings [62, 63].

Results

Seventeen individuals (providers $n = 5$, health administrators $n = 4$, office staff members $n = 3$, and navigators n = 5) participated in in-depth, face-to-face interviews (age = 44.7 ± 11.6 years, 82.4% female, 94.1% white, 13.3 ± 9.6 years work experience; Table 2). Below we present the fidelity of implementation followed by the themes

Table 2 Participant Demographic Characteristics (n = 17)

	Participants n (%)
Age (years)	44.7 ± 11.6
Gender	
Female	14 (82.4)
Male	3 (17.6)
Race	
White/Caucasian	16 (94.1)
Mixed	1 (5.9)
Position	
Navigator	5 (29.4)
Provider	5 (29.4)
Administrator	4 (23.5)
Office Staff	3 (17.6)
Work experience (years)	13.3 ± 9.6

addressing the role of the navigator, early successes of the program, and ongoing challenges of the program. Transcript identifiers are used with quotations indicating participant number and position.

Design

The Diabetes Navigation Program was a single-arm, repeated-measures pilot and feasibility study. Prospective participants were identified by providers at the Diabetes Endocrine Center. Providers referred patients who were not reaching glycemic targets or patients who needed help with barriers to self-care. All patients provided written informed consent and signed a release of protected health information. Participants meeting study inclusion criteria completed a baseline assessment protocol. Those enrolled received diabetes navigation services as needed. Participants completed follow-up assessments at 1-month and 6-months. The Diabetes Navigation Program was a 3-year study. A sample size of 150 was the recruitment goal.

Fidelity of implementation

As denoted in Table 3, the Work Plan for the Diabetes Navigation Program included activities to be accomplished in Year 1 along with anticipated dates, outcomes/results, evaluation/measurement, and partner responsible. The team successfully established the intake assessment, authorization for protected health information, and referral procedures as well as the Institutional Review Board application and consent process. Unfortunately, due to an impending merger between two health care systems, the navigators were not granted access to the EHR system and we had to continue with the fax referral system; medical chart information was sent to navigators via fax; thus this outcome was not achieved. A total of 49 patients were referred to the navigator in

Year 1. Ten patients refused services so exactly 80% of the patients referred were successfully engaged in navigation services; thereby hitting our targeted outcome in the Work Plan for Year 1.

The diabetes navigator had a caseload of 39 patients at year's end rather that the anticipated 50 patients (78% of target met). Thus, we did not hit our process outcome. The nurse navigator provided emotional support (59.0%, $n = 23$) to the patients, increased insurance coverage (53.8%, $n = 21$), food stamps and/or emergency food boxes (38.5%, $n = 15$), diabetes supplies (23.1%, $n = 9$), medical referrals (23.1%, n = 9), reduced hospital bills (17.9%, $n = 7$), diabetes education (15.4%, $n = 6$), legal referrals (12.8%, $n = 5$), permanent or temporary housing (10.3%, $n = 4$), and transportation (10.3%, n = 4), utility repairs (7.7%; $n = 3$). The navigator was able to address 90% of barriers for 35 of the 39 patients (89.7%). The manager of the navigator program coordinated all of the navigators and put in place protocols and policies to differentiate navigation services for the navigators who specialized in high-risk pregnancies as compared to the navigator who specialized in adult diabetes as compared to the navigator who specialized in children with diabetes. Finally, the navigators participated in continuing education unit courses and regular progress meetings with the Diabetes Endocrine Center staff, providers, and administrators. While the program successfully established intake and referral processes and engaged 80% of the referred patients, the program did not hit the patient enrollment target or gain access to the EHR. Further, the navigators were not able to resolve 90% of the barriers for four patients. Therefore, the Diabetes Navigation Program was implemented only somewhat successfully.

The role of the navigator
Theme 1: The navigator addresses sources of health disparities

All participants described the role of the diabetes navigator as someone who is knowledgeable about diabetes and able to identify and address health disparities. Common sources of health disparities discussed by the participants included housing issues, food insecurity, transportation barriers, and financial/insurance barriers. As articulated by one of the navigators:

"Navigation from the stance of a registered nurse is meeting clients where they are in their stage of development and health, and providing them with the tools they need to optimize outcomes. I think navigation involves assessing needs in their social life, in their medical life, mental health, social determinants of health issues, all of those things I think come into play...With our clients, we find that many have no housing or poor housing, substandard

Table 3 Summary of Work Plan for Year 1 of the Diabetes Navigation Program

GOAL: We will establish a Comprehensive Diabetes Patient Navigation Program for Rural Appalachians to improve health outcomes and lower health care expenditures for individuals with diabetes through the development and coordinated implementation of the Diabetes Patient Navigator Program to impact the health care delivery system, individual patients, and inform policy.

Objective One: Establish a Diabetes Patient Navigator Program that serves individuals with diabetes to improve health measures in diabetes clients by addressing barriers to health care and self-care activities

Evaluate Annually: # provider/staff trained to identify and refer patients with diabetes due to poor glycemic control; number of referrals received, % of referred individual who engage navigation services; number and type of barriers identified; number of barriers targeted for interventions; number of barriers resolved; repeated measures of patient health metrics including haemaglobin, blood pressure control (all available), depression symptoms, distress symptoms, self-care (intake, 6 m, 12 m); provider and patient satisfaction (annual). Patient admissions, readmissions and emergency department utilization, annual expenditures; patient improvement measures tracked.

Healthy People 2020: Improve glycemic control; improve blood pressure control; complete dental, eye, foot exams; increase number performing daily self-monitoring of glucose and getting formal diabetes education.

Activities Year One: October 2015–October 2016	Dates	Outcome/Results	Evaluation/Measurement	Partner Responsible
Year 1, Activity 1: Design intake, referral procedures, HIPAA compliant releases at Diabetes Endocrine Center (SYSTEM CHANGE)	May 2015–July 2015	• Intake and referral processes in place; staff trained • Navigator to serve Diabetes Endocrine Center • Obtain access EHR at both	• Workflow within health care practice is reformed to screen and refer patients to Diabetes Navigator • Number staff trained • Referrals made	Diabetes Navigators; Medical practice managers
Year 1, Activity 2: Submit protocol to IRB for approval; consent process established (EVALUATION)	August 2015–September 2015	• Consent forms and measurement tools selected • Data collection processes set	• IRB approval received	Principal Investigator
Year 1, Activity 3: Direct services provided to individuals referred to Diabetes Navigator. (INDIVIDUAL CHANGE)	October 2015–October 2016	• 80% of patient referred are successfully engaged in Navigation services • 90% barriers targeted for intervention that the consumer agreed to address with the Navigator are resolved.	• Process: number and types barriers identified and resolved. Goal to see 50 patients. • Health Outcomes: haemoglobin A1C, blood pressure, exams depression, distress, self-efficacy, satisfaction metrics 3 times year • Cost Outcomes: admissions, readmissions, and ED utilization rates tracked; annual expenditures	Diabetes Navigators
Year 1, Activity 4: Manager of Navigator Program facilitates the coordination of all navigation programs (SYSTEM CHANGE)	October 2015–October 2016	• Protocols and policies in place to differentiate types of navigation services and access • Best linkages of care for patients	• System integration increases the capacity and efficiency of service delivery; Single point of referral established	Diabetes Navigators
Years 1,2,3, Activity 5: Diabetes nurse navigators initiate clinical activity to become Certified Diabetes Educator	Jan 2015–April 2018	• Clinical hours accrued	• Certified Diabetes Educator earned at end of Year 3	Diabetes Navigators
Year 1, 2, 3; Activity 6: Diabetes Navigator and manager participate in consortium members meeting to discuss integration efforts, monitor challenges, improve practices; facilitate integration into Diabetes Institute; develop five year strategic plan.	October 2015–April 2018	• Consortium meetings held quarterly • Strategic planning sessions held • Integration of consortium into larger delivery system and Diabetes Institute	• 100% attendance • Steps identified to integrate with Diabetes Institute • Five year strategic plan written such that it situates to strategic initiatives of consortium partners; and adopted by consortium	Diabetes Navigators, Principal Investigator

housing. Some are in unsafe situations. Some have food insecurity. Some have difficulty with transportation. Some have educational barriers including an inability to read medical text or forms. Some have no insurance, no money to get things that aren't covered by Medicaid, a lot live in risky environments. Many have substance abuse."
[ID 9, Navigator].

Providers, administrators, and office staff from the Diabetes Endocrine Center stressed the complexity of diabetes management and explained that diabetes navigation filled in "gaps" or "holes" to standard clinical care. As the following administrator and provider shared:

"Diabetes is a pretty complex condition. There's obviously certain clinical, individualized types of needs somebody has with diabetes, but beyond that diabetes touches so many parts of your lives. To be able to manage diabetes, you have to sometimes have assistance beyond some of the clinical – standard clinical types of care. So, to me, diabetes navigation is filling in all the other holes left to manage diabetes beyond clinical care."
[ID 6, Health Administrator]

"I see Diabetes Navigation as helping stand in the gap between services as usual that are available through standard medical practice and the other aspects of our life that directly impact our quality of life, and our health, and our ability to make it day-to-day. And I see the Diabetes Navigators as helping folks navigate that intersection between what they need to do for their medical health, but also how that interfaces with their day-to-day lives and the multiple stressors they meet." [ID 12, Provider]

In addition, they discussed the navigators' ability to travel to and from patients' homes to identify and address barriers to diabetes management. These participants recognized that navigators provided services beyond what was conceivable at the Diabetes Endocrine Center, as demonstrated by the following two quotations:

"The navigators go to the patients' houses to see if they have anything in their house – like if they would need a refrigerator. They can go over there and look at their food, they can go over their food, what kind of living [arrangements], what kind of housing. They can help with a patient that is having trouble reading, trouble with transportation, trouble with food, trouble with electric. If they just need more information on nutrition and they don't have the transportation to get

here, the diabetes navigators can go to their home to help them there, or just meet them someplace."
[ID 3, Office Staff]

"A navigator who is trained in healthcare of some sort goes and identifies needs of diabetes patients, whether it be financial or transportation, food acquisition. Some way to improve their care in a way that we aren't able to in the clinic." [ID 17, Provider]

Early successes
Theme 2: The navigators are the eyes in the community and the patients' homes

All participants reported early successes with the Diabetes Navigation Program, from improved glycemic control to increased follow-up to learning about the patients' lives. For example, while only 17 of the 39 patients returned for a 6-month follow-up visit, these patients showed a significant improvement in A1C from baseline to 6-month follow-up via Wilcoxon Signed-Rank Test (mean change: -0.79% or -1.3 mmol/l, $Z = -2.131$, $p = 0.033$). Collectively, participants also acknowledged that navigation provided information about barriers that patients typically did not disclose during medical visits. For example, one navigator described a difficult home situation coupled with challenges administering insulin:

"I can tell you about one patient...she was referred because her blood sugars were out of control...I met her at the clinic she had bruising all over one side of her face and of course the first thing I did was ask her about the bruising. She was being abused by the brother that she was living with at the time. So number one thing was to get her out of that situation, but in doing that I discovered... I took her out to lunch while we were waiting to get her into a shelter and found out that she was not able to add together, the sliding scale together with the other dose. Plus, her eyesight was so poor she could not read what she was drawing up...So we were able to discover things that the clinics can't or don't have time to do."
[ID 10, Navigator]

Providers, in particular, valued the insight navigation afforded them regarding their patients' personal lives, as demonstrated by these two quotations:

"We depend very much on this outreach and many times it's important to understand the patients' circumstances so I view them as our eyes in the community and the patient's home because it helps us understand obstacles that people face and that they don't necessarily share during the medical interview and the history." [ID 2, Provider]

"I think the Diabetes Navigators can be really helpful in bringing the rest of that person into the room with the physician, that this person is not just diabetes with this A1C level, but this is a person who is also a caregiver and has these challenges and is going back to school, or doesn't have sufficient access to healthy food, or needs additional transportation supports to make it to their appointments or what have you. So they can help personify and also overcome some of those barriers." [ID 12, Provider]

Participants described seeing noticeable improvements in patients' self-care and glycemic control, which they attributed to navigators addressing these barriers via access to community resources and constant follow-up with patients. The most commonly discussed resources included enhanced insurance coverage, free or discounted medications, reduced medical bills, and increased food stamps. As one provider stated:

"I've had a couple of patients that really benefitted because they were able to either get more food stamps or they realized they were eligible for Medicaid or they were able to get some resources they may not have had before, which has helped them in other ways because there are a lot of social pieces to diabetes management. And that has helped me in some ways provide better care for my patients." [ID 17, Provider]

Further, providers, administrators, and office staff perceived that the frequent follow-up, in addition to the resources, encouraged patients to adhere to their self-care regimen (e.g., medication, blood glucose monitoring, clinic attendance). As expressed by the following provider and office staff member:

"I think sometimes what's really needed with patients is just knowing that somebody is going to be following up on a frequent basis with them instead of once every three months for appointments. And just having a conversation or looking at their blood sugar logs I think is an amazing way to help people stay on track. And so the navigators have really helped with that. Even going to the homes too and finding out what the family situation is like, what the home environment is like and giving us a little bit of insight into challenges." [ID 16, Provider]

"I've seen patients who've A1cs that have dropped because of the reminder or now that they can come to

their appointments like they should, or they can now afford their medication that they couldn't because of a program that maybe was related to them, or somebody just to remind them how important it is and why." [ID 4, Office Staff]

Ongoing challenges
Theme 3: Difficulties with cross-system integration of services

The Diabetes Endocrine Center and navigators serve the same population; however, the differences in organizational culture and vision contributed to systemic barriers. All participants identified the referral system, lack of access to EHR, patient documentation, and physical location as ongoing challenges to the program. The navigators were employed by the University and not the Diabetes Endocrine Center, and therefore, were not located in the center and did not have access to the EHR. These two logistical barriers contributed to challenges with the referral system and documentation of patient visits. To refer patients to the navigator, providers and staff at the center had to fill out a form and submit medical chart information via fax machine in order to protect sensitive patient data. This process created additional work and frustration for the providers and office staff, as one provider expressed:

"The thing that I find as a barrier for me with referring to navigation is I have to run off progress notes and not only fill out the form, but they want some documentation from the chart because the navigator doesn't have access to it. And that's ridiculous! And that is a barrier for me. Because I get busy and I don't have time to go and run off whatever they need. It needs to be more streamlined and easy to make the referral." [ID 16, Provider]

The fax referral system also led to noticeable delays in receiving referrals. Navigators often received referrals three to five days after the order was placed in the EHR. Moreover, navigators did not always receive medical chart information or the reason for the referral, which left them wanting more information. Navigators explained that they needed to know why providers were referring patients to them so that they could prepare and plan for patient intakes:

"They can be more specific in identifying their needs I think. It would be really nice because I remember getting a lot of referrals that were just a referral with nothing else written on it. I don't know if we could make it easier by making our referral more specific so that all they would have to do that...If you don't have a picture before you go in [navigation visit], it makes it twice as hard and twice as long to get that relationship established... It just makes it much more difficult. So I think that is a major thing. Making things really specific as to why they're doing this referral." [ID 10, Navigator]

The other main challenge identified by the providers, administrators, and office staff was infrequent documentation of navigation visits. They wanted more consistent updates detailing the navigators' progress with each patient, including an assessment of a patient's barriers and the plan to address each barrier. The following quotations from one provider and one administrator communicated these needs:

"When we started doing this, there was no communication back. I would refer someone and not know if they had even touched base with a navigator or what they were doing with them. And it was frustrating... I want to know what issues are identified and I want to know what our plans are to help with those issues. And if it's beyond what we can do for someone, then say it's beyond what we can do for someone. So we can better utilize the program for people we know can be helped." [ID 17, Provider]

"Making sure there is good communication between the navigator and the clinic so that the patient benefits the most from that in the sense that the entire healthcare team understands and knows all the different aspects of what is going on in their care. So it is important that the physician or the nurse practitioner understands and knows that these certain barriers have been taken care of because that might change how they address their care at their next appointment, whether things they choose to address or to congratulate the patient on and encourage them on. So I think communication, making sure that both ways is open and ongoing and documented appropriately." [ID 14, Administrator]

Also, providers and navigators differed on the frequency and types of documentation notes. Providers wanted frequent updates detailing the navigators' progress with each patient, following the SOAP (Subjective, Objective, Assessment, and Plan) note format [64]. However, the navigators collected information that was not typically discussed or observed in a clinic setting, and therefore did not conform to standard patient record documentation. As voiced by one of the navigators:

"I believe the challenges related to communication and availability of the navigator stem from the expectation that we would perform as if we were clinic employees adhering to standardized forms, reporting formats, and agency culture. Because we serve patients from multiple counties, we need the flexibility to communicate in a way that provides information that we feel the provider needs to know and is not usually asked in the clinic setting; information often related to social determinants: living conditions, anything leading to the inability of the patient's ability to adhere to the physician's directions. Often the format that providers use and prefer allows only for the gathering of information typically expected and gathered in a clinic setting. It is likely that the autonomy needed to best provide information for and about our clients can be challenging for stringently standardized environments and our non-formatted information was sometimes refused and not always provided to the physician." [ID 7, Navigator]

Further, patient documentation was faxed to the Diabetes Endocrine Center to be scanned into the EHR. Similar to the referral system, the fax documentation system resulted in delays in receiving and updating documentation of navigation visits. All participants agreed that access to the EHR would improve communication and timeliness of the documentation. The following quotations from one provider and one administrator communicated this need:

"I think the quicker the notes can be provided to the physician's office to be updated in the EHR I think the better off it is. I think a major gap right now, is you have navigators who do not have access to the EHR, so they have to rely on what's been faxed and a referral. So I see it as we have two separate models right now working." [ID 1, Administrator]

"Being able to communicate verbally is really, really helpful. But notes would be great too. And if they did have access to the EHR, we could see their notes because it will be in the chart. But right now you have to look for scanned-in documents on the chart. And it's less likely that you're going to bump cross it." [ID 16, Provider]

Finally, all participants expressed a desire to improve communication, and many suggested co-location as a potential solution to address the difficulties with referrals, EHR, and documentation:

"I think that if they were in the office we could just [say], 'Hey, do you have a minute to touch base with this person?' It would be easier...I think we would get better communication that way. Because then they could even come tell me, 'Hey, this is an issue with this patient I just found out about.' If the navigator was in the office more, we would be able to talk more in real-time." [ID 17, Provider]

"I think co-location and integration are important. I think they [navigators] need to be physically housed in the space so you can have those warm handoffs when you have someone who is in a situation...You can bring them in the room with you so that they can hear what is going on, they can be a part of the care team...where they're meeting with the team regularly and having an opportunity for feedback and information back and forth." [ID 13, Administrator]

Discussion

The purpose of this qualitative process evaluation was to assess the fidelity of implementation of the Diabetes Navigation Program in rural Appalachian Ohio as well as explore its early successes and ongoing challenges. The detailed description of the program and adherence to the activities listed in the Work Plan indicate that the Diabetes Navigation Program was implemented as intended. Overall, providers, administrators, staff, and navigators agreed that the navigation program was beneficial and necessary. They understood that the role of the navigator was to provide a variety of services to address patients' health disparities. Further, they agreed that these services filled in gaps in clinical care that providers, administrators, and staff could not address due to time constraints and logistical barriers. For example, navigators could travel to patients' homes to see their living conditions and what types of foods they had in their refrigerator. This task was not feasible for the providers. In the cancer literature, patients report that navigators fill in gaps in their psychosocial support [65]. As reported in the Work Plan and the interviews, the navigator's initial assessment of the patients' clinical and psychosocial well-being took a considerable amount of time and skill, which is not always conducive to a standard medical visit. However, this comprehensive assessment is well-suited to nurses as they are the medical team members with the most face-to-face time with patients. Early successes of the program focused on the navigators' ability to communicate information about barriers that patients typically did not disclose during medical visits. Providers described navigators as their "eyes to the community and the patients' homes" to help them provide more comprehensive diabetes care. All of the providers, administrators, staff, and navigators reported improvements in patients' glycemic control and diabetes self-care, which they attributed to

the navigators' ability to access new benefits and community resources as well as constant follow-up with patients. This was supported with preliminary data from 17 patients with baseline and 6-month follow-up data. Other diabetes navigation programs have shown improvements in A1C levels [35–42, 66]. Additional long-term follow-up data is needed to confirm these improvements in glycemic control and self-care with navigation services, particularly because of the high rate of attrition at 6-month follow-up observed after Year 1 in the study. High rates of attrition have been observed in other diabetes navigation programs [66], this is likely due to the high number of barriers to care. Currently, we are evaluating the clinical (e.g., glycemic control, diabetes self-care behaviors, diabetes distress, depressive symptoms) and health expenditure (e.g., emergency department visits, hospital admissions and readmissions) outcomes of the 3-year Diabetes Navigation Program. These data will be necessary to determine the value, effectiveness, replicability, and sustainability of the nurse-led Diabetes Navigation Program.

Ongoing challenges of the program included difficulties with cross-system integration of services. Differences in the organizational culture and vision of the specialty center and navigation office contributed to systemic barriers. Lack of access to the EHR and separate physical locations led to frustration with the referral system and patient documentation. In addition, navigation documentation did not conform to standard patient record documentation (e.g., SOAP note [64]). Thus, an agreed upon system for navigation documentation is necessary to improve efficiency and maintain participant satisfaction. The need for effective and clear referral and documentation processes has been reported in prior navigation research [15, 67–70]. While we were not able to provide access to the EHR or co-locate the navigator in the clinics, we were able to resolve the issues with the referral system and documentation of navigation visits. We revised the referral form to include the reason the provider was referring the patient, health disparities the provider would like the navigator to address, current A1C level, and blood pressure. For the documentation form, we included the patient barriers, the services provided, the diabetes education that was reinforced by the navigator, any progress that was made, the number of visits accompanied with dates, the next scheduled appointment, and the overall status of the case. These forms have been well received by the providers and navigators and we will continue to use them indefinitely (See Figs. 1 and 2). The process evaluation enabled the team to identify challenges to the referral system and documentation of navigation visits, and proactively address them in order to facilitate cross-system integration of services.

Diabetes Navigator Referral Form

Date_____   DOB: _____

Client Name: _____

Address: _____ City: _____ Zip: _____

Gender (Circle One)

M   F

Home Phone: _____ Cell: _____ Work: _____

Referring Provider Information

Referring Agency/Person: _____

Primary Care Provider: _____

Required Referral Information

Medical Info: A1C _____   BP _____

Please check known patient barriers you would like the navigator to address:

[ ] Transportation

[ ] Depression/Mental health referrals

[ ] Financial or other assistance related to insurance, food, housing, access to medication

[ ] Missed medical appointments

[ ] Assistance in understanding or following nutrition education already provided

 [ ] Assistance in understanding insulin or other medication adherence as prescribed

[ ] Other: _____

[ ] Client is aware of reason for referral

Caregiver's Name (If applicable): _____

Comments: _____

Fig. 1 Sample Provider Referral Form to Diabetes Navigator

Limitations

Study limitations include the homogeneity of the study sample with regards to setting, sample size, race/ethnicity, and self-reported data. The study was conducted at one endocrine specialty center located in rural Appalachian Ohio, with a small number of providers, administrators, office staff, and navigators. Further, the study sample was predominantly white, which is reflective of the racial and ethnic distribution in rural Appalachian Ohio (94.6% white [1]). Next, self-reported data were vulnerable to social desirability bias. To minimize bias, the researchers informed participants that their responses were confidential and could not be linked back to their personal identity. The researchers also emphasized the voluntary nature of participation and explicitly informed the participants that their responses had no bearing on their employment status. Also, we utilized nurse navigators in our program to address the medical complexities of diabetes and its complications. However, the salary of a registered nurse is substantially higher than a community health worker or peer. Thus, the sustainability of nurse-led navigation program may be difficult. In addition, resource limited areas tend to be health professional shortage areas and staffing a navigation program with

Diabetes Navigator Documentation Form

Patient Name: _____ DOB: _____ Gender: M F

Date Referral Received: _____ From: _____

Patient contact: Attempt 1 date:_____ Outcome: _____
              Attempt 2 date:_____ Outcome: _____
              Attempt 3 date:_____ Outcome: _____

Intake appointment date: _____ Attended DNKA Rescheduled: _____

Medical needs: A1C: _____ Blood pressure: _____

Social determinant needs identified:

Transportation	Housing
Depression/Mental Health	Medical bills
Insurance coverage	Utility repairs
Getting fresh, affordable food	Missed medical appointments
Paying for medications	Legal issues
Other: _____	Other: _____

Services provided:

Social Security Extra Help Program	MLP referral
HCAP	Cincy Smiles
PIPP	Food stamps
HEAP	Emergency food box
Other: _____	Other: _____

Education reinforced: _____

_____

Progress: _____

_____

Follow-up date: _____ Phone Meeting

Case open   Case closed   Referrals pending: _____

Signature Line: _____ Date_____

Fig. 2 Sample Diabetes Navigator Documentation Form

nurses may not be feasible. Along those lines, the Diabetes Navigation Program was designed and implemented via a partnership with Ohio University and the Diabetes Endocrine Center in a rural and underserved region in Appalachian Ohio. Most rural and underserved regions in the United States and other countries may not have specialty endocrine centers or universities to help coordinate a navigation program. These regions and countries would benefit greatly from partnerships with local county health departments or ministries. In addition, funding from rural health or global health programs would support additional personnel to provide navigation services and monitor outcomes. Finally, the Diabetes Navigation Program did not utilize a written curriculum to train the nurse navigators or include a formal assessment to assess the navigator's competency or skill set. Future programs should include written curriculum and competency-based assessments to ensure the integrity of the program.

Conclusions

Poverty, rural isolation, lack of public transportation, limited specialty providers, fragmentation of care, and a general lack of access to services continue to separate Appalachian families from the services they need. These findings highlight the importance of coordinating providers, health administrators, medical office staff, and navigators to address barriers to diabetes care in rural Appalachia. The qualitative nature of this process evaluation study allowed for an in-depth understanding of the successes and challenges of the Diabetes Navigation Program. These findings may be useful to other providers and researchers involved in designing and implementing patient navigation programs. For example, this study showed that navigators are able to report unrecognized barriers by traveling to and from patients' homes, access additional benefits and community resources, and serve as a consistent point of connection in between clinic appointments. This study also identified important challenges for providers and researchers to consider; specifically, a mutually beneficial referral and documentation system to facilitate open lines of communication. Finally, long-term follow-up assessing the clinical and health expenditure outcomes is needed to determine the feasibility, cost-effectiveness, and reproducibility of the Diabetes Navigation Program.

Acknowledgements
We thank the participants who shared their experiences and perceptions with us.

Funding
This work was supported by Health Resources & Services Administration (HRSA) Grant No. D04RH28409, The Ohio University Heritage College of Osteopathic Medicine, & The Ohio University Diabetes Institute.

Authors' contributions
EAB, JHL, SM, and AR provided substantial contributions to conception and design of the study; EAB acquired the data; EAB and LLJ conducted the qualitative data analysis; EAB and LLJ provided substantial contributions to the interpretation of data; EAB drafted the article; EAB, JHL, LLJ, SM, and AR revised the article critically for important intellectual content; and EAB, JHL, LLJ, SM, and AR gave final approval of the version of the article to be published.

Competing interests
The authors declare that they have no competing interests.

Author details
[1]Department of Family Medicine, Ohio University Heritage College of Osteopathic Medicine, Athens, OH 45701, USA. [2]The Diabetes Institute, Ohio University, Athens, OH 45701, USA. [3]Department of Pediatric Psychology, Nationwide Children's Hospital, Westerville, OH 43081, USA. [4]Department of Clinical Pediatrics, Ohio State University, Columbus, OH 43210, USA. [5]Community Service Programs, Ohio University Heritage College of Osteopathic Medicine, Athens, OH, USA. [6]Southeastern Ohio Legal Services, Athens, OH, USA.

References
1. County Economic Status and Distressed Areas in Appalachia [https://www.arc.gov/appalachian_region/CountyEconomicStatusandDistressed AreasinAppalachia.asp].
2. Johnson L, Milazzo L, Denham SA. Strengthening communities to prevent diabetes in rural Appalachia's vulnerable populations. Athens, Ohio: Voinovich School of Leadership and Public Affairs, Ohio University; 2011.
3. Johnson L, Denham SA. Diabetes: a family matter: evaluation year one implementation. Athens, Ohio: Voinovich School, Ohio University; 2010. p. 1–17.
4. Prevention CfDCa, National Diabetes Statistics Report, 2014. Atlanta, GA: U.S. Department of Health and Human Services, Centers for Disease Control and Prevention; 2014.
5. Ruhil A, Johnson L, Cook K, Trainer M, Beverly EA, Olson M, Wilson N, Berryman DE. What Does Diabetes Look Like in our Region: A Summary of the Regional Diabetes Needs Assessment Study. Athens, OH: The Diabetes Insitute; 2017.
6. Ohio 2015 BRFSS Annual Report. Columbus, OH: Chronic Disease Epidemiology and Evaluation Section, Bureau of Health Promotion, Ohio Department of Health; 2017.
7. Zaugg SD, Dogbey G, Collins K, Reynolds S, Batista C, Brannan G, Shubrook JH. Diabetes numeracy and blood glucose control: association with type of diabetes and source of care. Clin Diabetes. 2014;32(4):152–7.
8. de Groot M, Doyle T, Hockman E, Wheeler C, Pinkerman B, Shubrook J, Gotfried R, Schwartz F. Depression among type 2 diabetes rural Appalachian clinic attendees. Diabetes Care. 2007;30(6):1602–4.
9. Schwartz F, Ruhil AV, Denham S, Shubrook J, Simpson C, Boyd SL. High self-reported prevalence of diabetes mellitus, heart disease, and stroke in 11 counties of rural Appalachian Ohio. J Rural Health. 2009;25(2):226–30.
10. Brown KA, Holben DH, Shubrook JH, Schwartz FL. Glycemic control, food access and produce intake/behaviors of individuals with diabetes in rural Appalachian Ohio. J Acad Nutr Diet. 2012;112((9):A90.
11. Holben DH, Pheley AM. Diabetes risk and obesity in food-insecure households in rural Appalachian Ohio. Prev Chronic Dis. 2006;3(3):A82.
12. Freeman HP, Rodriguez RL. History and principles of patient navigation. Cancer. 2011;117(15 Suppl):3539–42.
13. Freeman HP. A model patient navigation program. Oncology Issues. 2004;19:44–6.
14. Wells KJ, Battaglia TA, Dudley DJ, Garcia R, Greene A, Calhoun E, Mandelblatt JS, Paskett ED, Raich PC, Patient Navigation Research P. Patient navigation: state of the art or is it science? Cancer. 2008;113(8):1999–2010.
15. Valaitis RK, Carter N, Lam A, Nicholl J, Feather J, Cleghorn L. Implementation and maintenance of patient navigation programs linking primary care with community-based health and social services: a scoping literature review. BMC Health Serv Res. 2017;17(1):116.
16. Freeman HP. Patient navigation: a community centered approach to reducing cancer mortality. J Cancer Educ. 2006;21(1 Suppl):S11–4.
17. Nguyen TU, Kagawa-Singer M. Overcoming barriers to cancer care through health navigation programs. Semin Oncol Nurs. 2008;24(4):270–8.
18. Dohan D, Schrag D. Using navigators to improve care of underserved patients: current practices and approaches. Cancer. 2005;104(4):848–55.
19. Manderson B, McMurray J, Piraino E, Stolee P. Navigation roles support chronically ill older adults through healthcare transitions: a systematic review of the literature. Health Soc Care Community. 2012;20(2):113–27.
20. Esperat MC, Flores D, McMurry L, Feng D, Song H, Billings L, Masten Y. Transformacion Para Salud: a patient navigation model for chronic disease self-management. Online J Issues Nurs. 2012;17(2):2.
21. Pesut B, Hooper B, Jacobsen M, Nielsen B, Falk M, O'Connor BP. Nurse-led navigation to provide early palliative care in rural areas: a pilot study. BMC Palliat Care. 2017;16(1):37.
22. Rice K, Gressard L, DeGroff A, Gersten J, Robie J, Leadbetter S, Glover-Kudon R, Butterly L. Increasing colonoscopy screening in disparate populations: results from an evaluation of patient navigation in the New Hampshire colorectal cancer screening program. Cancer. 2017;123:3356–66.
23. Wang ML, Gallivan L, Lemon SC, Borg A, Ramirez J, Figueroa B, McGuire A, Rosal MC. Navigating to health: evaluation of a community health center patient navigation program. Prev Med Rep. 2015;2:664–8.
24. Jolly SE, Navaneethan SD, Schold JD, Arrigain S, Konig V, Burrucker YK, Hyland J, Dann P, Tucky BH, Sharp JW, et al. Development of a chronic kidney disease patient navigator program. BMC Nephrol. 2015;16:69.
25. Trooskin SB, Poceta J, Towey CM, Yolken A, Rose JS, Luqman NL, Preston TW, Chan PA, Beckwith C, Feller SC, et al. Results from a geographically focused, community-based HCV screening, linkage-to-care and patient navigation program. J Gen Intern Med. 2015;30(7):950–7.
26. Balaban RB, Galbraith AA, Burns ME, Vialle-Valentin CE, Larochelle MR, Ross-Degnan D. A patient navigator intervention to reduce hospital readmissions among high-risk safety-net patients: a randomized controlled trial. J Gen Intern Med. 2015;30(7):907–15.
27. Battaglia TA, McCloskey L, Caron SE, Murrell SS, Bernstein E, Childs A, Jong H, Walker K, Bernstein J. Feasibility of chronic disease patient navigation in an urban primary care practice. J Ambul Care Manage. 2012;35(1):38–49.
28. McBrien KA, Ivers N, Barnieh L, Bailey JJ, Lorenzetti DL, Nicholas D, Tonelli M, Hemmelgarn B, Lewanczuk R, Edwards A, et al. Patient navigators for people with chronic disease: a systematic review. PLoS One. 2018;13(2):e0191980.
29. Darnell JS. Navigators and assisters: two case management roles for social workers in the affordable care act. Health Soc Work. 2013;38(2):123–6.
30. Freeman HP. The history, principles, and future of patient navigation: commentary. Semin Oncol Nurs. 2013;29(2):72–5.

31. Fischer SM, Sauaia A, Kutner JS. Patient navigation: a culturally competent strategy to address disparities in palliative care. J Palliat Med. 2007;10(5):1023–8.

32. Shlay JC, Barber B, Mickiewicz T, Maravi M, Drisko J, Estacio R, Gutierrez G, Urbina C. Reducing cardiovascular disease risk using patient navigators, Denver, Colorado, 2007-2009. Prev Chronic Dis. 2011;8(6):A143.

33. Goff SL, Pekow PS, White KO, Lagu T, Mazor KM, Lindenauer PK. IDEAS for a healthy baby--reducing disparities in use of publicly reported quality data: study protocol for a randomized controlled trial. Trials. 2013;14:244.

34. Scott LB, Gravely S, Sexton TR, Brzostek S, Brown DL. Examining the effect of a patient navigation intervention on outpatient cardiac rehabilitation awareness and enrollment. J Cardiopulm Rehabil Prev. 2013;33(5):281–91.

35. Billimek J, Guzman H, Angulo MA. Effectiveness and feasibility of a software tool to help patients communicate with doctors about problems they face with their medication regimen (EMPATHy): study protocol for a randomized controlled trial. Trials. 2015;16:145.

36. Corkery E, Palmer C, Foley ME, Schechter CB, Frisher L, Roman SH. Effect of a bicultural community health worker on completion of diabetes education in a Hispanic population. Diabetes Care. 1997;20(3):254–7.

37. Svoren BM, Butler D, Levine BS, Anderson BJ, Laffel LM. Reducing acute adverse outcomes in youths with type 1 diabetes: a randomized, controlled trial. Pediatrics. 2003;112(4):914–22.

38. Spencer MS, Rosland AM, Kieffer EC, Sinco BR, Valerio M, Palmisano G, Anderson M, Guzman JR, Heisler M. Effectiveness of a community health worker intervention among African American and Latino adults with type 2 diabetes: a randomized controlled trial. Am J Public Health. 2011;101(12):2253–60.

39. Thom DH, Ghorob A, Hessler D, De Vore D, Chen E, Bodenheimer TA. Impact of peer health coaching on glycemic control in low-income patients with diabetes: a randomized controlled trial. Ann Fam Med. 2013;11(2):137–44.

40. Prezio EA, Cheng D, Balasubramanian BA, Shuval K, Kendzor DE, Culica D. Community diabetes education (CoDE) for uninsured Mexican Americans: a randomized controlled trial of a culturally tailored diabetes education and management program led by a community health worker. Diabetes Res Clin Pract. 2013;100(1):19–28.

41. Carrasquillo O, Lebron C, Alonzo Y, Li H, Chang A, Kenya S. Effect of a community health worker intervention among Latinos with poorly controlled type 2 diabetes: the Miami healthy heart initiative randomized clinical trial. JAMA Intern Med. 2017;177(7):948–54.

42. Loskutova NY, Tsai AG, Fisher EB, LaCruz DM, Cherrington AL, Harrington TM, Turner TJ, Pace WD. Patient navigators connecting patients to community resources to improve diabetes outcomes. J Am Board Fam Med. 2016;29(1):78–89.

43. Laffel LM, Brackett J, Ho J, Anderson BJ. Changing the process of diabetes care improves metabolic outcomes and reduces hospitalizations. Qual Manag Health Care. 1998;6(4):53–62.

44. Gary TL, Batts-Turner M, Yeh HC, Hill-Briggs F, Bone LR, Wang NY, Levine DM, Powe NR, Saudek CD, Hill MN, et al. The effects of a nurse case manager and a community health worker team on diabetic control, emergency department visits, and hospitalizations among urban African Americans with type 2 diabetes mellitus: a randomized controlled trial. Arch Intern Med. 2009;169(19):1788–94.

45. Schoenberg NE, Ciciurkaite G, Greenwood MK. Community to clinic navigation to improve diabetes outcomes. Prev Med Rep. 2017;5:75–81.

46. Bowen DJ, Kreuter M, Spring B, Cofta-Woerpel L, Linnan L, Weiner D, Bakken S, Kaplan CP, Squiers L, Fabrizio C, et al. How we design feasibility studies. Am J Prev Med. 2009;36(5):452–7.

47. Linnan L, Steckler A. Process evaluation for public health interventions and research. San Francisco, CA: Jossey-Bass; 2002.

48. National Diabetes Statistics Report, 2017. Atlanta, GA: Centers for Disease Control and Prevention; 2017.

49. County Health Rankings [http://www.countyhealthrankings.org/app/ohio/2017/rankings/outcomes/overall].

50. Health Professional Shortage Areas (HPSAs). In. Columbus, OH: Ohio Department of Health; 2014.

51. Kroenke K, Spitzer RL, Williams JB. The PHQ-9: validity of a brief depression severity measure. J Gen Intern Med. 2001;16(9):606–13.

52. McGuire BE, Morrison TG, Hermanns N, Skovlund S, Eldrup E, Gagliardino J, Kokoszka A, Matthews D, Pibernik-Okanovic M, Rodriguez-Saldana J, et al. Short-form measures of diabetes-related emotional distress: the problem areas in diabetes scale (PAID)-5 and PAID-1. Diabetologia. 2010;53(1):66–9.

53. Weinger K, Butler HA, Welch GW, La Greca AM. Measuring diabetes self-care: a psychometric analysis of the self-care inventory-revised with adults. Diabetes Care. 2005;28(6):1346–52.

54. Sandelowski M. Sample size in qualitative research. Res Nurs Health. 1995;18(2):179–83.

55. Patton MQ. Qualitative evaluation and research methods. 2nd ed. Newbury Park: Sage; 1990.

56. Speziale HJ, Carpenter DR. Qualitative research in nursing: advancing the humanistic imperative. Philadelphia: Lippincott, Williams, & Wilkins; 2003.

57. Roper JM, Shapira J. Ethnography in nursing research. Thousand Oaks, California: Sage publications, Inc.; 2000.

58. Krueger RA, Casey MA. Focus groups: a practical guide for applied research. 3rd ed. Thousand Oaks, CA: Sage Publications, Inc.; 2000.

59. Krippendorf K. Content analysis: an introduction to its methodology. 2nd ed. Thousand Oaks, CA: Sage Publications, Inc.; 2004.

60. Denzin N. The research act: a theoretical introduction to sociological methods. 2nd ed. New York City: McGraw-Hill; 1978.

61. Trochim W, Donnelly JP, Arora K. Research methods: the essential Knowledge Base. 2nd ed. Boston, MA: Cengage Learning; 2016.

62. Miles M, Huberman A. Qualitative Data Analysis: An Expanded Sourcebook. 2nd ed. Thousand Oaks, California: SAGE Publications, Inc.; 1994.

63. Lincoln Y, Guba E. Naturalistic inquiry. New York: Sage Publications; 1985.

64. Jacobs L. Interview with Lawrence weed, MD- the father of the problem-oriented medical record looks ahead. Perm J. 2009;13(3):84–9.

65. Phillips S, Nonzee N, Tom L, Murphy K, Hajjar N, Bularzik C, Dong X, Simon MA. Patient navigators' reflections on the navigator-patient relationship. J Cancer Educ. 2014;29(2):337–44.

66. Horny M, Glover W, Gupte G, Saraswat A, Vimalananda V, Rosenzweig J. Patient navigation to improve diabetes outpatient care at a safety-net hospital: a retrospective cohort study. BMC Health Serv Res. 2017;17(1):759.

67. Spiro A, Oo SA, Marable D, Collins JP. A unique model of the community health worker: the MGH Chelsea community health improvement team. Fam Community Health. 2012;35(2):147–60.

68. Wolff JL, Rand-Giovannetti E, Palmer S, Wegener S, Reider L, Frey K, Scharfstein D, Boult C. Caregiving and chronic care: the guided care program for families and friends. J Gerontol A Biol Sci Med Sci. 2009;64((7):785–91.

69. Kramer A, Nosbusch JM, Rice J. Safe mom, safe baby: a collaborative model of care for pregnant women experiencing intimate partner violence. J Perinat Neonatal Nurs. 2012;26(4):307–16. quiz p 317–308

70. Anderson JE, Larke SC. Navigating the mental health and addictions maze: a community-based pilot project of a new role in primary mental health care. Ment Health Fam Med. 2009;6(1):15–9.

22

Comparison of health-related quality of Life (HRQOL) among patients with pre-diabetes, diabetes and normal glucose tolerance, using the 15D-HRQOL questionnaire in Greece: the DEPLAN study

Konstantinos Makrilakis[1][*] [iD], Stavros Liatis[1], Afroditi Tsiakou[1], Chryssoula Stathi[1], Eleftheria Papachristoforou[1], Despoina Perrea[2], Nicholas Katsilambros[1,2], Nikolaos Kontodimopoulos[3] and Dimitrios Niakas[1,3]

Abstract

Background: Diabetes mellitus is usually preceded by a pre-diabetic stage before the clinical presentation of the disease, the influence of which on persons' quality of life is not adequately elucidated. The purpose of this study was to compare the Health-Related Quality of Life (HRQOL) of persons with pre-diabetes with that of diabetes or normal glucose tolerance (NGT), using the validated HRQOL-15D questionnaire.

Methods: The HRQOL-15D scores of 172 people with pre-diabetes (108 with Impaired Fasting Glucose [IFG], 64 with Impaired Glucose Tolerance [IGT], aged 58.3 ± 10.3 years) and 198 with NGT (aged 54.4 ± 10.1 years) from the Greek part of the DEPLAN study (Diabetes in Europe - Prevention using Lifestyle, Physical Activity and Nutritional Intervention), were compared to 100 diabetes patients' scores (aged 60.9 ± 12.5 years, diabetes duration 17.0 ± 10.0 years, HbA1c 7.2 ± 1.2%), derived from the outpatient Diabetes Clinic of a University Hospital.

Results: The diabetes patients' HRQOL-15D score (0.8605) was significantly lower than the pre-diabetes' (0.9008) and the controls' (0.9092) ($p < 0.001$). There were no differences in the total score between the controls and the group with pre-diabetes. However, examination of individual parameters of the score showed that people with IGT had lower scores compared to the control group, as related to the parameters of "mobility" and "psychological distress". No differences were found in any component of the HRQOL-15D score between the control group and the IFG group, nor between the two groups with pre-diabetes (IFG vs. IGT).

Conclusions: Persons with pre-diabetes had a similar HRQOL score with healthy individuals, and a higher score than persons with diabetes. Specific components of the score, however, were lower in the IGT group compared to the controls. These findings help clarify the issue of HRQOL of persons with pre-diabetes and its possible impact on prevention.

Keywords: Diabetes mellitus, Pre-diabetes, Quality of life, HRQOL-15D questionnaire

* Correspondence: kmakrila@med.uoa.gr
[1]First Department of Propaedeutic Medicine, National and Kapodistrian University of Athens Medical School, Laiko General Hospital, 17 Ag. Thoma St, 11527 Athens, Greece
Full list of author information is available at the end of the article

Background

Diabetes mellitus (DM) is a chronic disease with serious complications, imposing a significant burden on the health status of affected individuals, both on physical and mental aspects [1, 2]. Its commonest form, Type 2 DM (T2D), usually follows distinct stages in its development: from normal glucose tolerance (NGT), to impaired glucose metabolism (pre-diabetes), and overt onset of the disease [3]. It is well established that the quality of life (QOL) of people with diabetes (total physical, mental, and social well-being) is adversely affected by the disease and its complications [4]. Concerning the QOL of persons with pre-diabetes, however, there is sparse and controversial data in the literature [5–8], possibly related to different methods of health-related QOL (HRQOL) measurement, small sample sizes or focus on selected populations (for example, elderly, instead of the general population) [9]. Especially in the Greek population, to our knowledge, no data exist at all on this matter.

Although people with pre-diabetes experience no symptoms and usually have no knowledge of their condition [10], there is evidence that around 10–20% of them already have some mild micro- or macro- vascular complications [11], which might confer some adverse impact on their HRQOL, or at least in some aspects of it [12]. The prevalence of DM in Greece remains high, and according to recent data [13] it accounts for 7.0% of the population (with 8.2% prevalence of T2D for people ≥15 years of age). On the other hand, pre-diabetes prevalence is not well studied, with some estimates from regional studies raising it to around 22% of the adult population [14].

The DEPLAN study (Diabetes in Europe - Prevention using Lifestyle, Physical Activity and Nutritional Intervention) [15] is a European Commission-funded multinational project, aiming to establish a model for the efficient identification of individuals at high risk for T2D in the community, in the primary care structure, in the EU member countries and to test the feasibility and cost-effectiveness of the translation of the intervention concepts learned from the prevention trials into existing health-care systems [16]. Data on the quality of life of subjects with pre-diabetes and NGT from the Greek part of this study [14, 17], based on the validated health-related quality of life [HRQOL]-15D questionnaire [18], were compared to respective data of patients with diabetes, derived from the outpatient Diabetes Clinic of the "Laiko" University Hospital, in Athens, Greece, in an effort to elucidate if any differences exist in the HRQOL among these groups.

Methods

Participants

The sample population of the present cross-sectional study consisted of persons with pre-diabetes (Impaired Fasting Glucose [IFG], Impaired Glucose Tolerance [IGT] or both) and people with NGT (that had provided data on their HRQOL in the Greek part of the DEPLAN study), as well as persons with known DM from the outpatient Diabetes Center of "Laiko" University hospital, in Athens, Greece. This study has been previously described in detail [14, 17]. In brief, the FINDRISC questionnaire [19] was distributed to around 7900 persons without known diabetes, aged 35–75 years, residing in the metropolitan area around Athens, in order to find people at high risk for developing T2D (a score ≥ 15 signifying high probability). Out of the 3240 completed questionnaires, 869 persons accepted to undergo an oral glucose tolerance test (OGTT), so as to identify people with unknown (screen-detected) diabetes and exclude them from further intervention. On the day of the OGTT, weight, height, waist circumference and blood pressure of the participants were measured and their medical histories recorded. Presence of co-morbidities (defined as hypertension and/or dyslipidemia) and vascular complications (any combination of coronary heart disease, stroke, peripheral arterial disease, nephropathy, retinopathy or neuropathy) were also recorded. Plasma glucose, total- and high density lipoprotein (HDL)-cholesterol and triglyceride levels were measured from fasting blood samples at a central accredited university research laboratory, using enzymatic assays. Low density lipoprotein (LDL)-cholesterol was calculated using the Friedewald formula [20].

According to the OGTT results, subjects were categorized as having normal glucose tolerance (NGT), impaired fasting glucose (IFG), impaired glucose tolerance (IGT) or diabetes. IFG was defined based on a fasting plasma glucose of 100–125 mg/dl, IGT as a 2-h plasma glucose between 140 and 199 mg/dl and (screen-detected) DM as a fasting plasma glucose ≥126 mg/dl and/or 2-h plasma glucose ≥200 mg/dl [3]. People with both IFG and IGT were considered as IGT. Persons with screen-detected DM from the DEPLAN cohort were not included in the present analysis. These people did not know they had DM before performing the OGTT and were thus thought they represented a special category of patients with diabetes (newly diagnosed), resembling more to the pre-diabetes group as regards to complications and QOL issues. The HRQOL data of the persons with pre-diabetes and the controls from the DEPLAN cohort were compared to respective data of people with known diabetes, derived from the outpatient Diabetes Center of "Laiko" University hospital.

The participants' HRQOL was recorded using the 15D questionnaire [18], a preference-based HRQOL instrument that has also been validated in the Greek population [21]. The reason that this measure was used in the present study is that this is the HRQOL instrument that had already been used in the DEPLAN study where the participants with pre-diabetes and NGT were derived from. License to use this HRQOL questionnaire had been centrally obtained from the Steering Committee of the original European DE-PLAN study and was used by all participating centers [15]. No other QOL measurements were available for the DEPLAN participants. The 15D-questionnaire contains 15 dimensions (questions): mobility, vision, hearing, breathing, sleeping, eating, speech, excretion, usual activities, mental function, discomfort and symptoms, depression, distress, vitality and sexual activity, each having five different levels of functional status. These dimensions can be presented as a 15-dimensional profile or as a one-index score. The 15D index score is obtained by weighing the dimensions with population-based preference weights based on an application of the multi-attribute utility theory. Obtained index scores vary between 0 and 1, where 0 represents a state of being dead and 1 represents perfect HRQOL [22]. Questionnaires were distributed to the participants and were self-filled, blindly to the investigators.

The study was approved by the cooperating hospital's ethics committee (Laiko General Hospital Ethics Review Board), and the Hellenic National Drug Organization. All participants signed an informed consent according to the general recommendations of the Declaration of Helsinki [23].

Statistical analysis

Continuous variables are presented as mean ± one-standard deviation, while qualitative variables as absolute and relative frequencies (%). Normal distribution of variables was tested with the Shapiro-Wilk test. Comparisons between 2 normally distributed continuous variables were performed with the calculation of the Student's t-test, whereas the Wilcoxon Mann-Whitney U-test was used for non-parametric variables. Associations between categorical variables were tested with the use of contingency tables and the calculation of the Chi-squared test. Pearson's correlation coefficient (r) or Spearman's rho (for non-normal distributions) were used for the evaluation of statistical correlations between variables. For comparisons of ≥3 variables, one-way analysis of variance (ANOVA) (for normally distributed variables), or the Kruskal-Wallis test (for non-normally distributed variables) was used. For controlling of confounding variables (such as age, gender, smoking, body mass index [BMI], hypertension, complications, co-morbidities) analysis of covariance (ANCOVA) was used. All reported p-values are derived from two-sided tests and compared to a significance level of 5%. Data were analyzed using the Statistical Package SPSS, version 23.0 (SPSS Inc., Chicago, IL).

Results

Out of the total 869 persons screened with an OGTT in the DEPLAN cohort, 383 (44.1%) had complete HRQOL data. The present analysis included 370 participants (mean age [±SD] 57.2 ± 11.0 years, 46% males), out of whom 172 had pre-diabetes (108 with IFG, 64 with IGT, aged 58.3 ± 10.3 years) and 198 had NGT (aged 54.4 ± 10.1 years). Thirteen individuals (age 64.2 ± 4.1 years, BMI 30.4 ± 6.4 kg/m^2) had screen-detected diabetes and, as explained above, due to their recent diagnosis and small number, precluding any meaningful statistical analysis as a separate group, were excluded from further analysis. The diabetes group in the present analysis was comprised of 100 persons (mean age 60.9 ± 12.5 years, DM duration 17.0 ± 10.0 years, HbA1c: 7.2 ± 1.2%) from the outpatient Diabetes Center of "Laiko" University hospital.

The demographic, clinical and laboratory characteristics of the study participants are presented in Table 1. As shown, people with diabetes were older, mostly males (59%), smoked less and had more frequently co-morbidities and vascular complications than the other two groups. Of note, individuals with pre-diabetes were more obese than the other two groups and had more co-morbidities than the NGT group (48.8% vs. 35.2%, respectively, $p = 0.008$), but the frequency of vascular complications did not differ between them (11.9% vs. 8.2%, respectively, $p > 0.05$).

Simple correlation analyses showed that the HRQOL-15D score was negatively correlated with age (Spearman's rho = − 0.13, $p = 0.010$), HDL-cholesterol (rho = − 0.11, $p = 0.030$), and BMI (rho = − 0.14, $p = 0.004$), and positively with LDL-cholesterol (rho = 0.10, $p = 0.050$). Specifically, within the group of patients with diabetes, there was a negative correlation of the HRQOL-15D score with DM duration (rho = − 0.34, $p = 0.001$) and a trend for a negative correlation with glycemic control (as measured by HbA1c) (rho = − 0.20, $p = 0.058$).

Table 2 shows the results of the comparison of the HRQOL-15D score (and its components) among the groups of NGT, pre-diabetes (IFG – IGT) and DM participants. Patients with diabetes had a lower total HRQOL-15D sore (0.8605) compared to the other two groups (0.9092 and 0.9008, for the NGT and pre-DM group, respectively, $p < 0.001$ by Kruskal-Wallis analysis), while IFG and IGT participants had similar scores (0.9043 and 0.8946, respectively). In *post-hoc* analyses, it was shown that there was a significant difference between the group of patients with diabetes and the NGT group ($p < 0.001$) as well as between the diabetes and the IFG group ($p = 0.007$). On the contrary, there were no statistically significant differences in the HRQOL score between any two of these three groups (NGT, IFG and IGT) (Fig. 1).

Table 1 Demographic, clinical and laboratory characteristics of participants (mean ± SD)

Variable	NGT	Pre-Diabetes			DM	P*
		IFG	IGT	All Pre-DM		
Number	198	108	64	172	100	–
Gender (male) [n (%)]	74 (37.4)	59 (54.6)	25 (39.1)	84 (48.8)	59 (59.0)	0.001
Age (years)	54.4 (10.1)	57.2 (10.1)	60.3 (10.5)	58.3 (10.3)	60.9 (12.5)	< 0.001
Weight (kg)	81.1 (15.6)	88.6 (13.6)	87.2 (14.7)	88.1 (14.0)	85.2 (20.4)	0.001
BMI (kg/m²)	29.4 (5.3)	31.5 (4.3)	32.2 (5.4)	31.7 (4.8)	29.6 (6.5)	< 0.001
Smoking (%)	56.6	58.3	53.1	56.4	37.1	0.007
Co-morbidities [n (%)]	69 (35.2)	48 (44.4)	36 (56.3)	84 (48.8)	74 (87.1)	< 0.001
Complications [n (%)]	5 (8.2)	7 (9.1)	8 (16.3)	15 (11.9)	26 (30.6)	< 0.001
SBP (mmHg)	119.3 (18.5)	129.5 (16.2)	128.0 (16.1)	128.9 (16.1)	134.9 (18.9)	< 0.001
DBP (mmHg)	75.9 (12.0)	78.9 (11.5)	77.4 (11.5)	78.3 (11.5)	74.9 (10.4)	NS
Cholesterol (mmol/L)	5.47 (0.97)	5.70 (0.97)	5.82 (1.01)	5.75 (0.99)	4.24 (1.08)	< 0.001
Triglycerides (mmol/L)	1.18 (0.57)	1.49 (0.88)	1.57 (0.71)	1.52 (0.36)	1.43 (0.74)	< 0.001
HDL-C (mmol/L)	1.20 (0.21)	1.22 (0.23)	1.25 (0.19)	1.23 (0.22)	1.22 (0.28)	NS
LDL-C (mmol/L)	3.72 (0.88)	3.82 (0.84)	3.86 (0.94)	3.84 (0.88)	2.35 (0.91)	< 0.001
DM duration (years)	–	–	–	–	17.0 (10.0)	–
HbA1c (%)	–	–	–	–	7.2 (1.2)	–

NGT Normal Glucose Tolerance, *DM* Diabetes mellitus, *SBP* Systolic blood pressure, *DBP* Diastolic blood pressure, *BMI* Body mass index, *NS* Non- significant, *Co-morbidities* Hypertension and/or dyslipidemia, *Complications* Any combination of coronary heart disease, stroke, peripheral arterial disease, nephropathy, retinopathy, neuropathy
P = Comparison among the 4 groups (NGT, IFG, IGT, DM) by Chi-squared or Kruskal-Wallis analysis

Table 2 Comparison of the HRQOL-15D score and its components among the DM patients, people with pre-DM (IFG – IGT) and NGT

	NGT	Pre-diabetes			DM	P*
		IFG	IGT	All pre-DM		
Mobility	0.9179	0.9122	0.8711	0.8969	0.8264	< 0.001
Vision	0.8688	0.8963	0.8938	0.8954	0.8333	NS
Hearing	0.9487	0.9562	0.9455	0.9522	0.9152	NS
Breathing	0.9150	0.8849	0.8862	0.8854	0.8473	0.044
Sleeping	0.8335	0.8385	0.8256	0.8338	0.8172	NS
Eating	0.9983	1.0000	0.9945	0.9980	0.9901	NS
Speech	0.9887	0.9880	0.9844	0.9867	0.9676	NS
Excretion	0.9433	0.9511	0.9234	0.9410	0.9048	NS
Usual activities	0.9214	0.9329	0.8956	0.9191	0.8226	< 0.001
Mental function	0.9153	0.9095	0.9068	0.9085	0.9007	NS
Discomfort and symptoms	0.8841	0.8779	0.8683	0.8743	0.8694	NS
Depression	0.8601	0.8627	0.8472	0.8569	0.8574	NS
Distress	0.7561	0.7333	0.6971	0.7205	0.7657	0.019
Vitality	0.8474	0.8150	0.8424	0.8246	0.8112	NS
Sexual activity	0.9000	0.8838	0.8895	0.8858	0.6642	< 0.001
Total score	0.9092	0.9043	0.8946	0.9008	0.8605	< 0.001

NGT Normal Glucose Tolerance, *IFG* Impaired Fasting Glucose, *IGT* Impaired Glucose Tolerance, *DM* Diabetes mellitus, *NS* Non-significant
P = Comparison among the 4 groups (NGT, IFG, IGT, DM) by Kruskal-Wallis analysis

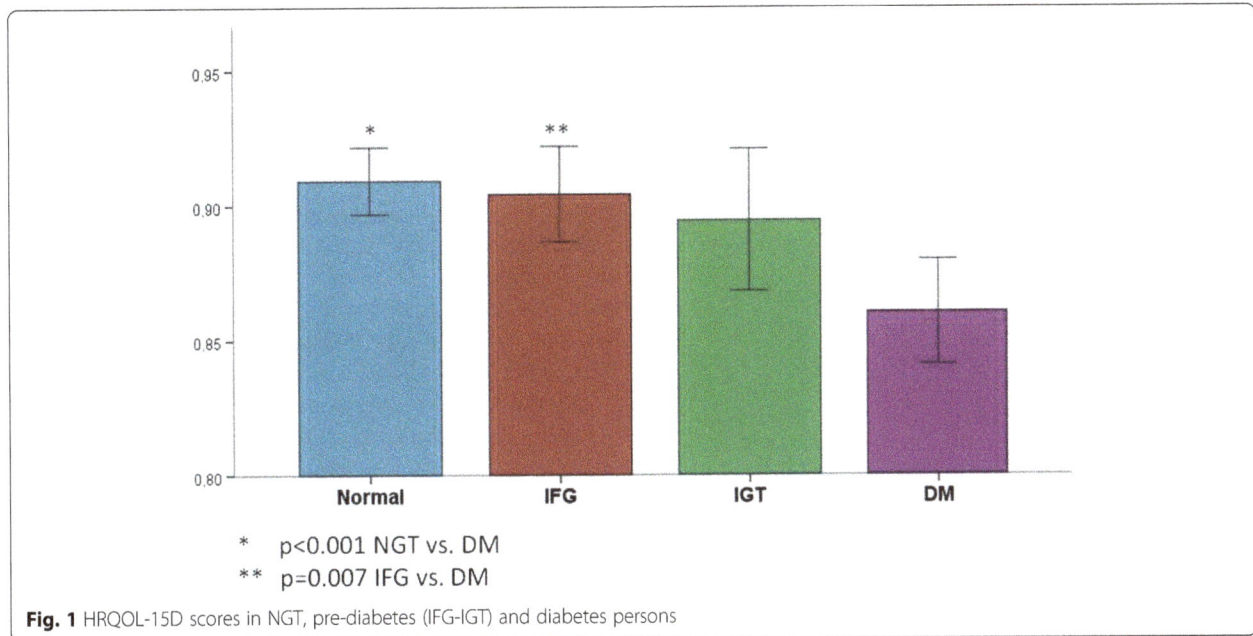

* p<0.001 NGT vs. DM
** p=0.007 IFG vs. DM

Fig. 1 HRQOL-15D scores in NGT, pre-diabetes (IFG-IGT) and diabetes persons

In a multifactorial analysis of covariance (ANCOVA), after controlling for age, gender, BMI and smoking (model 1, Table 3), the HRQOL-15D score was significantly associated with the glycemic status (NGT, pre-diabetes [IFG/IGT] or diabetes) ($p < 0.001$). Male gender ($p < 0.001$) and higher BMI ($p = 0.003$) were also significantly associated with a lower HRQOL score, and this model explained the variance of HRQOL score by 14% ($R^2 = 0.14$). When the presence, however, of co-morbidities and vascular complications were added to the model (model 2, Table 4), the relationship of the glycemic status with the HRQOL-15D score was attenuated and lost significance. Male gender still had a significant contribution to the model ($p < 0.001$), whereas the independent effect of vascular complications ($p = 0.004$) negated the effects of the glycemic status and of BMI (the model now explained the overall variance of the HRQOL score by 21.8% [$R^2 = 0.218$]).

The different components of the HRQOL-15D score were evaluated separately among the groups. As

Table 3 Analysis of covariance (ANCOVA) for the relationship between the HRQOL-15D score with glycemic status, controlling for age, gender, BMI and smoking (persons with pre-diabetes were considererd separately as IFG - IGT) (Model 1)

Variable	F	P
Age	0.72	NS
Gender (male)	20.05	< 0.001
BMI	8.53	0.003
Smoking (yes)	0.26	NS
Glycemic status	3.62	< 0.001

R^2 0.14, *BMI* Body mass index
Glycemic status: 1 = NGT, 2 = IFG, 3 = IGT, 4 = Diabetes

shown in Table 2, there were statistically significant differences for the components of "mobility", "breathing", "usual activities", "distress" and "sexual activity" among the groups as a whole. In *post-hoc* analyses, a statistically significant difference was found between the NGT and IGT groups as regarded to the components of "mobility" ($p = 0.042$) and "distress" ($p = 0.01$) (lower values for the IGT group), as well as between the IGT and DM groups as regarded to the components of "distress" ($p = 0.029$) (lower for the IGT group) and "sexual activity" ($p < 0.001$) (lower for the DM group). These associations were attenuated but persisted after adjustment for age, gender, BMI, presence of co-morbidities and complications. There were no differences in any component of the HRQOL-15D score between the two groups of the pre-diabetes participants (IFG and IGT), or the NGT vs. the IFG group (Fig. 2).

Discussion

There is a lot of interest in the past few decades in studies of health-related quality of life (HRQOL) and the impact of various diseases and disease-states upon it, which has led to the development and refinement of a number of generic and disease-specific HRQOL measures [24, 25]. It should be emphasized also that clinical variables alone do not comprehensively capture patients' perceptions of their health, which is in part due to the fact that HRQOL is influenced by many other factors, such as the existence of other health problems, social relationships, marital status, patient knowledge, treatment satisfaction and perceived ability to control one's disease [26].

Table 4 Analysis of covariance (ANCOVA) for the relationship between the HRQOL-15D score with glycemic status, controlling for age, gender, BMI, smoking, presence of co-morbidities and vascular complications (persons with pre-diabetes were considererd separately as IFG - IGT) (Model 2)

Variable	F	P
Age	2.08	NS
Gender (male)	19.07	< 0,001
BMI	3.48	NS
Smoking (yes)	1.28	NS
Co-morbidities	0.37	NS
Complications	6.39	0.004
Glycemic status	0.53	NS

R^2 0.218, *Co-morbidities* arterial hypertension and/or dyslipidemia, *Complications* any combination of coronary heart disease, stroke, peripheral arterial disease, nephropathy, retinopathy or neuropathy
Glycemic status: 1 = NGT, 2 = IFG, 3 = IGT, 4 = Diabetes

In the present study, the HRQOL of patients with diabetes was compared with that of pre-diabetes (IFG/IGT) and persons with normal glucose tolerance (NGT), using the HRQOL-15D questionnaire. It was found, that, in general, the HRQOL of patients with diabetes was significantly worse than that of the other two groups (owing mainly to the presence of vascular complications), while there were no significant differences in the overall HRQOL score between the NGT and the pre-diabetes groups. Examination, however, of the individual components of the HRQOL score showed significant differences between the NGT and the pre-diabetes group in certain aspects. In particular, the IGT group had lower scores compared to the NGT, as regarded to the components of "mobility" and "distress". No difference was noted in any of the 15 dimensions of the score between the NGT and IFG group, nor between the two groups of the pre-diabetes subjects (IFG vs. IGT).

The deterioration of the HRQOL in people with DM [4] and the contribution of vascular complications to that effect found in the present study is in line with previous reports in the literature [27, 28]. For people with pre-diabetes, however, there are only few published studies examining the relationship of their quality of life as regards to physical [5, 12] or psychological/mental parameters [7, 8, 10], sometimes with conflicting results, either because of the use of different HRQOL measurement methods (e.g. by recording only the physical health condition and not the psychological-mental), or because of the use of small sample sizes or because of focusing

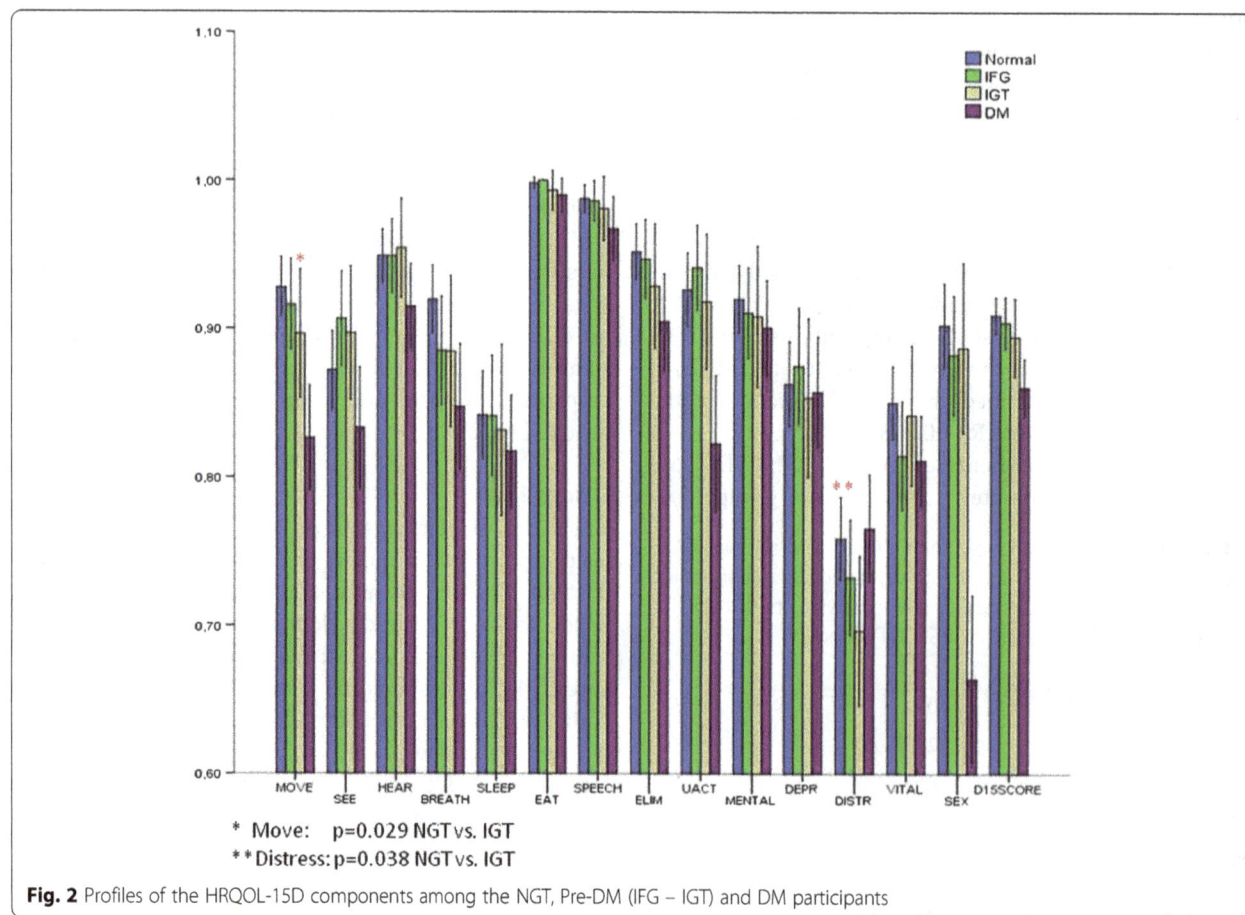

* Move: p=0.029 NGT vs. IGT
** Distress: p=0.038 NGT vs. IGT

Fig. 2 Profiles of the HRQOL-15D components among the NGT, Pre-DM (IFG – IGT) and DM participants

on specific population groups (e.g. the elderly) [6, 9, 29]. Specifically using the HRQOL-15D questionnaire, studies in people with pre-diabetes are extremely sparse [22].

Since these people (with pre-diabetes) usually have no symptoms and no major complications and very often no knowledge of their condition [10], their HRQOL should not be expected to be affected. The fact, however, that around 10–20% of them may already have some mild micro- or macro- vascular complications [11], could explain the findings of their affected HRQOL in some aspects of it. For example, limited joint action, prayer's sign and Dupuytren's contracture were more common in elderly IGT persons compared to controls [12].

In the present study, 'mobility' was found to be impaired in the group of pre-diabetes subjects with IGT (compared to those of the control group), which is broadly in line with findings in the literature [22, 30]. It is possible that mild, even subconscious abnormalities in physical functioning could explain this finding. In a recently published prospective study [22] using 3 different assessment tools of HRQOL (SF-36, SF-6D and 15D), and dividing the subjects into 5 groups (normal glucose tolerance, IFG, IGT, newly diagnosed diabetes and known diabetes), it was found that the deterioration of the glycemic status from the stage of normal glucose tolerance to the pre-diabetes and overt diabetes was associated with a worsening of HRQOL scores, as measured with all three questionnaires. Specifically for the 15D questionnaire, decreases in the components of "mobility" (similar to the present study), "breathing", "usual activities", "discomfort and symptoms", "vitality" and "sexual activity" were found, but not for the psychological dimensions of the questionnaire. These reductions - similar to the present study – did not occur in subjects with IFG but only in those with IGT or diabetes who exceeded the limits of minimal clinical significance [minimal (clinically) important differences (MIDs)] the study had set (i.e. the smallest change a patient or health professional can notice - for the 15D questionnaire MID was proposed at ≥0.02–0.03 units of the total score). A similar population study from Spain (Di@bet.es Study) [30], in 5047 individuals of the general population, using the SF-12 questionnaire, showed that women had worsening quality of life scores (relating both to physical and psychological parameters) with the deterioration of the glycemic status towards the pre-diabetes and diabetes states, while in men only physical parameters were affected (similarly in the present study male gender was independently associated with worsening HRQOL).

Other population studies from Australia (AusDiab study), using the quality of life short form-36 (SF-36) questionnaire, showed that people with IFG (especially women) [5] or IGT [31], had reduced values in mainly physical dimensions of quality of life, especially bodily pain and physical functioning, and in general health status [32]. On the contrary, in a population study in Western Finland (the Harmonica Project) in 1383 subjects, aged 45–70 years, no differences in HRQOL were detected (with the same questionnaire SF-36) in participants with pre-diabetes compared with non-diabetes subjects [6]. In this study, people with known cardiovascular disease were excluded in advance, which limits the generalization and validity of the results. In the largest population study to date [8], that included 55,882 people of the general population in Sweden (Västerbotten Intervention Program), using the Health Utility Weight [HUW] SF-6D questionnaire (that included the dimensions of physical functioning, role limitations, social function, bodily pain, mental health, and vitality), there was also a gradual decrease in HUWs with a progressive deterioration of the glycemic status from normal glucose tolerance to pre-diabetes and overt diabetes.

Another significant finding in the present study was that the "psychological distress" appeared to be highly affected in the group of pre-diabetes individuals with IGT (relative to normal, and surprisingly even to people with diabetes). Of note, the recording of this fact in the HRQOL-15D questionnaires was done before the participants were informed about the results of the OGTT tests that they belonged to the pre-diabetes group. Several studies in the literature have reported worsening of the psychological state in people with diabetes [2, 33], which may be caused by the impact of the diagnosis of diabetes itself, the psychological stress associated with the management of diabetes or the burden of diabetic complications [34], or even through physiological pathways, including inflammatory processes and reductions in neurotrophic function [35], which in turn may lead to reduced plasticity of neuronal networks and subsequently depression [36]. For pre-diabetes, however, the correlations that have been found are less robust. In initial studies, it was observed that depressive symptoms were more frequent in women with pre-diabetes [37], but a recent meta-analysis concluded that the risk for depression was not increased in impaired glucose metabolism compared to normal glucose metabolism or even undiagnosed diabetes subjects [38]. In the present study, "depression" did not differ between the groups of NGT, pre-diabetes or diabetes subjects.

The relationship between mental disorder and the affected glucose metabolism is likely to be bidirectional, as depressive symptoms or psychological distress may also lead to a higher risk of developing pre-diabetes (especially in men) [39] or diabetes [40]. Higher work distress has also been associated with prevalent diabetes and especially pre-diabetes in a German cohort, especially in men [41], which could also explain the findings of increased "distress" of participants with pre-diabetes in the present study, although no etiology of distress (e.g. work-related, social, family, etc) was elucidated.

There are several limitations of the present study. They include the relatively small sample size examined and the fact that it is a cross-sectional study, and thus cannot demonstrate cause and effect or the time frame in which indices of the HRQOL deteriorate. For this purpose, prospective studies are required, with a significant population sample and sufficient monitoring time. In such a relatively small study from Germany [7], there was a trend for a decline in the quality of life (only for physical parameters, as measured by the SF-12 questionnaire) within 7 years from the transition of NGT to pre-diabetes, but the association was statistically significant only for the subjects converting from NGT to diabetes.

Another limitation of this study is that the population examined is not necessarily representative of the general population, since the participants without diabetes selected themselves to participate in the study, while people with diabetes were derived from a large Diabetes University Center (Laiko Hospital), and thus the findings are not necessarily applicable to the general population. Also, the fact that the HRQOL-15D questionnaire is not specific for diabetes [25], may probably have as a result that the responses to it reflect problems associated with other conditions. The fact that it was applied only once may additionally preclude its ability to find fluctuations of HRQOL over time.

It has to be emphasized also, that there were many missing data regarding presence of vascular complications in the group of individuals with pre-diabetes (46 persons) and NGT (137 persons), which may have influenced the aforementioned comparisons.

On the other hand, strengths of the present study include the fact that the determination of the glycemic status was performed with a glucose tolerance test (OGTT) and was not self-reported, which enhances the reliability of the reported correlations. Also the HRQOL-15D questionnaire was completed by the participants of the DEPLAN cohort before they had learned the results of the OGTT, and thus their answers were not affected by the knowledge of their glycemic status. In addition, in a comparative evaluation of the HRQOL-15D questionnaire with other HRQOL assessment questionnaires in the Greek population [42], the 15D was found to be superior as regards to the assessment of vascular complications in diabetes (particularly for coronary heart disease and diabetic retinopathy). Furthermore, the exclusion of the few newly diagnosed (screen-detected) people with diabetes from the analysis, whose participation could cause distortion of the associations found, because of their actual position in-between the states of pre-diabetes and diabetes strengthens the findings of the study.

Conclusions

In conclusion, the quality of life of individuals with pre-diabetes was overall not significantly different from that of normal glucose tolerance subjects, whereas for participants with diabetes it was lower (mainly due to the presence of vascular complications). However, certain components of the quality of life were already affected in the pre-diabetic state of IGT (compared to the control group), specifically "mobility" and "psychological distress". Providing an understanding of the stages of diabetes where health status is diminished will allow prioritization of intervention efforts, and enable more effective targeting of policy and strategic interventions to improve health outcomes. Thus, quality of life issues (in particular physical and psychological-emotional issues) should be investigated when people with pre-diabetes are diagnosed in every-day routine clinical practice, since their identification could potentially lead to more effective overall management of their condition.

Abbreviations

DM: Diabetes mellitus; HRQOL: Health related quality of life; IFG: Impaired fasting glucose; IGT: Impaired glucose tolerance

Acknowledgements

We would like to thank the following Health Centers/individuals for helping implement the present study: the medical staff of the Health Center of Alimos (especially Dr. Ourania Zacharopoulou), the staff of the Center for the Elderly Agioi Anargyroi, the medical and nursing staff of the Health Center of Markopoulo (especially Mrs. R. Salonikioti), the medical and nursing staff of the Hellenic Telecommunications Company (especially Drs C. Pietris and C. Alexopoulos), the medical and nursing staff of the Hellenic Radiotelevision (especially Dr. M. Katsorida), the medical and nursing staff of the Bank of Greece (especially Drs V. Spandagos and P. Konstantopoulou), the medical staff of the Olympic Village complex (especially Dr. S. Tigas), the staff of the electrical equipment manufacturer "Pitsos-Bosch", the medical and nursing staff of the Health Center of Vari (especially Dr. M. Dandoulakis) and the medical and nursing staff of the Health Center of Vyronas (especially Dr. K. Kyriakopoulos).

Funding

This project was partly funded by the Commission of the European Communities, Directorate C – Public Health, grant agreement No. 2004310. Under the rules of the agreement, it was also partly co-funded by the private sector and in this case it was supported by an unrestricted educational grant from Bristol-Myers-Squibb, Greece.

Authors' contributions

KM designed the study, obtained the data, analyzed and interpreted the patient data and wrote the manuscript; SL designed the study, obtained the data and reviewed the first draft of the manuscript; AT, CS, EP obtained the data; DP analyzed the data; NK, NK and DN designed the study and provided critical revisions of important intellectual content to the manuscript. All authors revised the manuscript and approved the final version prior to the submission.

Competing interests

The authors declare that they have no competing interests.

Author details

[1]First Department of Propaedeutic Medicine, National and Kapodistrian University of Athens Medical School, Laiko General Hospital, 17 Ag. Thoma St, 11527 Athens, Greece. [2]Laboratory for Experimental Surgery and Surgical Research "Christeas Hall", University of Athens Medical School, Athens, Greece. [3]Hellenic Open University, Patras, Greece.

References

1. Wong E, Backholer K, Gearon E, Harding J, Freak-Poli R, Stevenson C, Peeters A. Diabetes and risk of physical disability in adults: a systematic review and meta-analysis. Lancet Diabetes Endocrinol. 2013;2:106–14.
2. Holt RIG, de Groot M, Golden SH. Diabetes and depression. Curr Diab Rep. 2014;14(6):491.
3. American Diabetes Association. Classification and diagnosis of diabetes. Diabetes Care. 2016;39(Suppl 1):S13–22.
4. Sikdar KC, Wang PP, MacDonald D, Gadag VG. Diabetes and its impact on health-related quality of life: a life table analysis. Qual Life Res. 2010;19(6):781–7.
5. Chittleborough CR, Baldock KL, Taylor AW, Phillips PJ. Health status assessed by the SF-36 along the diabetes continuum in an Australian population. Qual Life Res. 2006;15(4):687–94.
6. Seppälä T, Saxen U, Kautiainen H, Järvenpää S, Korhonen PE. Impaired glucose metabolism and health related quality of life. Prim Care Diabetes. 2013;7(3):223–7. https://doi.org/10.1016/j.pcd.2013.03.001.
7. Hunger M, Holle R, Meisinger C, Rathmann W, Peters A, Schunk M. Longitudinal changes in health-related quality of life in normal glucose tolerance, prediabetes and type 2 diabetes: results from the KORA S4/F4 cohort study. Qual Life Res. 2014;23(9):2515–20.
8. Neumann A, Schoffer O, Norström F, Norberg M, Klug SJ, Lindholm L. Health related quality of life for pre-diabetic states and type 2 diabetes mellitus: a cross-sectional study in Västerbotten Sweden. Health Qual Life Outcomes. 2014;12:150.
9. Hiltunen L, Keinänen-Kiukaanniemi S. Does glucose tolerance affect quality of life in an elderly population? Diabetes Res Clin Pract. 1999;46(2):161–7.
10. Tabák AG, Herder C, Rathmann W, Brunner EJ, Kivimäki M. Prediabetes: a high-risk state for diabetes development. Lancet. 2012;379(9833):2279–90.
11. Milman S, Crandall JP. Mechanisms of vascular complications in prediabetes. Med Clin North Am. 2011;95(2):309–25.
12. Cederlund RI, Thomsen N, Thrainsdottir S, Eriksson K-F, Sundkvist G, Dahlin LB. Hand disorders, hand function, and activities of daily living in elderly men with type 2 diabetes. J Diabetes Complicat. 2009;23(1):32–9.
13. Liatis S, Dafoulas GE, Kani C, Politi A, Litsa P, Sfikakis PP, Makrilakis K. The prevalence and treatment patterns of diabetes in the Greek population based on real-world data from the nation-wide prescription database. Diabetes Res Clin Pract. 2016;118:162–7.
14. Makrilakis K, Liatis S, Grammatikou S, Perrea D, Stathi C, Tsiligros P, Katsilambros N. Validation of the Finnish diabetes risk score (FINDRISC) questionnaire for screening for undiagnosed type 2 diabetes, dysglycaemia and the metabolic syndrome in Greece. Diabetes Metab. 2011;37(2):44–51.
15. Schwarz PEH, Lindström J, Kissimova-Scarbeck K, Szybinski Z, Barengo NC, Peltonen M, Tuomilehto J. The European perspective of type 2 diabetes prevention: diabetes in Europe - prevention using lifestyle, physical activity and nutritional intervention (DE-PLAN) project. Exp Clin Endocrinol Diabetes. 2008;116(3):167–72.
16. Cos FX, Barengo NC, Costa B, Mundet-Tudurí X, Lindström J, Tuomilehto JO. DEPLAN study group. Screening for people with abnormal glucose metabolism in the European DE-PLAN project. Diabetes Res Clin Pract. 2015;109(1):149–56.
17. Makrilakis K, Liatis S, Grammatikou S, Perrea D, Katsilambros N. Implementation and effectiveness of the first community lifestyle intervention programme to prevent type 2 diabetes in Greece. The DE-PLAN study. Diabet Med. 2010;27(4):459–65.
18. Sintonen H. The 15D instrument of health-related quality of life: properties and applications. Ann Med. 2001;33(5):328–36.
19. Lindström J, Tuomilehto J. The diabetes risk score: a practical tool to predict type 2 diabetes risk. Diabetes Care. 2003;26(3):725–31.
20. Friedewald WT, Levy RI, Fredrickson DS. Estimation of the concentration of low-density lipoprotein cholesterol in plasma, without use of the preparative ultracentrifuge. Clin Chem. 1972;18(6):499–502.
21. Anagnostopoulos F, Yfantopoulos J, Moustaki I, Niakas D. Psychometric and factor analytic evaluation of the 15D health-related quality of life instrument: the case of Greece. Qual Life Res. 2013;22(8):1973–86.
22. Väätäinen S, Keinänen-Kiukaanniemi S, Saramies J, Uusitalo H, Tuomilehto J, Martikainen J. Quality of life along the diabetes continuum: a cross-sectional view of health-related quality of life and general health status in middle-aged and older Finns. Qual Life Res. 2014;23(7):1935–44.
23. Williams JR. The declaration of Helsinki and public health. Bull. World Health Organ. 2008;86(8):650–2.
24. Greenfield S, Nelson EC. Recent developments and future issues in the use of health status assessment measures in clinical settings. Med Care. 1992; 30(5 Suppl):MS23–41.
25. El Achhab Y, Nejjari C, Chikri M, Lyoussi B. Disease-specific health-related quality of life instruments among adults diabetic: a systematic review. Diabetes Res Clin Pract. 2008;80(2):171–84.
26. Burroughs TE, Desikan R, Waterman BM, Gilin D, McGill J. Development and validation of the diabetes quality of life brief clinical inventory. Diab Spectr. 2004;17:41–9.
27. Wexler DJ, Grant RW, Wittenberg E, Bosch JL, Cagliero E, Delahanty L, et al. Correlates of health-related quality of life in type 2 diabetes. Diabetologia. 2006;49(7):1489–97.
28. Solli O, Stavem K, Kristiansen IS. Health-related quality of life in diabetes: the associations of complications with EQ-5D scores. Health Qual Life Outcomes. 2010;8:18.
29. Taylor LM, Spence JC, Raine K, Plotnikoff RC, Vallance JK, Sharma AM. Physical activity and health-related quality of life in individuals with prediabetes. Diabetes Res Clin Pract. 2010;90(1):15–21.
30. Marcuello C, Calle-Pascual AL, Fuentes M, Runkle I, Soriguer F, Goday A, et al. Evaluation of health-related quality of life according to carbohydrate metabolism status: a Spanish population-based study (Di@bet.es study). Int J Endocrinol. 2012;2012:872305.
31. Tapp RJ, Dunstan DW, Phillips P, Tonkin A, Zimmet PZ, Shaw JE. Association between impaired glucose metabolism and quality of life: results from the Australian diabetes obesity and lifestyle study. Diabetes Res Clin Pract. 2006; 74(2):154–61.
32. Tapp RJ, O'Neil A, Shaw JE, Zimmet PZ, Oldenburg BF. Is there a link between components of health-related functioning and incident impaired glucose metabolism and type 2 diabetes? The Australian diabetes obesity and lifestyle (AusDiab) study. Diabetes Care. 2010;33(4):757–62.
33. Holt RIG, Katon WJ. Dialogue on diabetes and depression: dealing with the double burden of co-morbidity. J Affect Disord. 2012;142(Suppl):S1–3.
34. Golden SH, Lazo M, Carnethon M, Bertoni AG, Schreiner PJ, Diez Roux AV, et al. Examining a bidirectional association between depressive symptoms and diabetes. JAMA. 2008;299(23):2751–9.
35. Krabbe KS, Nielsen AR, Krogh-Madsen R, Plomgaard P, Rasmussen P, Erikstrup C, et al. Brain-derived neurotrophic factor (BDNF) and type 2 diabetes. Diabetologia. 2007;50(2):431–8.
36. Castrén E, Rantamäki T. Role of brain-derived neurotrophic factor in the aetiology of depression: implications for pharmacological treatment. CNS Drugs. 2010;24(1):1–7.
37. Adriaanse MC, Dekker JM, Heine RJ, Snoek FJ, Beekman AJ, Stehouwer CD, et al. Symptoms of depression in people with impaired glucose metabolism or type 2 diabetes mellitus: the Hoorn study. Diabet Med. 2008;25(7):843–9.
38. Nouwen A, Nefs G, Caramlau I, Connock M, Winkley K, Lloyd CE, et al. Prevalence of depression in individuals with impaired glucose metabolism or undiagnosed diabetes: a systematic review and meta-analysis of the European depression in diabetes (EDID) research consortium. Diabetes Care. 2011;34(3):752–62.
39. Eriksson AK, Ekbom A, Granath F, Hilding A, Efendic S, Ostenson CG. Psychological distress and risk of pre-diabetes and type 2 diabetes in a prospective study of Swedish middle-aged men and women. Diabet Med. 2008;25(7):834–42.

40. Virtanen M, Ferrie JE, Tabak AG, Akbaraly TN, Vahtera J, Singh-Manoux A, et al. Psychological distress and incidence of type 2 diabetes in high-risk and low-risk populations: the Whitehall II cohort study. Diabetes Care. 2014;37(8): 2091-7.

41. Li J, Jarczok MN, Loerbroks A, Schöllgen I, Siegrist J, Bosch JA, et al. Work stress is associated with diabetes and prediabetes: cross-sectional results from the MIPH industrial cohort studies. Int J Behav Med. 2013;20(4):495-503.

42. Kontodimopoulos N, Pappa E, Chadjiapostolou Z, Arvanitaki E, Papadopoulos AA, Niakas D. Comparing the sensitivity of EQ-5D, SF-6D and 15D utilities to the specific effect of diabetic complications. Eur J Health Econ. 2012;13:111-20.

23

Identification of an obesity index for predicting metabolic syndrome by gender: the rural Chinese cohort study

Leilei Liu[1], Yu Liu[2], Xizhuo Sun[2], Zhaoxia Yin[2], Honghui Li[2], Kunpeng Deng[3], Xu Chen[1], Cheng Cheng[1], Xinping Luo[4], Ming Zhang[4], Linlin Li[1], Lu Zhang[1], Bingyuan Wang[1,4], Yongcheng Ren[1,4], Yang Zhao[1,4], Dechen Liu[1,4], Junmei Zhou[4], Chengyi Han[1], Xuejiao Liu[1], Dongdong Zhang[1], Feiyan Liu[4], Chongjian Wang[1] and Dongsheng Hu[1*]

Abstract

Background: To compare the accuracy of different obesity indexes, including waist circumference (WC), weight-to-height ratio (WHtR), body mass index (BMI), and lipid accumulation product (LAP), in predicting metabolic syndrome (MetS) and to estimate the optimal cutoffs of these indexes in a rural Chinese adult population.

Methods: This prospective cohort involved 8468 participants who were followed up for 6 years. MetS was defined by the International Diabetes Federation, American Heart Association, and National Heart, Lung, and Blood Institute criteria. The power of the 4 indexes for predicting MetS was estimated by receiver operating characteristic (ROC) curve analysis and optimal cutoffs were determined by the maximum of Youden's index.

Results: As compared with WHtR, BMI, and LAP, WC had the largest area under the ROC curve (AUC) for predicting MetS after adjusting for age, smoking, drinking, physical activity, and education level. The AUCs (95% CIs) for WC, WHtR, BMI, and LAP for men and women were 0.862 (0.851–0.873) and 0.806 (0.794–0.817), 0.832 (0.820–0.843) and 0.789 (0.777–0.801), 0.824 (0.812–0.835) and 0.790 (0.778–0.802), and 0.798 (0.785–0.810) and 0.771 (0.759–0.784), respectively. The optimal cutoffs of WC for men and women were 83.30 and 76.80 cm. Those of WHtR, BMI, and LAP were approximately 0.51 and 0.50, 23.90 and 23.00 kg/m^2, and 19.23 and 20.48 cm.mmol/L, respectively.

Conclusions: WC as a preferred index over WHtR, BMI, and LAP for predicting MetS in rural Chinese adults of both genders; the optimal cutoffs for men and women were 83.30 and 76.80 cm.

Keywords: Obesity index, Predict, Metabolic syndrome, Cohort study

Background

Metabolic syndrome (MetS) [1] is a cluster of metabolic abnormalities highly associated with type 2 diabetes mellitus [2], cardiovascular disease [3, 4], and all-cause mortality [5]. It is also a major and escalating public health and clinical challenge worldwide [6]. The increasing prevalence of MetS is observed all over the world and in China [7–10]. Therefore, the early prediction of MetS is essential to prevent potential severe-cardiometabolic consequences caused by MetS.

Obesity seems to be an underlying risk factor in the development of MetS [11, 12]. Waist circumference (WC) is used as a measure of abdominal obesity, and previous studies suggested that WC could be a powerful tool for predicting MetS [13, 14]. However, other obesity indexes such as weight-to-height ratio (WHtR), body mass index (BMI), and lipid accumulation product (LAP) have been found better predictors of MetS than WC [15–17]. As well, controversy remains as to the superiority and the optimal cutoffs of WC, WHtR, BMI, and LAP for predicting MetS [18, 19].

Many previous studies had a cross-sectional design and sample sizes were small, especially studies in China [20–22]. We used data from a large prospective cohort study to

---

* Correspondence: hud@szu.edu.cn
[1]Department of Epidemiology and Health Statistics, College of Public Health, Zhengzhou University, Zhengzhou, Henan, People's Republic of China
Full list of author information is available at the end of the article

compare the power of WC, WHtR, BMI, and LAP to identify an index for predicting MetS in rural Chinese adults and assess the optimal cutoffs of these indexes for predicting MetS for both genders.

Methods

Study design and participants

This prospective cohort study was conducted in rural areas around Luoyang City, Henan Province, in the middle of China. A total of 20,194 participants ≥18 years old were recruited by cluster sampling at baseline (July to August of 2007 and July to August of 2008), and 17,265 participants were followed up (July to August of 2013 and July to October of 2014) (response rate 85.5%).

For this study, we excluded participants with known MetS at baseline ($n = 6390$); incomplete data on anthropometric and laboratory measurements at baseline ($n = 199$); WC ≤ 65 cm for men and 58 cm for women ($n = 147$) (based on the calculation formula of LAP [23]); no follow-up examination or death during follow-up ($n = 2795$); and unknown MetS status at follow-up (2195). Finally, 8468 eligible participants (4085 men) without MetS at baseline were included in the present analysis to identify the baseline obesity indexes to predict the presence of MetS at follow-up.

The study was approved by the Ethics Committee of Zhengzhou University and all participants gave their written informed consent to participate before the start of the study.

Definition of metabolic syndrome

MetS at baseline and follow-up was diagnosed according to International Diabetes Federation (IDF), American Heart Association, and National Heart, Lung, and Blood Institute (AHA/NHLBI) criteria [24]. The criteria for MetS we used was the presence of 3 or more abnormal values among the following variables: WC (90 and 80 cm for men and women), triglycerides (TG) level (approximately 1.69 mmol/L), high-density lipoprotein-cholesterol (HDL-C) level (approximately 1.04 and 1.30 mmol/L for men and women), systolic blood pressure (SBP; 130 mmHg), diastolic blood pressure (DBP; 85 mmHg) and fasting plasma glucose (FPG; approximately 5.56 mmol/L).

Data collection and laboratory measurement

Demographic and anthropometric data for each participant were collected by trained investigators who used a standard questionnaire. In the present study, smokers were defined as currently smoking and/or having smoked at least 100 cigarettes during the lifetime; the others were considered non-smokers [25]. Drinking was defined as having consumed alcohol 12 or more times in the previous year. Education level was classified as high school or above and low education level. Physical activity

level was classified as low, moderate, and high physical activity level by the International Physical Activity Questionnaire scoring protocol [26].

Weight and height were measured twice to the nearest 0.5 kg and 0.1 cm, respectively, with participants wearing light clothing but no shoes, according to a standard protocol [27]. BMI is an index of general obesity that combines weight and height measurements and is calculated as weight in kilograms (kg) divided by height in meters squared (m^2) [28]. WC was measured twice at the mid-point between the lowest rib and the iliac crest to the nearest 0.1 cm [29], and WHtR was calculated by dividing WC (cm) by height (cm).

Blood pressure was measured by using an electronic sphygmomanometer (HEM-770AFuzzy, Omron, Japan) according to the AHA standardized protocol [30]. SBP and DBP were measured in triplicate and the results were averaged. Overnight fasting blood samples were collected for assessing levels of total cholesterol (TC), TG, HDL-C, and FPG by using an automatic biochemical analyzer (Hitachi 7080, Tokyo) with reagents from Wako Pure Chemical Industries (Osaka, Japan). Low-density lipoprotein-cholesterol (LDL-C) level was calculated by the Freidwald formula [31].

LAP was calculated by WC and TG concentration as *[WC (cm) – 65] × TG (mmol/L)* for men and *[WC (cm) - 58] × TG (mmol/L)* for women, as proposed by Kahn in 2005 [23].

Statistical analysis

The baseline data for study participants are described with number (percentage) or mean (standard deviation) for categorical or quantitative variables, respectively. Participants were divided into 2 groups by presence or absence of MetS and differences between the 2 groups were examined by t-tests for continuous variables and chi-square test for categorical variables.

Receiver operating characteristic (ROC) curves [18] were plotted to assess the performance of WC, WHtR, BMI, and LAP in MetS prediction by gender. The model was adjusted for age and the fully adjusted model for age, smoking, drinking, physical activity, and education level. The power of MetS prediction was quantified by the area under the ROC curve (AUC) [21, 22] with 95% confidence intervals (CIs), a larger AUC reflecting better predictive accuracy, and p-values for BMI, WHtR, and LAP were computed with WC as the reference measurement. The appropriate cutoffs of the indexes were determined by the maximum of Youden's index (sensitivity + specificity − 1, with the highest sensitivity and specificity combination).

All statistical analyses involved use of MedCalc 10.1.6.0 (MedCalc Software, Ostend, Belgium). The difference was considered statistically significant at p-value < 0.05 based on a 2-sided probability.

Results

The baseline characteristics of the study population by MetS status at follow-up are in Table 1. Compared to those without MetS men with MetS were younger, less of them were drinkers, and they had lower HDL-C levels. As expected they had higher BMI, LAP, SBP, DBP, TG, and FPG (p-value < 0.05). Compared to those without MetS women with MetS were older. As expected the anthropometric and biochemical differences were similar to those in men.

The predictive values for WC, WHtR, BMI, and LAP for MetS for both genders are in Table 2 and Fig. 1. WC, WHtR, BMI, and LAP were all associated with MetS for both genders even after adjusting for age, smoking, drinking, physical activity, and education level. In the unadjusted model (Model 1), WC had the highest AUC value for men and women (0.858, 95% CIs: 0.847–0.868 and 0.804, 95% CIs: 0.792–0.816). On age-adjusted analysis (Model 2), WC was the most accurate for both men and women (0.862, 95% CIs: 0.851–0.873 and 0.805, 95% CIs: 0.793–0.817) and had the highest accuracy in the fully adjusted model (Model 3) (0.862, 95% CIs: 0.851–0.873 and 0.806, 95% CIs: 0.794–0.817). The AUC values for WC, WHtR, BMI, and LAP were all significantly higher for men than women in the unadjusted or adjusted model. According to the results, WC possessed the best power for predicting MetS versus the other 3 indexes on unadjusted and adjusted analyses, with no significant differences between men and women by AUC value.

Table 3 shows the gender-specific optimal cutoffs of WC, WHtR, BMI, and LAP for predicting MetS. The Youden's index indicated that the appropriate cutoffs of WC for predicting MetS for men and women were 83.30 cm (sensitivity = 81.34%, specificity = 75.62 and Youden's index = 0.5696) and 76.80 cm (sensitivity = 74.01%, specificity = 72.81% and Youden's index = 0.4682). The Youden's index values were highest for WC for predicting MetS for both genders. Additionally, the optimal cutoffs of WHtR, BMI, and LAP for men and women were approximately 0.51 and 0.50, 23.90 and 23.00 kg/m^2, and 19.23 and 20.48 cm.mmol/L, respectively. The present results suggested that optimal cutoffs were higher for men than women for WC, lower for LAP and similar for WHtR and BMI.

Discussion

The present study suggested that WC had the highest accuracy and appropriate cutoffs for predicting MetS for both genders as compared with other obesity indexes such as WHtR, BMI, and LAP even after adjusting for age, smoking, drinking, physical activity, and education level.

In previous studies, the obesity index with the most power for predicting MetS has been widely debated. Among some cross-sectional studies, BMI, WC, and WHtR could similarly predict the presence of multiple metabolic risk factors in Chinese people [32]. However,

WHtR was a better index for screening MetS based on the IDF criteria as compared with BMI and LAP for both genders in a Xinjiang population [22]. In a population-based study in China [20], WHtR was the best predictor of MetS in men, but WHtR and WC were equally good predictors of MetS in women. In addition, LAP was a powerful tool for predicting MetS in undiagnosed Brazilian adults [17]. The HANDLS study [14] suggested that WC was the most powerful tool for predicting MetS among adults. Likewise, WC had the highest AUC value as compared with WHtR and LAP in a study of older men and women [33]. Additionally, in a study of adults in northeast China [34], WC was superior to BMI and WHtR in predicting MetS in men, but WHtR was superior to BMI and WC in predicting MetS in women. Among some cohort designs, the San Antonio Heart Study suggested that BMI and WC had equal power in predicting MetS in non-Hispanic whites and Mexican Americans [11]. In contrast, in an Iranian population in the north of Iran, LAP had strong and reliable diagnostic accuracy in predicting MetS, with better predictability than WC, WHtR, and BMI [35]. The Korean Genome and Epidemiology Study [36] suggested that WHtR was a better discriminator of MetS than WC and BMI. The most appropriate index and the accuracy for predicting MetS may depend on ethnicity, age, gender or the diagnostic criteria of MetS, given these inconsistent results.

The present study suggested that the cutoffs of WC for predicting MetS in rural Chinese men and women were 83.30 and 76.80 cm. A population-based study of Chinese people suggested that the optimal cutoffs of WC for men and women were 84.8 and 75.8 cm [21], which is similar to our findings, but lower than the IDF-suggested cutoffs for Chinese men and women of 90 and 80 cm [37]. As well, 2 population-based surveys conducted in China [32, 38] suggested higher WC cutoffs than those in our study. In addition, data from a cross-sectional study of 203 older Brazilians showed WC cutoffs of 90.90 cm for men and 80.20 cm for women [33]. The different ethnicities and race, cross-sectional design, and small sample size may lead to inconsistent results. Further study is needed to explore the application of current WC cutoffs to healthy people in the real world. WHtR cutoffs were 0.51 and 0.53 for Chinese men and women, respectively [32], and our results were the same as these findings and from other studies [34, 38]. The appropriate cutoffs of BMI we found among rural Chinese men and women were approximately 23.90 and 23.00 kg/m^2, which agreed with findings from population-based studies of Chinese adults [21, 32]. However, the cutoffs of LAP were lower than in previous research. The optimal cutoffs of LAP were previously found to be 34.7 and 27.3 cm.mmol/L for Chinese men and women, respectively [19], and 24.76 and 26.49 cm.mmol/L

Table 1 Baseline characteristics of study participants by metabolic syndrome (MetS) status at follow-up

Variables	Total ($n = 8468$)	With MetS ($n = 1825$)	Without MetS ($n = 6643$)	p-value
Men	4085 (48.24)	509 (12.46)	3576 (87.54)	
Age (years)	52.38 (13.07)	50.13 (12.77)	52.70 (13.08)	< 0.001
Smoking	2866 (70.16)	357 (70.14)	2509 (70.16)	0.991
Drinking	1063 (26.02)	173 (33.99)	890 (24.89)	< 0.001
Education level				0.228
High school or above	617 (15.10)	86 (16.90)	531 (14.85)	
Physical activity				0.079
Low	931 (22.79)	125 (24.56)	806 (22.54)	
Moderate	724 (17.72)	103 (20.24)	621 (17.37)	
High	2430 (59.49)	281 (55.21)	2149 (60.10)	
WC (cm)	79.59 (7.45)	88.33 (6.66)	78.34 (6.68)	< 0.001
WHtR	0.48 (0.05)	0.53 (0.04)	0.48 (0.04)	< 0.001
BMI (kg/m^2)	22.55 (2.49)	25.17 (2.46)	22.17 (2.26)	< 0.001
LAP (cm.mmol/L)	21.23 (17.02)	37.11 (20.08)	18.97 (15.25)	< 0.001
TC (mmol/L)	4.29 (0.85)	4.43 (0.86)	4.28 (0.85)	< 0.001
TG (mmol/L)	1.37 (0.66)	1.60 (0.75)	1.34 (0.65)	< 0.001
SBP (mmHg)	123.84 (17.88)	127.82 (19.14)	123.28 (17.62)	< 0.001
DBP (mmHg)	76.65 (10.69)	80.12 (11.13)	76.16 (10.54)	< 0.001
FPG (mmol/L)	5.44 (1.24)	5.59 (1.41)	5.42 (1.21)	0.009
HDL-C (mmol/L)	1.14 (0.25)	1.08 (0.22)	1.15 (0.25)	< 0.001
LDL-C (mmol/L)	2.53 (0.72)	2.62 (0.72)	2.52 (0.71)	0.004
Women	4383 (51.76)	1316 (30.03)	3067 (69.97)	
Age (years)	47.92 (12.45)	49.50 (11.23)	47.25 (12.88)	< 0.001
Smoking	13 (0.30)	4 (0.30)	9 (0.29)	0.953
Drinking	31 (0.71)	8 (0.61)	23 (0.75)	0.607
Education level				0.079
High school or above	337 (7.69)	87 (6.61)	250 (8.15)	
Physical activity				0.065
Low	1358 (30.98)	381 (28.95)	977 (31.86)	
Moderate	1035 (23.61)	316 (24.01)	719 (23.44)	
High	1990 (45.40)	619 (47.04)	1371 (44.70)	
WC (cm)	75.72 (7.85)	81.53 (7.86)	73.22 (6.39)	< 0.001
WHtR	0.49 (0.05)	0.53 (0.05)	0.48 (0.04)	< 0.001
BMI (kg/m^2)	22.75 (2.93)	24.75 (2.98)	21.89 (2.45)	< 0.001
LAP (cm.mmol/L)	23.10 (15.52)	32.73 (16.85)	18.98 (12.88)	< 0.001
TC (mmol/L)	4.40 (0.89)	4.56 (0.90)	4.33 (0.88)	< 0.001
TG (mmol/L)	1.28 (0.62)	1.42 (0.65)	1.22 (0.59)	< 0.001
SBP (mmHg)	120.47 (19.45)	125.18 (19.53)	118.46 (19.06)	< 0.001
DBP (mmHg)	75.73 (10.59)	79.15 (10.90)	74.27 (10.10)	< 0.001
FPG (mmol/L)	5.37 (1.11)	5.48 (1.26)	5.33 (1.04)	< 0.001
HDL-C (mmol/L)	1.27 (0.27)	1.23 (0.26)	1.29 (0.28)	< 0.001
LDL-C (mmol/L)	2.54 (0.74)	2.68 (0.75)	2.49 (0.73)	< 0.001

Abbreviations: *WC* waist circumference, *WHtR* waist-to-height ratio, *BMI* body mass index, *LAP* lipid accumulation product, *TC* total cholesterol, *TG* triglycerides, *SBP* systolic blood pressure, *DBP* diastolic blood pressure, *FPG* fasting plasma glucose, *HDL-C* high-density lipoprotein-cholesterol, *LDL-C* low-density lipoprotein-cholesterol
Data are number (percentage) or mean (standard deviation)

Table 2 AUC values for WC, WHtR, BMI, and LAP for predicting MetS by gender

Model	Variables	Men ($n = 4085$)		Women ($n = 4383$)	
		AUC (95% CIs)	p-value	AUC (95% CIs)	p-value
Model 1	WC	0.858 (0.847–0.868)	–	0.804 (0.792–0.816)	–
	WHtR	0.819 (0.807–0.831)	< 0.001	0.789 (0.776–0.801)	< 0.001
	BMI	0.821 (0.808–0.832)	< 0.001	0.781 (0.768–0.793)	< 0.001
	LAP	0.796 (0.783–0.808)	< 0.001	0.770 (0.758–0.783)	< 0.001
Model 2	WC	0.862 (0.851–0.873)	–	0.805 (0.793–0.817)	–
	WHtR	0.831 (0.820–0.843)	< 0.001	0.789 (0.776–0.801)	< 0.001
	BMI	0.823 (0.811–0.835)	< 0.001	0.790 (0.778–0.802)	0.012
	LAP	0.798 (0.785–0.810)	< 0.001	0.770 (0.758–0.783)	< 0.001
Model 3	WC	0.862 (0.851–0.873)	–	0.806 (0.794–0.817)	–
	WHtR	0.832 (0.820–0.843)	< 0.001	0.789 (0.777–0.801)	< 0.001
	BMI	0.824 (0.812–0.835)	< 0.001	0.790 (0.778–0.802)	0.010
	LAP	0.798 (0.785–0.810)	< 0.001	0.771 (0.759–0.784)	< 0.001

Abbreviations: *AUC* the area under the ROC curve, *WC* waist circumference, *WHtR* waist-to-height ratio, *BMI* body mass index, *LAP* lipid accumulation product
Model 1: unadjusted model
Model 2: adjusted for age
Model 3: adjusted for age, smoking, drinking, physical activity, and education level
*p-value indicates the statistical significance of other models compared with a model of WC

in the Kazakh adult population in Xinjiang [22]. Additionally, the HANDLS study [14] suggested that optimal cutoffs of various indexes may differ by gender, and we found this trend for WC and LAP but not WHtR and BMI.

The determinant (WC or WC plus TG) is a component of MetS, but in terms of considering the determinant as a potential confounder, we could not consider MetS as a cluster of metabolic abnormalities highly associated with type 2 diabetes mellitus and cardiovascular disease, which occurs together half the time than accidentally alone [24]. As well, although one study showed that confounding occurs in evaluating classification accuracy when a variable is

associated with both the marker and the binary outcome [39], many previous studies showed that only age and gender were potential confounders of the association of WC or LAP with MetS [17, 23, 35, 40–42]. We conducted the gender-specific study and adjusted for age in the present study, so the results do not have a bias of accuracy.

The primary purpose of this study was to define the baseline characteristics predicting the presence of MetS at follow-up based on a rural Chinese population. The sample size of this study was not determined specifically; 20,194 cohort members were recruited at baseline examination and followed up for 6 years currently. Therefore,

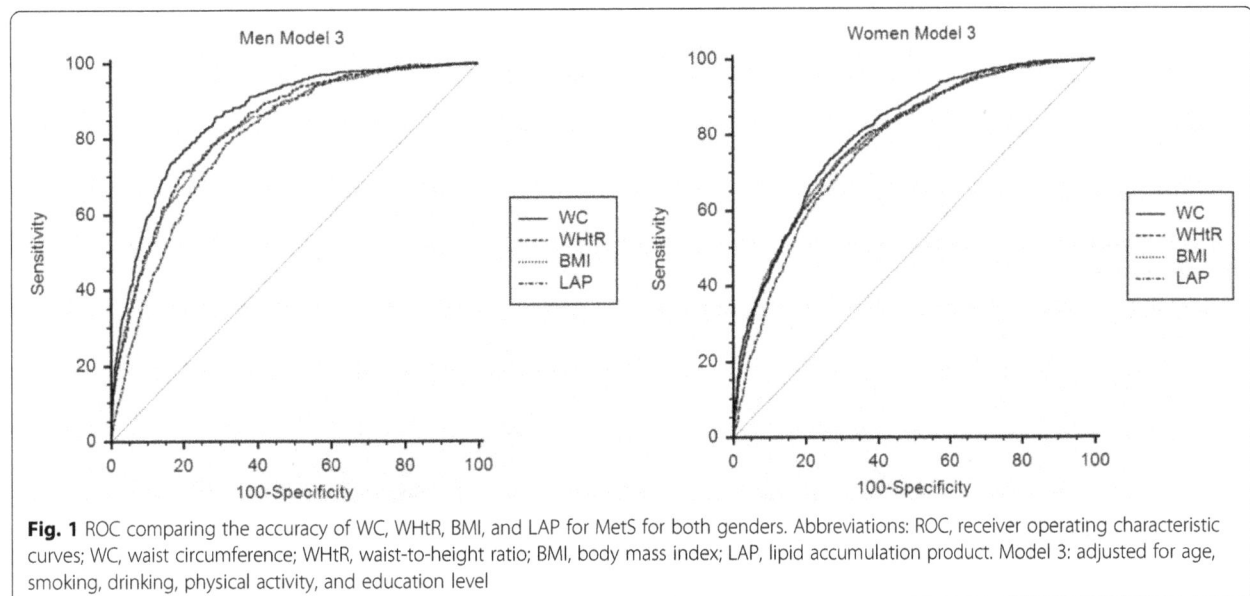

Fig. 1 ROC comparing the accuracy of WC, WHtR, BMI, and LAP for MetS for both genders. Abbreviations: ROC, receiver operating characteristic curves; WC, waist circumference; WHtR, waist-to-height ratio; BMI, body mass index; LAP, lipid accumulation product. Model 3: adjusted for age, smoking, drinking, physical activity, and education level

Table 3 Optimal cutoffs of WC, WHtR, BMI, and LAP for MetS prediction by gender

Variables	Cutoff	Sensitivity (%)	Specificity (%)	Youden's index
Men				
WC (cm)	83.30	81.34	75.62	0.5696
WHtR	0.51	73.08	76.43	0.4951
BMI (kg/m²)	23.90	72.69	76.99	0.4968
LAP (cm.mmol/ L)	19.23	84.28	61.94	0.4622
Women				
WC (cm)	76.80	74.01	72.81	0.4682
WHtR	0.50	74.39	69.61	0.4400
BMI (kg/m²)	23.00	71.28	70.33	0.4161
LAP (cm.mmol/L)	20.48	76.44	64.62	0.4106

Abbreviations: *WC* waist circumference, *WHtR* waist-to-height ratio, *BMI* body mass index, *LAP* lipid accumulation product

the sample size should be large enough to meet most of the study hypotheses for MetS conditions.

Many previous studies had limitations that included a cross-sectional design [32–34], but our study's strength lay in its prospective design. Furthermore, we used data from a large population-based-cohort of both genders as compared with previous studies with a small sample size [11, 19–21]. Additionally, we compared various indexes for predicting MetS among rural Chinese adults and provided corresponding AUC and cutoffs for these indexes in this analysis stratified by gender.

We are aware of several relevant limitations of our study besides the strengths we have mentioned. First, although we adjusted for age, smoking, drinking, physical activity, and education level, other confounders might have affected MetS, such as family history of disease, which were not included in the adjustment model. Second, participants were exclusively from rural areas in China, so our results may not be transferred to urban populations. Finally, 2929 participants were not followed up in this cohort, which could imply follow-up bias.

In conclusion, we provide longitudinal evidence for the power of WC, WHtR, BMI, and LAP in predicting MetS, and all 4 indexes were significantly associated with MetS for both genders even after adjusting for some known confounding variables. In addition, WC showed superior power for predicting MetS as compared with the other 3 indexes. The use of a simple index such as WC could contribute to the early prediction of MetS in rural Chinese people, as effective intervention to prevent and treat risks related to MetS. In addition, it may provide useful instruction for public health promotion to maintain optimal cutoffs of WC, BMI, WHtR, and LAP.

Nevertheless, from our results and those of previous research, controversy still remains as to which index has better accuracy for predicting MetS in different countries, ethnicities, and genders. Thus, further larger and prospective research is warranted to elucidate the association between the 4 obesity indexes and MetS and to define appropriate cutoffs in the adult Chinese population.

The WC cutoffs of 83.30 cm for men and 76.80 cm for women from our study are quite a lot different from the 90 cm for Asian American men and 80 cm for Asian American women used in the IDF and AHA/NHLBI criteria [24]. In Japan specific WC cutoffs of 85 cm for men and 90 cm for women were based on visceral fat quantitation on CT scan [43, 44]. Thus country and ethnic specific criteria based on good local data are an appropriate approach. If the cutoffs derived from our data are to be used in practice, we may need to use 83 cm or even 85 cm for men and 77 cm or even 75 cm for women for simplicity but these would still be different from those used for Asian American participants.

Conclusions

In summary, the present prospective cohort study found that WC at cutoffs 83.30 cm for men and 76.80 cm for women was superior to BMI, WHtR, and LAP for predicting MetS in rural Chinese adults. It is crucial for the early prediction and prevention of MetS to indentify an appropriate index and corresponding optimal cutoffs.

Abbreviations
AUC: the area under the ROC curve; BMI: body mass index; CIs: confidence intervals; DBP: diastolic blood pressure; FPG: fasting plasma glucose; HDL-C: high-density lipoprotein-cholesterol; LAP: lipid accumulation product; LDL-C: low-density lipoprotein-cholesterol; MetS: metabolic syndrome; ROC: receiver operating characteristic; SBP: systolic blood pressure; TC: total cholesterol; TG: triglycerides; WC: waist circumference; WHtR: weight-to-height ratio

Acknowledgments
We are indebted to all the subjects participating in this study.

Funding
This study was supported by the National Natural Science Foundation of China (No. 81373074, 81402752, and 81673260) and Science and Technology Development Foundation of Shenzhen (No. JCYJ20160307155707264).

Authors' contributions
LL1, LL2, MZ, CW, and DH. substantially contributed to the design and drafting of the study and the analysis and interpretation of the data. LL1, YL, XS, ZY, HL, and KD. contributed to the data analysis and discussion. XC, CC, XL2, LZ, BW, YR, YZ, and DL. made contributions to acquisition and interpretation of data. JZ, CH, XL1, DZ, FL, and DH. revised it critically for important intellectual content. All authors read and approved the final manuscript.

Competing interests

The authors declare that they have no competing interests.

Author details

[1]Department of Epidemiology and Health Statistics, College of Public Health, Zhengzhou University, Zhengzhou, Henan, People's Republic of China. [2]The Affiliated Luohu Hospital of Shenzhen University Health Sciences Center, Shenzhen, Guangdong, People's Republic of China. [3]Yantian Entry-exit Inspection and Quarantine Bureau, Shenzhen, Guangdong, People's Republic of China. [4]Department of Preventive Medicine, Shenzhen University Health Sciences Center, Shenzhen, Guangdong, People's Republic of China.

References

1. Eckel RH, Grundy SM, Zimmet PZ. The metabolic syndrome. Lancet. 2005; 365(9468):1415–28.
2. Grundy SM. Metabolic syndrome pandemic. Arterioscler Thromb Vasc Biol. 2008;28(4):629–36.
3. Grundy SM. Metabolic syndrome: connecting and reconciling cardiovascular and diabetes worlds. J Am Coll Cardiol. 2006;47(6):1093–100.
4. Mottillo S, Filion KB, Genest J, Joseph L, Pilote L, Poirier P, Rinfret S, Schiffrin EL, Eisenberg MJ. The metabolic syndrome and cardiovascular risk a systematic review and meta-analysis. J Am Coll Cardiol. 2010;56(14):1113–32.
5. Wu SH, Liu Z, Ho SC. Metabolic syndrome and all-cause mortality: a meta-analysis of prospective cohort studies. Eur J Epidemiol. 2010;25(6):375–84.
6. O'Neill S, O'Driscoll L. Metabolic syndrome: a closer look at the growing epidemic and its associated pathologies. Obesity reviews : an official journal of the International Association for the Study of Obesity. 2015;16(1):1–12.
7. Cai H, Huang J, Xu Y, Yang Z, Liu M, Mi Y, Liu W, Wang H, Qian D. Prevalence and determinants of metabolic syndrome among women in Chinese rural areas. PLoS One. 2012;7(5):e36936.
8. Song P, Yu J, Chang X, Wang M, An L: Prevalence and Correlates of Metabolic Syndrome in Chinese Children: The China Health and Nutrition Survey. Nutrients 2017, 9(1).
9. Mozumdar A, Liguori G. Persistent increase of prevalence of metabolic syndrome among U.S. adults: NHANES III to NHANES. Diabetes care 2011. 1999-2006;34(1):216–9.
10. Xi B, He D, Hu Y, Zhou D. Prevalence of metabolic syndrome and its influencing factors among the Chinese adults: the China health and nutrition survey in 2009. Prev Med. 2013;57(6):867–71.
11. Han TS, Williams K, Sattar N, Hunt KJ, Lean MEJ, Haffner SM. Analysis of obesity and Hyperinsulinemia in the development of metabolic syndrome: San Antonio heart study. Obes Res. 2002;10(9):923–31.
12. Yong-Woo Park M. PhD, Shankuan Zhu, MD, PhD, Latha Palaniappan, MD, Stanley, Heshka, PhD, Mercedes R. Carnethon, PhD, and Steven B. Heymsfield, MD: the metabolic syndrome: prevalence and associated risk factor findings in the US population from the third National Health and nutrition examination survey, 1988-1994. Arch Intern Med. 2003;24: 427–36.
13. Agredo-Zuniga RA, Aguilar-de Plata C, Suarez-Ortegon MF. Waist:height ratio, waist circumference and metabolic syndrome abnormalities in Colombian schooled adolescents: a multivariate analysis considering located adiposity. Br J Nutr. 2015;114(5):700–5.
14. Beydoun MA, Kuczmarski MT, Wang Y, Mason MA, Evans MK, Zonderman AB. Receiver-operating characteristics of adiposity for metabolic syndrome: the healthy aging in neighborhoods of diversity across the life span (HANDLS) study. Public Health Nutr. 2011;14(1): 77–92.
15. Sakurai M, Takamura T, Miura K, Kaneko S, Nakagawa H. BMI may be better than waist circumference for defining metabolic syndrome in Japanese women. Diabetes Care. 2008;31(3):e12.
16. Rodea-Montero ER, Evia-Viscarra ML, Apolinar-Jimenez E. Waist-to-height ratio is a better anthropometric index than waist circumference and BMI in predicting metabolic syndrome among obese Mexican adolescents. Int J Endocrinol. 2014;2014:195407.
17. Nascimento-Ferreira MV, Rendo-Urteaga T, Vilanova-Campelo RC, Carvalho HB, da Paz OG, Paes Landim MB, Torres-Leal FL. The lipid accumulation

18. product is a powerful tool to predict metabolic syndrome in undiagnosed Brazilian adults. Clin Nutr. 2017;36(6):1693–700.
18. Yang F, Lv JH, Lei SF, Chen XD, Liu MY, Jian WX, Xu H, Tan LJ, Deng FY, Yang YJ, et al. Receiver-operating characteristic analyses of body mass index, waist circumference and waist-to-hip ratio for obesity: screening in young adults in central south of China. Clin Nutr. 2006;25(6):1030–9.
19. Guo SX, Zhang XH, Zhang JY, He J, Yan YZ, Ma JL, Ma RL, Guo H, Mu LT, Li SG, et al. Visceral adiposity and anthropometric indicators as screening tools of metabolic syndrome among low income rural adults in Xinjiang. Sci Rep. 2016;6:36091.
20. Zhang ZQ, Deng J, He LP, Ling WH, Su YX, Chen YM. Comparison of various anthropometric and body fat indices in identifying cardiometabolic disturbances in Chinese men and women. PLoS One. 2013;8(8):e70893.
21. Zeng Q, He Y, Dong S, Zhao X, Chen Z, Song Z, Chang G, Yang F, Wang Y. Optimal cut-off values of BMI, waist circumference and waist:height ratio for defining obesity in Chinese adults. Br J Nutr. 2014;112(10):1735–44.
22. Zhang XH, Zhang M, He J, Yan YZ, Ma JL, Wang K, Ma RL, Guo H, Mu LT, Ding YS, et al. Comparison of anthropometric and Atherogenic indices as screening tools of metabolic syndrome in the Kazakh adult population in Xinjiang. Int J Environ Res Public Health. 2016;13(4):428.
23. Kahn HS. The "lipid accumulation product" performs better than the body mass index for recognizing cardiovascular risk: a population-based comparison. BMC Cardiovasc Disord. 2005;5:26.
24. Alberti KG, Eckel RH, Grundy SM, Zimmet PZ, Cleeman JI, Donato KA, Fruchart JC, James WP, Loria CM, Smith SC Jr, et al. Harmonizing the metabolic syndrome: a joint interim statement of the international diabetes federation task force on epidemiology and prevention; National Heart, Lung, and Blood Institute; American Heart Association; world heart federation; international atherosclerosis society; and International Association for the Study of obesity. Circulation. 2009;120(16):1640–5.
25. Wildman RP, Muntner P, Reynolds K, McGinn AP, Rajpathak S, Wylie-Rosett J, Sowers MR. The obese without cardiometabolic risk factor clustering and the normal weight with cardiometabolic risk factor clustering: prevalence and correlates of 2 phenotypes among the US population (NHANES 1999-2004). Arch Intern Med. 2008;168(15):1617–24.
26. Craig CL, Marshall AL, Sjostrom M, Bauman AE, Booth ML, Ainsworth BE, Pratt M, Ekelund U, Yngve A, Sallis JF, et al. International physical activity questionnaire: 12-country reliability and validity. Med Sci Sports Exerc. 2003; 35(8):1381–95.
27. Ulla Uusitalo AC, Liisa Palonen, Milorad Toša Zikic, et al.: Geographical variation in the major risk factors of coronary heart disease in men and women aged 35–64 years. Wld hlth statist quan 1988, 41:115–140.
28. Doak CM, Hoffman DJ, Norris SA, Campos Ponce M, Polman K, Griffiths PL. Is body mass index an appropriate proxy for body fat in children? Global Food Security. 2013;2(2):65–71.
29. Wang CJ, Li YQ, Wang L, Li LL, Guo YR, Zhang LY, Zhang MX, Bie RH. Development and evaluation of a simple and effective prediction approach for identifying those at high risk of dyslipidemia in rural adult residents. PLoS One. 2012;7(8):e43834.
30. Perloff D, Grim C, Flack J, Frohlich ED, Hill M, Mcdonald M, Morgenstern BZ. Human blood-pressure determination by Sphygmomanometry. Circulation. 1993;88(5):2460–70.
31. Bairaktari E, Hatzidimou K, Tzallas C, Vini M, Katsaraki A, Tselepis A, Elisaf M, Tsolas O. Estimation of LDL cholesterol based on the Friedewald formula and on apo B levels. Clin Biochem. 2000;33(7):549–55.
32. Liu Y, Tong G, Tong W, Lu L, Qin X. Can body mass index, waist circumference, waist-hip ratio and waist-height ratio predict the presence of multiple metabolic risk factors in Chinese subjects? BMC Public Health. 2011;11:35.
33. de Oliveira CC, Roriz AK, Ramos LB, Gomes Neto M. Indicators of adiposity predictors of metabolic syndrome in the elderly. Annals of nutrition & metabolism. 2017;70(1):9–15.
34. Yu J, Tao Y, Tao Y, Yang S, Yu Y, Li B, Jin L. Optimal cut-off of obesity indices to predict cardiovascular disease risk factors and metabolic syndrome among adults in Northeast China. BMC Public Health. 2016; 16(1):1079.
35. Motamed N, Razmjou S, Hemmasi G, Maadi M, Zamani F. Lipid accumulation product and metabolic syndrome: a population-based study in northern Iran, Amol. J Endocrinol Investig. 2016;39(4):375–82.
36. Ko KP, Oh DK, Min H, Kim CS, Park JK, Kim Y, Kim SS. Prospective study of optimal obesity index cutoffs for predicting development of multiple

metabolic risk factors: the Korean genome and epidemiology study. J Epidemiol. 2012;22(5):433–9.

37. Saito I. Epidemiological evidence of type 2 diabetes mellitus, metabolic syndrome, and cardiovascular disease in Japan. Circulation journal : official journal of the Japanese Circulation Society. 2012;76(5):1066–73.

38. Shao J, Yu L, Shen X, Li D, Wang K. Waist-to-height ratio, an optimal predictor for obesity and metabolic syndrome in Chinese adults. J Nutr Health Aging. 2010;14(9):782–5.

39. Janes H, Pepe MS. Adjusting for covariates in studies of diagnostic, screening, or prognostic markers: an old concept in a new setting. Am J Epidemiol. 2008;168(1):89–97.

40. Chiang JK, Koo M. Lipid accumulation product: a simple and accurate index for predicting metabolic syndrome in Taiwanese people aged 50 and over. BMC Cardiovasc Disord. 2012;12:78.

41. Tellechea ML, Aranguren F, Martinez-Larrad MT, Serrano-Rios M, Taverna MJ, Frechtel GD. Ability of lipid accumulation product to identify metabolic syndrome in healthy men from Buenos Aires. Diabetes Care. 2009;32(7):e85.

42. Taverna MJ, Martinez-Larrad MT, Frechtel GD, Serrano-Rios M. Lipid accumulation product: a powerful marker of metabolic syndrome in healthy population. Eur J Endocrinol. 2011;164(4):559–67.

43. Yuji M. Metabolic syndrome-definition and diagnostic criteria in Japan. J Atheroscler Thromb. 2005;12(6):301.

44. Yuji M. Metabolic syndrome-definition and diagnostic criteria in Japan. J Jpn Soc Intern Med. 2005;94:188–203.

24

The effects of single high-dose or daily low-dosage oral colecalciferol treatment on vitamin D levels and muscle strength in postmenopausal women

Mahmut Apaydin[1]*, Asli Gencay Can[2], Muhammed Kizilgul[1], Selvihan Beysel[1], Seyfullah Kan[1], Mustafa Caliskan[1], Taner Demirci[1], Ozgur Ozcelik[1], Mustafa Ozbek[1] and Erman Cakal[1]

Abstract

Introduction: Vitamin D deficiency is a common health problem. Vitamin D supplements are used to improve vitamin D status; however, there are contradictory data related to what doses to give and how often they should be given. Many studies have investigated the effects of vitamin D supplementation on muscle strength, but the results remain controversial. We aimed to compare the effects and safety of single high-dose with daily low-dose oral colecalciferol on 25(OH)D levels and muscle strength in postmenopausal women with vitamin D deficiency or insufficiency.

Methods and design: Sixty healthy postmenopausal women who had serum vitamin D levels < 20 ng/mL (50 nmol/L) were enrolled in the study. Group 1 ($n = 32$) was given daily oral dosages of 800 IU vitamin D3, and group 2 ($n = 28$) was given a single oral dose of 300,000 IU vitamin D3. Serum vitamin D levels and muscle strengths were measured at the beginning, 4th, and 12th week. Muscle strength tests were performed at 60° using a Biodex system 3 isokinetic dynamometer.

Results: Pretreatment vitamin D levels did not differ between the two groups (10.2 ± 4.4 ng/mL (25,4 ± 10,9 nmol/L); 9.7 ± 4.4 ng/mL (24,2 ± 10,9 nmol/L), $p > 0.05$). A significant increase in vitamin D levels was observed in both groups at 4 and 12 weeks after vitamin D3 treatment. The increase in the single-dose group was significantly higher than the daily low-dosage group at the 4th week (35.9 ± 9.6 ng/mL (89,6 ± 23,9 nmol/L), 16.9 ± 5.8 ng/mL (42,1 ± 14,4 nmol/L), $p = 0.01$). The increase in the single-dose group was significantly higher than in the daily low dosage group at the 12th week (23.4 ± 4.7 ng/mL (58,4 ± 11,7 nmol/L), 19.8 ± 7.2 ng/mL (49,4 ± 17,9 nmol/L), $p = 0.049$). The quadriceps muscle strength score increased significantly in the daily group at the 4th week ($p = 0.038$). The hamstring muscle strength score increased significantly in the daily group at the 12th week ($p = 0.037$).

Conclusion: Although daily administration routes are more effective in improving muscle strength, a single administration is more effective in increasing vitamin D levels.

Keywords: Vitamin D, Muscle strength, Postmenopausal women

* Correspondence: drmahmutapaydin@gmail.com
[1]Department of Endocrinology and Metabolism, Diskapi Training and Research Hospital, Ankara, Turkey
Full list of author information is available at the end of the article

Background

Vitamin D is a fat-soluble vitamin that is now known to play an important role in a variety of biologic functions including immune regulation, proliferation, differentiation, apoptosis, and angiogenesis, in addition to being the main hormone regulating calcium phosphate homeostasis and mineral bone metabolism [1]. Vitamin D deficiency is often undiagnosed and untreated because it has insidious or nonspecific signs and symptoms, and is a common health problem worldwide [2]. Many authors agree that a 25-hydroxyvitamin D3 (25(OH)D3) concentration less than 20 ng/mL (50 nmol/L) is defined as vitamin D deficiency; however, a 25(OH)D3 concentration between 21 and 29 ng/mL (50–74 nmol/L) is defined as vitamin D insufficiency [3]. The form of vitamin D therapy, the dose and dosing interval, and route of administration are not given much importance because there are no specific recommendations or guidelines in this regard [4]. It is well documented that increasing 25(OH)D3 serum levels in patients with vitamin D deficiency increases intestinal calcium absorption, decreases parathyroid hormone (PTH) levels, fall incidence and fracture risk, and increases muscle strength [5]. Serum 25(OH)D3 is accepted as the best indicator of vitamin D condition [6]. The cell nuclei of muscle cells express the vitamin D receptor (VDR) [7] and vitamin D has an impact on muscle cell contractility [8]. Vitamin D deficiency leads to disruption in muscular protein synthesis and consequently muscle mass, and finally muscle strength decreases as a result [9]. Vitamin D deficiency may lead to myopathy. Vitamin D supplementation is considered to have an influence on muscle fiber composition and morphology in vitamin D deficient older adults [10].

In a study conducted in 167 postmenopausal women, it was demonstrated that a serum 25(OH)D3 level higher than 20 ng/mL (50 nmol/L) was achieved with a vitamin D(3) dosage of 800 IU/d in 97.5% of women [11]. It is known that daily vitamin D supplementation reduces the frequency of falls and fractures in older women [12]. However, poor adherence to oral vitamin D replacement is a common clinical problem [13, 14]. Several studies about the pharmacokinetics, biochemical effects, efficacy, and safety proved that a single large dose of colecalciferol was safe, well tolerated, and effective [15–19]. In a systematic review of studies using large, single-dose, oral vitamin D supplementation in adult populations, a single vitamin D3 dose of ≥100,000 IU was shown to provide a perdurable effective means of increasing short-term vitamin D concentrations to > 20 ng/mL (50 nmol/L). However, larger vitamin D3 doses of ≥300,000 IU were required to achieve 25(OH)D3 concentrations > 30 ng/mL (75 nmol/L) and decreased plasma PTH concentrations [20]. Despite the presence of many studies on this topic, an accepted recommendation about the best dose and dose interval is still lacking.

Many studies have investigated the effects of vitamin D supplementation on muscle function but the results remain controversial. Some studies observed a favorable effect of vitamin D supplementation on muscle strength [21, 22], whereas others failed to show this beneficial effect [16, 23, 24]. A meta-analysis demonstrated that muscle strength could be improved by vitamin D supplementation [25]. On the contrary, another meta-analysis including 12 studies, which focused on older subjects with baseline 25(OH)D3 concentrations higher than (10 ng/mL) 25 nmol/L, indicated no beneficial effect of vitamin D supplementation on muscle strength [26].

The primary aim of this study was to evaluate and compare the effects and safety of single high- dose with daily low-dosage oral colecalciferol on 25(OH)D3 levels in older patients with vitamin D deficiency or insufficiency.

Methods

We enrolled 60 healthy, postmenopausal women aged 50–68 years whose vitamin D level was lower than 20 ng/mL (50 nmol/L). The participants, who were followed up by our clinic in Diskapi Training and Research Hospital, were consecutively randomized to the administration of daily 800 IU ($n = 32$) or a single oral bolus of 300,000 IU ($n = 28$) of vitamin D_3. Individuals who had granulomatous conditions, thyroid disease, malabsorption syndromes, liver disease, kidney disease, diabetes or postural instability (cerebellar disease, vestibular disease, vitamin B12 deficiency, drugs), and individuals taking anticonvulsants, calcium or vitamin D supplements, barbiturates, or steroids in any form were excluded. The study protocol was approved by the medical ethics committee of the Ankara Diskapi Training and Research Hospital, and all subjects gave written informed consent.

Design overview

Our study was a randomized clinical trial that lasted 3 months. The participants were collected in the spring and winter of 2015–2016 to minimize seasonal effects. Serum vitamin D levels and muscle strengths were measured at the beginning, and 4th and 12th weeks of treatment. The physiotherapist who assessed all functional endpoints was blinded to both regimens and the physiotherapist who performed the assessments was blinded to the treatment groups.

Analytical methods

Calcium and phosphate were measured using an enzyme method with an autoanalyzer (ADVIA 2400, Siemens Healthcare Diagnostics Inc., Tarrytown, NY, USA). iPTH and 25(OH)D were measured using an immunochemiluminescent assay (Siemens Advia Centaur XP, Siemens Healthcare Diagnostics Inc., Tarrytown, NY, USA).

Quadriceps (knee extensors) and hamstring (knee flexors) muscle strengths of each leg were measured in Biodex System 3 isokinetic dynamometer (Biodex, Shirley, NY) at the beginning, and 4th and 12th weeks of treatment. The patients were strapped into the chair with their knee flexed at 90°. The anatomic axis of the knee (lateral femoral condyle) was aligned with the axis of the dynamometer. The resistance pad was placed proximal to the medial malleolus. A seat belt harness was placed around the patient's chest and thigh for stabilization. The range of motion varied from 90° knee flexion to full extension. Maximal quadriceps and hamstring peak torques (Nm) were obtained through concentric isokinetic knee extension and flexion performed at the angular velocity of 60°/sn for 5 consecutive contractions. The highest peak torque value of these 5 contractions was recorded. The value of peak torque for each muscle was divided by body weight and the relative peak value (Nm/kg) was calculated. Isokinetic muscle strength was assessed using the relative peak value. All patients indicated that their right leg was dominant.

Statistical analysis
Statistical analysis was performed using the SPSS 18.0 (SPSS, Inc) software. Descriptive analyses are expressed as the mean ± standard deviation (SD) and percentages (%). Normality was tested using the Kolmogorov-Smirnov and Shapiro-Wilk W tests. The Chi-square test or Fisher's exact test, where appropriate, were used to compare categorical variables. Student's t-test was used for normally distributed continuous variables. The Mann-Whitney U test was used for continuous variables that were not normally distributed. The paired samples t-test was used for normally distributed continuous variables. $p < 0.05$ was considered as statistically significant.

Results
The clinical characteristics of study subjects are summarized in Table 1. There was no significant difference between the daily dosage and single-dose group according to age, body weight, height, and body mass index (BMI) ($p > 0.05$). There was no significant difference between the two groups in terms of sun exposure, physical activity, milk consumption, smoking habits, and clothing style ($p > 0.05$).

There was no difference in serum glucose, total cholesterol, low-density lipoprotein (LDL)-cholesterol, triglycerides, high-sensitivity C-reactive protein (hs-CRP) and thyroid-stimulating hormone (TSH) levels between the single-dose and daily-dosage groups at pretreatment,

4th, and 12th week ($p > 0.05$). Serum calcium and alkaline phosphatase and PTH levels were not different between the single-dose and daily-dosage groups at pretreatment, 4th, and 12th week (p > 0.05). The single-dose (9.7 ± 4.4; 35.9 ± 9.6 and 23.1 ± 4.7 ng/mL (24.2 ± 10.9; 89.6 ± 23.9 and 57.6 ± 11.7 nmol/L), $p < 0.001$) and daily-dosage groups (10.2 ± 4.4, 16.9 ± 5.8, and 19.8 ± 7.2 ng/ mL(25.4 ± 10.9; 42.1 ± 14.4 and 49.4 ± 17.9 nmol/L), $p < 0.001$) had lower pretreatment vitamin D levels than in the 4th and 12th week, respectively. Pretreatment vitamin D levels did not differ between the groups ($p > 0.05$). The vitamin D level was higher in the single-dose group than in the daily-dosage group at the 4th ($p = 0.001$) and 12th week ($p = 0.49$). The daily-dose group had lower pretreatment phosphorus levels than in 4th and 12th week ($p < 0.001$), whereas the single-dose group had higher phosphorus levels at the 4th week than at pretreatment and the 12th week ($p = 0.043$). Phosphorus levels were not different between two groups at pretreatment, 4th, and 12th week ($p > 0.05$). Pretreatment magnesium levels were not different between the two groups ($p > 0.05$). The pretreatment osteocalcin level was higher in the single-dose group than in the daily-dosage group ($p = 0.022$). The osteocalcin level was not different between the two groups at the 4th and 12th week ($p > 0.05$). The biochemical results of the single-dose and daily-dosage group at pretreatment, 4th, and 12th week are shown in Table 2.

The relative isokinetic peak values for knee extensor and flexor (both dominant and non-dominant) muscles did not differ between pretreatment, 4th, and 12th week in the single-dose group ($p > 0.05$). The pretreatment peak values for dominant knee extensors were lower as compared with the 4th week in the daily-dosage group (0.97 ± 0.4 vs. 1.06 ± 0.4 N/m/kg, respectively, $p = 0.03$). Pretreatment peak values for non-dominant knee flexors were lower as compared with the 12th week in daily-dosage group (0.32 ± 0.1 vs. 0.37 ± 0.1 Nm/kg, respectively, p = 0.03). The daily-dosage group had similar dominant knee flexors and non-dominant knee extensors between pretreatment, 4th, and 12th week ($p > 0.05$). The relative peak values for knee extensor and flexor (both dominant and non-dominant) muscles did not differ between the daily- dosage and single-dose group according to pretreatment, 4th, and 12th week ($p > 0.05$). The relative isokinetic peak values of the dominant and non-dominant knee extensor and flexor muscles are shown in Table 3. Muscle function tests measured at 1st month in daily dose group were similar between patients who achieved 25OHVitD$_3$ level of > 20 ng/mL (50 nmol/L) and patients with lower than 20 ng/mL (50 nmol/L).

All patients in both groups had baseline vitamin D levels lower than 20 ng/mL (50 nmol/L). Serum

Table 1 The clinical characteristics of the daily dosage group and the single-dose group

	Daily dosage group ($n = 32$)	Single-dose group ($n = 28$)	p value
Characteristics (mean ± SD)			
Age (years)	51.60 ± 5.80	51.58 ± 5.54	0.644
Height (cm)	160.40 ± 7.94	158.75 ± 5.10	0.152
Body weight, pretreatment (kg)	76.51 ± 12.51	72.04 ± 12.34	0.115
BMI, pretreatment (kg/m^2)	29.75 ± 5.31	28.61 ± 4.96	0.354
Body weight, 12th week, (kg)	74.51 ± 12.51	72.48 ± 12.84	0.544
BMI, 12th week, (kg/m^2)	29.07 ± 5.34	28.8 ± 5.24	0.855
Sun exposure (%)			0.255
< 1 h/d	0	3.6	
1–2 h/d	15.6	17.9	
2–4 h/d	56.3	39.3	
4–7 h/d	21.9	38.5	
> 7 h/d	6.3	0	
Physical activity (%)			0.377
< 1 h/d	0	3.6	
1–2 h/d	15.6	14.3	
2–4 h/d	50.0	39.3	
4–7 h/d	28.1	42.9	
> 7 h/d	6.3	0	
Milk consumption (%)			0.306
< 1 portion/d	21.9	22.2	
1–2 portion/d	46.9	63.0	
2–4 portion/d	31.3	14.8	
Smoking habits (%)			0.179
No	71.9	71.4	
Quit	15.6	3.6	
Yes	12.5	25.0	
Clothing style (%)			0.727
Western-style clothing	37.5	39.3	
Traditional	37.5	28.6	
Oriental-style clothing	25.0	32.1	

25-(OH)D levels greater than 20 ng/mL (50 nmol/L) were achieved in 96.7% of patients in the single large dose group at the end of 4th week, whereas it was 19.4% of patients in the daily low-dosage group ($p <$ 0.001) (Table 4). Serum 25-(OH)D levels greater than 30 ng/mL (75 nmol/L) were achieved in 63.3% of patients in single large dose group at the end of 4th week compared with 3.2% in the daily low-dosage group (p < 0.001). Serum 25-(OH)D levels greater than 20 ng/mL (50 nmol/l) were achieved in 63.3% of patients in the single large dose group at the end of 12th week, whereas it was 45.2% in the daily low-dosage group ($p >$ 0.05). The proportion of patients reaching vitamin D levels of 30 ng/mL

(75 nmol/L) were similar in both groups (6.7% vs. 6.5%, p > 0.05).

Discussion

25(OH)D3 levels increased significantly in both groups at weeks 4 and 12 week after vitamin D treatment. The increase in the single-dose group was significantly higher than in the daily low- dosage group at the 4th and 12th week.

In a study, it was demonstrated that a serum 25(OH)D3 level higher than 20 ng/mL (50 nmol/L) was achieved with a vitamin D(3) dosage of 800 IU/d in 97.5% of women. Approximately 50% of patients in the same study group reached vitamin D levels of 30 ng/mL

Table 2 The biochemical results of the single-dose and daily-dosage group at pretreatment, 4th, and 12th week

	Single-dose group				Daily-dosage group			
	Pretreatment	4th week	12th week	p	Pretreatment	4th week	12th week	p
Glucose (mg/dL)	88.2 ± 9.8	81.7 ± 17.4	92.4 ± 9.5	0.014	89.1 ± 7.5	85.3 ± 6.8	88.6 ± 18.0	0.016
Total cholesterol (mg/dL)	209.5 ± 37.4	209.1 ± 27.0	204.7 ± 35.4	0.569	203.6 ± 36.6	1999.1 ± 38.8	212.3 ± 33.6	0.763
Triglycerides (mg/dL)	136.5 ± 49.6	115.6 ± 43.7	128.7 ± 56.1	0.108	148.5 ± 72.7	146.6 ± 90.3	154.6 ± 61.9	0.601
LDL-cholesterol (mg/dL)	133.4 ± 32.3	137.5 ± 23.7	131.3 ± 26.7	0.411	125.6 ± 27.8	122.1 ± 31.1	134.5 ± 32.2	0.301
Calcium								
(mg/dL)	9.5 ± 0.4	9.5 ± 0.4	9.4 ± 0.5	0.507	9.4 ± 0.4	9.5 ± 0.5	9.6 ± 0.4	0.059
(mmol/L)	2.3 ± 0.1	2.3 ± 0.1	2.3 ± 0.1		2.3 ± 0.1	2.3 ± 0.1	2.4 ± 0.1	
Phosphorus (mg/dL)	3.5 ± 0.4	3.8 ± 0.4	3.6 ± 0.6	0.043	3.4 ± 0.5	3.9 ± 0.5	3.9 ± 0.5	< 0.001
Magnesium (mg/dL)	2.1 ± 0.2				2.2 ± 0.2			
iPTH (pg/ml)	55.1 ± 24.3	47.7 ± 19.1	50.7 ± 20.5	0.152	62.4 ± 24.9	55.9 ± 22.8	54.9 ± 20.6	0.081
Vitamin D								
(ng/mL)	9.7 ± 4.4	35.9 ± 9.6	23.1 ± 4.7	< 0.001	10.2 ± 4.4	16.9 ± 5.8	19.8 ± 7.2	< 0.001
(nmol/L)	24.2 ± 10.9	89.6 ± 23.9	57.6 ± 11.7		25.4 ± 10.9	42.1 ± 14.4	49.4 ± 17.9	
Osteocalcin (ng/ml)	21.2 ± 19.1	21.9 ± 7.5	20.5 ± 7.6	0.231	11.2 ± 8.3	22.0 ± 7.2	20.4 ± 5.5	0.008
Alkaline phosphatase (units/L)	72.5 ± 20.7	73.0 ± 23.1	73.6 ± 19.8	0.138	69.6 ± 17.6	68.1 ± 19.6	68.0 ± 19.1	0.051
TSH (mIU/L)	2.5 ± 1.5	2.8 ± 2.0	2.4 ± 1.5	0.580	2.2 ± 1.1	2.2 ± 1.3	2.2 ± 1.4	0.965
hs-CRP (mg/L)	3.3 ± 3.1	3.2 ± 3.2	2.4 ± 2.2	0.188	4.5 ± 4.9	4.1 ± 3.7	4.1 ± 3.9	0.376

(75 nmol/L) [11]. In the present study, 45.2% of patients reached serum 25(OH)D3 levels of more than 20 ng/mL (50 nmol/L) with daily 800 IU vitamin D replacement dosages, whereas only 6.5% of patients reached serum 25(OH)D3 levels higher than 30 ng/mL (75 nmol/L). This difference may be partly explained by the difference between baseline vitamin D levels in both studies (10.2 ng/mL (25.4 nmol/L) vs. 15.6 ng/mL (38.6 nmol/L)).

Vitamin D levels significantly increased at the 4th week when compared with baseline in a study conducted with single high dose of vitamin D (300,000 IU); however, vitamin D levels at the 12th week were similar at baseline [4]. A recent study demonstrated that a single dose of 250,000 IU of vitamin D3 concluded in a robust increase in plasma 25(OH)D3 after 5 days, but it decreased to baseline levels after 90 days. The authors proposed that a larger dose or more frequent dosing regimen might be required for long-term management of vitamin D insufficiency [27]. In our study, vitamin D levels increased significantly in the single high-dose group at the 4th and 12th weeks after vitamin D3 treatment; however, vitamin D levels decreased at the 12th week when compared with the 4th week in the single large-dose group. Maintenance doses with regular intervals would be reasonable in patients undergoing single large-dose vitamin D replacement.

Human skeletal muscles express vitamin D receptors (VDR) and genotypic variations for this receptor have been reported to be related to decreased muscle strength. It is known that vitamin D has an important role in muscle strength and function. This condition is more prominent in proximal muscles of lower extremity. Because of this, we evaluated knee muscles strength such as quadriceps and hamstrings. It is difficult to evaluate the hip muscles strengh with isokinetic device, therefore we selected the knee muscles [28]. Moreover, vitamin D deficiency-associated muscle weakness is predominantly of the proximal muscle groups and has an effect on daily living activities including walking and climbing stairs [10].

Table 3 Relative isokinetic peak torques (Nm/kg) of the knee extensor and flexor muscles

	Knee extension				p-value[a]	Knee flexion				p-value[a]
	Daily-dosage group		Single-dose group			Daily -dosage group		Single-dose group		
	Dominant	Non-dominant	Dominant	Non-dominant		Dominant	Non-dominant	Dominant	Non-dominant	
Pretreatment	0.97 ± 0.4	0.98 ± 0.4	1.02 ± 0.3	0.99 ± 0.4	0.62/0.89	0.34 ± 0.1	0.32 ± 0.1	0.36 ± 0.2	0.33 ± 0.2	0.62/0.81
4th week	1.06 ± 0.4	1.09 ± 0.4	1.05 ± 0.3	1.06 ± 0.3	0.95/0.78	0.37 ± 0.2	0.36 ± 0.2	0.39 ± 0.2	0.39 ± 0.2	0.69/0.59
12th week	1.03 ± 0.3	1.05 ± 0.4	1.13 ± 0.3	1.14 ± 0.3	0.35/0.36	0.37 ± 0.1	0.37 ± 0.1	0.39 ± 0.2	0.40 ± 0.2	0.69/0.55
p value	0.03[b]	0.21	0.20	0.05		0.18	0.03[c]	0.22	0.10	

Table 4 Percentage of patients that reach target serum 25 OH vitamin level based on treatment duration and replacement style

	Daily dose group	Single dose group	p
4th week Vitamin D < 20	23 (% 74.2)	0 (% 0)	< 0.001
Vitamin D ≥ 20	6 (% 19.4)	29 (% 96.7)	
4th week Vitamin D < 30	28 (% 90.3)	10 (33.3%)	< 0.001
Vitamin D ≥ 30	1 (% 3.2)	19 (63.3%)	
12th week Vitamin D < 20	12 (38.7%)	8 (26.7%)	0.360
Vitamin D ≥ 20	14 (45,2%)	19 (63.3%)	
12th week Vitamin D < 30	24 (77.4%)	25 (83.3%)	0.775
Vitamin D ≥ 30	2 (6.5%)	2 (6.7%)	

Marantes et al. observed no consistent association between 25(OH)D3 levels and any measurements related to muscle mass or strength in either men or women. The authors proposed that factors affecting neuromuscular function rather than muscle strength might be responsible for the association between low 25(OH)D3 and increased fall risk observed in other studies [29]. Several studies evaluated lower leg isometric muscle strength [16, 19, 23, 30–34]; however, only two demonstrated an improvement in isometric muscle strength after treatment [19, 31]. Pfeifer et al. found significantly increased quadriceps strength after 6 months of treatment with 800 IU/ day vitamin D3 [33]. Similarly, Moreira-Pfrimer et al. demonstrated an improvement in maximal isometric strength of hip flexors and knee extensors in vitamin D3-treated subjects (150,000 IU once a month during the first 2 months, followed by 90,000 IU once a month for the last 4 months) [19]. Handgrip strength after vitamin D replacement was evaluated in five studies, and none was able to show significant effects [23, 30, 32, 35, 36]. A recent meta-analysis reported muscle strength measures of 29 randomized controlled trials involving 5533 subjects [37]. The results demonstrated that vitamin D replacement had a small, but significantly positive impact on global muscle strength. A significant positive effect on lower limb muscle strength was observed, but handgrip muscle strength was not affected. Supplementation seemed to be more effective in patients who presented with a 25(OH)D3 levels < 12 ng/mL (30 nmol/L) and aged 65 years or over. The authors proposed that these results could explain the significant effect of vitamin D on falls determined in meta-analyses [38, 39]. Indeed, quadriceps strength was determined to be a significant predictor of fall incidence [40]. We found a significant improvement in dominant quadriceps and non-dominant hamstring muscle strengths in the daily vitamin D group. Non-dominant quadriceps and dominant hamstring muscle strengths were also increased but the differences were not statistically significant. The sample size of our study was not large enough to detect a significant difference. The differences in dose of oral vitamin D, patient population, treatment interval, and muscle strength assessment test have been considered to be responsible for the inconsistencies.

In our study, both replacement types were found to be safe but vitamin D levels were demonstrated to be higher after replacement with single large doses. However, the effect of daily low-dosage vitamin D replacement on muscle strength was better than single large-dose replacement. These findings might support the results of a randomized controlled trial which demonstrated high-dose colecalciferol leads to a higher risk of falls and fractures in older community-dwelling women [41]. Long-term studies with larger populations investigating skeletal development, bone health maintenance, and non-skeletal effects of vitamin D are required to clarify the best replacement dose and form for adequate vitamin D levels in the maintenance of health.

Being a single center stduy and a relatively small sample size were the limitations of the study. Being at lower threshold levels of vitamin D_3 which known to decrease fracture risk and falls at 1st and 3th of months of study could be another limitation of the study (referans), as it may make difficult to interpret the results of the study. Additionally, none of our patients was evaluated for vitamin D metabolites which has been demonstrated to be related to muscle function in recent studies. This is another limitation of our study.

Conclusion

Although daily administration routes are more effective in improving muscle strength, a single administration is more effective in increasing vitamin D levels.

Abbreviations

BMI: body mass index; CD: Celiac disease; DBP: diastolic blood pressure; EMA: anti endomysium antibody; ERS: endoplasmic reticulum stress; FPG: fasting plasma glucose; HC: hip circumference; HLD-C: HDL cholesterol; LDL-C: LDL-cholesterol; NIDDM: non-insulin dependent diabetes mellitus; PPPG: post-prandial plasma glucose; SBP: systolic blood pressure; T2DM: type 2 diabetes mellitus; TLR: Tool-like receptors; tTGA IgA: tissue transglutaminase antibody IgA; VA: villous atrophy; WC: waist circumference

Authors' contributions

MA: have made contributions to conception and design, acquisition of data, and analysis and interpretation of data. AGC, MK, SB: have made contributions to acquisition of data and interpretation of data. SK, MC, TD, OO: have made contributions to acquisition of data. MK, SB: performed the statistical analysis. MO, EC: have made contributions to conception, design, and interpretation of data. All authors read and approved the final manuscript.

Competing interests

The authors declare that they have no competing interest.

Author details

[1]Department of Endocrinology and Metabolism, Diskapi Training and Research Hospital, Ankara, Turkey. [2]Department of Physical Medicine and Rehabilitation, Diskapi Training and Research Hospital, Ankara, Turkey.

References

1. Plum LA, DeLuca HF. Vitamin D, disease and therapeutic opportunities. Nat Rev Drug Discov. 2010;9(12):941–55.
2. Bordelon P, Ghetu MV, Langan RC. Recognition and management of vitamin D deficiency. Am Fam Physician. 2009;80(8):841–6.
3. Holick MF, Chen TC. Vitamin D deficiency: a worldwide problem with health consequences. Am J Clin Nutr. 2008;87(4):1080S–6S.
4. Rossini M, et al. Dose-dependent short-term effects of single high doses of oral vitamin D(3) on bone turnover markers. Calcif Tissue Int. 2012;91(6):365–9.
5. Holick MF, et al. Evaluation, treatment, and prevention of vitamin D deficiency: an Endocrine Society clinical practice guideline. J Clin Endocrinol Metab. 2011;96(7):1911–30.
6. Holick MF. Optimal vitamin D status for the prevention and treatment of osteoporosis. Drugs Aging. 2007;24(12):1017–29.
7. Bischoff, H.A., et al., In situ detection of 1,25-dihydroxyvitamin D3 receptor in human skeletal muscle tissue. Histochem J, 2001. 33(1): p. 19–24.
8. Marcinkowska E. A run for a membrane vitamin D receptor. Biol Signals Recept. 2001;10(6):341–9.
9. Rinaldi I, et al. Correlation between serum vitamin D (25(OH)D) concentration and quadriceps femoris muscle strength in Indonesian elderly women living in three nursing homes. Acta Med Indones. 2007;39(3):107–11.
10. Ceglia L. Vitamin D and skeletal muscle tissue and function. Mol Asp Med. 2008;29(6):407–14.
11. Gallagher JC, et al. Dose response to vitamin D supplementation in postmenopausal women: a randomized trial. Ann Intern Med. 2012;156(6):425–37.
12. Trivedi DP, Doll R, Khaw KT. Effect of four monthly oral vitamin D3 (colecalciferol) supplementation on fractures and mortality in men and women living in the community: randomised double blind controlled trial. BMJ. 2003;326(7387):469.
13. Sanfelix-Genoves J, et al. Determinant factors of osteoporosis patients' reported therapeutic adherence to calcium and/or vitamin D supplements: a cross-sectional, observational study of postmenopausal women. Drugs Aging. 2009;26(10):861–9.
14. Diez A, et al. Observational study of treatment compliance in women initiating antiresorptive therapy with or without calcium and vitamin D supplements in Spain. Menopause. 2012;19(1):89–95.
15. Diamond TH, et al. Annual intramuscular injection of a megadose of colecalciferol for treatment of vitamin D deficiency: efficacy and safety data. Med J Aust. 2005;183(1):10–2.
16. Dhesi JK, et al. Vitamin D supplementation improves neuromuscular function in older people who fall. Age Ageing. 2004;33(6):589–95.
17. Leventis P, Kiely PD. The tolerability and biochemical effects of high-dose bolus vitamin D2 and D3 supplementation in patients with vitamin D insufficiency. Scand J Rheumatol. 2009;38(2):149–53.
18. Ilahi M, Armas LA, Heaney RP. Pharmacokinetics of a single, large dose of colecalciferol. Am J Clin Nutr. 2008;87(3):688–91.
19. Moreira-Pfrimer LD, et al. Treatment of vitamin D deficiency increases lower limb muscle strength in institutionalized older people independently of regular physical activity: a randomized double-blind controlled trial. Ann Nutr Metab. 2009;54(4):291–300.
20. Kearns MD, Alvarez JA, Tangpricha V. Large, single-dose, oral vitamin d supplementation in adult populations: a systematic review. Endocr Pract. 2014;20(4):341–51.
21. Janssen HC, Samson MM, Verhaar HJ. Vitamin D deficiency, muscle function, and falls in elderly people. Am J Clin Nutr. 2002;75(4):611–5.
22. Schacht E, Ringe JD. Alfacalcidol improves muscle power, muscle function and balance in elderly patients with reduced bone mass. Rheumatol Int. 2012;32(1):207–15.
23. Kenny AM, et al. Effects of vitamin D supplementation on strength, physical function, and health perception in older, community-dwelling men. J Am Geriatr Soc. 2003;51(12):1762–7.
24. Grady, D., et al., 1,25-Dihydroxyvitamin D3 and muscle strength in the elderly: a randomized controlled trial. J Clin Endocrinol Metab, 1991. 73(5): p. 1111–7.
25. Muir SW, Montero-Odasso M. Effect of vitamin D supplementation on muscle strength, gait and balance in older adults: a systematic review and meta-analysis. J Am Geriatr Soc. 2011;59(12):2291–300.
26. Stockton KA, et al. Effect of vitamin D supplementation on muscle strength: a systematic review and meta-analysis. Osteoporos Int. 2011;22(3):859–71.
27. Kearns MD, et al. The effect of a single, large bolus of vitamin D in healthy adults over the winter and following year: a randomized, double-blind, placebo-controlled trial. Eur J Clin Nutr. 2015;69(2):193–7.
28. Rejnmark L. Effects of vitamin D on muscle function and performance: a review of evidence from randomized controlled trials. Ther Adv Chronic Dis. 2011;2:25–37.
29. Marantes I, et al. Is vitamin D a determinant of muscle mass and strength? J Bone Miner Res. 2011;26(12):2860–71.
30. Janssen HC, Samson MM, Verhaar HJ. Muscle strength and mobility in vitamin D-insufficient female geriatric patients: a randomized controlled trial on vitamin D and calcium supplementation. Aging Clin Exp Res. 2010;22(1):78–84.
31. Pfeifer M, et al. Effects of a long-term vitamin D and calcium supplementation on falls and parameters of muscle function in community-dwelling older individuals. Osteoporos Int. 2009;20(2):315–22.
32. Bunout D, et al. Effects of vitamin D supplementation and exercise training on physical performance in Chilean vitamin D deficient elderly subjects. Exp Gerontol. 2006;41(8):746–52.
33. Bischoff HA, et al. Effects of vitamin D and calcium supplementation on falls: a randomized controlled trial. J Bone Miner Res. 2003;18(2):343–51.
34. Latham NK, et al. A randomized, controlled trial of quadriceps resistance exercise and vitamin D in frail older people: the frailty interventions trial in elderly subjects (FITNESS). J Am Geriatr Soc. 2003;51(3):291–9.
35. Brunner RL, et al. Calcium, vitamin D supplementation, and physical function in the Women's Health Initiative. J Am Diet Assoc. 2008;108(9):1472–9.
36. El-Hajj Fuleihan G, et al. Effect of vitamin D replacement on musculoskeletal parameters in school children: a randomized controlled trial. J Clin Endocrinol Metab. 2006;91(2):405–12.
37. Beaudart C, et al. The effects of vitamin D on skeletal muscle strength, muscle mass, and muscle power: a systematic review and meta-analysis of randomized controlled trials. J Clin Endocrinol Metab. 2014;99(11):4336–45.
38. Kalyani RR, et al. Vitamin D treatment for the prevention of falls in older adults: systematic review and meta-analysis. J Am Geriatr Soc. 2010;58(7):1299–310.
39. Murad MH, et al. Clinical review: the effect of vitamin D on falls: a systematic review and meta-analysis. J Clin Endocrinol Metab. 2011;96(10):2997–3006.
40. Scott D, et al. Investigating the predictive ability of gait speed and quadriceps strength for incident falls in community-dwelling older women at high risk of fracture. Arch Gerontol Geriatr. 2014;58(3):308–13.
41. Sanders KM, Stuart AL, Williamson EJ, Simpson JA, Kotowicz MA, Young D, et al. Annual high-dose oral vitamin D and falls and fractures in older women: a randomized controlled trial. JAMA. 2010;303(18):1815–22.

25

A modified M-stage classification based on the metastatic patterns of pancreatic neuroendocrine neoplasms: a population-based study

Xianbin Zhang[1,2]*[†] (iD), Jiaxin Song[3†], Peng Liu[1], Mohammad Abdul Mazid[1], Lili Lu[3], Yuru Shang[1], Yushan Wei[4], Peng Gong[5] and Li Ma[3,6]*

Abstract

Background: The present study aims to improve the M-stage classification of pancreatic neuroendocrine neoplasms (pNENs).

Methods: Two thousand six hundred sixty six pNENs were extracted from the Surveillance, Epidemiology, and End Results database to explore the metastatic patterns of pNENs. Metastatic patterns were categorized as single, two, or multiple (three or more) distant organ metastasis. The mean overall survival and hazard rate of different metastatic patterns were calculated by Kaplan-Meier and Cox proportional hazards models, respectively. The discriminatory capability of the modified M-stage classification was evaluated by Harrell's concordance index.

Results: The overall survival time significantly decreased with an increasing number of metastatic organs. In addition, pNENs with only liver metastasis had better prognosis when compared to other metastatic patterns. Thus, we modified the M-stage classification (mM-stage) as follows: mM_0-stage, tumor without metastasis; mM_1-stage, tumor only metastasized to liver; mM_2-stage, tumor metastasized to other single distant organ (lung, bone, or brain) or two distant organs; mM_3-stage, tumor metastasized to three or more distant organs. Harrell's concordance index showed that the modified M-stage classification had superior discriminatory capability than both the American Joint Committee on Cancer (AJCC) and the European Neuroendocrine Tumor Society (ENETS) M-stage classifications.

Conclusions: The modified M-stage classification is superior to both AJCC and ENETS M-stage classifications in the prognosis of pNENs. In the future, individualized treatment and follow-up programs should be explored for patients with distinct metastatic patterns.

Keywords: Metastasis, Survival, Prognosis, Pancreas, Cancer

Background

Pancreatic neuroendocrine neoplasms (pNENs) are relatively rare tumors. However, a recent population study showed that the incidence of pNENs increased more than 4-fold from 1973 to 2012 [1]. Moreover, pNENs are considered the most serious neuroendocrine neoplasms (NENs), due to the patients have a shorter median overall survival times (3.6 years) when compared to those with tumors located in lung (5.5 years), rectum (24.6 years), and appendix (more than 30.0 years) [1].

Cancer staging classification systems are used to codify the extent of cancer. They allow clinicians to quantify prognosis and plan treatment for individual patients. Two widely used tumor staging classification systems, which are proposed by the American Joint Committee on Cancer (AJCC) and the European Neuroendocrine Tumor Society (ENETS), describe M_0-stage as having no distant metastasis and M_1-stage as having at least one

* Correspondence: zhangxianbin@hotmail.com; mali_lele@sina.com
[†]Xianbin Zhang and Jiaxin Song contributed equally to this work.
[1]The First Affiliated Hospital of Dalian Medical University, Zhongshan 222, Dalian 116011, China
[3]Department of Epidemiology, Dalian Medical University, Lvshun West 9, Dalian 116044, China
Full list of author information is available at the end of the article

distant metastasis [2, 3]. However, several studies demonstrated that pNENs with liver metastasis have better prognosis than other metastatic patterns [4–6].

Therefore, we utilized the Surveillance, Epidemiology, and End Result (SEER) database to explore the prognosis of different metastatic patterns of pNENs and propose a modified M-stage classification. This modified M-stage classification proves to be superior to both AJCC and ENETS M-stage classifications in prognosis.

Methods
Study cohort
As published previously [3], we utilized the topography codes (C25.0 to C25.9) and histology codes (8150, 8151, 8152, 8153, 8154, 8155, 8156, 8157, 8240, 8241, 8242, 8243, 8244, 8245, 8246, and 8249) of the International Classification of Diseases for Oncology (third edition) to identify pNENs.

Outcomes and variables
The primary outcome was overall survival. Demographic data included age, sex, and race; tumor characteristics included tumor size, primary site, differentiation, 7th AJCC T-stage, and N-stage; treatment information included surgery and radiotherapy. Single organ metastasis was defined as the tumor spreading from pancreas to another single distant organ [7]. Similarly, two organ metastases were defined as the tumor spreading from pancreas to two distant organs. Tumors spreading from pancreas to three or more distant organs were defined as multiple metastases.

Inclusion and exclusion criteria
Patients microscopically diagnosed as pNENs were included in the present study. We excluded cases with unclear or incomplete information about metastasis. In addition, we also excluded cases without information about survival time.

Statistical analyses
To compare the constituent ratio of variables among patients, we broke the continuous variables (age, tumor size) into binary variables. Survival time was plotted using the Kaplan-Meier estimator and Cox proportional hazards model. The results were presented as mean and hazard ratio, respectively, each with a 95% confidence interval (CI). Harrell's concordance index was used to evaluate the discriminatory capability of the modified M stage classification. An index value of greater than 0.70 suggests the classification has an acceptable discriminatory capability [8]. Differences with $P \leq 0.05$ divided by the number of meaningful comparisons, Bonferroni correction, were considered to be significant. Differences with $P \leq 0.1$ divided by the number of meaningful comparisons, were considered to indicate a tendency. All statistical analyses were performed using SPSS 19.0 (IBM, New York, USA) or R (version 3.5.0).

Results
Patient characteristics
In total, 2666 patients (mean age 60.9 years ±13.6 years; 55.7% male, 78.8% white) were included in the present study (Fig. 1). Many patients (55.4%) underwent surgery, and some (4.7%) were treated with radiation. The constituent ratios of tumor size, location, differentiation, T-stage, and N-stage were significantly ($P < 0.05$) different between patients with and without metastasis (Table 1).

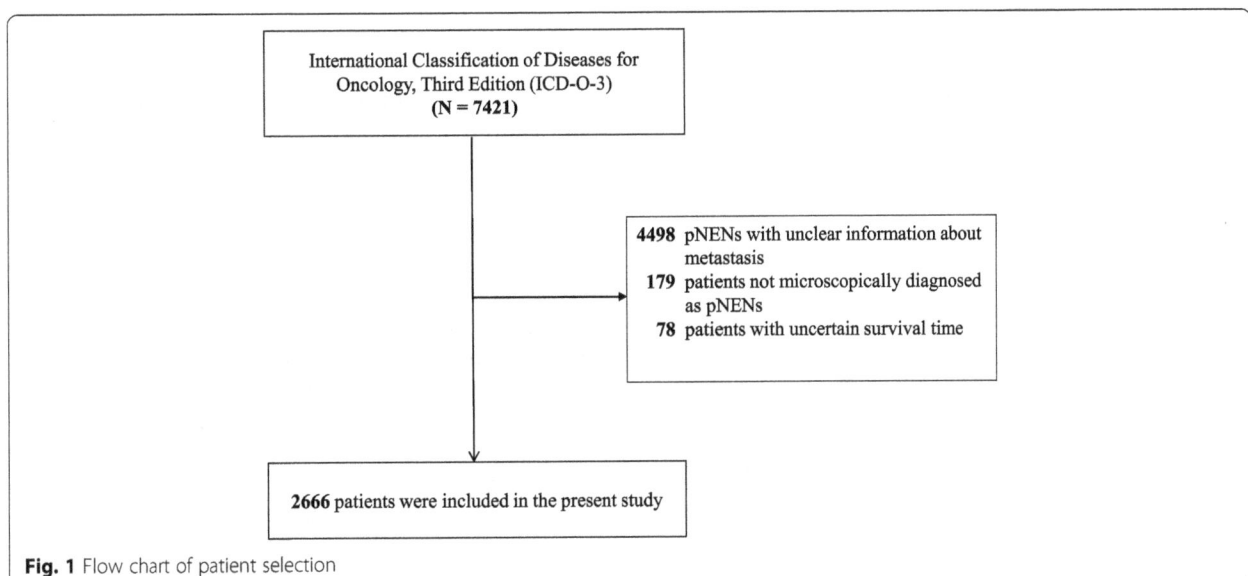

Fig. 1 Flow chart of patient selection

Table 1 Clinicopathological Characters

	Without Metastasis N = 1679	Metastasis N = 987	P
Age (years)			0.221[b]
≤ 60	793 (47.2%)	442 (44.8%)	
> 60	886 (52.8%)	545 (55.2%)	
Sex			0.338[a]
Male	924 (55.0%)	562 (56.9%)	
Female	755 (45.0%)	425 (43.1%)	
Race			0.011[a]
White	1314 (78.3%)	787 (79.7%)	
Black	191 (11.4%)	130 (13.2%)	
Other	174 (10.3%)	70 (7.1%)	
Size (cm)			< 0.001[b]
≤ 2	670 (39.9%)	68 (6.9%)	
> 2	934 (55.6%)	699 (70.8%)	
Unclear	75 (4.5%)	220 (22.3%)	
Primary Site			< 0.001[b]
Head	502 (29.9%)	258 (26.2%)	
Body	295 (17.6%)	106 (10.7%)	
Tail	542 (32.3%)	314 (31.8%)	
Other	340 (20.2%)	309 (31.3%)	
Differentiation			< 0.001[b]
Well	1043 (62.1%)	189 (19.1%)	
Moderately	221 (13.2%)	86 (8.7%)	
Poorly	64 (3.8%)	95 (9.6%)	
Undifferentiated	17 (1.0%)	28 (2.8%)	
Unclear	334 (19.9%)	589 (59.7%)	
T-sage			< 0.001[b]
T_1	602 (35.9%)	37 (3.7%)	
T_2	538 (32.0%)	276 (28.0%)	
T_3	389 (23.2%)	271 (27.5%)	
T_4	67 (4.0%)	102 (10.3%)	
Tx	83 (4.9%)	301 (30.5%)	
N-stage			< 0.001[b]
N_0	1247 (74.3%)	463 (46.9%)	
N_1	401 (23.9%)	338 (34.3%)	
Nx	31 (1.8%)	186 (18.8%)	
Surgery			< 0.001[b]
Yes	1313 (78.2%)	164 (16.6%)	
No	339 (20.2%)	813 (82.4%)	
Unclear	27 (1.6%)	10 (1.0%)	
Radiation			< 0.001[b]
Yes	52 (3.1%)	74 (7.5%)	
No	1609 (95.8%)	905 (91.7%)	
Unclear	18 (1.1%)	8 (0.8%)	

[a]Chi-square test; [b]Kruskal-Wallis test

Metastatic patterns and survival

At the time of diagnosis, 1679 (62.98%) patients showed no metastasis. As shown in Fig. 2a, single organ metastases comprised 850 (31.88%) patients, including 817 liver (30.64%), 22 lung (0.83%), nine bone (0.34%), and two brain (0.07%) cases. One hundred and twelve patients (4.20%) showed two-organ metastases, including 52 liver plus bone (1.95%), 53 liver plus lung (1.99%), four bone plus lung (0.15%), two liver plus brain (0.08%), and one bone plus brain (0.04%) cases. Twenty-five patients (0.94%) presented multiple organ metastases, including 19 cases of liver plus lung plus bone (0.71%), three cases of liver plus lung plus brain (0.11%), and three cases of liver plus lung plus brain plus bone (0.11%).

To assess survival time of different metastatic patterns, we compared the survival time of patients without metastasis to those with single distant organ metastasis, two-organ metastases, and multiple organ metastases. As the number of metastatic organs increased, survival time was significantly ($P < 0.001$) reduced (Fig. 2b). In addition, patients with only liver metastasis had a longer survival time than did other single-organ metastases (Fig. 2c), whereas patients with bone, lung or two-organ metastasis had similar mean survival time (bone, 18.32 months ± 5.27 months; lung, 17.77 months ± 3.54 months, two organs metastases, 15.79 months ± 1.70 months).

Modified M-stage classification and discriminatory capability

Thus, based on the observed metastatic patterns and survival times, we modified the M-stage classification (mM-stage) as shown in Table 2. Tumor without metastasis was defined as mM_0-stage. Tumor spread from pancreas only to liver was defined as mM_1-stage. Tumor spreading from pancreas to other single distant organ or to two distant organs was defined as mM_2-stage. Tumor spreading to three or more distant organs was defined as mM_3-stage.

To evaluate survival time among mM-stage classifications, survival curves were plotted using the Kaplan-Meier estimator and then compared with the log-rank test. We observed that all survival curves were well separated (Fig. 2d). Patients with advanced mM stages (mM_1, mM_2, mM_3) had significantly ($P < 0.001$) shorter survival times than patients with mM_0-stage (Fig. 2e). Moreover, the modified M-stage classification was an independent prognostic factor for pNENs, after adjusting for other clinical and pathological characteristics (Table 3).

To explore discriminatory capability of the modified M-stage classification, Harrell's concordance index was calculated. The mM-stage classification had a better discriminatory capability (Harrell's concordance index, 0.712; 95% CI, 0.692–0.732) than AJCC M-stage and

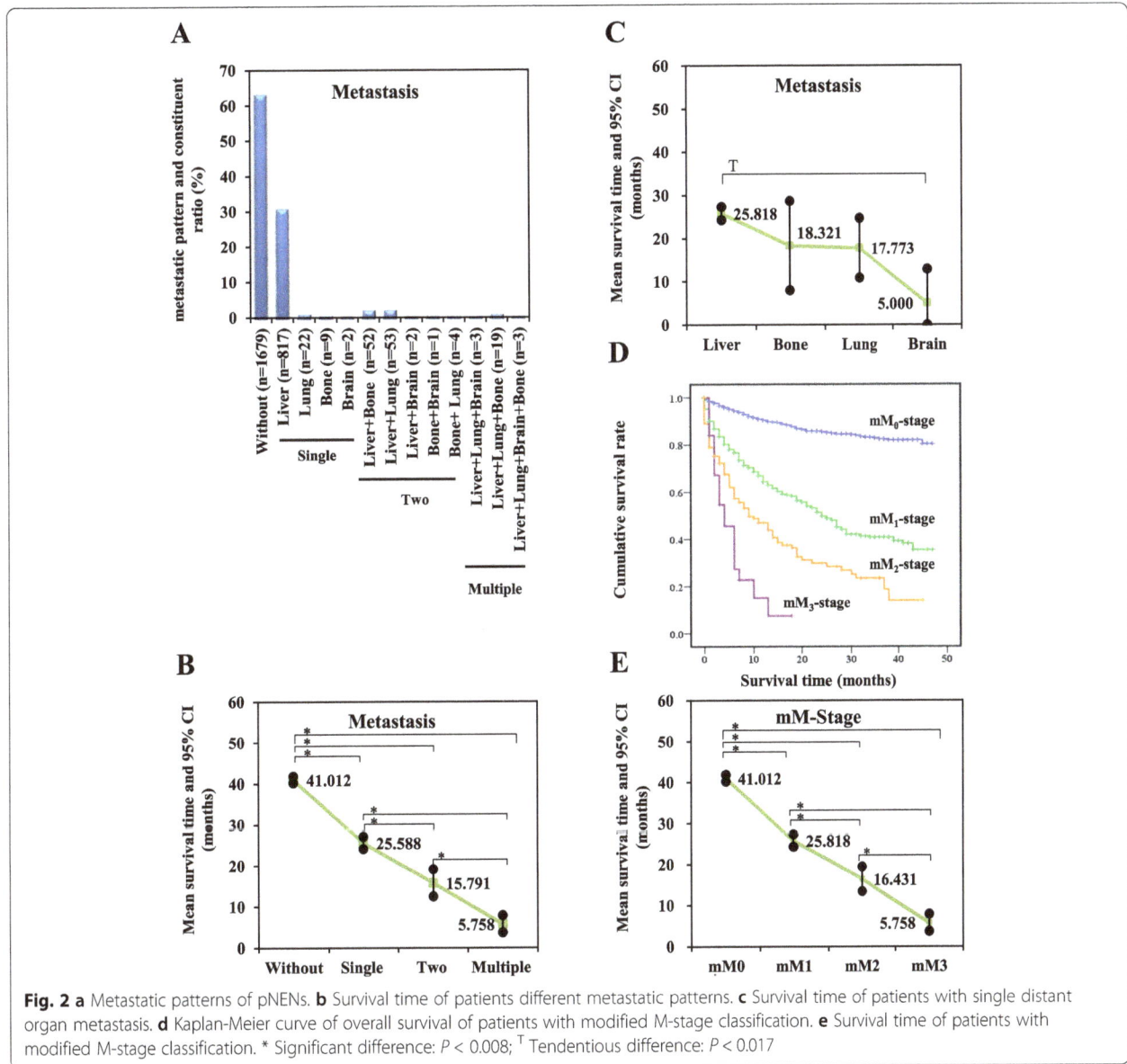

Fig. 2 a Metastatic patterns of pNENs. **b** Survival time of patients different metastatic patterns. **c** Survival time of patients with single distant organ metastasis. **d** Kaplan-Meier curve of overall survival of patients with modified M-stage classification. **e** Survival time of patients with modified M-stage classification. * Significant difference: $P < 0.008$; ^{T} Tendentious difference: $P < 0.017$

ENETS M-stage (Harrell's concordance index, 0.697; 95% CI, 0.678–0.717).

Discussion

In agreement with previous studies [9–11], the present study also demonstrated that nearly one quarter of patients (37.02%, 987/2666) presenting metastasis at the time of pNEN diagnosis. In addition, liver metastasis was the majority metastatic pattern, followed by lung, bone and brain metastasis. The hematogenous mode of metastasis might contribute to the metastatic pattern, which we have observed in the present study. Unsually, carcinoma cells seed in the liver via the portal venous system. Then, these cells would spread to lung via the inferior vena cava and pulmonary arteries. Finally, the carcinoma cells from lung metastases would seed in other organs via arterial blood [12].

Table 2 Definition of M-stage classifications

AJCC and ENTES M-stage classifications	Modified M-stage classifications
M_0-stage, no distant metastasis	mM_0-stage, no distant metastasis
M_1-stage, distant metastasis	mM_1-stage, only liver metastasis
	mM_2-stage, other single distant organ or two organs metastases
	mM_3-stage, three or more organs metastases

AJCC American Joint Committee on Cancer; *ENETS* European Neuroendocrine Tumor Society

Table 3 Independent Prognostic Factors

	Univariate		Multivariate	
	HR and 95% CI	P-value	HR and 95% CI	P-value
Age (years)				
≤ 60	Reference		Reference	
> 60	1.875 (1.595–2.204)	< 0.001	1.744 (1.479–2.055)	< 0.001
Sex				
Male	Reference		Reference	
Female	0.808 (0.691–0.945)	0.008	0.850 (0.726–0.996)	0.044
Race				
White	Reference		Reference	
Black	1.345 (1.082–1.670)	0.007	1.247 (0.998–1.558)	0.052
Other	0.715 (0.527–0.970)	0.031	0.767 (0.565–1.043)	0.090
Size (cm)				
≤ 2	Reference		Reference	
> 2	2.889 (2.241–3.724)	< 0.001	1.322 (1.009–1.731)	0.043
Unclear	6.799(5.110–9.047)	< 0.001	1.547(1.129–2.119)	0.007
Primary Site			a	
Head	Reference			
Body	0.684(0.530–0.884)	0.004		
Tail	0.682(0.556–0.836)	< 0.001		
Other	1.128(0.929–1.368)	0.223		
Differentiation				
Well	Reference		Reference	
Moderately	1.557 (1.095–2.215)	0.014	1.049 (0.735–1.498)	0.791
Poorly	7.414 (5.608–9.803)	< 0.001	3.349 (2.498–4.489)	< 0.001
Undifferentiated	9.494 (6.113–14.743)	< 0.001	3.166 (2.000–5.011)	< 0.001
Unclear	5.136 (4.179–6.311)	< 0.001	1.626 (1.290–2.048)	< 0.001
T-stage			a	
T_1	Reference			
T_2	3.434(2.474–4.766)	< 0.001		
T_3	3.353(2.399–4.688)	< 0.001		
T_4	7.082(4.867–10.306)	< 0.001		
Tx	9.288(6.696–12.882)	< 0.001		
N-stage				
N_0	Reference		Reference	
N_1	1.679 (1.415–1.993)	< 0.001	1.304 (1.092–1.557)	0.003
Nx	3.732 (3.019–4.613)	< 0.001	1.452 (1.152–1.829)	0.002
Surgery				
Yes	Reference		Reference	
No	8.556 (6.941–10.548)	< 0.001	3.901 (3.013–5.050)	< 0.001
Unclear	1.991 (0.812–4.883)	0.133	1.487 (0.601–3.680)	0.391
Radiation			a	
Yes	Reference			
No	1.984(1.511–2.603)	< 0.001		
Unclear	0.939(0.420–2.098)	0.878		

Table 3 Independent Prognostic Factors (Continued)

	Univariate		Multivariate	
	HR and 95% CI	P-value	HR and 95% CI	P-value
mM-stage				
mM$_0$-stage	Reference		Reference	
mM$_1$-stage	4.520 (3.789–5.393)	< 0.001	1.643 (1.339–2.016)	< 0.001
mM$_2$-stage	8.199(6.380–10.537)	< 0.001	2.249(1.704–2.968)	< 0.001
mM$_3$-stage	16.356 (10.266–26.059)	< 0.001	5.034 (3.110–8.150)	< 0.001

[a]variables excluded by multivariate forward stepwise cox regression

The present study found that with an increasing number of metastatic organs, there was a significant decrease in survival time. In addition, pNENs with liver metastasis had longer overall survival than other single-organ metastatic patterns. However, AJCC and ENETS classify both pNENs with liver metastasis and pNENs with the other metastasitic patterns as M$_1$-stage. Our modified M-stage classification distinguishes that tumor spreading from pancreas only to liver should be separated from the other metastatic patterns, and that it is necessary to design individualized treatment and follow-up programs for patients with lung, bone, or brain metastasis.

Usually, pancreatic resection is not performed when the pancreatic malignant tumor has spread to other organs [13]. However, considering the indolent behavior of pNENs and the high frequency of liver metastasis, several clinicians suggested surgical management could give rise to benefit to pNENs with liver metastasis [4, 14]. Birnbaum et al. pancreatic resection could slow down tumor growth and reduce hormone production [14], possibly resulting in considerable benefit for patients with liver metastasis [4].

Consistent with previous studies, the tumor size, primary site, differentiation, AJCC T-stage and AJCC N-stage were identified as predictors of distant organ metastasis (Additional file 1: Table S1). Unfortunately, SEER database did not record Ki-67 status and graded the primary tumor only on the basis of morphological description (ICD-O-3) in the pathology report. Thus, we failed to evaluate the predictive role of Ki-67 status and WHO 2010 grading classification (NET G1, NET G2, NET G3 and NEC) in distant organ metastasis.

It seems the primary tumor site is a particularly useful predictor because it is available before any operation occurs. Hao et al. reported that compared to tumors located in the head and neck of the pancreas, tumors in the body and tail showed a decreased risk of liver metastasis in pancreatic adenocarcinoma [15]. In contrast, the present study showed that pNENs located in the pancreatic tail are actually 1.728 times more likely ($P < 0.001$) to develop metastasis, as compared to tumors located in the pancreatic head. This may be due to the fact that patients with pNENs, especially non-functioning pNENs,

in the tail of the pancreas are less likely to experience obstructive signs and hormonal symptoms until tumors spread to the peritoneum, spleen, and distant organs [16, 17]. Thus, at the time of diagnosis, distant organ metastases exist in most of these patients.

Some limitations of the present study should be noted. First, the SEER database only provides information on pNEN metastasis to liver, lung, bone, and brain. The frequency of pNEN metastasis might be underestimated. Second, Hlatky et al. noted that multiple metastatic lesions may be related to a short survival time [18]. However, the SEER database did not collect data on the number of metastatic lesions in each distant organ.

Conclusions

In conclusion, this is the first population-based study to investigate the metastatic patterns and predictors in advanced pNENs. We found significant differences in survival time across different metastatic patterns. Thus, the modified M-stage classification show a better discriminatory capability than the AJCC and ENETS M-stage classifications. In the future, clinicians should determine individualized treatment and follow-up programs for pNENs with different metastatic patterns.

Abbreviations
AJCC: American Joint Committee on Cancer; ENETS: European Neuroendocrine Tumor Society; OS: Overall survival; pNENs: Pancreatic neuroendocrine neoplasms; SD: Standard deviation; SEER: Surveillance, Epidemiology, and End Result

Acknowledgments
We thank the Surveillance, Epidemiology, and End Results (SEER) program providing the original data. We also thank Prof. Wenli Zhang and Prof. Houli Zhang gave us critical comments during the revision of the manuscript.

Funding
This work was supported by the National Natural Science Foundation of China [grant number 81473504, 81200989]; China Scholarship Council [grant number 201608080195]. The funders had no any role in the manuscript.

Authors' contributions
XZ identified the pNENs from SEER database, designed the study and wrote the manuscript; XZ, JS, MM, PL, LL, YS analyzed and interpreted the data; YW is responsible for the statistical analyses; PG and LM contributed to conception, design and funding. All authors have been involved in revising and proofreading of the manuscript. All authors listed have approved the manuscript.

Competing interests
The authors declare that they have no competing interests.

Author details
[1]The First Affiliated Hospital of Dalian Medical University, Zhongshan 222, Dalian 116011, China. [2]Institute for Experimental Surgery, Rostock University Medical Center, Schillingallee 69a, 18057 Rostock, Germany. [3]Department of Epidemiology, Dalian Medical University, Lvshun West 9, Dalian 116044, China. [4]Department of Evidence-based Medicine and Statistics, the First Affiliated Hospital of Dalian Medical University, Zhongshan 222, Dalian 116011, China. [5]Department of General Surgery, the Shenzhen University General Hospital and Shenzhen University School of Medicine, Xueyuan 1098, Shenzhen 518055, China. [6]Department of Epidemiology, Dalian Medical University, Zhongshan Road 222, Dalian 116011, China.

References
1. Dasari A, Shen C, Halperin D, et al. Trends in the incidence, prevalence, and survival outcomes in patients with neuroendocrine tumors in the United States. JAMA Oncol. 2017;3:1335–42.
2. Panzuto F, Boninsegna L, Fazio N, et al. Metastatic and locally advanced pancreatic endocrine carcinomas: analysis of factors associated with disease progression. J Clin Oncol. 2011;29:2372–7.
3. Zhang X, Lu L, Shang Y, et al. The number of positive lymph node is a better predictor of survival than the lymph node metastasis status for pancreatic neuroendocrine neoplasms: a retrospective cohort study. Int J Surg. 2017;48:142–8.
4. Jin K, Xu J, Chen J, et al. Surgical management for non-functional pancreatic neuroendocrine neoplasms with synchronous liver metastasis: a consensus from the Chinese study Group for Neuroendocrine Tumors (CSNET). Int J Oncol. 2016;49:1991–2000.
5. Garcia-Carbonero R, Rinke A, Valle JW, et al. ENETS consensus guidelines for the standards of care in neuroendocrine neoplasms. Systemic therapy 2: chemotherapy. Neuroendocrinology. 2017;105:281–94.
6. Chamberlain RS, Canes D, Brown KT, et al. Hepatic neuroendocrine metastases: does intervention alter outcomes? Am Coll Surg. 2000;190:432–45.
7. Vatandoust S, Price TJ, Karapetis CS. Colorectal cancer: metastases to a single organ. World J Gastroenterol. 2015;21:11767–76.
8. Bando E, Makuuchi R, Tokunaga M, et al. Impact of clinical tumor–node–metastasis staging on survival in gastric carcinoma patients receiving surgery. Gastric Cancer. 2017;20:448–56.
9. Niederle MB, Hackl M, Kaserer K, et al. Gastroenteropancreatic neuroendocrine tumours: the current incidence and staging based on the WHO and European neuroendocrine tumour society classification: an analysis based on prospectively collected parameters. Endocr Relat Cancer. 2010;17:909–18.
10. Lawrence B, Gustafsson BI, Chan A, et al. The epidemiology of gastroenteropancreatic neuroendocrine tumors. Endocrinol Metab Clin N Am. 2011;40:1–18.
11. Pavel M, Costa F, Capdevila J, et al. ENETS consensus guidelines update for the management of distant metastatic disease of intestinal, pancreatic, bronchial neuroendocrine neoplasms (NEN) and NEN of unknown primary site. Neuroendocrinology. 2016;103:172–85.
12. Weiss L, Grundmann E, Torhorst J, et al. Haematogenous metastatic patterns in colonic carcinoma: an analysis of 1541 necropsies. J Pathol. 1986;150:195–203.
13. Partelli S, Bartsch DK, Capdevila J, et al. ENETS consensus guidelines for standard of care in neuroendocrine tumours: surgery for small intestinal and pancreatic neuroendocrine tumours. Neuroendocrinology. 2017;105:255–65.
14. Birnbaum DJ, Turrini O, Vigano L, et al. Surgical management of advanced pancreatic neuroendocrine tumors: short-term and long-term results from an international multi-institutional study. Ann Surg Onco. 2015;22:1000–7.
15. S D LW, GY B, et al. Risk factors of liver metastasis from advanced pancreatic adenocarcinoma: a large multicenter cohort study. World J Surg Oncol. 2017;15:120.
16. Freelove R, Walling AD. Pancreatic cancer: diagnosis and management. Am Fam Physician. 2006;73:485–92.
17. Zhang X, Ma L, Bao H, et al. Clinical, pathological and prognostic characteristics of gastroenteropancreatic neuroendocrine neoplasms in China: a retrospective study. BMC Endocr Disord. 2014;14:54.
18. Hlatky R, Suki D, Sawaya R. Carcinoid metastasis to the brain. Cancer. 2004;101:2605–13.

26

IL-10/STAT3 is reduced in childhood obesity with hypertriglyceridemia and is related to triglyceride level in diet-induced obese rats

Yuesheng Liu[1], Dong Xu[2], Chunyan Yin[1], Sisi Wang[1], Min Wang[1] and Yanfeng Xiao[1*]

Abstract

Background: The prevalence of childhood obesity and obesity-related metabolic disorder such as dyslipidemia has sharply increased in the past few decades. Chronic low-grade inflammation is associated with the development of comorbidities and poor prognosis in obesity. This study aims to evaluate interleukin-10 (IL-10) in childhood obesity with hypertriglyceridemia.

Method: We evaluated IL-10 and signal transducer and activator of transcription 3 (STAT3) mRNA expression in adipose tissue (AT) as well as serum IL-10 in 62 children of 3 groups and in high-fat diet (HFD) induced obese rat. Expression of IL-10 and STAT3 protein in AT of diet-induced obese rats were examined over feed period.

Results: Adipose IL-10 and STAT3 mRNA expression and serum IL-10 reduced in obese children with hypertriglyceridemia and in HFD obese rats. The protein expression of IL-10 and STAT3 decreased in AT of obese rats compared with the control rats at end time. Expression of IL-10 mRNA was negatively correlated to TG and LDL-C levels, and positively correlated to HDL-C, adiponectin and serum IL-10 levels.

Conclusions: IL-10 expression and its downstream JAK-STAT pathway are down-regulated in obese children with hypertriglyceridemia and in HFD obese rats.

Keywords: Childhood obesity, High-fat diet, IL-10, JAK-STAT, Triglyceride

Background

In the past few decades, with the rapid economic growth and shifts in diet and lifestyle, the prevalence of overweight and obesity has also sharply increased in children and adolescents in both developed and developing countries [1–3]. In 2010, the overweight and obesity combined prevalence had reached 19.2% among Chinese children and adolescents aged 7–18 years [4]. As the prevalence of obesity and associated disease continues to rise, social costs also escalate rapidly [5]. Childhood obesity is strongly associated with several metabolic abnormalities such as dyslipidemia, hypertension, impaired fasting glucose, and metabolic syndrome (MetS) [6–8]. Low serum high-density lipoprotein

cholesterol (HDL-C) levels, increased low-density lipoprotein cholesterol (LDL-C), high triglycerides (TG) levels are frequent metabolic disorders in childhood obesity and hypertriglyceridemia is the most frequent [9]. These health problems not only affect metabolism and psychosocial conditions in the short term, but also lead to an increased risk of cardiovascular disease in adulthood. Therefore, it is important to determine effective measures for the prevention of obesity and obesity-related hypertriglyceridemia in children.

Obesity may be accompanied by chronic low-grade inflammation with unclear triggers [10]. Alterations of adipokines secreted by adipose tissue (AT) and several further cytokines are thought to contribute to a low-grade inflammation [11]. Some studies have indicated that the pro-inflammatory cytokines, such as IL-6, could promote lipolysis [12, 13]. Besides, a lot of adipose tissue-related

* Correspondence: xiaoyanfeng0639@sina.com
[1]Department of Pediatrics, The Second Affiliated Hospital of Xi'an Jiaotong University, 157 Xiwu Road, Xi'an, Shaanxi 710061, People's Republic of China
Full list of author information is available at the end of the article

anti-inflammatory factors have been suggested to be involved in the pathogenesis of systemic inflammation in obesity. IL-10 is known as one of the most important anti-inflammatory and immunosuppressive cytokines that mainly acts on monocytes. The main source of IL-10 in vivo appears to be immune cells, such as monocytes, macrophages, and different T-cell subsets [14]. Previous study has shown that monocyte subsets display lower IL-10 expression during childhood obesity [15]. STAT3 is one of the downstream pathway gene of IL-10. JAK-STAT3 pathway is associated with on the development of obesity-associated disorders such as leptin resistance and insulin resistance [16]. However, the regulation and role of IL-10 and JAK-STAT3 pathway in adipose tissue are not completely understood in childhood obesity. Are these factors alterant in childhood obesity and obesity-related disorder?

In the present study, we observed that childhood obesity with hypertriglyceridemia were accompanied by a predominant inflammatory state with a decrease of IL-10 expression in SAT. In addition, we conducted a diet induced obese rat study to validate it. Our hypothesis is that decrease of IL-10 in AT is associated with triglyceride metabolism, which could contribute to the pathogenesis of childhood obesity. Clarifying the role of IL-10 in lipid metabolism may provide a new therapeutic strategies in obesity-association disorders.

Methods
Study population
Sixty-two children undergoing surgery for nonmalignant and non-inflammatory diagnose were recruited. According to the BMI reference norm for Chinese children and adolescences, subjects were considered to be obese when the BMI exceeded 95th percentile of the norm [17]. BMI standard deviation score (SDS-BMI) were calculated according to WHO BMI-for-age (5–19 years) [18].Subjects were diagnosed with hypertriglyceridemia (serum TG level > 1.7 mmol/L) according to the new International Diabetes Federation definition for Chinese people [19]. The study protocol was approved by the Ethical Committee of Xi'an Jiaotong University. Written informed consent was obtained from all guardians of children participating in the study. The study was conducted according to the Declaration of Helsinki.

Adipose tissue and blood sample
Immediately after skin incision and subcutaneous tissue exposure during the surgery, AT were separated bluntly, washed in cold PBS, and stored at liquid nitrogen for quantitative real-time PCR (qRT-PCR). Fasting venous blood sample from each participant was collected and stored at – 80 °C for biochemical measurements.

Animals
One hundred forty-four male clean Sprague-Dawley rats from the age of 3 weeks after weaned were purchased in Animal Experimental Center of Xi'an Jiaotong University. Rats were housed under a 12:12 h light-dark cycle with well ventilation and constant temperature (26 ± 1 °C). Animals were adapted to laboratory lighting and feeding condition for 1 week before experiment. Rats were allowed free access to food and drinking water. After adaptation, rats were randomly divided into two groups. The control group ($n = 48$) was given normal diet (ND). The other group ($n = 96$) were fed with high-fat diet (HFD). The HFD was prepared by mixing 2 g cholesterol and 15 g lard oil with 83 g ND. The HFD consists of 44.9% fat, 35.1% carbohydrate as starch, 20.0% protein as casein as the energy sources while the ND contained 20.8% fat, 60.9% carbohydrate, 18.3% protein. The body weight and food intake of each rat were measured once and twice per week. Rats with weight 20% higher than average weight of control group were regarded of obese rats. Obesity evaluation was conducted in 8th, 16th, 20th and 24th week, respectively. 12 ND rats and 12 HFD obese rats were sacrificed under anesthesia by an intraperitoneal injection of chloral hydrate in 8th, 16th, 20th week, respectively. In 24th week, all of the remaining rats ($n = 16$) were sacrificed in the same way, while non-obesity HFD rats were excluded. All animal experiment protocols were approved by the Ethics Committee of the Xi'an Jiaotong University and were performed according to the Institutional Animal Care and Use Committee of Xi'an Jiaotong University. All experimental procedures conformed to the European Guidelines for the care and use of Laboratory Animals (directive 2010/63/EU).

Biochemical measurements
Fasting blood glucose (FBG), total cholesterol (TC), triglycerides (TG), high-density lipoprotein cholesterol (HDL-C) and low-density lipoprotein cholesterol (LDL-C) were measured enzymatically using an autoanalyzer (Hitachi 747). Plasma free fatty acids (FFA) concentrations were determined using a commercial enzymatic kit (Applygen). Fasting Insulin was assayed by RIA (BeiFang systems). Plasma levels of leptin and adiponectin were also measured by Elisa kits (Excell). Serum IL-10 concentrations were measured using Elisa kits (Wuhan Boster Biotechnology Inc.).

Immunohistochemistry
After rats were sacrificed, perirenal and epididymal AT were quickly removed, weighed, frozen immediately in liquid nitrogen, and kept at – 80 °C for the analysis of mRNA expression or fixed with 4% paraformaldehyde for histological examination. AT sections (5 μm) were stained with IL-10 and P-STAT3 (Immunoway) respectively. The

protein–antibody immune complexes were detected with horseradish peroxidase-conjugated secondary antibodies and enhanced chemiluminescence reagents (Millipore). The average optical density (AOD) of each protein in sections were detected by Image-Pro plus 6.0.

RNA isolation and quantitative real-time PCR

Total RNA was isolated using Trizol reagent (Invitrogen). Then cDNA was synthesized using a high-capacity Reverse Transcription kit (Takara) and diluted in DNase-free water before use. QRT-PCR was performed on an ABI HT7500 PCR machine using the comparative Ct-method with SYBR Green PCR kit (Takara). Relative mRNA expression levels of target genes were normalized to GAPDH. The following primers were used: IL-10 (human), 5'-TGTCATCG ATTTCTTCCCTGT-3' and 5'-GGCTTTGTAGATGCCT TTCTCT-3'; IL-10 (rat), 5'-CAGACCCACATGCTCCGA GA-3' and 5'-CAAGGCTTGGCAACCCAAGTA-3'; STA T3 (human), 5'-TTTGAGACAGAGGTGTACCACCAA G-3' and 5'-ACCACAGGATTGATGCCCAAG-3'; STA T3 (rat) 5'-TGTGACACCAACGACCTGC-3' and 5'-TCC ATGTCAAACGTGAGCGA-3'; GAPDH (human), 5' -A ATGGACAACTGGTCGTGGAC-3' and 5' -CCCTCCA GGGGATCTGTTTG-3'; GAPDH (rat), 5' -GGTGGACC TCATGGCCTACA-3' and 5' -CTCTCTTGCTCTCAGT ATCCTTGCT-3'.

Statistical analysis

The data was expressed as the mean ± standard error. Differences between the two groups were analyzed with a Student's t-test. Differences between the serum lipids at the different feed periods were assessed using a two-way ANOVA. Pearson's correlations between IL-10 and other parameters were calculated. The differences were considered statistically significant at $p < 0.05$. All analyses were performed by SPSS 22.0 (SPSS Inc.).

Results

Inflammation and metabolic disorders associated with childhood obesity

The clinical features of non-obese controls ($n = 31$), obese children without hypertriglyceridemia ($n = 17$) and obese children with hypertriglyceridemia ($n = 14$) are shown in Table 1. Anthropometric evaluation showed that BMI, SDS-BMI, waist circumference, waist-hip Ratio and SBP of obese children with/without hypertriglyceridemia were higher than non-obese children. For biochemical measurements, obese children with/without hypertriglyceridemia also showed an increase in fasting insulin, HOMA-IR, TG, FFA and LDL-C, and concomitant reduction in HDL-C levels.

Table 1 Clinical features of study groups

	Non-obese ($n = 31$)	Obese without hypertriglyceridemia ($n = 17$)	Obese with hypertriglyceridemia ($n = 14$)
Sex (male/female)	21/10	11/6	9/5
Age (years)	8.14 ± 1.69	8.72 ± 2.36	8.59 ± 1.78
BMI (kg/m²)	15.13 ± 1.19	22.19 ± 2.77*	22.85 ± 2.19*
SDS-BMI	−0.52 (−1.41, 0.38)	2.59 (2.02, 3.08)*	2.66 (1.99,3.39)*
Waist circumference (cm)	55.48 ± 3.84	71.52 ± 11.59*	71.65 ± 9.3*
Waist-hip Ratio	0.88 ± 0.06	0.92 ± 0.05*	0.92 ± 0.05*
SBP (mmHg)	95 ± 7	100 ± 7*	103 ± 9*
DBP (mmHg)	59 ± 6	62 ± 5	61 ± 10
FBG (mmol/L)	4.67 ± 0.40	4.72 ± 0.42	4.76 ± 0.63
Fasting insulin (μU/mL)	5.04 ± 3.34	12.96 ± 4.36*	13.03 ± 5.07*
HOMA-IR	0.96 ± 0.41	2.59 ± 1.21*	2.67 ± 1.10*
TC (mmol/L)	3.43 ± 0.66	3.80 ± 0.36	3.71 ± 0.79
TG (mmol/L)	0.86 ± 0.40	0.87 ± 0.32*	2.79 ± 0.95*,**
FFA (μmol/L)	367.22 ± 50.79	416.62 ± 44.72*	445.36 ± 60.38*
HDL-C (mmol/L)	1.37 ± 0.19	1.15 ± 0.11*	1.04 ± 0.14*
LDL-C (mmol/L)	1.67 ± 0.48	2.11 ± 0.47	2.33 ± 0.13*,**
Leptin (ng/mL)	10.56 ± 8.99	30.80 ± 15.11*	26.02 ± 10.89*
Adiponectin (μg/mL)	3.35 ± 1.20	2.73 ± 1.33*	2.57 ± 1.09*,**
leptin-to-adiponectin ratio (ng/μg)	3.45 ± 2.11	11.56 ± 5.90*	14.71 ± 9.18*,**

BMI body mass index, *SDS-BMI* standard deviation scores BMI, *SBP* systolic blood pressure, *DBP* diastolic blood pressure, *FBG* fasting blood glucose, *TC* total cholesterol, *TG* triglycerides, *FFA* free fatty acids, *HDL-C* high-density lipoprotein cholesterol, *LDL-C* low-density lipoprotein cholesterol. *$p < 0.05$ vs. Non-obese. **$p < 0.05$ vs. Obese without hypertriglyceridemia

Adiponectin and leptin were measured to characterize inflammation status. Obese children with/without hypertriglyceridemia showed an increase of leptin and leptin-to-adiponectin ratio, and a decrease in adiponectin (Table 1). Moreover, we observed that obese children with hypertriglyceridemia showed a decrease in adiponectin compared with children without hypertriglyceridemia (Table 1).

IL-10 decreased in adipose tissue and serum of obese children with hypertriglyceridemia

QRT-PCR and Elisa showed that IL-10 mRNA in AT and serum IL-10 levels were similar between non-obese and obese group (Additional file 1: Table S1). However, when compared with the non-obese and the obese without hypertriglyceridemia group, IL-10 mRNA expression in AT and serum IL-10 levels were lower in obese children with hypertriglyceridemia (Fig. 1a, b). Furthermore, the expression of IL-10 mRNA in AT was negatively correlated to TG and LDL-C levels, and positively correlated to HDL-C, adiponectin and serum IL-10 levels in this cohort (Fig. 1c-g).

Serum lipids is increased in HFD obese rats

Physical appearance and body weights of rats were measured to confirm the HFD-induced obese phenotype.

Rats fed with HFD with the end body weight 20% higher than that in the ND group were considered as obese rats (obesity rate was 86.2%). Obese rats were significantly larger in size, with yellow pelage (Fig. 2a). Rats fed with HFD showed a significant increase in mean body weight as compared to the ND rats after 8th week (Fig. 2b). After 20th week, serum FFA and TG in HFD obese rats were significantly higher than those in ND rats, remarkably in 24th week. Serum TC level was significantly higher compared with ND rats in 24th week (Table 2). Serum lipids is increased in HFD obese rats in 24th week.

IL-10 is reduced in HFD obese rats

In HFD obese rats, the serum IL-10 concentrations was reduced in 24th week (Fig. 2c). When compared with controls, IL-10 mRNA expression in AT was lower in HFD obese rats in 24th week (Fig. 2d). Immunohistochemical staining showed that IL-10 protein expression was reduced in HFD obese rats in 24th week (Fig. 2e). Moreover, the AOD of IL-10 protein expression in AT of HFD rats was significantly reduced compared with ND rats (Fig. 2f). QRT-PCR and immunohistochemical staining showed that the expression of IL-10 in AT was reduced in HFD obese rats. According to the sorting of

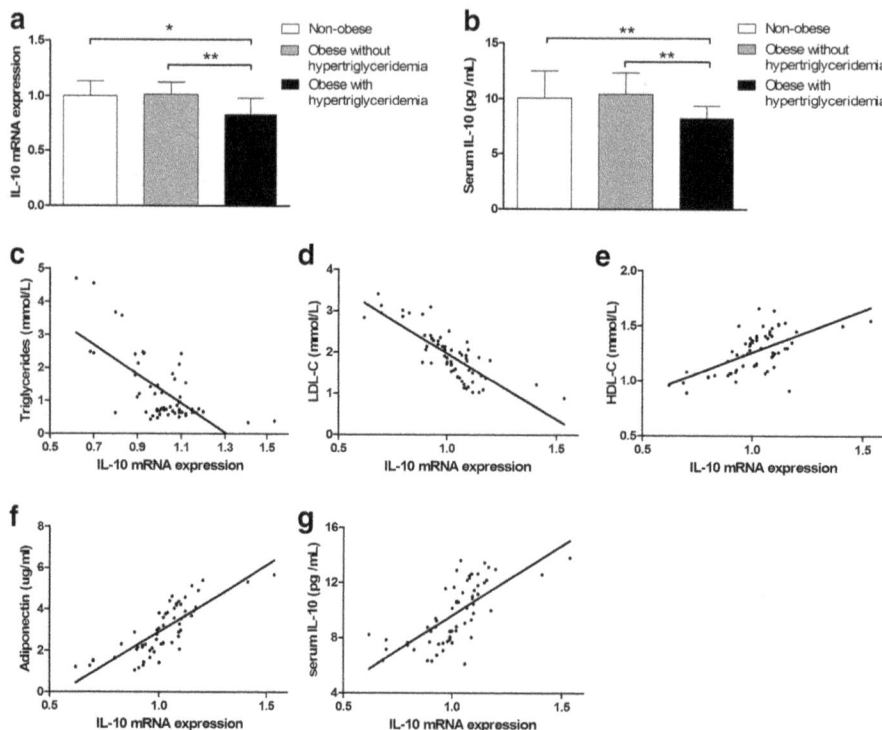

Fig. 1 Evaluation of mRNA expression in adipose tissue and serum levels of IL-10. **a** Adipose IL-10 mRNA expression and (**b**) serum IL-10 decreased in obese children with hypertriglyceridemia ($n = 14$). $*P < 0.01$ vs. non-obese controls ($n = 31$). $**P < 0.01$ vs. obese without hypertriglyceridemia ($n = 17$). IL-10 mRNA expression was negatively correlated to (**c**) TG and (**d**) LDL-C levels, and positively correlated to (**e**) HDL-C, (**f**) Adiponectin and (**g**) serum IL-10 levels. The data are presented as mean ± SD

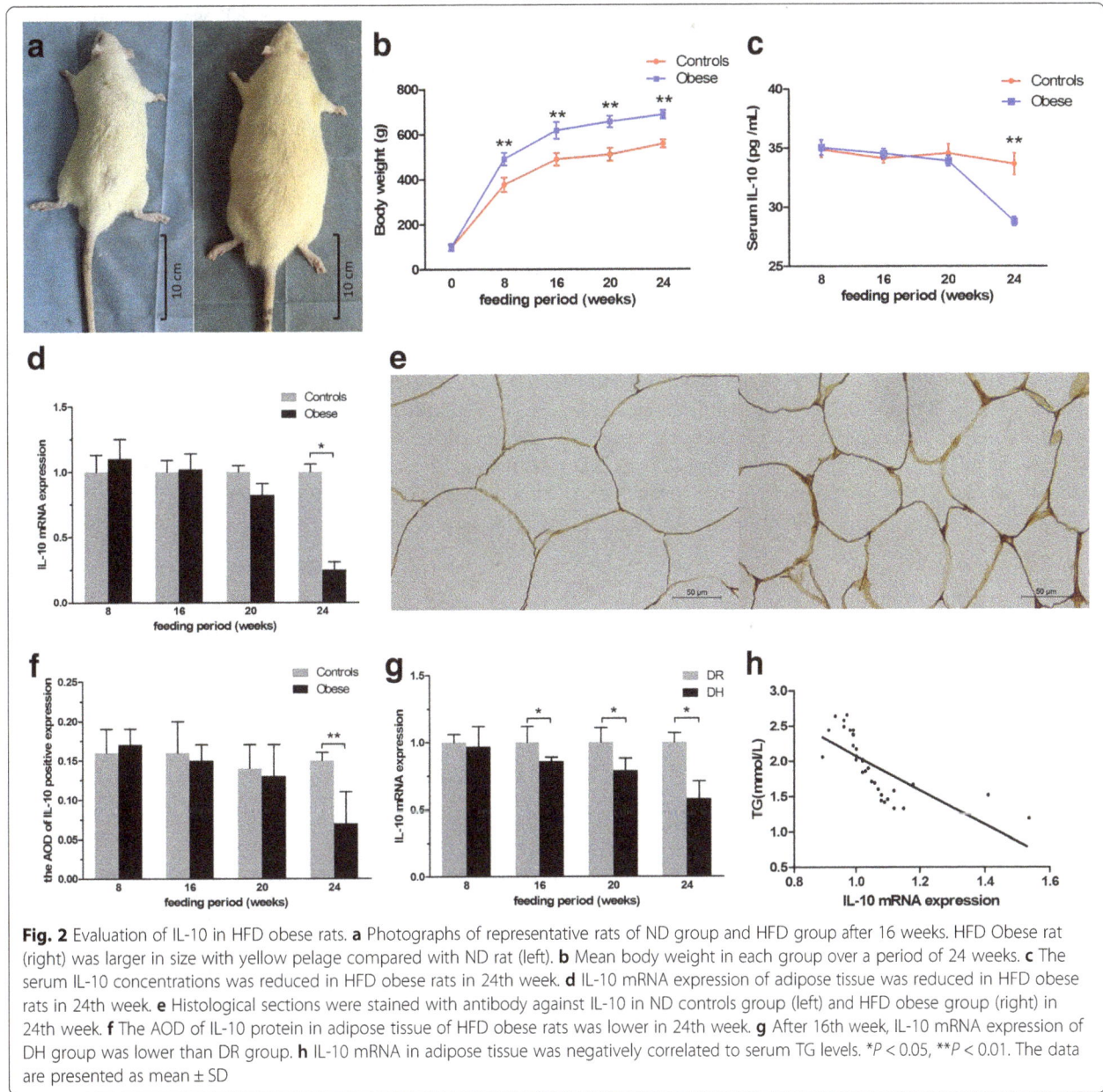

Fig. 2 Evaluation of IL-10 in HFD obese rats. **a** Photographs of representative rats of ND group and HFD group after 16 weeks. HFD Obese rat (right) was larger in size with yellow pelage compared with ND rat (left). **b** Mean body weight in each group over a period of 24 weeks. **c** The serum IL-10 concentrations was reduced in HFD obese rats in 24th week. **d** IL-10 mRNA expression of adipose tissue was reduced in HFD obese rats in 24th week. **e** Histological sections were stained with antibody against IL-10 in ND controls group (left) and HFD obese group (right) in 24th week. **f** The AOD of IL-10 protein in adipose tissue of HFD obese rats was lower in 24th week. **g** After 16th week, IL-10 mRNA expression of DH group was lower than DR group. **h** IL-10 mRNA in adipose tissue was negatively correlated to serum TG levels. *$P < 0.05$, **$P < 0.01$. The data are presented as mean ± SD

Table 2 Serum lipids of ND and HFD rats

week	TG(mmol/L)		TC(mmol/L)		FFA(μmol/L)	
	ND	HFD	ND	HFD	ND	HFD
8	1.64 ± 0.23	1.77 ± 0.44	1.29 ± 0.26	1.27 ± 0.53	305.23 ± 8.35	307.43 ± 11.87
16	1.51 ± 0.31	1.79 ± 0.31	1.25 ± 0.12	1.30 ± 0.44	310.56 ± 7.42	315.95 ± 4.20
20	1.76 ± 0.34	2.06 ± 0.11[a]	1.33 ± 0.42	1.37 ± 0.59	308.73 ± 11.64	321.89 ± 6.12[a]
24	1.61 ± 0.29	2.67 ± 0.94[a,b]	1.36 ± 0.31	1.76 ± 0.53[a,b]	302.64 ± 10.14	329.32 ± 4.15[a,b]

TG triglyceride, *TC* total cholesterol, *FFA* free fatty acids. [a] $p < 0.05$ vs. ND. [b] $p < 0.05$ vs. 8th week. 8th, 16th, 20th week $n = 12$, 24th week n = 16

TG increments, HFD rats at the top 1/3 ($n = 4$) of TG were considered as diet-induce hypertriglyceridemia (DH) group and HFD rats at the lower 1/3 (n = 4) of TG were considered as diet-induce hypertriglyceridemia resistance (DR) group. After 16th week, IL-10 mRNA expression of DH rats was lower than DR rats. Additionally, IL-10 mRNA in AT was negatively correlated to serum TG levels (Fig. 2h).

STAT3 is reduced in obese children with hypertriglyceridemia and HFD obese rats

QRT-PCR showed that when compared with the non-obese and the obese without hypertriglyceridemia group, STAT3 mRNA expression were lower in obese children with hypertriglyceridemia (Fig. 3a). Immunohistochemical staining showed that P-STAT3 protein expression was reduced in HFD obese rats when compared with ND rats (Fig. 3d, e). QRT-PCR showed the similar results that

STAT3 mRNA expression of AT was reduced in HFD obese rats in 24th week when compared with ND rats (Fig. 3f). In addition, STAT3 mRNA expression in AT was positively correlated to IL-10 expression, and negatively correlated to TG levels both in children and rats (Fig. 3b, c, g, h).

Discussion

Obesity is a chronic and persistent low inflammatory condition triggered by the immune response and by the metabolic regulator molecules. The mechanisms behind this association are still unclear. However, it is possible that the key inflammatory regulators also play important role in regulating inflammatory responses. IL-10 is anti-inflammatory cytokine and contributed with low inflammatory condition in childhood obesity [20, 21]. However, the effect of IL-10 on pathogenesis of childhood obesity and related disorder is unclear.

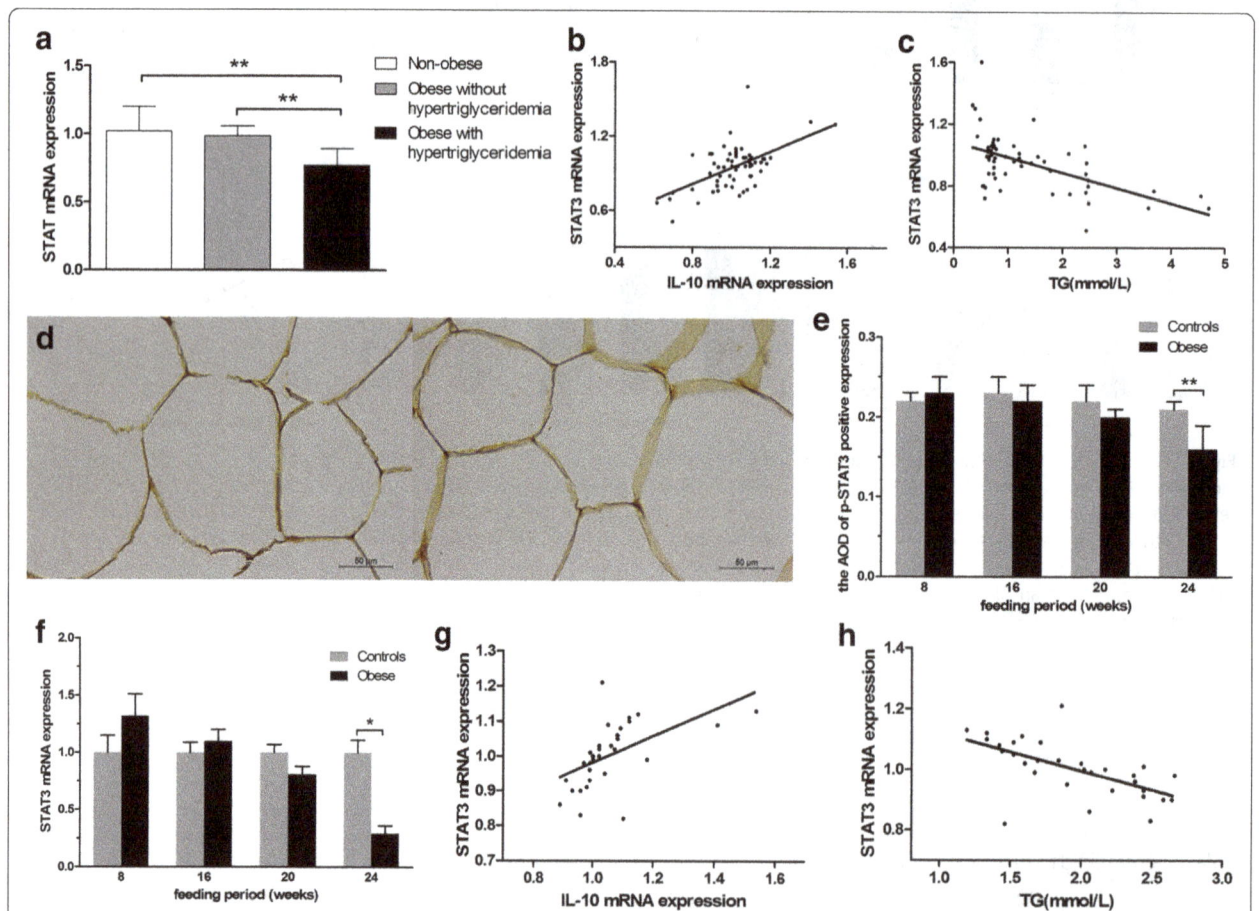

Fig. 3 Evaluation of STAT3 expression. **a** STAT3 mRNA expression were reduced in obese children with hypertriglyceridemia. **b** Adipose STAT3 mRNA expression was positively correlated to IL-10 expression in adipose tissue of children. **c** Adipose STAT3 mRNA expression was negatively correlated to serum TG levels in children. **d** Histological sections were stained with antibody against P-STAT3 in ND controls group (left) and HFD obese group (right) in 24th week. **e** The AOD of P-STAT3 protein in adipose tissue of HFD obese rats was lower in 24th week. **f** STAT3 mRNA expression of adipose tissue was lower in HFD obese rats in 24th week. **g** Adipose STAT3 mRNA expression was positively correlated to IL-10 expression in rats. **h** Adipose STAT3 mRNA expression was negatively correlated to serum TG levels in rats. *$P < 0.05$, **$P < 0.01$. The data are presented as mean ± SD

In the present study, we evaluated the adipose and circulating IL-10 levels and their association with the childhood obesity and obesity–related hypertriglyceridemia in both a cross-sectional study of humans and in a rat study. Clinical and laboratorial characteristics of obese children with or without hypertriglyceridemia and controls showed that obese children with hypertriglyceridemia have lower adiponectin and higher leptin-to-adiponectin ratio when compared to the controls and children without hypertriglyceridemia. These results are consistent with the adult cohort that adiponectin level is lower in hypertriglyceridemia and independent relation to hypertriglyceridemia [22] which indicated higher grade of inflammatory status and adipose tissue physiology. Previous study reported that in obese women the prevalence of the metabolic syndrome was associated with low circulating IL-10 levels [23]. Moreover, IL-10 expression was not reduced in obesity with normal blood triglycerides adult cohort [24], which is similar to our observation. However, we innovatively demonstrated that obese children with hypertriglyceridemia showed lower adipose and serum IL-10 compared to obese children without hypertriglyceridemia and non-obese children. Thus, IL-10 in adipose tissue and circulation is down-regulated in obese children with hypertriglyceridemia.

Previous study reported that increased IL-10 in patients with lymphoproliferative disorder causes elevated triglycerides, low LDL-C and HDL-C deficiency, and IL-10 is thus a potent modulator of lipoprotein levels [25]. HDL-C decreased significantly in IL-10-deficient mice compared to WT mice [26], consistent with effects of systemic inflammation in decreasing HDL-C [27]. We evidenced that mRNA expression of IL-10 in SAT of children was negatively correlated to TG and LDL-C levels, and positively correlated to HDL-C. Coincide with the human study, the negative correlation between adipose IL-10 and serum TG was indicated in rats study. Lipid abnormalities occur in autoimmune and inflammatory disorders with incompletely understood mechanism, but the inflammatory cytokines have been implicated to play an important role [27]. Several cytokines that induce lipolysis, including TNF, IFN-α, and IFN-γ, produce a marked decrease in hormone-sensitive lipase (HSL) mRNA [28]. IL-1 effect on serum TG levels is attributable to enhanced hepatic FA synthesis and TG secretion [29]. Thus, dysregulation of IL-10 is directly or indirectly associated with pathogenesis of obesity-related hypertriglyceridemia.

It is appropriate to use high energy and high fat diet to induce obesity model in obese rats, which have been widely used to study the pathogenesis and progression of obesity because they have the similar gene expression profiling with obese humans [30, 31]. To observe the adipose and circulating IL-10 levels and their association with obesity, we established a high-fat diet induced

obesity rat model with aggravated lipids disorders, of which serum TG, FFA and TC were increased. Consistent with previous study, we observed showed that serum IL-10 was reduced in obese rats induced by HFD [32]. HFD-induced obesity is accompanied by inflammatory status of IL-10 down-regulation in tissue. In heart tissue, IL-10 was found to be down-regulated in HFD rats and up-regulated in HFD-exercise groups [33]. We focused on adipose tissue and evidenced that the levels of IL-10 decreased in adipose tissue of obese rats after a long HFD feed period (in 24th week). Interestingly, after dividing the obese rats into subgroup according to the TG increments ranking, we observed that IL-10 mRNA expression of diet-induce hypertriglyceridemia rats was lower than hypertriglyceridemia resistance rats in the earlier feed period (in 16th week) along with weight gain in HFD rats. Adipose tissue dysfunction with chronic inflammation is considerably associated with the development of insulin resistance, type 2 diabetes, and cardiovascular diseases [34]. Dysfunction of adipocytes, changes in metabolic profile or immune cells profile have been indicated in obesity [35, 36], which may result in the alteration of IL-10 expression and chronic inflammation in AT.

Recent studies have demonstrated that IL-10 can exert anti-inflammatory effects through the JAK-STAT3 pathway: After IL-10 binding to the receptor on the target cell membrane, the tyrosine kinase 2 (Tyk2), which is a subtype of the JAK protein family coupled with the IL-10 receptor, is further activated; Stimulation of Tyk2 with IL-10 leads to activation of STAT3 by its SH2 domain tyrosine phosphorylation [14, 37, 38]. One of the primary determinants of plasma TG is lipoprotein and the various proteins, such as apoC-II, apoC-III, ANGTPL3, that regulate lipoprotein. [39–41] Overexpression of apolipoprotein A-I significantly increased the phosphorylation of STAT3 as well as its upstream JAK2 kinase, which increased serum TG, TC and HDL-C levels [42]. It is reported that interleukin-10 gene transfer inhibits atherogenesis in ApoE-deficient mice through a STAT3-dependent anti-inflammatory pathway [43]. Present study has shown that adipose STAT3 expression was decreased in obese children with hypertriglyceridemia and in HFD obese rats. Moreover, STAT3 mRNA expression in AT was positively correlated to IL-10 expression, and negatively correlated to TG levels. We therefore concluded that IL-10/JAK-STAT pathway is associated with obesity-related hypertriglyceridemia, and the pathogenesis mechanism require further study.

We recognize that our research has some limitations. In the present study, the clinical sample size for evaluation of IL-10 expression was still small and a larger sample cohort is needed for verification. In addition, we observed and hypothesized that IL-10 participated in triglyceride metabolism associated with JAK-STAT pathway in HFD obese rats. However, the molecular regulation mechanisms of these potential regulators in childhood obesity still require to be investigated in vivo or vitro.

Conclusion

We highlight the decrease of IL-10 expression and its downstream JAK-STAT pathway in obese children with hypertriglyceridemia and in HFD obese rats, which indicated that IL-10 might have a protective effect on the lipid metabolic disorders, particularly hypertriglyceridemia. We believe that these alternations exacerbate the inflammatory process and dysfunction in adipose tissue, contributing to dyslipidemia. Thenceforward, the observation of IL-10 as key cytokine in obesity-related metabolic disorders opens perspectives for designing new therapeutic strategies in to treat childhood obesity and its consequences.

Abbreviations

AOD: Average optical density.; CHD: Coronary heart disease; DBP: Diastolic blood pressure; FBG: Fasting blood glucose; FFA: Free fatty acids; HDL-C: High-density lipoprotein cholesterol; HFD: High-fat diet; HSL: Hormone sensitive lipase; JAK: Janus Kinase; LDL-C: Low-density lipoprotein cholesterol; ND: Normal diet; SAT: Subcutaneous adipose tissue; SBP: Systolic blood pressure; STAT: Signal transducers and activators of transcription; TC: Total cholesterol; TG: Triglyceride; TG: Triglycerides

Funding

This study was supported by the National Natural Science Foundation of China (No. 81673187).

Authors' contributions

DX and YX designed and supervised the study. YL, CY and SW collected and analyzed the data. DX, YL, SW and MW contributed in the samples collection and animal experiment. YL organized and wrote the manuscript. YL and YX revised the manuscript critically. All authors approved the final version for submission.

Competing interests

The authors declare that they have no competing interests.

Author details

[1]Department of Pediatrics, The Second Affiliated Hospital of Xi'an Jiaotong University, 157 Xiwu Road, Xi'an, Shaanxi 710061, People's Republic of China. [2]Tongji Hospital, Tongji Medical College, Huazhong University of Science and Technology, Wuhan, Hubei 430030, People's Republic of China.

References

1. Malik VS, Willett WC, Hu FB. Global obesity: trends, risk factors and policy implications. Nat Rev Endocrinol. 2013;9(1):13–27.
2. Low S, Chin MC, Deurenberg-Yap M. Review on epidemic of obesity. Ann Acad Med Singap. 2009;38(1):57–65.
3. Lee AM, Gurka MJ, DeBoer MD. Trends in metabolic syndrome severity and lifestyle factors among adolescents. Pediatrics. 2016;137(3):9.
4. Sun H, Ma Y, Han D, Pan C-W, Xu Y: Prevalence and trends in obesity among China's children and adolescents, 1985-2010. PLoS One. 2014;9(8):e105469.
5. Cox AJ, West NP, Cripps AW. Obesity, inflammation, and the gut microbiota. Lancet Diabetes Endocrinol. 2015;3(3):207–15.
6. Daniels SR. The consequences of childhood overweight and obesity. Future Child. 2006;16(1):47–67.
7. Kopelman P. Health risks associated with overweight and obesity. Obes Rev. 2007;8(Suppl 1):13–7.
8. Lloyd LJ, Langley-Evans SC, McMullen S. Childhood obesity and risk of the adult metabolic syndrome: a systematic review. Int J Obesity. 2012;36(1):1–11.
9. Cook S, Kavey REW. Dyslipidemia and pediatric obesity. Pediatr Clin N Am. 2011;58(6):1363.
10. van Greevenbroek MMJ, Schalkwijk CG, Stehouwer CDA. Obesity-associated low-grade inflammation in type 2 diabetes mellitus: causes and consequences. Neth J Med. 2013;71(4):174–87.
11. Skurk T, Alberti-Huber C, Herder C, Hauner H. Relationship between adipocyte size and adipokine expression and secretion. J Clin Endocr Metab. 2007;92(3):1023–33.
12. van Hall G, Steensberg A, Sacchetti M, Fischer C, Keller C, Schjerling P, Hiscock N, Moller K, Saltin B, Febbraio MA, et al. Interleukin-6 stimulates lipolysis and fat oxidation in humans. J Clin Endocrinol Metab. 2003;88(7):3005–10.
13. Watt MJ, Carey AL, Wolsk-Petersen E, Kraemer FB, Pedersen BK, Febbraio MA. Hormone-sensitive lipase is reduced in the adipose tissue of patients with type 2 diabetes mellitus: influence of IL-6 infusion. Diabetologia. 2005;48(1):105–12.
14. Sabat R, Grutz G, Warszawska K, Kirsch S, Witte E, Wolk K, Geginat J. Biology of interleukin-10. Cytokine Growth Factor Rev. 2010;21(5):331–44.
15. Mattos RT, Medeiros NI, Menezes CA, Fares RCG, Franco EP, Dutra WO, Rios-Santos F, Correa-Oliveira R, Gomes JAS. Chronic low-grade inflammation in childhood obesity is associated with decreased IL-10 expression by monocyte subsets. PLoS One. 2016;11(12):14.
16. Wunderlich CM, Hovelmeyer N, Wunderlich FT. Mechanisms of chronic JAK-STAT3-SOCS3 signaling in obesity. Jak-Stat. 2013;2(2):e23878.
17. Ji CY. Report on childhood obesity in China (1) - body mass index reference for screening overweight and obesity in Chinese school-age children. Biomed Environ Sci. 2005;18(6):390–400.
18. Hawcutt DB, Bellis J, Price V, Povall A, Newland P, Richardson P, Peak M, Blair J. Growth hormone prescribing and initial BMI SDS: increased biochemical adverse effects and costs in obese children without additional gain in height. PLoS One. 2017;12(7):e0181567.
19. Federation ID. The IDF consensus worldwide definition of the metabolic syndrome. Belgium: International Diabetes Federation; 2006.
20. Medeiros NI, Mattos RT, Menezes CA, Fares RCG, Talvani A, Dutra WO, Rios-Santos F, Correa-Oliveira R, Gomes JAS. IL-10 and TGF-beta unbalanced levels in neutrophils contribute to increase inflammatory cytokine expression in childhood obesity. Eur J Nutr. 2017. https://doi.org/10.1007/s00394-017-1515-y.
21. Rodrigues KF, Pietrani NT, Bosco AA, Campos FMF, Sandrim VC, Gomes KB. IL-6, TNF-alpha, and IL-10 levels/polymorphisms and their association with type 2 diabetes mellitus and obesity in Brazilian individuals. Archives of endocrinology and metabolism. 2017;61(5):438–46.
22. Tanyansky DA, Firova EM, Shatilina LV, Denisenko AD. Adiponectin: lowering in metabolic syndrome and independent relation to hypertriglyceridemia. Kardiologiya. 2008;48(12):20–5.
23. Esposito K, Pontillo A, Giugliano F, Giugliano G, Marfella R, Nicoletti G, Giugliano D. Association of low interleukin-10 levels with the metabolic syndrome in obese women. J Clin Endocr Metab. 2003;88(3):1055–8.
24. Pereira S, Teixeira L, Aguilar E, Oliveira M, Savassi-Rocha A, Pelaez JN, Capettini L, Diniz MT, Ferreira A, Alvarez-Leite J. Modulation of adipose tissue inflammation by FOXP3+Treg cells, IL-10, and TGF-beta in metabolically healthy class III obese individuals. Nutrition. 2014;30(7-8):784–90.
25. Moraitis AG, Freeman LA, Shamburek RD, Wesley R, Wilson W, Grant CM, Price S, Demosky S, Thacker SG, Zarzour A, et al. Elevated interleukin-10: a

new cause of dyslipidemia leading to severe HDL deficiency. J Clin Lipidol. 2015;9(1):81–90.

26. Mallat Z, Heymes C, Ohan J, Faggin E, Leseche G, Tedgui A. Expression of interleukin-10 in advanced human atherosclerotic plaques - relation to inducible nitric oxide synthase expression and cell death. Arterioscl Throm Vas. 1999;19(3):611–6.

27. Khovidhunkit W, Kim MS, Memon RA, Shigenaga JK, Moser AH, Feingold KR, Grunfeld C. Effects of infection and inflammation on lipid and lipoprotein metabolism: mechanisms and consequences to the host. J Lipid Res. 2004;45(7):1169–96.

28. Doerrler W, Feingold KR, Grunfeld C. Cytokines induce catabolic effects in cultured adipocytes by multiple mechanisms. Cytokine. 1994;6(5):478–84.

29. Feingold KR, Soued M, Adi S, Staprans I, Neese R, Shigenaga J, Doerrler W, Moser A, Dinarello CA, Grunfeld C. Effect of INTERLEUKIN-1 on lipid-metabolism in the rat - similarities to and differences from tumor-necrosis-FACTOR. Arterioscler Thromb. 1991;11(3):495–500.

30. Li SY, Zhang HY, Hu CC, Lawrence F, Gallagher KE, Surapaneni A, Estrem ST, Calley JN, Varga G, Dow ER, et al. Assessment of diet-induced obese rats as an obesity model by comparative functional genomics. Obesity. 2008;16(4):811–8.

31. Buettner R, Scholmerich J, Bollheimer LC. High-fat diets: modeling the metabolic disorders of human obesity in rodents. Obesity. 2007;15(4):798–808.

32. Schaalan MF, Ramadan BK, Abd Elwahab AH. Synergistic effect of carnosine on browning of adipose tissue in exercised obese rats; a focus on circulating irisin levels. J Cell Physiol. 2018;233(6):5044–57.

33. Kesherwani V, Chavali V, Hackfort BT, Tyagi SC, Mishra PK. Exercise ameliorates high fat diet induced cardiac dysfunction by increasing interleukin 10. Front Physiol. 2015;6:7.

34. Romacho T, Elsen M, Rohrborn D, Eckel J. Adipose tissue and its role in organ crosstalk. Acta Physiol. 2014;210(4):733–53.

35. Bluher M. Adipose tissue inflammation: a cause or consequence of obesity-related insulin resistance? Clin Sci. 2016;130(18):1603–14.

36. Sun K, Kusminski CM, Scherer PE. Adipose tissue remodeling and obesity. J Clin Invest. 2011;121(6):2094–101.

37. Stark George R, Darnell Jr James E. The JAK-STAT pathway at twenty. Immunity. 2012;36(4):503–14.

38. Niemand C, Nimmesgern A, Haan S, Fischer P, Schaper F, Rossaint R, Heinrich PC, Muller-Newen G. Activation of STAT3 by IL-6 and IL-10 in primary human macrophages is differentially modulated by suppressor of cytokine signaling 3. *Journal of immunology (Baltimore, Md : 1950)*. 2003;170(6):3263–72.

39. Wolska A, Dunbar RL, Freeman LA, Ueda M, Amar MJ, Sviridov DO, Remaley AT. Apolipoprotein C-II: new findings related to genetics, biochemistry, and role in triglyceride metabolism. Atherosclerosis. 2017;267:49–60.

40. Xu Y-X, Redon V, Yu H, Querbes W, Pirruccello J, Liebow A, Deik A, Trindade K, Wang X, Musunuru K, et al. Role of angiopoietin-like 3 (ANGPTL3) in regulating plasma level of low-density lipoprotein cholesterol. Atherosclerosis. 2018;268:196–206.

41. Jin J-L, Guo Y-L, Li J-J. Apoprotein C-III: a review of its clinical implications. Clin Chim Acta. 2016;460:50–4.

42. Yin K, Tang SL, Yu XH, Tu GH, He RF, Li JF, Xie D, Gui QJ, Fu YC, Jiang ZS, et al. Apolipoprotein A-I inhibits LPS-induced atherosclerosis in ApoE(−/−) mice possibly via activated STAT3-mediated upregulation of tristetraprolin. Acta Pharmacol Sin. 2013;34(6):837–46.

43. Yoshioka T, Okada T, Maeda Y, Ikeda U, Shimpo M, Nomoto T, Takeuchi K, Nonaka-Sarukawa M, Ito T, Takahashi M, et al. Adeno-associated virus vector-mediated interleukin-10 gene transfer inhibits atherosclerosis in apolipoprotein E-deficient mice. Gene Ther. 2004;11(24):1772–9.

The product of fasting plasma glucose and triglycerides improves risk prediction of type 2 diabetes in middle-aged Koreans

Joung-Won Lee[1,2], Nam-Kyoo Lim[1] and Hyun-Young Park[1*]

Abstract

Background: Screening for risk of type 2 diabetes mellitus (T2DM) is an important public health issue. Previous studies report that fasting plasma glucose (FPG) and triglyceride (TG)-related indices, such as lipid accumulation product (LAP) and the product of fasting glucose and triglyceride (TyG index), are associated with incident T2DM. We aimed to evaluate whether FPG or TG-related indices can improve the predictive ability of a diabetes risk model for middle-aged Koreans.

Methods: 7708 Koreans aged 40–69 years without diabetes at baseline were eligible from the Korean Genome and Epidemiology Study. The overall cumulative incidence of T2DM was 21.1% (766 cases) in men and 19.6% (797 cases) in women. Therefore, the overall cumulative incidence of T2DM was 20.3% (1563 cases). Multiple logistic regression analysis was conducted to compare the odds ratios (ORs) for incident T2DM for each index. The area under the receiver operating characteristic curve (AROC), continuous net reclassification improvement (cNRI), and integrated discrimination improvement (IDI) were calculated when each measure was added to the basic risk model for diabetes.

Results: All the TG-related indices and FPG were more strongly associated with incident T2DM than WC in our study population. The adjusted ORs for the highest quartiles of WC, TG, FPG, LAP, and TyG index compared to the lowest, were 1.64 (95% CI, 1.13–2.38), 2.03 (1.59–2.61), 3.85 (2.99–4.97), 2.47 (1.82–3.34), and 2.79 (2.16–3.60) in men, and 1.17 (0.83–1.65), 2.42 (1.90–3.08), 2.15 (1.71–2.71), 2.44 (1.82–3.26), and 2.85 (2.22–3.66) in women, respectively. The addition of TG-related parameters or FPG, but not WC, to the basic risk model for T2DM (including age, body mass index, family history of diabetes, hypertension, current smoking, current drinking, and regular exercise) significantly increased cNRI, IDI, and AROC in both sexes.

Conclusions: Adding either TyG index or FPG into the basic risk model for T2DM increases its prediction and reclassification ability. Compared to FPG, TyG index was a more robust T2DM predictor in the stratified sex and fasting glucose level. Therefore, TyG index should be considered as a screening tool for identification of people at high risk for T2DM in practice.

Keywords: TyG index, Type 2 diabetes mellitus, Risk model

* Correspondence: mdhypark@gmail.com
[1]Division of Cardiovascular Diseases, Center for Biomedical Sciences, Korea National Institute of Health, 187 Osongsaengmyeng 2-ro, Osong-eup, Heungdeok-gu, Cheongju-si, Chungcheongbuk-do 361-951, South Korea
Full list of author information is available at the end of the article

Background

Type 2 diabetes mellitus (T2DM) is one of the most prevalent non-communicable diseases in the middle-aged population worldwide, largely because of recent changes in diet and lifestyle [1, 2]. In the Korean National Health and Nutrition Examination Surveys (KNHANES), the prevalence of diabetes among adults aged 30 and over was found to have slightly increased, from 12.4% in 2011 to 13.0% in 2014 [3, 4]. According to an estimate by the International Diabetes Federation, 46.3% of cases of diabetes in Koreans aged 20–79 were undiagnosed in 2015 [5]. However, lifestyle intervention can reduce the risk of incident T2DM and mortality in individuals at high risk of diabetes [6, 7]. Therefore, it is important to screen high-risk individuals for T2DM regularly to ensure early diagnosis. For this reason, risk models for diabetes have been proposed in previous studies, and, recently, T2DM risk prediction models have been reported in Korea [8–14].

Obesity is the most significant risk factor for incident T2DM [15, 16]. Body mass index (BMI) has been used as a surrogate marker for obesity and included as one of the variables in most risk models for T2DM [9, 11–14]. However, BMI does not reflect central obesity. Lee et al. selected waist circumference (WC) instead of BMI in their diabetes risk model considering its association with diabetes [10]. In the systematic review, more than 30% of the diabetes risk models stating its components included both BMI and WC [8]. To improve the prediction ability of a risk model for incident T2DM, blood parameters are also frequently included [8].

Also, the increase of fasting plasma glucose (FPG) in the normal range is associated with increased incident T2DM [17]. Of these, serum triglyceride (TG) has been used to identify people at high risk for T2DM, alongside obesity [18]. In addition, lipid accumulation product (LAP) and the product of fasting plasma glucose and triglyceride (TyG index), composite indices including TG, have been proposed as predictors of T2DM [19, 20]. In particular, TyG index has been used as a marker of insulin resistance [19]. Although the simple diabetes risk model is convenient for self-assessment, more accurate prediction models that include blood parameters are also required to facilitate more accurate clinical consultations [8]. In Korea, most people are registered with the National Health Insurance (NHI), which provides biannual medical check-ups for middle-aged people, including the measurement of key blood parameters [21]. Therefore, risk models for incident T2DM that are based on the data obtained from these medical check-ups would be of great use for

the prediction of risk of future T2DM. To date, few studies have been undertaken in Korea that compare the predictive ability for incident T2DM of the simple model and composite models, which include blood test results [11, 22]. Recently, a risk model for T2DM that included blood test results was proposed based on cohort data, and its reclassification ability was significantly improved when glycated hemoglobin (HbA$_{1c}$) was included [11]. However, HbA$_{1c}$ is not assessed in the routine health examination and this study did not consider reclassification ability when other blood test results apart from HbA$_{1c}$ were included in the T2DM risk model [23].

Therefore, in the present study, we aimed to identify which of the TG-related indices that can be derived from general check-up data would improve the prediction ability of the simple T2DM risk model in middle-aged Koreans.

Methods

Study population

The Korean Genome and Epidemiology Study (KoGES) consists of a gene-environment model and population-based studies [24]. KoGES: Ansan and Ansung study is an ongoing prospective cohort study conducted in urban (Ansan) and rural (Ansung) areas in Korea with biennial follow-ups, which started in 2001. 10038 people underwent an initial examination, and 9001 subjects were included after exclusion of 1037 who refused to participate or died. Thirty-five participants were not suitable for the present study because of their age, and subjects with a history of diabetes at baseline or incomplete data were also excluded. Finally, 7708 people aged 40 to 69 years remained eligible for the current study. Written informed consent was obtained from all subjects. The Institutional Review Board of the Korean Centers for Disease Control and Prevention approved the study protocol.

Measurements and surveys

Height and weight were measured to the nearest 0.1 cm and 0.1 kg using a digital stadiometer and a scale, respectively. Resting blood pressure while sitting was measured by trained technicians using a standard mercury sphygmomanometer. Blood samples were collected after fasting for at least 8 h. The Friedewald formula was used to indirectly estimate low-density lipoprotein cholesterol levels in subjects with plasma TG < 400 mg/dl [25]. Diabetes was defined by FPG > 126 mg/dl, 2 h post-challenge plasma glucose > 200 mg/dl, HbA$_{1c}$ > 6.5%, or prescription for anti-diabetic medication [26]. Subjects were questioned by trained interviewers regarding their socio-demographics, family history of diabetes, and lifestyle factors including smoking and alcohol consumption. The subjects' smoking and alcohol consumption status was subdivided according to their past and present habits. Regular exercise was defined as subjects' exercise was over 90 min as the sum of moderate and vigorous physical activity a day [27].

LAP and TyG index were calculated as follows:

$$\text{LAP for men} = [WC(cm)\text{-}65] \times TG(mmol/L)$$
$$\text{LAP for women} = [WC(cm)\text{-}58] \times TG(mmol/L)$$
$$\text{TyG index} = \ln[TG(mg/dl) \times FPG(mg/dl)/2]$$

Statistical analysis

Data are expressed as numbers and proportions for discrete variables and mean ± SD for continuous variables, and were analyzed using Chi-square and Student's t-tests, respectively.

Based on the maximized Youden index, we calculated sex-specific cut-off points of each index for T2DM. Multiple logistic regression analysis was conducted and adjusted for age, BMI, hypertensive status, family history of diabetes, current smoking and alcohol consumption status, and regular exercise. The basic model was derived from the published diabetes risk model for middle-aged Koreans and included the variables listed above [10, 11]. We tested multicollinearity for all covariates based on the variable inflation factor (VIF). The area under the receiver operating characteristic curve (AROC) was calculated for each risk model of incident T2DM, indicating the diagnostic power of each model for incident T2DM during the follow-up period [28]. Differences in AROC between the basic model and each composite model were analyzed using the method of DeLong et al. [29]. Pencina et al. have suggested category-based net reclassification improvement (NRI) and integrated discrimination improvement (IDI) for calculating the usefulness of a new marker in prediction models [30]. The category-based NRI measures the accuracy of reclassification based on how well the subjects are reclassified as upwards for events and downwards for non-events. However, the category-based NRI can be affected by the number and choice of categories [31]. The continuous (category-free) NRI (cNRI) is an expanded method to solve limitation of the categories. They also proposed the IDI that calculates the extent of average sensitivity and '1-specificity' when a new marker is added to the basic model [30]. We calculated the cNRI and IDI to compare the prediction and reclassification abilities of each measure when added to the basic model of diabetes.

Macros were used to calculate cNRI and IDI, and data analysis was performed using SAS 9.4 and MedCalc [32].

Results

Baseline characteristics

Table 1 indicates the baseline characteristics of the study subjects. The ages of the subjects were 51.4 ± 8.6 years for men and 52.0 ± 8.9 years for women. The prevalence of hypertension was higher in men than in women (29.5% vs. 27.0%, P = 0.0149). By contrast, the percentage of subjects with a family history of diabetes was higher in women than in men (11.0% vs. 9.2%, P = 0.0067). There were also significant differences in anthropometric indices between sexes. Mean BMI and WC were 24.1 ± 2.9 kg/m^2 and 83.3 ± 7.6 cm in men, and 24.7 ± 3.2 kg/m^2 and 81.2 ± 9.5 cm in women, respectively. Mean TG, FPG, LAP, and TyG index were 170.8 ± 111.6 mg/dl, 84.5 ± 9.0 mg/dl, 38.1 ± 34.0, and 8.7 ± 0.5 in men, and 140.9 ± 75.6 mg/dl, 81.1 ± 7.7 mg/dl, 39.0 ± 30.6, and 8.5 ± 0.5 in women, respectively. TG-related indices also showed significant differences between the sexes, with the exception of LAP.

Table 1 Characteristics of the study population at baseline

Variables	Men (n = 3636)	Women (n = 4072)	P-value
Age, years	51.4 ± 8.6	52.0 ± 8.9	0.0011
Current Smoker, n(%)	1753 (48.2)	142 (3.5)	<.0001
Current Drinker, n(%)	2580 (71.0)	1085 (26.7)	<.0001
Hypertension, n(%)	1074 (29.5)	1101 (27.0)	0.0149
Family history of diabetes, n(%)	333 (9.2)	449 (11.0)	0.0067
Regular exercise, n(%)	1712 (47.1)	1654 (40.6)	<.0001
BMI, kg/m^2	24.1 ± 2.9	24.7 ± 3.2	<.0001
WC, cm	83.3 ± 7.6	81.2 ± 9.5	<.0001
TG, mg/dl	170.8 ± 111.6	140.9 ± 75.6	<.0001
TyG index	8.7 ± 0.5	8.5 ± 0.5	<.0001
LAP	38.1 ± 34.0	39.0 ± 30.6	0.1925
SBP, mmHg	121.2 ± 16.6	119.9 ± 19.1	0.0029
DBP, mmHg	81.6 ± 10.8	78.5 ± 11.6	<.0001
FPG, mg/dl	84.5 ± 9.0	81.1 ± 7.7	<.0001
2hPG, mg/dl	110.5 ± 32.0	117.2 ± 28.3	<.0001
Total cholesterol, mg/dl	190.3 ± 34.6	188.9 ± 33.9	0.0670
HDL-C, mg/dl	43.8 ± 10.0	46.0 ± 10.0	<.0001
LDL-C, mg/dl	112.4 ± 34.2	114.7 ± 30.7	0.0017
HbA$_{1c}$, mg/dl	5.6 ± 0.3	5.5 ± 0.4	0.1636

P values are from t-tests or chi-square tests for analysis of variance for continuous variables and categorical variables

Abbreviations: *BMI* body mass index, *WC* waist circumference, *TG* triglycerides; TyG index, the product of fasting glucose and triglycerides; *LAP* lipid accumulation product, *SBP* systolic blood pressure, *DBP* diastolic blood pressure, *FPG* fasting plasma glucose, *HDL-C* high-density lipoprotein cholesterol, *LDL-C* low density lipoprotein cholesterol, *HbA$_{1c}$* glycated hemoglobin

Incidence of T2DM according to each index category

During the 10 year follow-up, the overall cumulative incidence of T2DM was 21.1% (766 cases) in men and 19.6% (797 cases) in women. Table 2 shows the overall cumulative incidence of T2DM, categorized by quartiles for each index. In men, the cumulative incidences of T2DM across the quartiles of TyG index were (lowest-highest) 13.3 and 31.5% and those of FPG were 12.9 and 35.9% and those of WC were 16.4 and 27.7%. In women, the values for TyG index were 11.1 and 30.9% and those FPG were 13.9 and 28.4% and those WC were 13.4 and 24.5%. The increase in the cumulative incidence of T2DM with higher category of WC was less marked than that with increasing TyG index or FPG.

Cut-off points of each index for predicting T2DM

Table 3 shows the AROC values and cut-off points of the indices for predicting T2DM. The AROCs for WC, TG, FPG, LAP, and TyG index were 0.579, 0.592, 0.660, 0.602, and 0.623 in men 0.576, 0.627, 0.599, 0.623, and 0.644 in women respectively. The cut-off points for predicting T2DM were 84.00 cm, 172.00 mg/dl, 87.00 mg/dl, 30.50, and 8.86 in men and 78.17 cm, 122.00 mg/dl, 84.00 mg/dl, 35.84, and 8.52 in women for WC, TG, FPG, LAP, and TyG index, respectively.

Odds ratios for incident T2DM for each composite predictive model

Table 4 shows the odds ratio (OR) for incident T2DM in higher quartiles compared to the first quartile of each index. The unadjusted ORs for all TG-related indices for incident T2DM were higher than that of WC. These trends were similar after adjustment for age, BMI, hypertensive status, family history of diabetes, smoking, alcohol consumption status and regular exercise. When the highest quartile for each index was compared to the lowest, the adjusted ORs of WC, TG, FPG, LAP, and TyG index were 1.64 (95% confidence interval (CI), 1.13–2.38), 2.03 (1.59–2.61), 3.85 (2.99–4.97), 2.47 (1.82–3.34), and 2.79 (2.16–3.60) in men, and 1.17 (0.83–1.65),

Table 2 Number of incident type 2 diabetes cases according to the quartiles for each measure

Categories	Men (n = 3636)		Women (n = 4072)	
	Quartile	Diabetes (%)	Quartile	Diabetes (%)
WC (cm)	Q1 (< 78.0)	143 (16.4)	Q1 (< 74.0)	128 (13.4)
	Q2 (78.0–83.2)	162 (17.6)	Q2 (74.0–80.6)	198 (18.1)
	Q3 (83.3–88.2)	207 (22.3)	Q3 (80.7–87.8)	222 (22.2)
	Q4 (≥88.3)	254 (27.7)	Q4 (≥87.9)	249 (24.5)
TG (mg/dl)	Q1 (< 106.0)	137 (15.2)	Q1 (< 92.5)	126 (12.4)
	Q2 (106.0–142.9)	167 (18.4)	Q2 (92.5–121.9)	136 (13.6)
	Q3 (143.0–200.9)	196 (21.5)	Q3 (122.0–165.9)	225 (21.9)
	Q4 (≥201.0)	266 (29.0)	Q4 (≥166.0)	310 (30.3)
FPG (mg/dl)	Q1 (< 78.0)	106 (12.9)	Q1 (< 76.0)	133 (13.9)
	Q2 (78.0–82.9)	132 (14.7)	Q2 (76.0–79.9)	143 (16.3)
	Q3 (83.0–89.9)	190 (19.5)	Q3 (80.0–84.9)	206 (18.3)
	Q4 (≥90.0)	338 (35.9)	Q4 (≥85.0)	315 (28.4)
LAP	Q1 (< 16.7)	137 (15.1)	Q1 (< 18.8)	126 (12.4)
	Q2 (16.7–29.4)	140 (15.4)	Q2 (18.8–30.7)	167 (16.4)
	Q3 (29.5–49.1)	212 (23.3)	Q3 (30.8–50.1)	190 (18.7)
	Q4 (≥49.2)	277 (30.5)	Q4 (≥50.2)	314 (30.8)
TyG index	Q1 (< 8.4)	121 (13.3)	Q1 (< 8.2)	113 (11.1)
	Q2 (8.4–8.6)	153 (16.8)	Q2 (8.2–8.4)	140 (13.8)
	Q3 (8.7–9.0)	206 (22.7)	Q3 (8.5–8.7)	229 (22.5)
	Q4 (≥9.1)	286 (31.5)	Q4 (≥8.8)	315 (30.9)

Abbreviations: *WC* waist circumference, *TG* triglycerides, *FPG* fasting plasma glucose, *LAP* lipid accumulation product, *TyG index* the product of fasting glucose and triglycerides

Table 3 The area under the ROC curve (AROC) and cut-off points for indices to predict type 2 diabetes

Index	AROC (95% CI)	Cut-off point	Sensitivity (%)	Specificity (%)	Youden index
Men					
WC (cm)	0.579 (0.563–0.595)	84.00	56.01	57.11	0.13
TG (mg/dl)	0.592 (0.576–0.608)	172.00	46.74	67.84	0.15
FPG (mg/dl)	0.660 (0.645–0.676)	87.00	51.31	72.89	0.24
LAP	0.602 (0.586–0.618)	30.50	62.79	55.54	0.18
TyG index	0.623 (0.607–0.638)	8.86	52.09	66.59	0.19
Women					
WC (cm)	0.576 (0.561–0.592)	78.17	69.26	43.54	0.13
TG (mg/dl)	0.627 (0.612–0.642)	122.00	66.37	54.41	0.21
FPG (mg/dl)	0.599 (0.584–0.614)	84.00	39.52	75.69	0.15
LAP	0.623 (0.607–0.637)	35.84	57.59	61.59	0.19
TyG index	0.644 (0.629–0.659)	8.52	67.25	55.85	0.23

Abbreviations: *AROC* area under the receiver operating characteristic curve, *WC* waist circumference, *TG* triglycerides, *FPG* fasting plasma glucose, *LAP* lipid accumulation product, TyG index, the product of fasting glucose and triglycerides

2.42 (1.90–3.08), 2.15 (1.71–2.71), 2.44 (1.82–3.26), and 2.85 (2.22–3.66) in women, respectively. The calculated VIF for all covariates in the multivariate model, were below 5.0, indicating no severe multicollinearity among covariates [33].

Effects of the addition of each index to the basic model of T2DM on cNRI, IDI, and AROC

Table 5 shows the reclassification and discrimination abilities when each measure was added to the basic model of diabetes. The AROCs for the addition of TyG index or FPG to the basic model were larger than those for the other indices in both sexes. The cNRI for TG, FPG, LAP, and TyG index were 22.7% ($P < 0.0001$), 48.0% ($P < 0.0001$), 23.6% ($P < 0.0001$), and 38.7% ($P < 0.0001$) in men, and 28.6% ($P < 0.0001$), 21.3% ($P < 0.0001$), 21.3% ($P < 0.0001$), and 36.0% ($P < 0.0001$) in women, respectively. By contrast, the addition of WC made cNRI only 5.6% ($P = 0.1689$), in men and – 2.3% ($P = 0.5666$), in women. The IDI was also higher when TG-related indices or FPG was added than when WC was added to the basic model of T2DM in both sexes.

Discussion

We showed that the predictive ability of the simple T2DM risk model was increased when TG-related indices or FPG was added. Recently, several diabetes risk models have been proposed to screen high-risk groups, some of which included blood parameters. WC was included as one of the components in the model because increased WC increases T2DM risk [8]. However, WC is not easily used in

practice because of measurement inaccuracy [34]. Among the TG-related indices analyzed in the present study, the AROC and reclassification ability of TyG index were higher than for TG or LAP. Although the inclusion of LAP also improved the predictive ability of the risk model for incident diabetes, this required the additional inclusion of WC, while this was not required to demonstrate improvements in the risk model by the inclusion of TG or TyG index [20]. Most studies that used TyG index to predict incident T2DM used it as a surrogate for insulin resistance, and reported that its predictive ability is better than that of the homeostasis model of assessment (HOMA-IR) [19, 35, 36]. However, Abbasi and Reaven showed that the correlation between insulin-mediated glucose uptake (IMGU) and TyG index is not better than that between IMGU and TG or HOMA-IR [37, 38]. Nevertheless, it was noted that TyG index is a practical measure for use in T2DM prediction because of its cost-efficiency [37]. Moreover, the use of HbA_{1c} has been recommended for diagnosis and screening of patients. Lim et al. added HbA_{1c} to a diabetes risk model and demonstrated an increase in predictive ability for T2DM in a middle-aged Korean cohort, while Ahn et al. also demonstrated through longitudinal validation analysis that adding FPG or HbA_{1c} to the simple diabetes risk model also improves its predictive ability [11, 22]. Thus, in general, the predictive ability of a diabetes risk model that includes laboratory parameters such as TG, FPG, or HbA_{1c} is better than that of the simple diabetes risk model [11, 14, 22].

Table 4 Multiple logistic regression analyses for each measure in predicting type 2 diabetes (odds ratios and 95% confidence intervals)

Categories	Unadjusted					Adjusted[a]				
	WC ORs (95% CI)	TG ORs (95% CI)	FPG ORs (95% CI)	LAP ORs (95% CI)	TyG index ORs (95% CI)	WC ORs (95% CI)	TG ORs (95% CI)	FPG ORs (95% CI)	LAP ORs (95% CI)	TyG index ORs (95% CI)
Men										
Q1	Ref.	Ref.	Ref.	Ref.	Ref.	Ref.	Ref.	Ref.	Ref.	Ref.
Q2	1.09 (0.85–1.39)	1.26 (0.99–1.62)	1.16 (0.88–1.53)	1.03 (0.79–1.33)	1.32 (1.02–1.70)	1.07 (0.81–1.40)	1.21 (0.94–1.55)	1.18 (0.89–1.56)	1.04 (0.79–1.36)	1.26 (0.97–1.64)
Q3	1.46 (1.15–1.85)	1.54 (1.21–1.95)	1.64 (1.27–2.12)	1.71 (1.35–2.18)	1.91 (1.49–2.45)	1.35 (1.00–1.83)	1.39 (1.08–1.79)	1.68 (1.29–2.19)	1.70 (1.28–2.25)	1.82 (1.41–2.36)
Q4	1.95 (1.55–2.46)	2.29 (1.82–2.88)	3.78 (2.96–4.82)	2.47 (1.96–3.11)	2.99 (2.36–3.79)	1.64 (1.13–2.38)	2.03 (1.59–2.61)	3.85 (2.99–4.97)	2.47 (1.82–3.34)	2.79 (2.16–3.60)
Women										
Q1	Ref.	Ref.	Ref.	Ref.	Ref.	Ref.	Ref.	Ref.	Ref.	Ref.
Q2	1.43 (1.12–1.82)	1.11 (0.86–1.44)	1.20 (0.93–1.55)	1.39 (1.08–1.78)	1.28 (0.98–1.66)	1.14 (0.88–1.48)	1.02 (0.78–1.33)	1.18 (0.91–1.53)	1.26 (0.97–1.64)	1.19 (0.91–1.55)
Q3	1.86 (1.46–2.36)	1.98 (1.56–2.51)	1.38 (1.09–1.75)	1.63 (1.27–2.07)	2.32 (1.82–2.97)	1.27 (0.95–1.69)	1.69 (1.32–2.16)	1.32 (1.04–1.68)	1.35 (1.03–1.78)	1.97 (1.53–2.53)
Q4	2.10 (1.66–2.66)	3.07 (2.44–3.87)	2.45 (1.95–3.06)	3.15 (2.51–3.97)	3.59 (2.83–4.55)	1.17 (0.83–1.65)	2.42 (1.90–3.08)	2.15 (1.71–2.71)	2.44 (1.82–3.26)	2.85 (2.22–3.66)

[a]Adjusted for age, body mass index, status of hypertension, family history of diabetes, smoking status, alcohol consumption, and regular exercise

Abbreviations: *ORs* odds ratios, *WC* waist circumference, *TG* triglycerides, *FPG* fasting plasma glucose, *LAP* lipid accumulation product, *TyG index*, the product of fasting glucose and triglycerides

Table 5 Reclassification and discrimination results associated with the risk prediction of incident type 2 diabetes according to each measure

Parameter	Men						Women					
	AROC	p-value*	cNRI	p-value	IDI	p-value	AROC	p-value*	cNRI	p-value	IDI	p-value
Basic model[a]	0.615						0.621					
Basic model + WC	0.619	0.1176	0.056	0.1689	0.002	0.0140	0.621	0.3233	−0.023	0.5666	0.000	1.0000
Basic model + TG	0.632	<.0001	0.227	<.0001	0.007	<.0001	0.652	<.0001	0.286	<.0001	0.019	<.0001
Basic model + FPG	0.692	<.0001	0.480	<.0001	0.064	<.0001	0.652	<.0001	0.214	<.0001	0.018	<.0001
Basic model + LAP	0.634	<.0001	0.236	<.0001	0.007	<.0001	0.644	<.0001	0.213	<.0001	0.016	<.0001
Basic model + TyG index	0.656	<.0001	0.387	<.0001	0.023	<.0001	0.666	<.0001	0.360	<.0001	0.029	<.0001

[a]Basic model: age, body mass index, status of hypertension, family history of diabetes, smoking status, alcohol consumption, and regular exercise
*P-value for AROC means vs. Basic model
Abbreviations: AROC area under the receiver operating characteristic curve, WC waist circumference, TG triglycerides, LAP lipid accumulation product, TyG index the product of fasting glucose and triglycerides, cNRI continuous net reclassification improvement, IDI Integrated Discrimination Improvement

The advantages of the simple diabetes risk model are that it is inexpensive and patients can use it for self-assessment [8]. Weighed against the improved predictive accuracy obtained by the addition of HbA_{1c} and the Oral Glucose Tolerance Test (OGTT) to the T2DM risk model, there are substantial practical constraints on screening the whole population using such measurements [22]. As an effective alternative, a two-pronged approach to screening has been proposed [22, 39]. This approach consists of using the non-laboratory score for the general population and using the laboratory score for patients in a higher-risk group for T2DM. For screening as part of the Korean NHI program, TG-related indices or FPG are more suitable as one of the components of the T2DM risk model than OGTT or HbA_{1c}, given that these measurements are not currently included in primary screening measurements in Korea [23]. To the best of our knowledge, there is no TyG index criterion yet. On the other hand, several studies conducted in Europe and Asian have shown that the risk of incident T2DM was increased with increasing TyG index [40–42]. Some researchers have proposed a cut-off value of TyG index of 8.8 for incident T2DM and insulin resistance [41, 42]. The subjects in the present study were classified by the cut-off value of TyG index of 8.8. The adjusted odds ratio (95% CI) of incident T2DM in the subjects with TyG index ≥8.8 was 1.95 (1.73–2.20) compared to the counterparts. We also have proposed sex-specific cut-off points of TyG index (≥ 8.86 in men, ≥ 8.52 in women) as predictors of T2DM based on the maximized Youden index. Compared to the counterparts, the adjusted odds ratio (95% CI) of incident T2DM in the men with TyG index ≥8.86 and in the women with TyG index ≥8.52 were 2.01 (1.69–2.39) and 2.16 (1.82–2.56), respectively (Appendix 1). Considering NIH's

universe coverage, the health promotion that offered the general health check-ups for 17.6 million Koreans in 2016, and its following examination rate (77.7%), there should be less burden caused by blood tests than other countries [43]. Therefore, TyG index is recommended as a screening tool for the prediction of T2DM. Although TyG index predicts incident T2DM well, its usefulness is inconsistent, when compared to fasting glucose [38, 44]. For predicting T2DM risk, TyG index was not better than FPG or OGTT in Isfahan Diabetes Prevention Study [38]. Wang et al. reported that TyG index, LAP, and visceral adiposity were not superior to FPG or WC alone as diabetes predictors among Chinese [44]. In the Vascular-Metabolic CUN cohort, Navarro-Gonzalez et al. compared the prediction ability of TyG index and FPG for onset T2DM [35]. Association between indexes and their discrimination for onset T2DM were different depending on the fasting glucose subgroup. When the highest quartile for each index was compared to the lowest, the hazard ratios (HRs) of TyG index and FPG were 3.0 and 7.3 in the impaired fasting glucose group. On the other hand, TyG index showed stronger association with onset DM than FPG in the normal fasting glucose group (HRs: 6.8 vs. 4.6). The discrimination of TyG index for onset T2DM was also better than that of FPG in the normal fasting glucose group (AROC: 0.75 vs. 0.66). In the present study, we found the association between some metabolic syndrome (MetS) components and incident T2DM (Appendix 2). Therefore, we compared the discrimination of each index for incident T2DM in the stratified MetS components (Appendix 3). In the elevated FPG group, the discrimination of FPG (AROC: 0.506) for incident T2DM was inferior to that of other indices. On the other hand, TyG index was a more robust discrimination index than other indices in the group stratified by sex and MetS components. Our findings indicate that TyG index is not only a better predictor for incident diabetes than WC, LAP, and TG, but it also has a better reclassification ability. On the other hand, association between FPG and its(their) reclassification ability for incident T2DM were different depending on sex. The present study used community-based long-term prospective cohort data. Therefore, the temporal relationship between each measure and incident diabetes is clear. Our findings indicate that TyG index is not only a better predictor for incident diabetes than WC, LAP, and TG, but it also has a better reclassification ability. It was also noted that association between FPG and its reclassification ability for incident T2DM were different depending on sex. There were, however, a few limitations to this study. Firstly, even though KoGES is designed to include subjects who live both in rural and urban areas, the data are not representative of the entire Korean population [45]. Secondly, dietary intake was not included in the analysis. Moreover, Baik et al. had reported that the usefulness of dietary information in cardiovascular disease risk prediction models [46]. However, dietary information has been excluded from the questionnaire in medical check since 2009. Finally, our results were not validated using a separate Korean dataset. Therefore, additional studies are required to validate our data.

Conclusions

In conclusion, TG-related indices and FPG were more accurate than WC in the prediction of incident T2DM. In the subgroup categorized by sex and fasting glucose level, TyG index was a more robust predictor for onset T2DM than other indexes. Therefore, TyG index can be a useful screening tool for incident T2DM in middle-aged Koreans.

Appendix 1

Table 6 Multiple logistic regression analyses for cutoff-points of TyG index in predicting type 2 diabetes (odds ratios and 95% confidence intervals)

Cutoff-points	Men		Women	
	Unadjusted	Adjusted[a]	Unadjusted	Adjusted[a]
	ORs (95% CI)	ORs (95% CI)	ORs (95% CI)	ORs (95% CI)
TyG index ≥8.8[b]	2.05 (1.75–2.41)	1.93 (1.62–2.29)	2.41 (2.05–2.83)	2.03 (1.71–2.41)
TyG index ≥8.86/8.52[c]	2.13 (1.82–2.51)	2.01 (1.69–2.39)	2.57 (2.18–3.02)	2.16 (1.82–2.56)

[a]Adjusted for age, body mass index, status of hypertension, family history of diabetes, smoking status, alcohol consumption, and regular exercise, [b]TyG index ≥8.8 cm, Lee et al. [42], [c]TyG index ≥8.86 cm for men ≥8.52 for women in the present study
Abbreviations: ORs odds ratios; TyG index, the product of fasting glucose and triglycerides

Appendix 2

Table 7 Multiple logistic regression analyses for each MetS component in predicting type 2 diabetes (odds ratios and 95% confidence intervals)

Components of MetS[a]	Men		Women	
	Unadjusted	Adjusted [h]	Unadjusted	Adjusted [h]
	ORs (95% CI)	ORs (95% CI)	ORs (95% CI)	ORs (95% CI)
Central obesity[b]	1.71 (1.42–2.06)	1.35 (1.10–1.65)	1.56 (1.33–1.83)	1.16 (0.97–1.38)
Elevated TG[c]	1.70 (1.45–2.00)	1.57 (1.31–1.87)	2.26 (1.93–2.64)	1.90 (1.60–2.26)
Low HDL-C[d]	1.14 (0.96–1.34)	1.01 (0.84–1.22)	1.53 (1.28–1.83)	1.21 (1.00–1.47)
Elevated FPG[e]	5.43 (4.09–7.21)	5.16 (3.85–6.92)	3.65 (2.39–5.57)	3.55 (2.29–5.50)
Elevated BP[f]	1.79 (1.52–2.10)	1.47 (1.24–1.75)	1.65 (1.41–1.93)	1.29 (1.09–1.54)
MetS[g]	2.22 (1.86–2.66)	2.24 (1.87–2.69)[i]	2.22 (1.88–2.61)	2.03 (1.70–2.41)[i]

[a]Modified NCEP-ATP III criteria [47] with the Korean cut-off for WC, [b]WC ≥ 90 cm for men ≥85 for women, Lee et al. [48], [c]TG ≥ 150 mg/dl, [d]HDL-C < 40 mg/dl for men < 50 mg/dl for women, [e]FPG ≥ 100 mg/dl, [f]Systolic blood pressure ≥ 130 mmHg or diastolic blood pressure ≥ 85 mmHg, [g]Number of MetS components ≥3, [h]Adjusted for other components of MetS, age, family history of diabetes, smoking status, alcohol consumption, and regular exercise, [i]Adjusted for age, family history of diabetes, smoking status, alcohol consumption, and regular exercise
Abbreviations: MetS Metabolic syndrome, ORs odds ratios, TG triglyceride, HDL-C high-density lipoprotein cholesterol, FPG fasting plasma glucose, BP blood pressure, WC, waist circumference

Appendix 3

Table 8 The area under the ROC curve (AROC) for indices to predict type 2 diabetes stratified by MetS components

MetS components[a]	Central obesity[b]		Elevated TG[c]		Low HDL-C[d]		Elevated FPG[e]		Elevated BP[f]	
Subgroup	No	Yes	No	Yes	No	Yes	No	Yes	No	Yes
Index	AROC	AROC	AROC	AROC	AROC	AROC	AROC	AROC	AROC	AROC
Men	($n = 2929$)	($n = 707$)	($n = 1970$)	($n = 1666$)	($n = 2326$)	($n = 1310$)	($n = 3423$)	($n = 213$)	($n = 2092$)	($n = 1544$)
WC	0.553	0.532	0.535	0.569	0.570	0.584	0.571	0.573	0.565	0.559
TG	0.589	0.534	0.546	0.559	0.598	0.574	0.588	0.591	0.572	0.588
FPG	0.648	0.680	0.637	0.676	0.661	0.666	0.621	0.506	0.649	0.661
LAP	0.584	0.537	0.546	0.582	0.598	0.599	0.595	0.604	0.582	0.591
TyG index	0.618	0.569	0.605	0.607	0.631	0.605	0.607	0.586	0.602	0.620
Women	($n = 2680$)	($n = 1392$)	($n = 2754$)	($n = 1318$)	($n = 1276$)	($n = 2796$)	($n = 3983$)	($n = 89$)	($n = 2639$)	($n = 1433$)
WC	0.556	0.519	0.536	0.564	0.520	0.583	0.576	0.506	0.570	0.545
TG	0.610	0.626	0.567	0.559	0.611	0.622	0.629	0.596	0.614	0.621
FPG	0.590	0.598	0.581	0.617	0.550	0.616	0.586	0.566	0.598	0.587
LAP	0.601	0.625	0.553	0.590	0.565	0.630	0.623	0.570	0.608	0.609
TyG index	0.628	0.643	0.595	0.596	0.621	0.643	0.641	0.597	0.633	0.634

[a]Modified NCEP-ATP III criteria [47] with the Korean cut-off for WC, [b]WC ≥ 90 cm for men ≥85 for women, Lee et al. [48], [c]TG ≥ 150 mg/dl, [d]HDL-C < 40 mg/dl for men < 50 mg/dl for women, [e]FPG ≥ 100 mg/dl, [f] Systolic blood pressure ≥ 130 mmHg or diastolic blood pressure ≥ 85 mmHg
Abbreviations: MetS Metabolic syndrome, TG triglyceride, HDL-C high-density lipoprotein cholesterol, FPG fasting plasma glucose, BP blood pressure, AROC area under the receiver operating characteristic curve, WC waist circumference, LAP lipid accumulation product, TyG index, the product of fasting glucose and triglycerides

Abbreviations
AROC: Area under the receiver operating characteristic curve; BMI: Body mass index; CI: Confidence interval; cNRI: Continuous net reclassification improvement; FPG: Fasting plasma glucose; HbA$_{1c}$: Glycated hemoglobin; HRs: Hazard ratios; IDI: Integrated discrimination improvement; IMGU: Insulin-mediated glucose uptake; KNHANES: Korea National Health and Nutrition Examination; KNIH: Korea National Institute of Health; KoGES: Korean Genome and Epidemiology Study; LAP: Lipid accumulation product; NHI: National Health Insurance; OGTT: Oral Glucose Tolerance Test; ORs: Odds ratios; T2DM: Type 2 diabetes mellitus; TG: Triglyceride; TyG index: Product of fasting glucose and triglyceride; VIF: Variable inflation factor; WC: Waist circumference

Acknowledgements
Epidemiologic data used in this study were from the Korean Genome and Epidemiology Study (KoGES) of the Korea Centers for Disease Control & Prevention, Republic of Korea.

Funding
This study was supported by an intramural grant of the Korea National Institute of Health, Korea 4800–4845-302 (2017-NI63001–00). The funders had no role in the design of the study and collection, analysis, and interpretation of data and in writing the manuscript.

Authors' contributions
JWL carried out the data analysis and wrote the manuscript. NKL contributed to study design and advised statistical analyses. HYP contributed to study design and critically reviewed the paper. All authors read and approved the final manuscript.

Competing interests
The authors declare that they have no competing interest.

Author details
[1]Division of Cardiovascular Diseases, Center for Biomedical Sciences, Korea National Institute of Health, 187 Osongsaengmyeng 2-ro, Osong-eup, Heungdeok-gu, Cheongju-si, Chungcheongbuk-do 361-951, South Korea. [2]Department of Public Health Sciences, Graduate School, Korea University, Seoul, South Korea.

References
1. Esteghamati A, Gouya MM, Abbasi M, Delavari A, Alikhani S, Alaedini F, Safaie A, Forouzanfar M, Gregg EW. Prevalence of diabetes and impaired fasting glucose in the adult population of Iran: National Survey of risk factors for non-communicable diseases of Iran. Diabetes Care. 2008; 31(1):96–8.
2. Kim DJ. The epidemiology of diabetes in Korea. Diabetes Metab J. 2011; 35(4):303–8.
3. Ministry of Health and Welfare of Korea KCfDCaP. Korea health statistics 2011: Korea National Health and Nutrition Examination Survey (KNHANES V-2). Seoul: Ministry of Health and Welfare of Korea; 2012.
4. Ministry of Health and Welfare of Korea KCfDCaP. Korea health statistics 2014: Korea National Health and Nutrition Examination Survey (KNHANES VI-2). Sejong: Ministry of Health and Welfare of Korea; 2015.
5. Federation ID. IDF Diabetes Atlas. 7th ed; 2015.
6. Li G, Zhang P, Wang J, An Y, Gong Q, Gregg EW, Yang W, Zhang B, Shuai Y, Hong J. Cardiovascular mortality, all-cause mortality, and diabetes incidence after lifestyle intervention for people with impaired glucose tolerance in the Da Qing diabetes prevention study: a 23-year follow-up study. Lancet Diabetes Endocrinol. 2014;2(6):474–80.

7. Tuomilehto J, Schwarz P, Lindström J. Long-term benefits from lifestyle interventions for type 2 diabetes prevention time to expand the efforts. Diabetes Care. 2011;34(Supplement 2):S210–4.

8. Noble D, Mathur R, Dent T, Meads C, Greenhalgh T. Risk models and scores for type 2 diabetes: systematic review. Bmj. 2011;343:d7163.

9. Chien K, Cai T, Hsu H, Su T, Chang W, Chen M, Lee Y, Hu F. A prediction model for type 2 diabetes risk among Chinese people. Diabetologia. 2009; 52(3):443–50.

10. Lee Y-H, Bang H, Kim HC, Kim HM, Park SW, Kim DJ. A simple screening score for diabetes for the Korean population development, validation, and comparison with other scores. Diabetes Care. 2012;35(8):1723–30.

11. Lim N-K, Park S-H, Choi S-J, Lee K-S, Park H-Y. A risk score for predicting the incidence of type 2 diabetes in a middle-aged Korean cohort. Circ J. 2012; 76(8):1904–10.

12. Lindström J, Tuomilehto J. The diabetes risk score. Diabetes Care. 2003;26(3): 725–31.

13. Mann DM, Bertoni AG, Shimbo D, Carnethon MR, Chen H, Jenny NS, Muntner P. Comparative validity of 3 diabetes mellitus risk prediction scoring models in a multiethnic US cohort the multi-ethnic study of atherosclerosis. Am J Epidemiol. 2010;171(9):980–8.

14. Wilson PW, Meigs JB, Sullivan L, Fox CS, Nathan DM, D'Agostino RB. Prediction of incident diabetes mellitus in middle-aged adults: the Framingham offspring study. Arch Intern Med. 2007;167(10):1068–74.

15. Consultation WE: Waist circumference and waist-hip Ratio 2011.

16. Ko G, Chan J, Woo J, Lau E, Yeung V, Chow C, Wai H, Li J, So W, Cockram C: Simple anthropometric indexes and cardiovascular risk factors in Chinese. Int J Obes Relat Metab Disord 1997, 21(11):995–1001.

17. Janghorbani M, Amini M. Normal fasting plasma glucose and risk of prediabetes and type 2 diabetes: the Isfahan diabetes prevention study. Rev Diabet Stud. 2011;8(4):490.

18. Zhang M, Gao Y, Chang H, Wang X, Liu D, Zhu Z, Huang G. Hypertriglyceridemic-waist phenotype predicts diabetes: a cohort study in Chinese urban adults. BMC Public Health. 2012;12(1):1081.

19. Lee S-H, Kwon H-S, Park Y-M, Ha H-S, Jeong SH, Yang HK, Lee J-H, Yim H-W, Kang M-I, Lee W-C. Predicting the development of diabetes using the product of triglycerides and glucose: the Chungju metabolic disease cohort (CMC) study. PLoS One. 2014;9(2):e90430.

20. Kahn HS. The lipid accumulation product is better than BMI for identifying diabetes a population-based comparison. Diabetes Care. 2006;29(1):151–3.

21. Song YJ. The south Korean health care system. JMAJ. 2009;52(3):206–9.

22. Ahn CH, Yoon JW, Hahn S, Moon MK, Park KS, Cho YM. Evaluation of non-laboratory and laboratory prediction models for current and future diabetes mellitus: a cross-sectional and retrospective cohort study. PLoS One. 2016; 11(5):e0156155.

23. Korean National Health Insurance Service: National Health Insurance [http://www.nhis.or.kr/static/html/wbd/g/a/wbdga0606.html].

24. Kim Y, Han B-G. Cohort profile: the Korean genome and epidemiology study (KoGES) consortium. Int J Epidemiol. 2016;46(2):e20–e20.

25. Friedewald WT, Levy RI, Fredrickson DS. Estimation of the concentration of low-density lipoprotein cholesterol in plasma, without use of the preparative ultracentrifuge. Clin Chem. 1972;18(6):499–502.

26. Association AD. Diagnosis and classification of diabetes mellitus. Diabetes Care. 2010;33(Supplement 1):S62–9.

27. Park SK, Ryoo J-H, Oh C-M, Choi J-M, Choi Y-J, Lee KO, Jung JY. The risk of type 2 diabetes mellitus according to 2-hour plasma glucose level: the Korean genome and epidemiology study (KoGES). Diabetes Res Clin Pract. 2017. https://www.ncbi.nlm.nih.gov/pubmed/?term=The+risk+of+type+2+diabetes +mellitus+according+to+2-hour+plasma+glucose+level%3A+the+Korean +genome+and+epidemiology+study.

28. Zweig MH, Campbell G. Receiver-operating characteristic (ROC) plots: a fundamental evaluation tool in clinical medicine. Clin Chem. 1993;39(4):561–77.

29. DeLong ER, DeLong DM, Clarke-Pearson DL. Comparing the areas under two or more correlated receiver operating characteristic curves: a nonparametric approach. Biometrics. 1988;44(3):837–45.

30. Pencina MJ, D'Agostino RB, D'Agostino RB, Vasan RS. Evaluating the added predictive ability of a new marker: from area under the ROC curve to reclassification and beyond. Stat Med. 2008;27(2):157.

31. Pencina MJ, D'Agostino RB, Steyerberg EW. Extensions of net reclassification improvement calculations to measure usefulness of new biomarkers. Stat Med. 2011;30(1):11–21.

32. Kennedy K, Pencina M. A SAS macro to compute added predictive ability of new markers predicting a dichotomous outcome. In: SouthEeast SAS Users Group Annual Meeting Proceedings: 2010; 2010.

33. Vatcheva KP, Lee M, McCormick JB, Rahbar MH. Multicollinearity in regression analyses conducted in epidemiologic studies. Epidemiol. 2016; 6(227). https://doi.org/10.4172/2161-1165.1000227. https://www.omicsonline.org/open-access/multicollinearity-in-regression-analyses-conducted-in-inepidemiologic-studies-2161-1165-1000227.php?aid=69442.

34. Sebo P, Beer-Borst S, Haller DM, Bovier PA. Reliability of doctors' anthropometric measurements to detect obesity. Prev Med. 2008;47(4): 389–93.

35. Navarro-González D, Sánchez-Íñigo L, Pastrana-Delgado J, Fernández-Montero A, Martinez JA. Triglyceride–glucose index (TyG index) in comparison with fasting plasma glucose improved diabetes prediction in patients with normal fasting glucose: the vascular-metabolic CUN cohort. Prev Med. 2016;86:99–105.

36. Vasques ACJ, Novaes FS, MdS d O, JRM S, Yamanaka A, Pareja JC, Tambascia MA, MJA S, Geloneze B. TyG index performs better than HOMA in a Brazilian population: a hyperglycemic clamp validated study. Diabetes Res Clin Pract. 2011;93(3):e98–e100.

37. Abbasi F, Reaven G. Statin-induced diabetes: how important is insulin resistance? J Intern Med. 2015;277(4):498–500.

38. Janghorbani M, Almasi SZ, Amini M. The product of triglycerides and glucose in comparison with fasting plasma glucose did not improve diabetes prediction. Acta Diabetol. 2015:1–8.

39. Wannamethee S, Papacosta O, Whincup P, Thomas M, Carson C, Lawlor D, Ebrahim S, Sattar N. The potential for a two-stage diabetes risk algorithm combining non-laboratory-based scores with subsequent routine non-fasting blood tests: results from prospective studies in older men and women. Diabet Med. 2011;28(1):23–30.

40. Zheng R, Mao Y. Triglyceride and glucose (TyG) index as a predictor of incident hypertension: a 9-year longitudinal population-based study. Lipids Health Dis. 2017;16(1):175.

41. Navarro-González D, Sánchez-Íñigo L, Fernández-Montero A, Pastrana-Delgado J, Martinez JA. TyG index change is more determinant for forecasting type 2 diabetes onset than weight gain. Medicine. 2016;95(19)

42. Lee DY, Lee ES, Kim JH, Park SE, Park C-Y, Oh K-W, Park S-W, Rhee E-J, Lee W-Y. Predictive value of triglyceride glucose index for the risk of incident diabetes: a 4-year retrospective longitudinal study. PLoS One. 2016;11(9): e0163465.

43. National Health Insurance Service. 2016 National health screening statistical yearbook http://www.nhis.or.kr/menu/boardRetriveMenuSet.xx?menuId=F3328.

44. Wang B, Zhang M, Liu Y, Sun X, Zhang L, Wang C, Linlin L, Ren Y, Han C, Zhao Y. Utility of three novel insulin resistance-related lipid indexes for predicting type 2 diabetes mellitus among people with normal fasting glucose in rural China. J Diab. 2018. https://www.ncbi.nlm.nih.gov/pubmed/29322661.

45. Shin C, Abbott R, Lee H, Kim J, Kimm K. Prevalence and correlates of orthostatic hypotension in middle-aged men and women in Korea: the Korean health and genome study. J Hum Hypertens. 2004;18(10):717–23.

46. Baik I, Cho N, Kim S, Shin C. Dietary information improves cardiovascular disease risk prediction models. Eur J Clin Nutr. 2013;67(1):25.

47. Third Report of the National Cholesterol Education Program. (NCEP) expert panel on detection, evaluation, and treatment of high blood cholesterol in adults (adult treatment panel III) final report. Circulation. 2002;106(25): 3143–421.

48. Lee SY, Park HS, Kim DJ, Han JH, Kim SM, Cho GJ, Kim DY, Kwon HS, Kim SR, Lee CB. Appropriate waist circumference cutoff points for central obesity in Korean adults. Diabetes Res Clin Pract. 2007;75(1):72–80.

Short stature as a presenting symptom of attenuated Mucopolysaccharidosis type I: case report and clinical insights

Ana Maria Martins[1], Kristin Lindstrom[2], Sandra Obikawa Kyosen[1], Maria Veronica Munoz-Rojas[3], Nathan Thibault[3] and Lynda E. Polgreen[4*]

Abstract

Background: Mucopolysaccharidosis type I (MPS I) results in significant disease burden and early treatment is important for optimal outcomes. Recognition of short stature and growth failure as symptoms of MPS I among pediatric endocrinologists may lead to earlier diagnosis and treatment.

Case presentation: A male patient first began experiencing hip pain at 5 years of age and was referred to an endocrinologist for short stature at age 7. Clinical history included recurrent respiratory infections, sleep apnea, moderate joint contractures, mild facial dysmorphic features, scoliosis, and umbilical hernia. Height was more than -2 SD below the median at all time points. Growth velocity was below the 3rd percentile. Treatment for short stature included leuprolide acetate and recombinant human growth hormone. The patient was diagnosed with MPS I and began enzyme replacement therapy with laronidase at age 18.

Conclusions: The case study patient had many symptoms of MPS I yet remained undiagnosed for 11 years after presenting with short stature. The appropriate path to MPS I diagnosis when patients present with short stature and/or growth failure plus one or more of the common signs of attenuated disease is described. Improved awareness regarding association of short stature and growth failure with attenuated MPS I is needed since early identification and treatment significantly decreases disease burden.

Keywords: MPS I diagnosis, MPS I signs and symptoms, Growth delay, Physician awareness, Early diagnosis, Short stature

Background

Mucopolysaccharidosis type I (MPS I) is a life-threatening, autosomal recessive disease caused by deficiency of α-L-iduronidase (IDUA), a lysosomal enzyme responsible for metabolizing the glycosaminoglycans (GAGs) dermatan and heparan sulfate [1]. MPS I has an estimated incidence of 1/100,000 live births with a spectrum of phenotypes that range from severe (Hurler syndrome) to attenuated (Hurler-Scheie and Scheie syndromes) disease, depending on neurocognitive involvement and the rate of disease progression [2–4].

MPS I results in significant disease burden, disability, and premature death from respiratory and cardiac disease if left untreated, as well as neurodegeneration in the severe phenotype [2]. Treatment options include enzyme replacement with laronidase (recombinant human IDUA; Aldurazyme®) for patients with attenuated MPS I [5–8] and hematopoietic stem cell transplantation (HSCT), with or without laronidase, for patients with severe MPS I [9–13]. Treatment outcomes depend on phenotype and age at initiation of treatment [6, 14, 15]. Early treatment, prior to irreversible damage, can delay, stabilize, or prevent disease, and is associated with substantially improved patient outcomes [5, 6, 10, 16–22]. Unfortunately, there may be considerable delays in the diagnosis of MPS I, especially for patients with attenuated disease [16, 23–25]. In a study of the diagnostic

* Correspondence: lpolgreen@labiomed.org
[4]Los Angeles Biomedical Research Institute at Harbor-UCLA Medical Center, 1124 West Carson Street, Liu Research Building, Torrance, CA 90502, USA
Full list of author information is available at the end of the article

history of MPS I patients, approximately 20% of a population of 60 patients with attenuated MPS I had delays of 5 years or longer in diagnosis, and consulted between 4 and 5 specialists before receiving an MPS I diagnosis [25]. Similarly, for 18 patients with MPS I (13 of whom had attenuated disease) whose symptoms were noted at 18 months, the mean age at biochemical diagnosis was 75 months [26]. While pilot programs for MPS I NBS are in progress around the world [27], they are not universally available, and diagnostic delay persists. There has been no significant improvement in reducing the delay in diagnosis of MPS I as of 2017 [28]. Thus, it remains likely that children with undiagnosed MPS I will be referred to specialists, including endocrinologists, for their care, and awareness of the early clinical signs and symptoms remains important.

Short stature and skeletal sequelae known as dysostosis multiplex are key features among patients with MPS I [15, 24, 29–31], but MPS may be under recognized in patients presenting with short stature, particularly in patients with attenuated disease. Regardless of age and gender, children with MPS have severely disordered growth with percentile values for both longitudinal and transversal parameters (e.g., body length, trunk length, lower extremity length, shoulder breadth, and hip breadth) much lower than reference chart norms [32, 33].

Children with short stature (height less than 2 standard deviations below the mean, i.e., near the third percentile) and/or growth failure (growth rate below age-appropriate growth velocity) are often referred to pediatric endocrinologists [34, 35]. While there are multiple monogenic causes of short stature [35], attenuated MPS I should be considered in the differential diagnosis of patients with growth retardation in conjunction with any of the signs and symptoms of MPS I (Table 1), joint contractures, (particularly of hands, with claw hand deformity, although other joints can be affected), carpal tunnel syndrome (with

Table 1 Common presenting/early symptoms in patients with attenuated MPS I [24, 51]

- Growth delay (normal birth weight, but growth failure or short stature)
- Joint contractures (primarily in hands/claw hand deformity), joint pain and stiffness, restricted mobility
- Carpal tunnel syndrome (trigger digits)
- Recurrent hernias (umbilical and/or inguinal)
- Corneal clouding
- Hepatosplenomegaly
- Skeletal abnormalities/dysostosis multiplex (e.g., kyphosis, scoliosis, hip dysplasia, flattened vertebral bodies, oar-shaped ribs, short thickened clavicles, bullet-shaped phalanges, dysplastic femoral heads, flattened acetabula, coxa valga and genu valgum deformities)
- Ear/nose/throat symptoms (recurrent ear infections, noisy breathing, sleep apnea, enlarged tongue, hearing loss)
- Heart murmur (valve abnormalities)
- Surgical history of multiple hernia repairs, PE tubes, tonsillectomy, adenoidectomy

All symptoms may not be present in the same patient, but are usually progressive. See Fig. 2 for the path to diagnosis

trigger digits), umbilical and inguinal hernias, corneal clouding, hepatosplenomegaly, frequent respiratory infections, sleep apnea, cardiac valve abnormalities, and extensive surgical history. The constellation of radiologic abnormalities of ribs, extremities and spine known as dysostosis multiplex are more pronounced in severe MPS I but can develop in patients with attenuated disease at a later age. However, even patients with severe MPS I are still misdiagnosed and treated for other disorders, such as rickets [36], while patients with attenuated disease can go undiagnosed or misdiagnosed [37, 38].

A real-world case report is presented to highlight the existence of undiagnosed MPS I patients in pediatric endocrinology clinics, and describe the appropriate path to MPS I diagnosis when patients present with short stature and/or growth failure plus one or more of the common signs of attenuated disease as described in Table 1 and Fig. 3.

Case presentation

A male patient first began experiencing hip pain at 5 years of age and was diagnosed with bilateral Legg-Calve-Perthes disease by an orthopedic surgeon (see Table 2 Timeline). The patient was not tested for juvenile idiopathic arthritis. The patient experienced recurrent upper airway tract infections during childhood and was hospitalized multiple times between 5 and 7 years of age for wheezing. He was first seen by a pediatric endocrinologist at 7 years of age due to his short stature, was treated with leuprolide acetate (3.75 mg/month) between the ages of 13 and 16 years, and recombinant human growth hormone (0.1UI/kg/day), although the patient was not labeled as growth hormone deficient (GHD), between 14 and 18 years of age. Longitudinal growth curves and growth velocity for the patient between the ages of 10 and 21 are shown in Figs. 1 and 2. Height was more than − 2 SD below the median at all time points. Growth velocity was below the 3rd percentile prior to starting growth hormone. Final height of 159 cm was reached at 20 years of age.

The patient experienced sleep apnea throughout his teenage years, and at 17 years 9 months of age was referred to a metabolic disease center by a pneumologist (pulmonologist) who had seen the patient and suspected MPS. Upon examination, the patient was found to have moderate joint contractures, mild facial dysmorphic features (coarsening of features), scoliosis, and an umbilical hernia. His height at examination was 154 cm, with a z-score of − 2.94. Weight was 43.7 kg, and head circumference was 56.5 cm. Alpha-iduronidase activity on dried blood spot testing was 0.62 μmol/L/h (normal reference range 2.5–16.7), and genotype analysis revealed 2 pathogenic *IDUA* missense variants, c.1148G > A (p.R383H) and c.1598C > G (p.P533R), confirming the

Table 2 Timeline of assessments, diagnoses and treatment

Patient age	Symptom(s)	Assessments/diagnoses	Treatment(s)
5–7 years	Hip pain, recurrent respiratory infections	Orthopedist assessment and diagnosis of bilateral Legg-Calve-Perthes disease	unknown
7–18 years	Short stature: see Figs. 1 and 2	Pediatric endocrinologist assessment	Leuprolide acetate (3.75 mg/month) ages 13–16 Growth hormone (0.1UI/kg/day) ages 14–18
18 years	Short stature, moderate joint contractures, mild facial dysmorphic features (coarsening of features), scoliosis, and an umbilical hernia	Referred to metabolic disease center by treating pulmonologist. enzyme activity screening for MPS I positive; genetic analysis positive for MPS I	Enzyme replacement therapy with laronidase (weekly 0.58 mg/kg infusions) initiated

diagnosis of MPS I. The patient began ERT with laronidase (0.58 mg/kg/week) at age 18.

Discussion and conclusions

The case study demonstrates that endocrinologists may not consider MPS I in cases of short stature, even when there are signs and symptoms suggestive of MPS I. Red-flag signs and symptoms for attenuated MPS I (Table 1) exist in the absence of parameters indicating juvenile idiopathic arthritis [39, 40]. The case presentation highlights the diagnostic journey of a patient with attenuated MPS I and short stature followed for over 10 years in a pediatric endocrinology clinic. A strength of this case is the duration of care and longitudinal growth data, although in some instances, assessments

and clinical management information were unavailable. This patient had many of the signs and symptoms of attenuated MPS I, yet was not diagnosed until nearly 11 years after presenting to the pediatric endocrinologist with short stature. While not all of the signs listed in Table 1 may be apparent at the initial patient presentation to the endocrinologist, they are likely to develop over time when untreated, or be documented in patient clinical records and history. It is important to note that assessment of bone age in children with growth delay is typically done with an X-ray of the left hand and wrist; thus, pediatric endocrinologists are ideally situated to identify early phalangeal abnormalities (i.e., bullet shaped phalanges) typical of MPS I. A path to MPS I diagnosis when indicating signs are present is shown in Fig. 3.

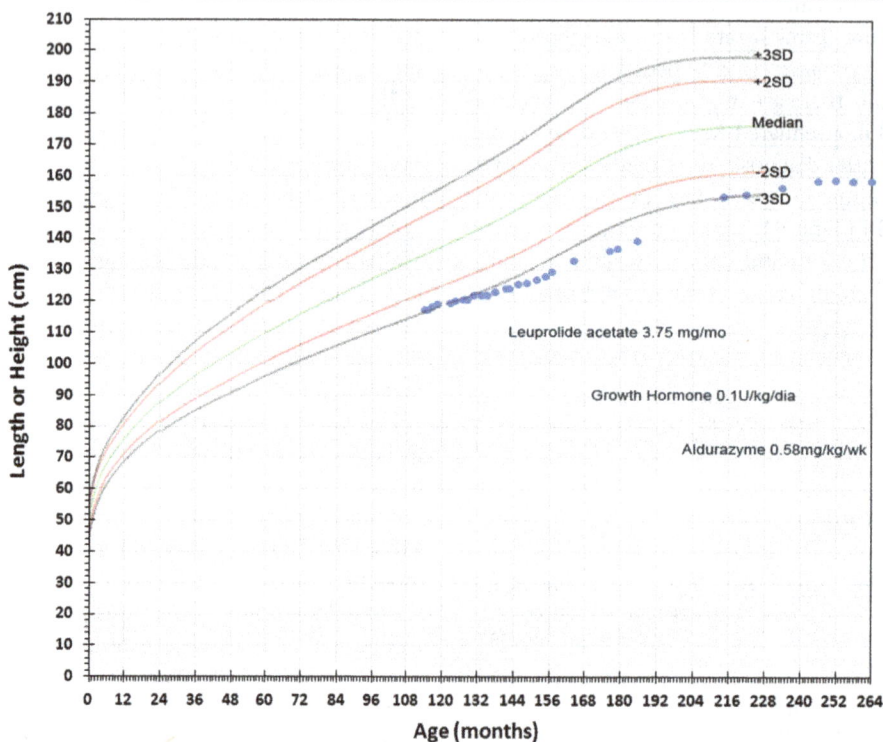

Fig. 1 Longitudinal Growth for Patient with Attenuated MPS I from Case Study. Height of case study patient by age is shown by the blue markers with timing and duration of leuprolide acetate, growth hormone and laronidase treatments indicated. WHO Child Growth Standards are indicated

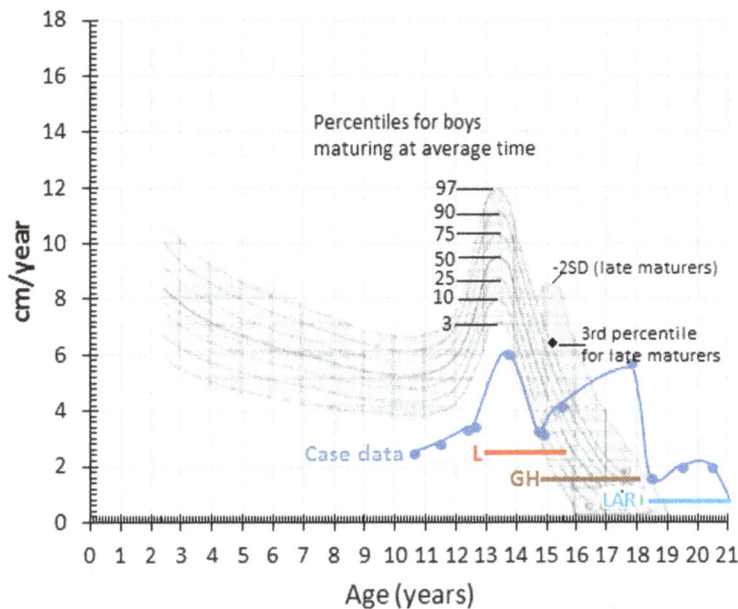

Fig. 2 Growth Velocity of Patient with Attenuated MPS I from Case Study Relative to Growth Standards. Growth velocity by age is shown by the blue markers with timing and duration of leuprolide acetate (L), growth hormone (GH) and laronidase (LAR) treatments indicated. Treatment doses are the same as shown in Fig. 1. Percentiles for boys maturing at average time or for late maturers are shown as adapted from Tanner JM and Davies PS. Clinical longitudinal standards for height and height velocity for North American children [50]

There is considerable overlap of presenting symptoms among the MPS disorders, therefore, screening identified in Fig. 3 should take into account other MPS disorders where short stature is common. Upon consideration of an MPS disorder, a urine GAG (uGAG) test (that may include analyses to determine abnormal GAG pattern,

such as electrophoresis or tandem mass spectrometry) can determine the presence of lysosomal storage material. Results of the uGAG test as indicated in Fig. 3 can warrant referral to a geneticist or metabolic disease specialist, who can initiate appropriate enzyme and genetic testing to confirm or rule out an MPS diagnosis. Several

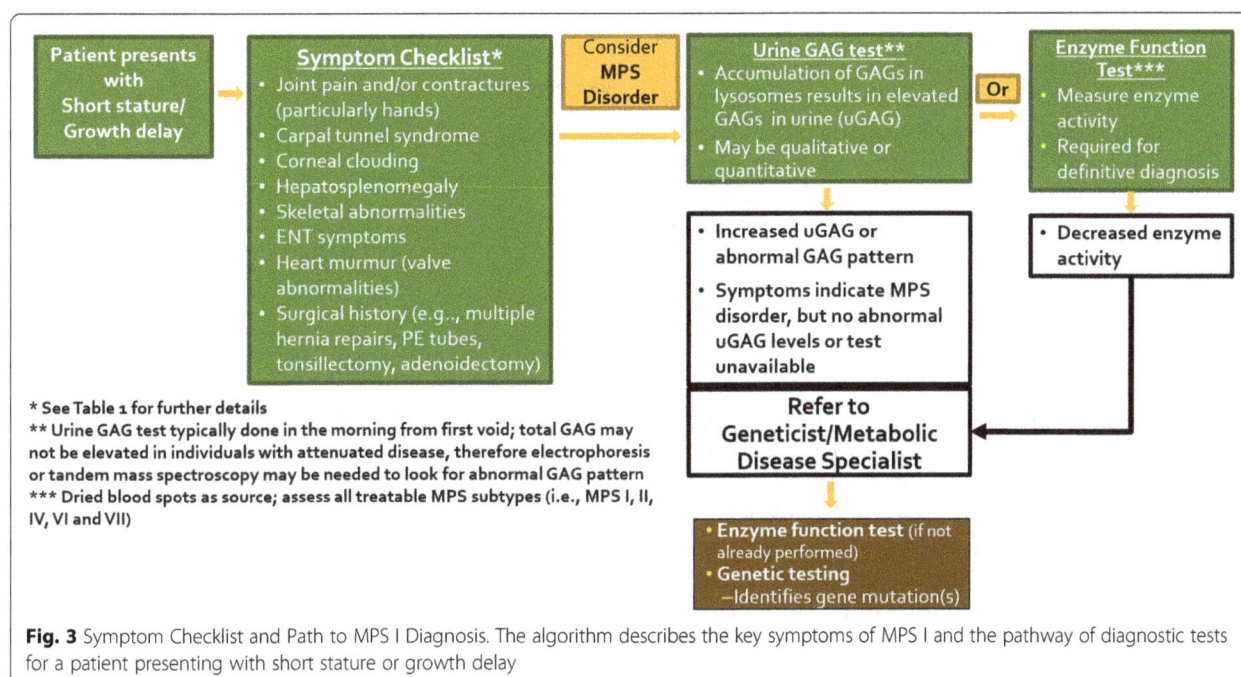

Fig. 3 Symptom Checklist and Path to MPS I Diagnosis. The algorithm describes the key symptoms of MPS I and the pathway of diagnostic tests for a patient presenting with short stature or growth delay

barriers can exist for appropriate referrals of pediatric patients to metabolic specialists and geneticists, including cost and insurance, wait times, and location [41, 42] and improvements in accessibility for lysosomal storage disease assays may be needed [43].

Studies suggest that increased awareness for endocrinologists may be helpful to highlight the possibility of attenuated MPS in patients presenting with short stature [37, 38]. In a retrospective assessment of outpatient medical records of patients with short stature of unknown etiology in a pediatric endocrinology service, follow-up screening of 23 patients revealed previously undiagnosed MPS in 3 patients [37]. In another study, 135 physicians with expertise in pediatrics and endocrinology from seven countries (United States, Canada, Italy, Germany, Spain, Mexico, and Brazil) participated in a blinded review of cases for pediatric or adolescent patients with MPS I [38]. Depending on the case reviewed, only 22% to 58% of physicians took steps towards a correct MPS I diagnosis. Juvenile idiopathic arthritis was the most common incorrect diagnosis made. A key distinction in the diagnosis of MPS I is the absence of biochemical parameters diagnostic of juvenile idiopathic arthritis. While algorithms exist that include MPS I in the differential diagnosis of juvenile arthritis for pediatric rheumatologists [39, 40], growth specialists and endocrinologists may be among the physicians encountering individuals with undiagnosed MPS disorders, and similar guidelines could prove helpful for recognizing the red-flag signs and symptoms of MPS I and other MPS disorders. A proposed algorithm that includes short stature as a presenting sign in attenuated MPS I has recently been published [44].

The mechanism behind short stature in patients with MPS I is not completely known, but is most likely a secondary characteristic resulting from structural, metabolic, and endocrine abnormalities. Structurally, skeletal abnormalities limit longitudinal growth and final height, but alone cannot explain short stature in patients with MPS I. Pituitary and thyroid dysfunction, GHD, precocious puberty, and pubertal failure have all been reported in patients with MPS I [32, 45]. However, it is important to note that in the absence of GHD, hGH treatment of patients with MPS has not been proven to be effective.

Enzyme replacement therapy with laronidase has resulted in increased growth velocity in pediatric patients [46], particularly in prepubescent children with MPS I [20]. In sibling studies, improved musculoskeletal outcomes were noted in the younger sibling who began ERT in infancy [5, 18, 19]. Retrospective studies indicate that early initiation of laronidase can stabilize existing skeletal disease, and prevent or delay clinical manifestations if initiated prior to symptom onset [5, 19–22].

Patients with attenuated MPS I that were less than 10 years of age at treatment initiation remained closer to age-matched norms for several disease parameters, including height, compared with patients that were ≥ 10 years of age at the start of treatment [22]. There is disagreement regarding the benefits of administration of recombinant human growth hormone, and this is an area of active study [47].

In summary, short stature is a common presenting sign of attenuated MPS I, and may be the symptom that drives clinical care in these patients [36, 48, 49]. Since pediatric endocrinologists are typically the first physician to whom patients with short stature are referred [35], they can play a pivotal role in improving the health and quality of life of patients with attenuated MPS I. Early diagnosis of MPS I and initiation of treatment is critically important as it improves patient outcomes and reduces disease burden [5, 6, 8, 19, 22]. MPS I should be considered in any patient with short stature and/or growth failure plus one or more of the common signs described in Table 1. The path to diagnosis (Fig. 2) includes urine GAG test, referral to geneticist (or metabolic disease specialist), and appropriate enzyme and genetic testing. Improving the ability of pediatric endocrinologists to recognize the disease manifestations of MPS I can lead to earlier diagnosis and treatment for individuals with MPS I.

Abbreviations
GAG: Glycosaminoglycans; GHD: Growth hormone deficient; hGH: Human growth hormone; HSCT: Hematopoeitic stem cell transplant; IDUA: α-L-iduronidase; MPS I: Mucopolysaccharidosis type I; uGAG: Urinary glycosaminoglycans

Acknowledgments
The authors thank the individual and their family whose case was presented in this manuscript.

Funding
Funding was provided by Sanofi Genzyme. Patrice C. Ferriola (KZE PharmAssociates, LLC) provided assistance in preparation of the manuscript and was funded by Sanofi Genzyme.

Authors' contributions
AMM and SK provided patient data; LP, KL, AMM and SK were involved in assessing and interpreting data; MVMR and NT initiated the study, and all authors participated in manuscript development and writing. All authors read and approved the final manuscript.

Author's information
Not applicable.

Competing interests

- LP received research support from Sanofi Genzyme, Shire, and Horizon. Received research grants from the MPS1 Foundation and NIH.
- AMM received grants and speaker honoraria from Sanofi Genzyme.
- SK received Travel Grants from Sanofi Genzyme
- MVMR and NT are employees of Sanofi Genzyme
- KL received fees from Biomarin and Alexion for lectures

Author details

¹Universidade Federal de São Paulo, São Paulo, Brazil. ²Phoenix Children's Hospital, Phoenix, AZ, USA. ³Sanofi Genzyme, Cambridge, MA, USA. ⁴Los Angeles Biomedical Research Institute at Harbor-UCLA Medical Center, 1124 West Carson Street, Liu Research Building, Torrance, CA 90502, USA.

References

1. Muenzer J. Overview of the mucopolysaccharidoses. Rheumatology (Oxford). 2012;50(Suppl 5):v4–12.
2. Moore D, Connock MJ, Wraith E, Lavery C. The prevalence of and survival in Mucopolysaccharidosis I: hurler, hurler-Scheie and Scheie syndromes in the UK. Orphanet J Rare Dis. 2008;3:24–30.
3. Neufeld E, Muenzer J. The mucopolysaccharidoses. In: Schriver C, Beaudet A, Sly W, Valle DCB, Kinzler K, Vogelstein B, editors. The metabolic and molecular basis of inherited disease. New York: McGraw Hill; 2001. p. 3421–52.
4. Thomas JA, Beck M, Clarke JT, Cox GF. Childhood onset of Scheie syndrome, the attenuated form of mucopolysaccharidosis I. J Inherit Metab Dis. 2010;33(4):421–7.
5. Al-Sannaa NA, Bay L, Barbouth DS, Benhayoun Y, Goizet C, Guelbert N, et al. Early treatment with laronidase improves clinical outcomes in patients with attenuated MPS I: a retrospective case series analysis of nine sibships. Orphanet J Rare Dis. 2015;10(1):131–9.
6. Muenzer J. Early initiation of enzyme replacement therapy for the mucopolysaccharidoses. Mol Genet Metab. 2014;111(2):63–72.
7. Tolar J, Orchard PJ. Alpha-L-iduronidase therapy for mucopolysaccharidosis type I. Biologics. 2008;2(4):743–51.
8. Clarke LA, Wraith JE, Beck M, Kolodny EH, Pastores GM, Muenzer J, et al. Long-term efficacy and safety of laronidase in the treatment of mucopolysaccharidosis I. Pediatrics. 2009;123(1):229–40.
9. Aldenhoven M, Jones SA, Bonney D, Borrill RE, Coussons M, Mercer J, et al. Hematopoietic cell transplantation for mucopolysaccharidosis patients is safe and effective: results after implementation of international guidelines. Biol Blood Marrow Transplant. 2015;21(6):1106–9.
10. Aldenhoven M, Wynn RF, Orchard PJ, O'Meara A, Veys P, Fischer A, et al. Long-term outcome of hurler syndrome patients after hematopoietic cell transplantation: an international multicenter study. Blood. 2015;125(13):2164–72.
11. Grewal SS, Wynn R, Abdenur JE, Burton BK, Gharib M, Haase C, et al. Safety and efficacy of enzyme replacement therapy in combination with hematopoietic stem cell transplantation in hurler syndrome. Genet Med. 2005;7(2):143–6.
12. Yasuda E, Mackenzie W, Ruhnke K, Shimada T, Mason RW, Zustin J, et al. Molecular genetics and metabolism report long-term follow-up of post hematopoietic stem cell transplantation for hurler syndrome: clinical, biochemical, and pathological improvements. Mol Genet Metab Rep. 2015;2:65–76.
13. Eisengart JB, Rudser KD, Tolar J, Orchard PJ, Kivisto T, Ziegler RS, et al. Enzyme replacement is associated with better cognitive outcomes after transplant in hurler syndrome. J Pediatr. 2012;162(2):375–80 e1.
14. Giugliani R. Mucopolysacccharidoses: From understanding to treatment, a century of discoveries. Genet Mol Biol. 2012;35(4 (suppl)):924–31.
15. Muenzer J, Wraith JE, Clarke LA. Mucopolysaccharidosis I: management and treatment guidelines. Pediatrics. 2009;123(1):19–29.
16. D'Aco K, Underhill L, Rangachari L, Arn P, Cox GF, Giugliani R, et al. Diagnosis and treatment trends in mucopolysaccharidosis I: findings from the MPS I registry. Eur J Pediatr. 2012;171(6):911–9.
17. de Ru MH, Boelens JJ, Das AM, Jones SA, van der Lee JH, Mahlaoui N, et al. Enzyme replacement therapy and/or hematopoietic stem cell transplantation at diagnosis in patients with mucopolysaccharidosis type I: results of a European consensus procedure. Orphanet J Rare Dis. 2011;6:55–62.
18. Gabrielli O, Clarke LA, Bruni S, Coppa GV. Enzyme-replacement therapy in a 5-month-old boy with attenuated presymptomatic MPS I: 5-year follow-up. Pediatrics. 2009;125(1):e183–7.
19. Gabrielli O, Clarke LA, Ficcadenti A, Santoro L, Zampini L, Volpi N, et al. 12 year follow up of enzyme-replacement therapy in two siblings with attenuated mucopolysaccharidosis I: the important role of early treatment. BMC Med Genet. 2016;17(1):19.
20. Sifuentes M, Doroshow R, Hoft R, Mason G, Walot I, Diament M, et al. A follow-up study of MPS I patients treated with laronidase enzyme replacement therapy for 6 years. Mol Genet Metab. 2007;90(2):171–80.
21. Laraway S, Breen C, Mercer J, Jones S, Wraith JE. Does early use of enzyme replacement therapy alter the natural history of mucopolysaccharidosis I? Experience in three siblings. Mol Genet Metab. 2013;109(3):315–6.
22. Laraway S, Mercer J, Jameson E, Ashworth J, HensmanDip P, Jones SA. Outcomes of long-term treatment with Laronidase in patients with Mucopolysaccharidosis type I. J Pediatr. 2016;178:219–26 e1.
23. Beck M, Arn P, Giugliani R, Muenzer J, Okuyama T, Taylor J, et al. The natural history of MPS I: global perspectives from the MPS I registry. Genet Med. 2014;16(10):759–65.
24. Vijay S, Wraith JE. Clinical presentation and follow-up of patients with the attenuated phenotype of mucopolysaccharidosis type I. Acta Paediatr. 2005;94(7):872–7.
25. Bruni S, Lavery C, Broomfield A. The diagnostic journey of patients with mucopolysaccharidosis I: a real-world survey of patient and physician experiences. Mol Genet Metab Rep. 2016;8:67–73.
26. Vieira T, Schwartz I, Munoz V, Pinto L, Steiner C, Ribeiro M, et al. Mucopolysaccharidoses in Brazil: what happens from birth to biochemical diagnosis? Am J Med Genet A. 2008;146A(13):1741–7.
27. Parini R, Broomfield A, Cleary MA, De Meirleir L, Di Rocco M, Fathalla WM, et al. International working group identifies need for newborn screening for mucopolysaccharidosis type I but states that existing hurdles must be overcome. Acta Paediatr. 2018.
28. Kuiper GA, Meijer OLM, Langereis EJ, Wijburg FA. Failure to shorten the diagnostic delay in two ultra-orphan diseases (mucopolysaccharidosis types I and III): potential causes and implications. Orphanet J Rare Dis. 2018;13(1):2.
29. Morishita K, Petty RE. Musculoskeletal manifestations of mucopolysaccharidoses. Rheumatology (Oxford). 2011;50(Suppl 5):v19–25.
30. Rozdzynska-Swiatkowska A, Jurecka A, Cieslik J, Tylki-Szymanska A. Growth patterns in children with mucopolysaccharidosis I and II. World J Pediatr. 2015;11(3):226–31.
31. Tylki-Szymanska A, Rozdzynska A, Jurecka A, Marucha J, Czartoryska B. Anthropometric data of 14 patients with mucopolysaccharidosis I: retrospective analysis and efficacy of recombinant human alpha-L-iduronidase (laronidase). Mol Genet Metab. 2009;99(1):10–7.
32. Polgreen LE, Miller BS. Growth patterns and the use of growth hormone in the mucopolysaccharidoses. J Pediatr Rehabil Med. 2010;3(1):25–38.
33. Rogers DG, Nasomyont N. Growth hormone treatment in a patient with hurler-Scheie syndrome. J Pediatr Endocrinol Metab. 2014;27(9–10):957–60.
34. Barstow C, Rerucha C. Evaluation of short and tall stature in children. Am Fam Physician. 2015;92(1):43–50.
35. Wit JM, Oostdijk W, Losekoot M, van Duyvenvoorde HA, Ruivenkamp CA, Kant SG. Mechanisms In Endocrinology: novel genetic causes of short stature. Eur J Endocrinol. 2016;174(4):R145–73.
36. Ayuk A, Obu H, Ughasoro M, Ibeziako N. Unresolving short stature in a possible case of mucopolysccharidosis. Ann Med Health Sci Res. 2014;4(Suppl 1):S38–42.
37. Franco J, Espinosa G, Garcia F. Screening for mucopolysaccaridoses in patients with short stature of unknown etiology. MGM. 2016;117:S47.
38. Thibault N, Cabral JM, Munoz Rojas MV, Bruni S. Awareness of MPS I Among Pediatric Endocrinologists. 14th International Sumposium on MPS and Rlated Disorders; July14–17; Bonn, Germany 2016.

39. Cimaz R, Coppa GV, Kone-Paut I, Link B, Pastores GM, Elorduy MR, et al. Joint contractures in the absence of inflammation may indicate mucopolysaccharidosis. Pediatr Rheumatol Online J. 2009;7:18–25.

40. Cimaz R, Vijay S, Haase C, Coppa GV, Bruni S, Wraith E, et al. Attenuated type I mucopolysaccharidosis in the differential diagnosis of juvenile idiopathic arthritis: a series of 13 patients with Scheie syndrome. Clin Exp Rheumatol. 2006;24(2):196–202.

41. Delikurt T, Williamson GR, Anastasiadou V, Skirton H. A systematic review of factors that act as barriers to patient referral to genetic services. Eur J Hum Genet. 2015;23(6):739–45.

42. Beene-Harris RY, Wang C, Bach JV. Barriers to access: results from focus groups to identify genetic service needs in the community. Community Genet. 2007;10(1):10–8.

43. Verma J, Thomas DC, Kasper DC, Sharma S, Puri RD, Bijarnia-Mahay S, et al. Inherited Metabolic Disorders: Efficacy of Enzyme Assays on Dried Blood Spots for the Diagnosis of Lysosomal Storage Disorders. JIMD Rep. 2016.

44. Tylki-Szymanska A, De Meirleir L, Di Rocco M, Fathalla WM, Guffon N, Lampe C, et al. Easy-to-use algorithm would provide faster diagnoses for mucopolysaccharidosis type I and enable patients to receive earlier treatment. Acta Paediatr. 2018;107(8):1402–8.

45. Gardner CJ, Robinson N, Meadows T, Wynn R, Will A, Mercer J, et al. Growth, final height and endocrine sequelae in a UK population of patients with hurler syndrome (MPS1H). J Inherit Metab Dis. 2011;34(2):489–97.

46. Kakkis ED, Muenzer J, Tiller GE, Waber L, Belmont J, Passage M, et al. Enzyme-replacement therapy in mucopolysaccharidosis I. N Engl J Med. 2001;344(3):182–8.

47. Polgreen LE, Thomas W, Orchard PJ, Whitley CB, Miller BS. Effect of recombinant human growth hormone on changes in height, bone mineral density, and body composition over 1-2 years in children with hurler or hunter syndrome. Mol Genet Metab. 2014;111(2):101–6.

48. Clarke LA, Hollak CE. The clinical spectrum and pathophysiology of skeletal complications in lysosomal storage disorders. Best Pract Res Clin Endocrinol Metab. 2015;29(2):219–35.

49. Gadve SS, Sarma D, Saikia UK. Short stature with umbilical hernia - not always due to cretinism: a report of two cases. Indian J Endocrinol Metab. 2012;16(3):453–6.

50. Tanner JM, Davies PS. Clinical longitudinal standards for height and height velocity for north American children. J Pediatr. 1985;107(3):317–29.

51. Pastores GM, Arn P, Beck M, Clarke JT, Guffon N, Kaplan P, et al. The MPS I registry: design, methodology, and early findings of a global disease registry for monitoring patients with Mucopolysaccharidosis type I. Mol Genet Metab. 2007;91(1):37–47.

Permissions

List of Contributors

Wimonrut Boonsatean
Faculty of Nursing Science, Rangsit University, Pathum Thani 12000, Thailand

Anna Carlsson, Irena Dychawy Rosner and Margareta Östman
Faculty of Health and Society, Malmö University, SE 205 06 Malmö, Sweden

Danting Li, Hongmei Xue, Jieyi Zhang, Mengxue Chen and Guo Cheng
Department of Nutrition, Food Safety and Toxicology, West China School of Public Health, Sichuan University, No.16, Section 3, Renmin Nan Road, Chengdu 610041, Sichuan, China

Haoche Wei
Center of Growth, Metabolism and Aging, Collage of Life Sciences, Sichuan University, Chengdu, China

Yunhui Gong
Department of Obstetrics and Gynecology, West China Second University Hospital, Sichuan University, Chengdu, China

Rıfat Emral
Department of Endocrinology and Metabolic Diseases, Ankara University, Faculty of Medicine, İbn-i Sina Hospital, Academic Region M1/09, Samanpazarı, 06100 Ankara, Turkey

Tamer Tetiker
Faculty of Medicine, Department of Endocrinology and Metabolic Diseases, Çukurova University, Adana, Turkey

Ibrahim Sahin
Endocrinology and Metabolism Department, Inonu University School of Medicine, Malatya, Turkey

Ramazan Sari
Division of Endocrinology and Metabolism, School of Medicine, Akdeniz University, Antalya, Turkey

Ahmet Kaya
Division of Endocrinology and Metabolism, Meram School of Medicine, Necmettin Erbakan University, Konya, Turkey

İlhan Yetkin
Division of Endocrinology and Metabolism, School of Medicine, Gazi University, Ankara, Turkey

Sefika Uslu Cil
Medical Department, Novo Nordisk, Istanbul, Turkey

Neslihan Başcıl Tütüncü
Division of Endocrinology and Metabolism, School of Medicine, Baskent University, Ankara, Turkey

Tao Tao, Peihong Wu and Yuying Wang
Department of Endocrinology and Metabolism, Renji Hospital, School of Medicine, Shanghai Jiaotong University, 160 Pujian Road, Shanghai 200127, China

Wei Liu
Department of Endocrinology and Metabolism, Renji Hospital, School of Medicine, Shanghai Jiaotong University, 160 Pujian Road, Shanghai 200127, China Shanghai Key laboratory for Assisted Reproduction and Reproductive Genetics, Center for Reproductive Medicine, Renji Hospital, School of Medicine, Shanghai Jiaotong University, 160 Pujian Road, Shanghai 200127, China

Khadijeh Nasri, Mehri Jamilian and Elham Rahmani
Endocrinology and Metabolism Research Center, Arak University of Medical Sciences, Arak, Iran

Fereshteh Bahmani and Zatollah Asemi
Research Center for Biochemistry and Nutrition in Metabolic Diseases, Kashan University of Medical Sciences, Kashan, IR, Iran

Maryam Tajabadi-Ebrahimi
Faculty member of Science department, Science Faculty, Islamic Azad University, Tehran Central Branch, Tehran, Iran

Klemens Wallner, Isaac Awotwe and Christopher McCabe
Department of Emergency Medicine Research Group, Department of Emergency Medicine, University of Alberta, 8303 - 112 Street, Edmonton, AB T6G 2T4, Canada

Rene G. Pedroza and James M. Piret
Michael Smith Laboratories and Department of Chemical and Biological Engineering, University of British Columbia, 2185 East Mall, Vancouver, BC V6T 1Z4, Canada

Peter A. Senior
Clinical Islet Transplant Program, Alberta Diabetes Institute, University of Alberta, 2000 College Plaza, 8215 - 112 Street, Edmonton, AB T6G 2C8, Canada

Department of Medicine, University of Alberta, Edmonton, Canada

A. M. James Shapiro
Clinical Islet Transplant Program, Alberta Diabetes Institute, University of Alberta, 2000 College Plaza, 8215 - 112 Street, Edmonton, AB T6G 2C8, Canada
Department of Medicine, University of Alberta, Edmonton, Canada
Department of Surgery, University of Alberta, Edmonton, AB, Canada

Ji Yeon Shin, Tae Hwa Kim, Eun Heui Kim, Min Jin Lee, Jong Ho Kim, Yun Kyung Jeon, Sang Soo Kim and In Joo Kim
Department of Internal Medicine, Pusan National University College of Medicine, Busan 49241, South Korea

Bo Hyun Kim
Department of Internal Medicine, Pusan National University College of Medicine, Busan 49241, South Korea
Biomedical Research Institute, Pusan National University Hospital, Busan 49241, South Korea
Division of Endocrinology and Metabolism, Department of Internal Medicine, Pusan National University Hospital, 305 Gudeok-ro, Seo-gu, Busan 602-739, South Korea

Young Keum Kim
Department of Pathology, Pusan National University Hospital and Pusan National University School of Medicine, Busan 49241, South Korea

Khalid Al-Rubeaan, Yousuf Al Farsi, Hamid AlQumaidi, Basim M. Al-Malki, Khalid A. Naji and Khalid Al-Shehri
University Diabetes Center, College of Medicine, King Saud University, Riyadh, Riyadh 11415, Saudi Arabia

Nahla Bawazeer
Nutrition Department, University Diabetes Center, King Saud University, Riyadh, Saudi Arabia

Amira M. Youssef
Registry Department, University Diabetes Center, King Saud University, Riyadh, Saudi Arabia

Abdulrahman A. Al-Yahya and Fahd I. Al Rumaih
College of Medicine, King Saud University, Riyadh, Saudi Arabia

Karunee Kwanbunjan, Pornpimol Panprathip and Somchai Puduang
Department of Tropical Nutrition and Food Science, Faculty of Tropical Medicine, Mahidol University, Bangkok 10400, Thailand

Chanchira Phosat
Department of Nutrition, Faculty of Public Health, Mahidol University, Bangkok 10400, Thailand

Noppanath Chumpathat
Faculty of Nursing, Huachiew Chalermprakiet University, Samut Prakan 10540, Thailand

Naruemon Wechjakwen
Faculty of Public Health, Nakhonratchasima Rajabhat University, Nakhon Ratchasima 30000, Thailand

Ratchada Auyyuenyong
Department of Food Business and Nutrition, Faculty of Agriculture, Ubon Ratchathani Rajabhat University, Ubon Ratchathani 34000, Thailand

Ina Henkel and Florian J. Schweigert
Institute of Nutritional Science, University of Potsdam, 14558 Potsdam, Germany

J. Lawton, M. Blackburn and D. Rankin
Usher Institute of Population Health Sciences and Informatics, University of Edinburgh, Edinburgh, UK

J. Allen, M. Tauschmann and R. Hovorka
Wellcome Trust-MRC Institute of Metabolic Science, University of Cambridge, Cambridge, UK
Department of Paediatrics, University of Cambridge, Cambridge, UK

F. Campbell
Leeds Children's Hospital, Leeds, UK

D. Elleri
Royal Hospital for Sick Children, Edinburgh, UK

L. Leelarathna and H. Thabit
Manchester Diabetes Centre, Central Manchester University Hospitals NHS Foundation Trust, Manchester Academic Health Science Centre, Manchester, UK

Jiannong Jiang, Qiang Wang, Jun Zong and Leiyan Zhang
Department of Orthopedics, The Affiliated Yixing Hospital of Jiangsu University, Yixing 214200, China

Heping Zhu
Department of Orthopedics, The Affiliated Yixing Hospital of Jiangsu University, Yixing 214200, China
Department of Orthopedics, The Second Affiliated Hospital of Soochow University, Suzhou 215004, China

Youjia Xu
Department of Orthopedics, The Second Affiliated Hospital of Soochow University, Suzhou 215004, China

Liang Zhang
Department of Orthopedics, Northern Jiangsu People's Hospital, Yangzhou 225001, China

Tieliang Ma
Central Laboratory, The Affiliated Yixing Hospital of Jiangsu University, Yixing 214200, China

Jieun Jang, Sang Ah Lee and Young Choi
Department of Public Health, Graduate School, Yonsei University, Seoul, Republic of Korea
Institute of Health Services Research, Yonsei University, Seoul, Republic of Korea

Jaeyong Shin and Eun-Cheol Park
Institute of Health Services Research, Yonsei University, Seoul, Republic of Korea
Department of Preventive Medicine and Institute of Health Services Research, Yonsei University College of Medicine, 50 Yonsei-ro, Seodaemun-gu, Seoul 120-752, Republic of Korea

Youngsook Kim
Department of Anesthesia, Indiana University School of Medicine, Indianapolis 46202, USA

Jia Liu and Jiajun Zhao
Department of Endocrinology, Shandong Provincial Hospital Affiliated to Shandong University, Jinan, Shandong 250021, China
Shandong Clinical Medical Center of Endocrinology and Metabolism, Jinan, Shandong 250021, China
Institute of Endocrinology and Metabolism, Shandong Academy of Clinical Medicine, Jinan, Shandong 250021, China

Dongmei Zheng
Department of Endocrinology, Shandong Provincial Hospital Affiliated to Shandong University, Jinan, Shandong 250021, China
Shandong Clinical Medical Center of Endocrinology and Metabolism, Jinan, Shandong 250021, China
Institute of Endocrinology and Metabolism, Shandong Academy of Clinical Medicine, Jinan, Shandong 250021, China
Department of Endocrinology and Metabolism, Shandong Provincial Hospital Affiliated to Shandong University, Jingwu Road 324, Jinan, Shandong 250021, China

Ling Gao
Shandong Clinical Medical Center of Endocrinology and Metabolism, Jinan, Shandong 250021, China
Institute of Endocrinology and Metabolism, Shandong Academy of Clinical Medicine, Jinan, Shandong 250021, China

Qiang Li
Department of Endocrinology and Metabolism, the Second Affiliated Hospital of Harbin Medical University, Harbin, Heilongjiang 150086, China

Xulei Tang
Department of Endocrinology, the First Hospital of Lanzhou University, Lanzhou, Gansu 730000, China

Zuojie Luo
Department of Endocrinology, the First Affiliated Hospital of Guangxi University, Nanning, Guangxi 530021, China

Zhongshang Yuan
Department of Biostatistics, School of Public Health, Shandong University, Jinan, Shandong 250021, China

Stela Carpini, Sofia Helena Valente de Lemos-Marini and Gil Guerra-Junior
Department of Pediatrics, Faculty of Medical Sciences (FCM), State University of Campinas (Unicamp), São Paulo, Brazil

Annelise Barreto Carvalho
Post-Graduate Program in Child and Adolescent Health, FCM, Unicamp, São Paulo, Brazil

Andréa Trevas Maciel-Guerra
Department of Medical Genetics, FCM, Unicamp, Rua Tessalia Vieira de Camargo, 126, Campinas, SP 13083-887, Brazil

Daniel K. Langlois, William D. Schall and N. Bari Olivier
Department of Small Animal Clinical Sciences, College of Veterinary Medicine, Michigan State University, East Lansing, MI 48824, USA

Michele C. Fritz
Department of Small Animal Clinical Sciences, College of Veterinary Medicine, Michigan State University, East Lansing, MI 48824, USA
Present address: College of Human Medicine, Michigan State University, East Lansing, MI 48824, USA

Rebecca C. Smedley
Veterinary Diagnostic Laboratory, College of Veterinary Medicine, Michigan State University, East Lansing, MI 48824, USA

Paul G. Pearson
Pearson Pharma Partners, Inc., Los Angeles, California 91362, USA

Marc B. Bailie
Integrated Non-Clinical Development Solutions, Inc., Ann Arbor, MI 48103, USA

Stephen W. Hunt III
Millendo Therapeutics, Inc., Ann Arbor, MI 48104, USA

Peter H. Kann and Simona Bergmann
Division of Endocrinology and Diabetology, Philipp's University Marburg, D-35033 Marburg, Germany

Martin Bidlingmaier
Endocrine Laboratory, Medizinische Klinik und Poliklinik IV, Ludwig-Maximilians University, 80336 Munich, Germany

Christina Dimopoulou and Günter K. Stalla
Neuroendocrinology, Max-Planck-Institute for Psychiatry, 80804 Munich, Germany

Birgitte T. Pedersen
Epidemiology, Novo Nordisk A/S, 2860 Søborg, Denmark

Matthias M. Weber
Endocrinology and Metabolism, Johannes Gutenberg University Hospital, 55131 Mainz, Germany

Stefanie Meckes-Ferber
Clinical, Medical and Regulatory Department, Novo Nordisk Pharma GmbH, 55127 Mainz, Germany

Nikolai Paul Pace and Alex Felice
Centre for Molecular Medicine and Biobanking, University of Malta, Msida, Malta

Johann Craus
Department of Obstetrics and Gynaecology, University of Malta, Msida, Malta

Josanne Vassallo
Department of Medicine, University of Malta, Msida, Malta

Haileab Fekadu Wolde, Asrat Atsedeweyen, Addisu Jember, Tadesse Awoke, Malede Mequanent and Adino Tesfahun Tsegaye
Department of Epidemiology and Biostatistics, Institute of Public Health, College of Medicine and Health Sciences, University of Gondar, Gondar, Ethiopia

Shitaye Alemu
Department of Internal Medicine, School of Medicine, College of Medicine and Health Sciences, University of Gondar, Gondar, Ethiopia

Masoud Behzadifar
Social Determinants of Health Research Center, Lorestan University of Medical Sciences, Khorramabad, Iran

Rahim Sohrabi
Iranian Social Security Organization, Zanjan Province Health Administration, Zanjan, Iran.

Roghayeh Mohammadibakhsh, Sharare Taheri Moghadam and Masood Taheri Mirghaedm
Department of Health Services Management, School of Health Management and Information Sciences, Iran University of Medical Sciences, Tehran, Iran

Morteza Salemi
Social Determinants in Health Promotion Research Center, Hormozgan University of Medical Sciences, Bandar Abbas, Iran

Meysam Behzadifar
Health Management and Economics Research Center, Iran University of Medical Sciences, Tehran, Iran

Hamid Reza Baradaran
Endocrine Research Center Institute of Endocrinology and Metabolism, Iran University of Medical Sciences, Tehran, Iran

Nicola Luigi Bragazzi
School of Public Health, Department of Health Sciences (DISSAL), University of Genoa, Genoa, Italy

Zhigang Wu
Department of Andrology, The First Affiliated Hospital of Wenzhou Medical University, Wenzhou 325000, Zhejiang Province, China

Hongwei Wang, Fubiao Ni, Jiao Luo and Bicheng Chen
Hepatobiliary and pancreatic surgery laboratory, The First Affiliated Hospital of Wenzhou Medical University, Wenzhou 325000, Zhejiang Province, China

Ziqiang Xu and Yong Cai
Department of Transplantation, The First Affiliated Hospital of Wenzhou Medical University, Wenzhou 325000, Zhejiang Province, China

Xuan Jiang and Hongxing Fu
School of Pharmacy, Wenzhou Medical University, Wenzhou 325000, Zhejiang Province, China

Chengyang Liu
Department of Surgery, Perelman School of Medicine at the University of Pennsylvania, Philadelphia, PA 19104-5160, USA

Zhixian Yu and Wenwei Chen
Department of Urology, the First Affiliated Hospital of Wenzhou Medical University, Wenzhou 325000, Zhejiang Province, China

Laura L. Jensen
Department of Family Medicine, Ohio University
Heritage College of Osteopathic Medicine, Athens,
OH 45701, USA

Elizabeth A. Beverly
Department of Family Medicine, Ohio University
Heritage College of Osteopathic Medicine, Athens,
OH 45701, USA
The Diabetes Institute, Ohio University, Athens, OH
45701, USA

Jane Hamel-Lambert
Department of Pediatric Psychology, Nationwide
Children's Hospital, Westerville, OH 43081, USA
Department of Clinical Pediatrics, Ohio State
University, Columbus, OH 43210, USA

Sue Meeks
Community Service Programs, Ohio University
Heritage College of Osteopathic Medicine, Athens,
OH, USA

Anne Rubin
Southeastern Ohio Legal Services, Athens, OH, USA

**Konstantinos Makrilakis, Stavros Liatis, Afroditi
Tsiakou, Chryssoula Stathi and Eleftheria
Papachristoforou**
First Department of Propaedeutic Medicine, National
and Kapodistrian University of Athens Medical
School, Laiko General Hospital, 17 Ag. Thoma St,
11527 Athens, Greece

Nicholas Katsilambros
First Department of Propaedeutic Medicine, National
and Kapodistrian University of Athens Medical
School, Laiko General Hospital, 17 Ag. Thoma St,
11527 Athens, Greece
Laboratory for Experimental Surgery and Surgical
Research "Christeas Hall", University of Athens
Medical School, Athens, Greece

Dimitrios Niakas
First Department of Propaedeutic Medicine, National
and Kapodistrian University of Athens Medical
School, Laiko General Hospital, 17 Ag. Thoma St,
11527 Athens, Greece
Hellenic Open University, Patras, Greece

Despoina Perrea
Laboratory for Experimental Surgery and Surgical
Research "Christeas Hall", University of Athens
Medical School, Athens, Greece

Nikolaos Kontodimopoulos
Hellenic Open University, Patras, Greece

**Leilei Liu, Xu Chen, Cheng Cheng, Linlin Li, Lu
Chengyi Han, Zhang, Xuejiao Liu, Dongdong Zhang,
Chongjian Wang and Dongsheng Hu**
Department of Epidemiology and Health Statistics,
College of Public Health, Zhengzhou University,
Zhengzhou, Henan, People's Republic of China

**Bingyuan Wang, Yongcheng Ren, Yang Zhao and
Dechen Liu**
Department of Epidemiology and Health Statistics,
College of Public Health, Zhengzhou University,
Zhengzhou, Henan, People's Republic of China
Department of Preventive Medicine, Shenzhen
University Health Sciences Center, Shenzhen,
Guangdong, People's Republic of China

Yu Liu, Xizhuo Sun, Zhaoxia Yin and Honghui Li
The Affiliated Luohu Hospital of Shenzhen University
Health Sciences Center, Shenzhen, Guangdong,
People's Republic of China

Kunpeng Deng
Yantian Entry-exit Inspection and Quarantine Bureau,
Shenzhen, Guangdong, People's Republic of China

**Xinping Luo, Ming Zhang, Junmei Zhou and Feiyan
Liu**
Department of Preventive Medicine, Shenzhen
University Health Sciences Center, Shenzhen,
Guangdong, People's Republic of China

**Mahmut Apaydin, Muhammed Kizilgul, Selvihan
Beysel, Seyfullah Kan, Mustafa Caliskan, Taner
Demirci, Ozgur Ozcelik, Mustafa Ozbek and Erman
Cakal**
Department of Endocrinology and Metabolism, Diskapi
Training and Research Hospital, Ankara, Turkey

Asli Gencay Can
Department of Physical Medicine and Rehabilitation,
Diskapi Training and Research Hospital, Ankara,
Turkey

Peng Liu, Mohammad Abdul Mazid and Yuru Shang
The First Affiliated Hospital of Dalian Medical
University, Zhongshan 222, Dalian 116011, China

Xianbin Zhang
The First Affiliated Hospital of Dalian Medical
University, Zhongshan 222, Dalian 116011, China
Institute for Experimental Surgery, Rostock University
Medical Center, Schillingallee 69a, 18057 Rostock,
Germany

Jiaxin Song and Lili Lu
Department of Epidemiology, Dalian Medical
University, Lvshun West 9, Dalian 116044, China

Li Ma
Department of Epidemiology, Dalian Medical University, Lvshun West 9, Dalian 116044, China
Department of Epidemiology, Dalian Medical University, Zhongshan Road 222, Dalian 116011, China

Yushan Wei
Department of Evidence-based Medicine and Statistics, the First Affiliated Hospital of Dalian Medical University, Zhongshan 222, Dalian 116011, China

Peng Gong
Department of General Surgery, the Shenzhen University General Hospital and Shenzhen University School of Medicine, Xueyuan 1098, Shenzhen 518055, China

Yuesheng Liu, Chunyan Yin, Sisi Wang, Min Wang and Yanfeng Xiao
Department of Pediatrics, The Second Affiliated Hospital of Xi'an Jiaotong University, 157 Xiwu Road, Xi'an, Shaanxi 710061, People's Republic of China

Dong Xu
Tongji Hospital, Tongji Medical College, Huazhong University of Science and Technology, Wuhan, Hubei 430030, People's Republic of China

Nam-Kyoo Lim and Hyun-Young Park
Division of Cardiovascular Diseases, Center for Biomedical Sciences, Korea National Institute of Health, 187 Osongsaengmyeng 2-ro, Osong-eup, Heungdeok-gu, Cheongju-si, Chungcheongbuk-do 361-951, South Korea

Joung-Won Lee
Division of Cardiovascular Diseases, Center for Biomedical Sciences, Korea National Institute of Health, 187 Osongsaengmyeng 2-ro, Osong-eup, Heungdeok-gu, Cheongju-si, Chungcheongbuk-do 361-951, South Korea
Department of Public Health Sciences, Graduate School, Korea University, Seoul, South Korea

Ana Maria Martins and Sandra Obikawa Kyosen
Universidade Federal de São Paulo, São Paulo, Brazil

Kristin Lindstrom
Phoenix Children's Hospital, Phoenix, AZ, USA

Maria Veronica Munoz-Rojas and Nathan Thibault
Sanofi Genzyme, Cambridge, MA, USA

Lynda E. Polgreen
Los Angeles Biomedical Research Institute at Harbor-UCLA Medical Center, 1124 West Carson Street, Liu Research Building, Torrance, CA 90502, USA

Index